# Novel Developments in Granular Computing:
## Applications for Advanced Human Reasoning and Soft Computation

JingTao Yao
*University of Regina, Canada*

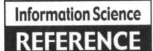

**INFORMATION SCIENCE REFERENCE**

Hershey · New York

| Director of Editorial Content: | Kristin Klinger |
| Director of Book Publications: | Julia Mosemann |
| Acquisitions Editor: | Lindsay Johnston |
| Development Editor: | Heather Probst |
| Publishing Assistant: | Myla Harty |
| Typesetter: | Thomas Foley |
| Production Editor: | Jamie Snavely |
| Cover Design: | Lisa Tosheff |
| Printed at: | Yurchak Printing Inc. |

Published in the United States of America by
Information Science Reference (an imprint of IGI Global)
701 E. Chocolate Avenue
Hershey PA 17033
Tel: 717-533-8845
Fax: 717-533-8661
E-mail: cust@igi-global.com
Web site: http://www.igi-global.com/reference

Library of Congress Cataloging-in-Publication Data


Novel developments in granular computing : applications for advanced human reasoning and soft computation / JingTao Yao, editor.
    p. cm.
  Includes bibliographical references and index.
  Summary: "This book investigages granular computing (GrC), which emerged as one of the fastest growing information processing paradigms in computational intelligence and human-centric systems"--Provided by publisher.
  ISBN 978-1-60566-324-1 (hardcover) -- ISBN 978-1-60566-325-8 (ebook)  1.
Granular computing. 2. Soft computing. I. Yao, JingTao.
  QA76.9.S63N693 2010
  006.3--dc22
                        2009043366


British Cataloguing in Publication Data
A Cataloguing in Publication record for this book is available from the British Library.

All work contributed to this book is new, previously-unpublished material. The views expressed in this book are those of the authors, but not necessarily of the publisher.

# Editorial Advisory Board

# Table of Contents

# Detailed Table of Contents

**Chapter 1**
*Yiyu Yao, University of Regina, Canada*

In this chapter, a view of granular computing as a paradigm of human-inspired problem solving and information processing, covering human-oriented studies and machine-oriented studies is explored. The triarchic theory, namely, a philosophy of structured thinking, a methodology of structured problem solving, and a computation paradigm of structured information processing is detailed. The stress on multilevel, hierarchical structures makes granular computing a human-inspired and structured approach to problem solving.

**Chapter 2**
*Hung Son Nguyen, Warsaw University, Poland*
*Andrzej Jankowski, Institute of Decision Processes Support and*
    *AdgaM Solutions Sp. z o.o., Poland*
*James F. Peters, University of Manitoba, Canada*
*Andrzej Skowron, Warsaw University, Poland*
*Jarosław Stepaniuk, Białystok University of Technology, Poland*
*Marcin Szczuka, Warsaw University, Poland*

This chapter outlines some issues of process mining from data and domain knowledge as well as approximate reasoning about changes along trajectories of approximated processes. A rough-granular approach is proposed for modeling the discovery process. The need for developing rough granular computing based on interactions among granules as well as learning strategies for approximation of functions characterizing changes, and approximation of trajectories of complex dynamical systems are also emphasized in this chapter.

# Chapter 3

This chapter explores the technology of hyperboxes and fuzzy sets as a fundamental conceptual vehicle of information granulation. In particular, a new algorithm for pattern classification based on novel representation of class sets as a difference of two types of fuzzy sets is presented, i.e., the union of hyperboxes belonging to the given class and the union of hyperboxes belonging to different classes. It has been shown that, compared to the standard hyperbox paving approaches, the proposed algorithm results in a more efficient generation of complex topologies that are necessary to describe the pattern classes.

# Chapter 4

This chapter focuses mainly on rough set algebras characterized by a dual pair of lower and upper approximation operators in both of crisp and fuzzy environments. It reviews the definitions of generalized crisp rough sets, rough fuzzy sets and fuzzy rough sets, and then presents the essential properties of the corresponding lower and upper approximation operators. The approximation operators are characterized by axioms, and as an example, the connection between fuzzy rough set algebras and fuzzy topological spaces are established.

# Chapter 5

This chapter proposes a taxonomy of types of granularity and discusses for each leaf type how the entities or instances relate within its granular level and between levels. It gives guidelines to a modeler to better distinguish between the types of granularity in the design phase and the software developer to improve on implementations of granularity.

This chapter presents a study of granular computing from an interval computing perspective. It is shown that extended interval computation enables us to find estimates in feasible time.

This chapter proposes a new understanding for data mining, namely, domain-oriented data-driven data mining (3DM), and analyses its relationship with granular computing. It also discusses the granular computing based data mining in the views of rough set and fuzzy set, and introduces some applications of granular computing in data mining.

This chapter introduces a new framework to represent socio-technical conflicts during negotiation. It is argued that conflict situations result from different sets of view points (perceptions) about issues under negotiation, therefore, reasoning about conflict dynamics is made possible with nearness relations and tolerance perceptual near sets used in defining measures of nearness. This approach provides a new way of representing and reasoning about conflicts in the context of requirements engineering using near set theory.

This chapter presents a dynamic approximation method of target concepts based on a granulation order, which consists of the positive approximation and converse approximation. Two algorithms for rule extracting called MABPA and REBCA are designed and applied to hierarchically generate decision rules from a decision table. It also proposes measures to evaluate the certainty, consistency and support of a decision-rule set extracted from a decision table. These three measures may be helpful in determining which rule extraction technique should be chosen in a practical decision problem.

This chapter presents a study on design and implementation of granular models with clearly defined semantics, i.e., linguistic models. It shows that fuzzy sets of context plays an important role in shaping up modeling activities and help handle dimensionality issues decomposing the original problem into a series of sub-problems guided by specific contexts. It presents a context-based clustering approach that forms a viable vehicle to build information granules when considering their further usage in some input-output mapping. By bringing the concept of conditional clustering along with the granular neuron as some aggregation mechanism, it shows that granular models are easily assembled into a web of connections between information granules and these architectural considerations.

This chapter Liu presents a study on the semantics of rough logic. It also discusses related operations and related properties of semantics based on rough logic as well as related reasoning of the semantics.

This chapter proposes and investigates a granular rough entropy method in the area of image clustering. The proposed rough entropy clustering algorithm results in a robust new approach into rough entropy computation.

This chapter discusses the basic components of a granular structure, the modeling of classification in terms of these components as well as the top-down, bottom-up strategies for searching classification solutions within different granule networks.

This chapter presents a research to discover perceptual information granules that are in some sense near each other with near set theory. It argues that the near set theory can provide a basis for observation, comparison and classification of perceptual granules. It further suggests that every family of perceptual granules is a dual chopped lattice.

This chapter focuses on the applications of granular computing in various aspects and phases of the object-oriented software development process, including user requirement specification and analysis, software system analysis and design, algorithm design, structured programming, software testing, and system deployment design. The importance and usefulness of granular computing as a human-centered problem solving strategy in object-oriented software development process are highlighted.

This chapter tries to systematically connect granular computing with formal concepts. Granular spaces generated by ideal-filter, congruence relations and tolerance relations and their properties are studied.

This chapter shows how concepts of rough sets can be used to model static and dynamic nonlinear systems. The granular modeling methodology introduced here gives rule-based models associated with a functional representation that can uniformly approximate continuous functions with a certain degree of accuracy. Experiments and examples testify that granular models with function approximation and estimation capabilities can model continuous linear and nonlinear systems.

# Chapter 18

This chapter introduces a model named Granular Semantic Tree (GST) for Web search. The model more conveniently represents associations among concepts than the traditional Word Sense Disambiguation methods. Fuzzy logic is used to determine the most appropriate concepts related to queries based on contexts and users' preferences.

This chapter provides arguments for the claim that the Dominance-based Rough Set Approach (DRSA) is a proper way of handling monotonically ordered data in granular computing. DRSA in the context of ordinal classification, its fuzzy extension, and a rough probabilistic model of DRSA have been presented.

# Preface

## 1. GRANULAR COMPUTING

Granular computing (GrC) has emerged as one of the fastest growing information processing paradigms in computational intelligence and human-centric systems.

In recent years, the research on granular computing has attracted many researchers and practitioners. The concept of granular computing was initially called information granularity or information granulation related to the research of fuzzy sets (Zadeh 1979). The term granular computing first appeared within literature in 1997 in Zadeh's paper where it was defined as "*a subset of computing with words*" (Zadeh, 1997). It is a generally accepted that 1997 is considered as the year of the birth of granular computing (Yao, 2007). We have experienced the emergence and growth of granular computing research in the past decade (Bargiela, A. & Pedrycz, W., 2006; Yao, 2005; Yao & Yao, 2002; Yao YY, 2005; Zadeh, 2006). Although the term granular computing is new (just over ten years mark), the basic notions and principles of granular computing occurred under various forms in many disciplines and fields (Yao, 2004, Zadeh, 1997). Similar views are shared by research in belief functions, artificial intelligence, cluster analysis, chunking, data compression, databases, decision trees, divide and conquer, fuzzy logic, interval computing, machine learning, structured programming, quantization, quotient space theory, and rough set theory.

Granular computing is often loosely defined as an umbrella term to cover any theories, methodologies, techniques, and tools that make use of granules in complex problem solving (Yao YY, 2005). Zadeh considers granular computing as basis for computing with words, i.e., computation with information described in natural language (Zadeh, 1997; Zadeh, 2006). Yao views granular computing as a complementary and dependant triangle: structured thinking in philosophical perspective, structured problem solving in methodological perspective and structured information processing in computational perspective (Yao, 2005; Yao, 2007).

An important fuzzy aspect in granular computing is to view granular computing as human-centric intelligent systems. Human-centered information processing was initiated with the introduction of fuzzy sets. The insights have led to the development of the granular computing paradigm (Bargiela and Pedrycz 2008, Zadeh 1997). Shifting from machine-centered approaches to human-centered approaches is considered one of the trends in GrC research.

The basic ingredients of granular computing are granules such as subsets, classes, objects, clusters, and elements of a universe. These granules are composed of finer granules that are drawn together by distinguishability, similarity and functionality (Zadeh, 1997). Based on complexity, abstraction level and size, granules can be measured in different levels. The problem domain, i.e., the universe, exists at the highest and coarsest granule. Granules at the lowest level are composed of elements or basic particles of the particular model that is used (Yao 2007).

Granulation is one of the key issues in granular computing for problem solving. The original meaning of granulation from dictionaries, such as the Merriam-Webster's Dictionary, is the act or process of forming something into granules. It is a process of making a larger object into smaller ones. Zadeh (1996) adopted this idea to decompose a universe to granules and pointed out "*granulation involves a decomposition of whole into parts. Conversely, organization involves an integration of parts into whole.*" Based on this definition, there will be two operations in granular computing, i.e., granulation and organization. It is suggested that a broad view of granulation in granular computing is easy to understand and manageable for granular computing research and applications (Yao 2005). Granulation involves the process of two directions in problem solving: construction and decomposition. The construction involves the process of forming a larger and higher level granule with smaller and lower level sub-granules. The decomposition involves the process of dividing a larger granule into smaller and lower level granules. The former is a bottom-up process and the latter a top-down process. The reason for a more general and broad view of granulation is that construction and decomposition are tightly related. When one chooses a particular granulation in an application, the benefits and efficiency of one direction is correlated to its opposite direction. If we consider a decomposition operation without the consideration of construction we may end up with a very efficient decomposition operation and a very inefficient construction.

In order to conduct granulation, it is crucial to understand relationships amongst granules. We may classify granular relationships into two groups: interrelationship and intrarelationship (Yao 2005). Decomposition concerns breaking down a larger granule into smaller granules from which a larger granule can still be formed with construction. Construction concerns grouping smaller granules that share similarity, indistinguishability, and functionality to a larger granule. The relationship involved in the former granulation is considered as interrelationship, the latter intrarelationship. In other words, interrelationship is the basis of grouping small objects together while intrarelationship is the foundation of dividing a granule into smaller ones. Refinement and coarsening are additional types of relationships (Yao & Yao, 2002). A granule $o_1$ is defined as a refinement of another granule $o_2$, or equivalently, $o_2$ is a coarsening of $o_1$, if every sub-granule or object of $o_1$ is contained in some sub-granules of $o_2$. Partitions and coverings are two simple and commonly used granulations of a universe. A partition of a universe is a collection of its non-empty and pairwise disjoint subsets whose union is the universe. It forms a covering if it is not disjoint. The subsets are called covering granules in a covering, and partition granules in a partition.

## 2. RECENT DEVELOPMENTS IN GRANULAR COMPUTING

Representative and influential research in granular computing were identified recently (Yao, 2006; Yao, 2007). We will briefly summarize the findings here.

## 2.1 Philosophic and Fundamental Views of Granular Computing

The triarchic theory is a representative research on the foundations of granular computing (Yao YY, 2008). Defining granular computing is one of the important research tasks for this community. Instead of simply defining what granular computing research is, Y.Y. Yao views the scope of granular computing from three perspectives, namely, the philosophical perspective, methodological perspective and computational perspective. It is argued that with each perspective focusing on different aspects of granular structures, the three perspectives working together will provide a more general and complementary view of granular computing. The philosophical perspective concerns structured thinking. The methodological perspective concerns structured problem solving. The computational perspective concerns structured information processing. Granular computing also focuses on the application of its theory to knowledge-intensive systems. The representation and processes of a system are two things to consider. Representation of a system describes the granules and granular structures within the application domain.

## 2.2 Human-Centered and Fuzzy Information Processing

Human-centered information processing was initiated with the introduction of fuzzy sets. The insights have led to the development of the granular computing paradigm (Bargiela & Pedrycz, 2008; Zadeh, 1997). Shifting from machine-centered approaches to human-centered approaches is considered one of trends in granular computing research (Yao YY, 2008). Bargiela and Pedrycz's (2008) research adopt granular computing into a structured combination of algorithmic and non-algorithmic information processing that mimics human, intelligent synthesis of knowledge from information. By integrating various different agents in which each pursues its own agenda, exploits its environment, develops its own problem solving strategy and establishes required communication strategies, one may form a more effective human-centered information system (Pedrycz, 2008). In fact, each agent may encounter a diversity of problem-solving approaches and realize their processing at the level of information granules that is the most suitable from their local points of view. To this level, the hybrid model raises a fundamental issue of forming effective interaction linkages between the agents so that they fully broadcast their findings and benefit from interacting with others.

## 2.3 Rough-Granular Computing

Rough set theory plays an important role in granular computing. A recent work by Skowron studies the formation of granules with different criteria from a rough computing point of view (Skowron & Stepaniuk, 2007). When searching for optimal solutions satisfying some constraints, one of the challenges is that these constraints are often vague and imprecise. In addition, specifications of concepts and dependencies between these involving in the constraints are often incomplete. Granules are constructed in computations aiming at solving such optimization tasks. General optimization criterion based on the minimal length principle was used. In searching for (sub-)optimal solutions, it is necessary to construct many compound granules using some specific operations such as generalization, specification or fusion. It is suggested that these criteria can be based on the minimal length principle, can express acceptable risk degrees of granules, or can use some utility functions (Skowron & Stepaniuk, 2007).

## 2.4 Dominance-Based Rough Set Approach

The dominance-based rough set approach is another representation of rough set-based granular computing methodology. It extends the classical rough set approach by utilizing background knowledge about ordinal evaluations of objects and about monotonic relationships between these evaluations (Slowinski, Greco & Matarazzo, 2007) The indiscernibility or tolerance relation among objects, which is used in the classical rough set approach, has been replaced by the dominance relation: the only relation uncontested in multi attribute pair-wise comparisons when attribute scales are ordered. In addition, the fuzzy-rough approximations taking into account monotonic relationships between memberships to different sets may be applied to case-based reasoning.

## 2.5 Other Important Research Directions

Topological views of granular computing are also attracting some researchers. For instance, Zhu (2007) studies covering-based rough sets from the topological view.

Yager (2007) adopted granular computing on information fusion applications. In particular, fuzzy sets are used to provide a granular representation of uncertain information about a variable of interest.

Zhang & Zhang (2004) proposed a theoretical framework of a fuzzy reasoning model under quotient space structure. The quotient space structure is introduced into fuzzy sets to construct fuzzy set representations of different grain-size spaces and their relationships.

Liu et al. studied granular computing from a rough logic aspect (Liu, Sun & Wang, 2007). The granulation is based on the meaning of a rough logical formula in a given information system. It is suggested that the practicability of the granulations will offer a new idea for studying the meaning of classical logic and the meaning of other nonstandard logic.

## 3. THE MOST CITED GRANULAR COMPUTING PAPERS AND CALL FOR CHAPTERS

In (Yao, 2007) and (Yao, 2008), the most influential research papers on the topic of granular computing were identified. We defined a granular computing paper as a paper that contains granular computing related terms, for instance, "granular computing", "information granularity", "information granulation" or "granular computation". We used the Web of Science of ISI to locate granular computing papers that are indexed by ISI. We searched by Topic which is defined as the words or phrases within article titles, keywords, or abstracts in Web of Science. Top highly cited granular computing papers retrieved from Web of Science on Oct 1, 2007 are listed below in the Additional Reading section.

As stated in Wohlin's article (Wohlin, 2008),

*"Citations are a common way of judging the most influential work in different fields. The most cited articles often provide new insights, open a new avenue of research, or provide a significant summary of the state-of-the-art in an area. Citations are a way to show how researchers build their work on existing research to evolve research further. Basically, they are the backbone of research and hence articles and authors being cited frequently deserve acknowledgment for their contribution."*

One of the goals of this book is to seek for research papers from authors of the most influential papers in order to see recent development of granular computing research. We invited these most influential authors to contribute a chapter together with a public call for papers. Eight chapters in the book are authored by the most influential authors in granular computing. We underline the authors who contributed to this book.

## 4. CHAPTER SUMMARY

In the chapter *"Human-Inspired Granular Computing"* authored by Yiyu Yao, a view of granular computing as a paradigm of human-inspired problem solving and information processing, covering human-oriented studies and machine-oriented studies is explored. The triarchic theory, namely, a philosophy of structured thinking, a methodology of structured problem solving, and a computation paradigm of structured information processing is detailed. The stress on multilevel, hierarchical structures makes granular computing a human-inspired and structured approach to problem solving.

The chapter entitled "*Discovery of Process Models from Data and Domain Knowledge: A Rough-Granular Approach*" by Hung Son Nguyen, Andrzej Jankowski, James F. Peters, Andrzej Skowron, Jarosław Stepaniuk, and Marcin Szczuka outlines some issues of process mining from data and domain knowledge as well as approximate reasoning about changes along trajectories of approximated processes. A rough-granular approach is proposed for modeling the discovery process. The need for developing rough granular computing based on interactions among granules as well as learning strategies for approximation of functions characterizing changes, and approximation of trajectories of complex dynamical systems are also emphasized in this chapter.

The third chapter entitled "*Supervised and Unsupervised Information Granulation: A Study in Hyperbox Design*" authored by Andrzej Bargiela and Witold Pedrycz explores the technology of hyperboxes and fuzzy sets as a fundamental conceptual vehicle of information granulation. In particular, a new algorithm for pattern classification based on novel representation of class sets as a difference of two types of fuzzy sets is presented, i.e., the union of hyperboxes belonging to the given class and the union of hyperboxes belonging to different classes. It has been shown that, compared to the standard hyperbox paving approaches, the proposed algorithm results in a more efficient generation of complex topologies that are necessary to describe the pattern classes.

The next chapter "*On Characterization of Relation Based Rough Set Algebras*" authored by Wei-Zhi Wu and Wen-Xiu Zhang focuses mainly on rough set algebras characterized by a dual pair of lower and upper approximation operators in both of crisp and fuzzy environments. It reviews the definitions of generalized crisp rough sets, rough fuzzy sets and fuzzy rough sets, and then presents the essential properties of the corresponding lower and upper approximation operators. The approximation operators are characterized by axioms, and as an example, the connection between fuzzy rough set algebras and fuzzy topological spaces are established.

The chapter entitled "*A Top-Level Categorization of Types of Granularity*" authored by C. Maria Keet proposes a taxonomy of types of granularity and discusses for each leaf type how the entities or instances relate within its granular level and between levels. It gives guidelines to a modeler to better distinguish between the types of granularity in the design phase and the software developer to improve on implementations of granularity.

The chapter entitled "*From Interval Computations to Constraint-Related Set Computations: Towards Faster Estimation of Statistics and ODEs under Interval, p-Box, and Fuzzy Uncertainty*" by Martine Ceberio, Vladik Kreinovich, Andrzej Pownuk, and Barnabás Bede presents a study of granular computing from an interval computing perspective. It is shown that extended interval computation enables us to find estimates in feasible time.

The chapter entitled "*Granular Computing Based Data Mining in the Views of Rough Set and Fuzzy Set*" authored by Guoyin Wang, Jun Hu, Qinghua Zhang, Xianquan Liu, and Jiaqing Zhou proposes a new understanding for data mining, namely, domain-oriented data-driven data mining (3DM), and analyses its relationship with granular computing. It also discusses the granular computing based data mining in the views of rough set and fuzzy set, and introduces some applications of granular computing in data mining.

The chapter entitled "*Near Sets in Assessing Conflict Dynamics within a Perceptual System Framework*" by Sheela Ramanna and James F. Peters introduces a new framework to represent socio-technical conflicts during negotiation. It is argued that conflict situations result from different sets of view points (perceptions) about issues under negotiation, therefore, reasoning about conflict dynamics is made possible with nearness relations and tolerance perceptual near sets used in defining measures of nearness. This approach provides a new way of representing and reasoning about conflicts in the context of requirements engineering using near set theory.

The chapter entitled *"Rule Extraction and Rule Evaluation Based on Granular Computing"* authored by Jiye Liang, Yuhua Qian, and Deyu Li presents a dynamic approximation method of target concepts based on a granulation order, which consists of the positive approximation and converse approximation. Two algorithms for rule extracting called MABPA and REBCA are designed and applied to hierarchically generate decision rules from a decision table. It also proposes measures to evaluate the certainty, consistency and support of a decision-rule set extracted from a decision table. These three measures may be helpful in determining which rule extraction technique should be chosen in a practical decision problem.

The chapter entitled *"Granular Models: Design Insights and Development Practices"* authored by Witold Pedrycz and Athanasios Vasilakos presents a study on design and implementation of granular models with clearly defined semantics, i.e., linguistic models. It shows that fuzzy sets of context plays an important role in shaping up modeling activities and help handle dimensionality issues decomposing the original problem into a series of sub-problems guided by specific contexts.

It presents a context-based clustering approach that forms a viable vehicle to build information granules when considering their further usage in some input-output mapping. By bringing the concept of conditional clustering along with the granular neuron as some aggregation mechanism, it shows that granular models are easily assembled into a web of connections between information granules and these architectural considerations.

The chapter entitled *"Semantic Analysis of Rough Logic"* by Qing Liu presents a study on the semantics of rough logic. It also discusses related operations and related properties of semantics based on rough logic as well as related reasoning of the semantics.

The chapter entitled *"Rough Entropy Clustering Algorithm in Image Segmentation"* authored by Dariusz Małyszko and Jarosław Stepaniuk proposes and investigates a granular rough entropy method in the area of image clustering. The proposed rough entropy clustering algorithm results in a robust new approach into rough entropy computation.

The chapter entitled *"Modeling Classification by Granular Computing"* by Yan Zhao discusses the basic components of a granular structure, the modeling of classification in terms of these components as well as the top-down, bottom-up strategies for searching classification solutions within different granule networks.

The chapter entitled *"Discovering Perceptually Near Information Granules"* authored by James F. Peters presents a research to discover perceptual information granules that are in some sense near each other with near set theory. It argues that the near set theory can provide a basis for observation, comparison and classification of perceptual granules. It further suggests that every family of perceptual granules is a dual chopped lattice.

The chapter entitled *"Granular Computing in Object-Oriented Software Development Process"* by Jianchao Han focuses on the applications of granular computing in various aspects and phases of the object-oriented software development process, including user requirement specification and analysis, software system analysis and design, algorithm design, structured programming, software testing, and system deployment design. The importance and usefulness of granular computing as a human-centered problem solving strategy in object-oriented software development process are highlighted.

The chapter entitled *"Granular Computing in Formal Concept Analysis"* authored by Yuan Ma, Zhangang Liu, and Xuedong Zhang tries to systematically connect granular computing with formal concepts. Granular spaces generated by ideal-filter, congruence relations and tolerance relations and their properties are studied.

The chapter entitled *"Granular Synthesis of Rule-Based Models and Function Approximation using Rough Sets"*, authored by Carlos Pinheiro, Fernando Gomide, Otávio Carpinteiro, and Isaías Lima shows how concepts of rough sets can be used to model static and dynamic nonlinear systems. The granular modeling methodology introduced here gives rule-based models associated with a functional representation that can uniformly approximate continuous functions with a certain degree of accuracy. Experiments and examples testify that granular models with function approximation and estimation capabilities can model continuous linear and nonlinear systems.

The chapter entitled *"A Genetic Fuzzy Semantic Web Search Agent Using Granular Semantic Trees for Ambiguous Queries"*, authored by Yan Chen and Yan-Qing Zhang introduces a model named Granular Semantic Tree (GST) for Web search. The model more conveniently represents associations among concepts than the traditional Word Sense Disambiguation methods. Fuzzy logic is used to determine the most appropriate concepts related to queries based on contexts and users' preferences.

Last but not least the chapter entitled *"Dominance-based Rough Set Approach to Granular Computing"* authored by Salvatore Greco, Benedetto Matarazzo, and Roman Słowiński provides arguments for the claim that the Dominance-based Rough Set Approach (DRSA) is a proper way of handling monotonically ordered data in granular computing. DRSA in the context of ordinal classification, its fuzzy extension, and a rough probabilistic model of DRSA have been presented.

*JingTao Yao*
*University of Regina, Canada*

## REFERENCES

Bargiela, A., & Pedrycz, W. (2006). The roots of granular computing. In *Proceedings of the IEEE International Conference on Granular Computing* (pp. 806-809). Washington, DC: IEEE Press.

Bargiela, A., & Pedrycz, W. (2008). Toward a theory of granular computing for human-centred information processing. *IEEE Transactions on Fuzzy Systems. 16*(2), 320-330.

Liu, Q. Sun, H., & Wang, Y. (2007). Granulations based on semantics of rough logical formulas and its reasoning. In *Proceedings of the International Conference on Rough Sets, Fuzzy Sets, Data Mining and Granular Computing*, (LNCS 4482, pp. 419-426).

Pedrycz, W. (2008). Granular computing in multi-agent systems. In *Proceedings of the 3rd International Conference on Rough Sets and Knowledge Technology*, (LNCS 5009, pp. 3-17).

Skowron, A., & Stepaniuk, J. (2007). Modeling of high quality granules. In *Proceeding. of the International Conference on Rough Sets and Intelligent Systems Paradigms*, (LNCS 4585, pp. 300-309).

Slowinski, R., Greco S., & Matarazzo, B. (2007). Dominance-based rough set approach to reasoning about ordinal data. In *Proceedings of International Conference on Rough Sets and Intelligent Systems Paradigms*, (LNCS 4585, pp. 5-11).

Wohlin, C. (2008). An analysis of the most cited articles in software engineering journals - 2001. *Information and Software Technology, 50*(1-2), 3-9.

Yager, R. A. (2007). On the soundness of altering granular information. *International Journal Approximate Reasoning, 45*(1), 43-67.

Yao, J. T. (2005). Information granulation and granular relationships. In *Proceedings of the IEEE Conference on Granular Computing* (pp. 326-329). Washington, DC: IEEE Press.

Yao, J.T. (2007). A ten-year review of granular computing. In *Proceedings of the IEEE International Conference on Granular Computing* (pp. 734-739). Washington, DC: IEEE Press

Yao, J. T. (2008). Recent Developments in Granular Computing: A Bibliometrics Study. In Proceedings of the IEEE International Conference on Granular Computing (pp.74-79). Washington, DC: IEEE Press.

Yao, J. T., & Yao, Y. Y. (2002). Induction of classification rules by granular computin , In *Proceedings of the Third International Conference on Rough Sets and Current Trends in Computing*. (LNAI 2475, pp. 331-338). Berlin, Germany: Springer.

Yao, Y. Y. (2004). Granular computing. *Computer Science, 31*(10.A), 1-5.

Yao, Y. Y. (2005). Perspectives of granular computing. In *Proceedings of IEEE International Conference on Granular Computing*, (vol. 1,(pp. 85-99). Washington, DC: IEEE Press.

Yao, Y. Y (2007). The art of granular computing. In *Proceedings of International Conference on Rough Sets and Emerging Intelligent Systems Paradigms* (RSEISP'07), (LNAI 4585, pp. 101-112).

Yao, Y.Y. (2008). Granular computing: past, present, and future. In *Proceedings of the 3rd International Conference on Rough Sets and Knowledge Technology*, (LNCS 5009, pp. 27-28).

Zadeh, L. A. (1996). Key roles of information granulation and fuzzy logic in human reasoning, Concept formulation and computing with words. In *Proceedings of the IEEE 5th International Fuzzy Systems*, (pp 1.)

Zadeh, L. A. (1979). Fuzzy sets and information granularity. In M. Gupta, R.K. Ragade, & R.R. Yager (eds). *Advances in Fuzzy Set Theory and Applications* (pp.3-18). Amsterdam: North-Holland Publishing Company.

Zadeh, L. A. (1997), Towards a theory of fuzzy information granulation and its centrality in human reasoning and fuzzy logic. *Fuzzy Sets and Systems, 90*(2), 111-127.

Zadeh, L. A. (2006). Generalized theory of uncertainty (GTU) -principal concepts and ideas. *Computational Statistics & Data Analysis, 51*(1), 15-46.

Zhang, L., & Zhang, B. (2004). The quotient space theory of problem solving, *Fundamenta Informaticae, 59*(2-3), 287-298.

Zhu W. (2007). Topological approaches to covering rough sets. *Information Sciences, 177*(6), 1499-1508.

## ADDITIONAL READING

Al-Khatib, W., Day, Y.F., Ghafoor, A., et al. (1999). Semantic modeling and knowledge representation in multimedia databases. IEEE Transactions on Knowledge and Data Engineering 11(1), 64-80.

Greco, S., Matarazzo, B., & Slowinski, R. (2000). Extension of the rough set approach to multicriteria decision support. INFOR 38(3), 161-195.

Greco, S., Matarazzo, B., Slowinski, & R. (2001). Rough sets theory for multicriteria decision analysis. European Journal of Operational Research, 129(1), 1-47.

Hata, Y., Kobashi, S., Hirano, S., et al. (2000). Automated segmentation of human brain MR images aided by fuzzy information granulation and fuzzy inference. IEEE Transactions on Systems, Man and Cybernetics Part C-Applications And Reviews 30(3), 381-395.

Hirota, K., & Pedrycz, W. (1999). Fuzzy relational compression. IEEE Transactions on Systems, Man and Cybernetics Part B-Cybernetics, 29(3), 407-415.

Hirota, K., Pedrycz, W. (1999). Fuzzy computing for data mining. In Proceedings of the IEEE, 87 (9), 1575-1600.

Pal, S. K., & Mitra, P. (2002). Multispectral image segmentation using the rough-set-initialized EM algorithm. IEEE Transactions on Geoscience and Remote Sensing, 40(11), 2495-2501.

Pal, S. K., Mitra, P. (2004). Case generation using rough sets with fuzzy representation. IEEE Transactions on Knowledge and Data Engineering, 16(3): 292-300.

Pedrycz, W. (2001). Fuzzy equalization in the construction of fuzzy sets. Fuzzy Sets and Systems, 119(2), 329-335.

Pedrycz, W., & Gudwin, R. R. (1997). Gomide FAC, Nonlinear context adaptation in the calibration of fuzzy sets. Fuzzy Sets and Systems 88(1), 91-97.

Pedrycz, W., Vasilakos, A. V. (1999). Linguistic models and linguistic modeling. IEEE Transactions on Systems Man, and Cybernetics Part B-Cybernetics, 29(6), 745-757.

Peters, J. F., Skowron, A., Synak, P., et al. (2003). Rough sets and information granulation. Lecture Notes in Artificial Intelligence, (2715, pp. 370-377).

Skowron, A., & Stepaniuk, J. (2001). Information granules: Towards foundations of granular computing. International Journal of Intelligent Systems 16(1), 57-85.

Slowinski, R, Greco, S, Matarazzo, B. (2002). Rough set analysis of preference-ordered data. Lecture Notes in Artificial Intelligence, (2475, pp. 44-59).

Yao, Y. Y. (2001). Information granulation and rough set approximation, International Journal of Intelligent Systems, 16(1), 87-104.

Yao, Y. Y. (2003). Probabilistic approaches to rough sets. Expert Systems 20(5), 287-297.

Zadeh, L. A. (1997). Toward a theory of fuzzy information granulation and its centrality in human reasoning and fuzzy logic. Fuzzy Sets And Systems, 90(2), 111-127.

# Acknowledgment

I would like to thank all authors who contributed a chapter in this book as well as the reviewers who helped to improve the quality of chapters. I would like to thank IGI Global for providing a great channel for delivering the set of excellent work on recent development on granular computing research. Thanks to Heather Probst and Julia Mosemann, Editors of IGI Global for their assistance and patience during the lengthy editing period. Thanks to my colleagues, students and friends at the University of Regina for providing all possible support for my editing work. Special thanks go to Editorial Advisory Board Dr. Lotfi A. Zadeh, Dr. Nick Cercone, Dr. Jerzy W. Grzymala-Busse, Dr. Pawan Lingras, Dr. Vijay V. Raghavan, and Dr. Ning Zhong. Without everyone's effort, it is impossible to see the completion of this book.

*JingTao Yao*
*Editor*

# Chapter 1
# Human–Inspired Granular Computing

**Yiyu Yao**
*University of Regina, Canada*

## ABSTRACT

*In this chapter, I explore a view of granular computing as a paradigm of human-inspired problem solving and information processing, covering human-oriented studies and machine-oriented studies. By exploring the notion of multiple levels of granularity, one can identify, examine and formalize a special family of principles, strategies, heuristics, and methods that are commonly used by humans in daily problem solving. The results may then be used for human and machine problem solving, as well as for implementing human-inspired approaches in machines and systems. The triarchic theory of granular computing unifies both types of studies from three perspectives, namely, a philosophy of structured thinking, a methodology of structured problem solving, and a computation paradigm of structured information processing. The stress on multilevel, hierarchical structures makes granular computing a human-inspired and structured approach to problem solving.*

## 1. INTRODUCTION

In two recent papers, J.T. Yao (2007, 2008) presents a ten-year review of granular computing by analyzing published papers collected from the ISI's *Web of Science* and the *IEEE Digital Library*. The objective is to "study the current status, the trends and the future direction of granular computing and identify prolific authors, impact authors, and the most impact papers in the past decade." The results from such a citation analysis shed new lights on the current research in granular computing. For example, it is found that the current research is dominated by fuzzy sets and rough sets, and the number of granular computing publications has a linear growth rate. According to a study by Crane (1972), this indicates that members

DOI: 10.4018/978-1-60566-324-1.ch001

of the granular computing community have less interaction with each other and with researchers in other areas. To promote granular computing as a field of study, J.T. Yao (2007) makes several recommendations. We must first search for and adopt a set of common terminologies and notations so that we can easily find granular computing papers and increase effective exchange of ideas. We need to interact and communicate with each other and with researchers in other fields.

An immediate task is to establish a conceptual framework of granular computing, within which many views, interpretations, and theories can be developed and examined. Although a well-accepted definition and formulation of granular computing does not exist yet, recent results show a great diversity of research and a convergence to a unified framework. Initiatives include granular computing as a way of problem solving (Yao, 2004a, 2004b, 2007a; Zhang and Zhang, 2007), granular computing as a paradigm of information processing (Bargiela and Pedrycz, 2002, 2008), artificial intelligence perspectives on granular computing (Yao, 2008b, Zhang and Zhang, 2007), connections between granular computing and systems theory (Yao, 2008b), a general theory of granularity (Hobbs, 1985; Keet, 2006, 2008), and a triarchic theory of granular computing (Yao, 2000, 2004a, 2004b, 2005, 2006, 2007a, 2008a, 2008b). Granular computing is evolving from a set of simple concepts and notions into a field of interdisciplinary and cross-disciplinary study. It draws results from many fields and synthesizes them into an integrated whole (Yao, 2007a, 2008b).

One purpose of this chapter is to examine a view of granular computing as a paradigm of human-inspired problem solving and information processing with multiple levels of granularity. I classify research of granular computing into human-oriented and machine-oriented studies, and discuss two purposes of granular computing, one for humans and the other for machines. Another purpose is to outline the triarchic theory of granular computing with three components integrated. The studies of philosophy of granular computing promote structured thinking, the studies of methodology promote structured problem solving, and the studies of computation promote structured information processing. The classification of the two types of studies and the identification of the two purposes help clarify some confusion about the goals and scopes of granular computing.

The view of granular computing as a paradigm of human-inspired computing with multiple levels of granularity is not really new; it simply weaves together powerful ideas from several fields, including human problem solving, computer programming, cognitive science, artificial intelligence, and many others. By revisiting, reinterpreting and combing these ideas, we obtain new insights into granular computing. In the rest of the chapter, I will explain this view with reference to works that have significant influences on my thinking; and hope this will help in appreciating the principles and ideas of granular computing.

## 2. GRANULAR COMPUTING AS HUMAN-INSPIRED PROBLEM SOLVING

Several important characteristics of human problem solving may be considered as a starting point for approaching granular computing. First, humans tend to organize and categorization is essential to mental life (Pinker, 1997). Results of such organizations are some types of structures. For example, hierarchical structures seem to be a reasonable choice. Second, humans tend to form multiple versions of the same world (Bateson, 1978) and to have several kinds of data presentations in the brain (Pinker, 1997). For a particular problem, we normally have several versions of descriptions and understanding (Minsky, 2007). Third, we consider a problem at multiple levels of granularity. This allows us to focus on solving a problem at the most appropriate level of granularity by ignoring unimportant and irrelevant details

(Hobbs, 1985). Fourth, we can readily switch between levels of granularity at different stages of problem solving (Hobbs, 1985); we can also easily switch from one description to another. At the present stage, we may not be ready to define all these characteristics quantitatively. They may only be explained to humans qualitatively through a set of rules of thumb. With the efforts of granular computing researchers, we expect to formalize some or all of them.

Let us now consider three specific issues in the study of granular computing as human-inspired problem solving.

First, granular computing focus on a special class of approaches to problem solving; this classes is characterized by multiple levels of granularity. Regarding human intelligence, Minsky (2007) points out that humans have many "Ways to Think." We can easily switch among them and create new "Ways to Think" if none of them works. It is easy to convince us that humans have many approaches to problem solving. The use of multiple levels of granularity and abstraction is only one of them. It may be more realistic for the study of granular computing not to cover the whole spectrum of approaches to human problem solving. Therefore, I restrict study of granular computing to human-inspired and granularity-based way of problem solving.

Second, the study of granular computing has two goals. One is to understand the nature, the underlying principles and mechanisms of human problem solving, and the other is to apply them in the design and implementation of human-inspired machines and systems. They in turn lead to two classes of research on granular computing, namely human-oriented studies and machine-oriented studies. These two types of studies are relatively independent and mutually support each other. The former focuses on human problem solving and the latter on machine problem solving.

Third, the study of granular computing serves two purposes. On the one hand, an understanding of the underlying principles of human problem solving may help more people to consciously apply these principles. Once we articulate and master these principles, we become a better problem solver. I use the phrase "granular computing for humans" to denote this aspect. On the other hand, an understanding human problem solving is a prerequisite of building machines having the similar power. The human brain is perhaps the only device that represents the highest level of intelligence for problem solving. Unlocking the mechanisms of human brain may provide the necessary hints on designing intelligent machines. Results from human-oriented studies may serve as a solid basis for machine-oriented studies. Once we have a full understanding of human problem solving, we can design machines and systems based on the same principles. I use the phrase "granular computing for machines" to denote the second aspect. In summary, granular computing is for both humans and machines.

To conclude this section, I look at granular computing again in the light of a conceptual framework by Golhooly (1989) on problem solving. According to Gilhooly, there are three angles from which one may approach the topic of problems solving. The normative approaches deal with the best means for solving various types of problems; the psychological studies attempt to understand and analyze problem-solving processes in humans and other animals; computer science, or more specifically artificial intelligence, approaches focus on machine problem solving. The cognitive science integrate both human and machine problem solving from an information-processing point of view. It covers information and knowledge processing in the abstract, in human brains and in machines. Based on these results, Gilhooly suggests developing "a comparative cognitive science of problem solving in which the differing information-processing procedures followed by human and machine may be compared and contrasted, with a view to developing general principles applicable both to natural and artificial problem solving." It offers three perspectives on problem solving, namely, the psychological (or human) perspective, the machine perspective, and the interaction of human and machine perspectives. If we view granular computing as human-inspired problem solving, the comparative cognitive science framework is also instructive to the study of granular computing.

The interaction of human and machine perspectives consider bidirectional influences. Machine analogies contribute to psychological approaches to human thinking, which leads to the machine-inspired information-processing approach to the study of human intelligence. Conversely, human-inspired problem solving may contribute a great deal to machine problem solving. While research on the former is abundant, there is still a lack of study on the latter. Since human problem solving processes are rarely known in detail, and hence are not described in precise terms and in a formal way, we have only rather general influences from human problem solving to machine problem solving (Gilhooly, 1989). Granular computing attempts to fill this gap by focusing on human-inspired approaches to machine problem solving.

## 3. HUMAN-ORIENTED AND MACHINE-ORIENTED STUDIES

For human-oriented studies of granular computing, we focus on a particular way of human problem solving that uses multiple levels of granularity. We attempt to identify, extract and formalize such a class of principles, strategies, heuristics and methods. The main objective is to understand and unlock the underlying working principle of granular thinking, and to develop new theories and methods for human problem solving. On the evidence and results from human-oriented studies, the machine-oriented studies focus on the application of granular computing in the design and implementation of human-inspired machines and systems.

For machine-oriented studies of granular computing, we assume that the principles of human problem solving apply equally to machines. The principles of human problem solving may be applied either directed or indirectly to intelligent machines. It may be true that one can build special machines and systems for solving particular types of problem, independent of human problem solving. However, without an understanding of human problem solving, we cannot expect a high likelihood of building a general problem solving machine or system that has the human-level capacity. Machines may solve a problem in a different manner as humans; they must employ the same underlying principles.

Granular computing integrates human-oriented and machine-oriented studies, relying on the dependency of the latter on the former. Particularly, granular computing involves the following sequence of tasks:

(1) to understand the underlying principles and mechanisms of human problem solving, with emphasis on multiple levels of granularity,
(2) to extract a set of principles of granular computing,
(3) to develop formal methodology, theories and models of granular computing,
(4) to empower everyone with principles of granular computing,
(5) to design human-inspired machines and systems for problem solving.

Therefore, the task (1) emphasizes the role of multiple levels of granularity and limits the scope of granular to a special class of approaches to problem solving. Results from (2) may be intuitive, qualitative, schematic, subjective, incomplete, philosophical, and/or relative vague; they are represented as heuristics, common-sense rules and/or rules of thumb and explained in natural languages. Results from (3) may be interpreted as the next level articulation and precision of the results from (2), and inevitably less general and more restrictive. Results from (2) and (3) may be directly applied to granular computing for humans, namely, task (4). While results from (3) can be directly applied to granular computing for machines, namely, task (5), results from (2) play only a guiding role.

A main stream of research of granular computing focuses on tasks (3) and (5), with very little attention to other tasks. This seems to be paradoxical. On the one hand, it is well recognized that granular computing is motivated by the ways in which humans solve problems (Yao, 2008b). On the other hand, we have not started a systematic and full-scale study of human problem solving in granular computing, although there are extensive studies in other fields such as cognitive science, psychology, education, and many more. We over emphasize granular computing for machines and fail to appreciate the power of granular computing for humans.

Some misunderstandings about granular computing may stem from a confusion of granular computing for humans and granular computing for machines. Many questions, doubts, and criticisms of granular computing are only applicable to (5), where formal, precise and concrete models are necessary. As granular computing for humans, namely, (4), its principles can be explained at more abstract levels and in an informal manner, relying heavily on human intuition, understanding and power. It may take times before we can have some breakthroughs in precisely defining all aspects of human problem solving. However, this should not discourage us to pursue.

The idea of separating and integrating human-oriented and machine-oriented studies is influenced by results and lessons from the fields of artificial intelligence (AI) and computer programming. Let us first consider artificial intelligence. Several decades ago, Samuel (1962) identified two fundamentally different approaches to artificial intelligence. One approach focuses the problem and not the device that solves it. That is, the specific mechanisms of the brain are not considered. The other approach focuses on the studies on devices that solve the problem and the emulation of such devices. Some researchers consider that building an intelligent machine is the primary goal of AI, and that finding out about the nature of intelligence is the second goal (Schank, 1987). Consequently, they have led to different approaches to artificial intelligence.

The earlier advances in AI, such as theorem proving, computer chess, and so on, depend crucially on a deep understanding of how humans solve the same problems (Newell and Simon, 1972). Successful intelligent systems are built based on the same principles. However, a lack of consideration by AI researchers about the human mind and natural intelligence has perhaps negatively affected the development of artificial intelligence (Hawkins, 2004; Schank, 1987). In the last few years, many researchers began to reconsider the role of the studies of brain science and natural intelligence for artificial intelligence. A fully exploration on this account and many references can be found in another paper (Yao, 2008b). It seems that understanding the nature of intelligence is the primary goal of AI, which in turn supports the goal of building intelligent machines. In the context to granular computing, human-oriented studies should be considered as the primary focus.

The National Academy of Engineering (2008) lists "reverse-engineer the brain" as one of the 14 grand challenges for engineering for the 21st century. The following excerpt from its document supports the above argument:

*While some of thinking machines have mastered specific narrow skills-playing chess, for instance-- general-purpose artificial intelligence (AI) has remained elusive.*

*Part of the problem, some experts now believe, is that artificial brains have been designed without much attention to real ones. Pioneers of artificial intelligence approached thinking the way that aeronautical engineers approached flying without much learning from birds. It has turned out, though, that the secrets about how living brains work may offer the best guide to engineering the artificial variety. Discovering those secrets by reverse-engineering the brain promises enormous opportunities for reproducing intelligence the way assembly lines spit out cars or computers.*

*Figuring out how the brain works will offer rewards beyond building smarter computers. Advances gained from studying the brain may in return pay dividends for the brain itself. Understanding its methods will enable engineers to simulate its activities, leading to deeper insights about how and why the brain works and fails.*

We may pose a similar challenge to granular computing. That is, a grand challenge for granular computing is to reverse-engineer the mechanisms of human problem solving. It is of significant value to both human and machine problem solving

Consider now the problem of computer programming. Programming is a complex and difficult problem solving task. Many methodologies and principles have been proposed and effectively applied. It is one of best examples that we may use to explain and articulate principles of human problem solving. It also supports the view of "granular computing for humans." Programming methodologies empower programmers rather than machines, namely, programming methodologies are for humans. Research on this angle of granular computing may be more fruitful at the present stage. In previous papers (Yao, 2004a, 2007a), I argue that the principles and methodologies of computer programming may be easily adopted for granular computing.

The division of granular computing for humans and for machines is also related to a programming paradigm known as the literate programming proposed by Knuth (1984). It represents a change of attitude: the task of programming is changed from instructing a computer what to do into explaining to human beings what we want a computer to do (Knuth, 1984). A program in WEB, a system for literate programming, is the source for two different system routines: one to produce a document that describes the program clearly for human beings, and the other to produce a machine-executable program. The explanations of a program are a salient feature of literate programming. Borrowing the ideas of literate programming to granular computing, one may focus on explaining to human beings about human problem solving. Once we can explain the principles of human problem solving clearly, we may be able to design systems that adopt the same principles.

There are several benefits from separating human-oriented and machine-oriented studies and from separating granular computing for humans and for machines. First, they identify clearly the scopes and goals of granular computing. Second, they enable us to recognize the importance of granular computing for humans, an aspect that has been overlooked so far. Third, they make us to ask the right questions and to tackle the right problems with respect to different tasks of granular computing. Fourth, they help us to envision different stages of study on granular computing with both long-term and short-term perspectives.

## 4. GRANULAR COMPUTING FOR HUMANS

My previous effort concentrated on granular computing for humans (Yao, 2004a, 2005, 2007a). An assumption of such studies is that there is a set of common principles underlying human problem solving, independent of particular problem domains and specific problems. Consider, for example, scientific research that is a typical task of problem solving. Although scientists in different disciplines study different subject matters and use different formulations, they all employ remarkably common structures for describing problems and apply common principles, strategies, and heuristics for problem solving (Beveridge, 1967; Martella *et al.*, 1999). On the other hand, these common principles are examined in relative isolation, expressed in discipline dependent concepts and notions, buried in technical details, and scattered in many places. Granular computing aims at extracting the common discipline-independent principles, strategies and heuristics that have been applied either explicitly or implicitly in human problem.

I list the following specific goals about studying the principles of granular computing and their usages (Yao, 2007a):

- to make implicit principles explicit,
- to make invisible principles visible,
- to make discipline-specific principles discipline-independent,
- to make subconscious effects conscious.

The principles of granular computing serve as a guide in the problem solving process, and may not guarantee a good solution. However, by making these principles explicit, visible and disciplinary-independent to everyone, we increase the probability of arriving at a good solution. If we can precisely and clearly describe the principles of granular computing, we can empower more people to effectively use them in problem solving. There is evidence from psychology and cognitive sciences that shows the benefits from our awareness of these rules and our conscious effort in using them. For example, the conscious access hypothesis states, "consciousness might help to mobilize and integrate brain functions that are otherwise separate and independent" (Baars, 2002). If we can change from subconscious behaviors into a systematic conscious effort in applying the principles of granular computing, it is more feasible that we become better problem solvers.

The central ideas of granular computing for humans derive from several studies in computer science. In the context of structured programming, Dijkstra (EWD237, EWD245) makes a compelling and beautiful argument that promotes a conscious effort at exploiting good structures as a useful thinking aid. Specifically, when one makes a conscious effort at using good structures and principles, it is more feasible to produce a correct program. Influenced by Dijkstra's ideas, I single out two crucial issues about granular computing for humans. One is the extraction of structures and principles of granular computing, and the other is to promote a conscious effort in using these principles.

In the context of computer education, Wing (2006) points out the importance of computational thinking, in addition to the classical three Rs (reading, writing, and arithmetic). She argues that computational thinking represents a universally applicable attitude and skill set that can be learned and used by everyone, not just computer scientists. In some sense, it represents a view of computational thinking for humans. For this reason, I choose the phrase "granular computing for humans," with an understanding that granular computing has a large overlap with computational thinking.

Dijkstra attempts to convince programmers to make a conscious effort in using good structures and principles of structured programming, and Wing attempts to make computational thinking, originally developed in computer science, as a universally applicable attitude and skill set to everyone. In several papers (Yao, 2004a, 2005, 2007a), I suggest that some of the basic principles of computer programming and computational thinking, such as top-down design, step-wise refinement, multiple levels of abstraction, and so on, are some of the important ingredients of the methodology of granular computing. Granular computing for humans is therefore aims at a methodology applicable to many fields and to everyone.

There is evidence supporting the viewpoint of granular computing for everyone. Leron (1983) and Friske (1985) demonstrate that the principles of structured programming are equally applicable in developing, teaching and communicating mathematical proofs. Recently, several authors (Han and Dong, 2007; Xie et al., 2008; Zhu, 2008) apply ideas of granular computing to software engineering and system modeling. In another paper (Yao, 2007b), I argue that scientists may employ the principles of granular computing in structured scientific writing. Some authors (Sternberg and Frensch, 1991) show that principles of granular computing have, in fact, been used in reading, writing, arithmetic, and a wide range of tasks. It may be the time to study granular thinking as an effective and applicable methodology for humans.

## 5. GRANULAR COMPUTING FOR MACHINES

Granular computing for machines deals with more specific and concrete theories and methods. Central issues are to represent information and knowledge at multiple levels of granularity, to process it based on such a multilevel granular structure, to reasoning at multiple levels of abstraction, and to explore variable levels of schematic and approximate solutions of problems, from qualitative and symbolic to quantitative and numeric. Depending on particular applications, the high-level principles of granular computing may be implemented differently.

The major research effort on granular computing for machines focuses on an information processing perspective (Bargiela and Pedrycz, 2002, 2008; Lin *et al.*, 2002; Pedrycz, et al., 2008; Yao, 2007a). Three areas related to granular compting are the rough set model (Pawlak, 1998), the fuzzy set model (Zadeh, 1997), and artificial intelligence. The notion of information and knowledge granulation plays an essential role. Rough set theory studies a particular type of granulation known as partitions. Each block of a partition is called a granule. The multilevel granular structure is the lattice formed by all equivalence classes and unions of equivalence classes (Yao, 2004a). Normally, such a structure is defined based on different subsets of attributes in an information table. The model thus provides an effective means for analyzing information tables based on various granulations. In fuzzy set theory, a granule is interpreted as a fuzzy set that quantitatively defines a natural language word. It provides a framework of computing with words and approximate reasoning with granules. Artificial intelligence studies knowledge representation, abstraction, reasoning, learning, problem solving, and many more topics. The notions of granularity and abstraction have been investigated many authors (Yao, 2008a). The results from these fields, though limited, establish groundwork of granular computing.

Instead of giving a full account of granular computing for machines, I will address a few fundamental issues related to the notion of multiple levels of granularity. For describing and understanding a problem, we need to explore multiple representations in terms of multiple views and multiple levels of abstraction; for finding the most suitable solutions to problem, we need to examine the space of multiple approximate solutions; in the process of problem solving, we need to employ multiple strategies. In other words, a key to granular computing for machines is to represent and work with different levels of granularity in every stages of problem solving.

One step in machine problem solving is to choose most suitable and accurate representations of the problem. Furthermore, machines must be able to understand and operate on such representations. We consider two levels of representations in terms of multiview and multilevel, as shown in Figure 1. For a problem, we may view it from many different angles, and associate a representation with a particular view. A representation normally makes certain features explicit at the expense of hiding others (Marr, 1982). With each view capturing particular aspects of the problem, the consideration of multiple views may, to some extent, avoid limitations of a single view-level representation (Bateson, 1978; Chen and Yao, 2008). For each view, we may consider multiple levels of abstractions, which each representing the problem at a particular level of details. The multiple levels of abstraction require us to further divide a view-level representation into multiple representations.

In Figure 1, we consider a framework of representations with two levels of granularity: at the view-level, we have multiple representations for different views; within each view, we also have multiple representations for different level of abstraction. In general, one may consider many-level granularity for representation. As another note on representation, one may use different representation languages and schemes in different views and at different levels in each view. Representation schemes and approaches used by humans may provide hints to obtaining good machine representations.

Another crucial task in machine problem solving is to design criteria for evaluating a solution. Due to resource constraints, such as space and time, we may only be able to, or need to, obtain approximate and sub-optimal solutions instead of the optimal solution. For example, in some cases we may only need a qualitative characterization of solutions. This requires a multiple level organization of the space of approximate solutions so that a machine can stop at the appropriate level. The space of approximate solutions reflects the granularity of solutions. When more resources are available, or when new requirements are given, it is possible to search solutions at further levels of accuracy. Finally, the solution space may be related to the problem of representations, so that a particular level of approximate solutions is obtained at the most suitable levels of abstraction and within most suitable views.

With multiple representations of a problem and a multilevel organization of approximate solutions, it comes naturally in the problem solving process to use multiple strategies. In general, problem representation, criteria on solutions, and problem solving strategies work together. It is necessary to choose the most appropriate strategies for obtaining required solutions under particular representation. Furthermore, when one combination fails, it is necessary to search for others; such a switch should also be relatively simple and easy.

To a large extent, the above discussions are based on the Minsky's study on human minds. According to Minsky (2007), human minds are versatile, and some of their features are summarized as follows:

- We can see things from many different points of view; we can rapidly switch among views.

*Figure 1. Multiview and multilevel granular structures*

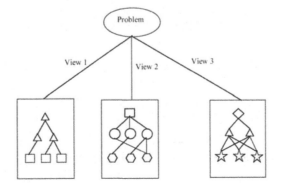

- We have multiple descriptions of things; we develop good ways to organize these representations; we can quickly switch among them.
- We have many ways to ways to think; when one of the ways fails, we can easily switch to another.
- We can learn and create new ways to think.

The requirements of multiple representations, multiple criteria on solutions, and multiple strategies are inspired by humans. Granular computing for machine needs to implement these human-inspired ideas and notions in machines.

# 6. THE TRIARCHIC THEORY OF GRANULAR COMPUTING

The discussions of the last two sections provide a context for studying granular computing. The triarchic theory is a unified view that stresses the study of granular computing as a new field in its wholeness, rather than scattered pieces. The triarachic theory can be described by the granular computing triangle as shown in Figure 2. By focusing on multiple level hierarchical structures, the theory integrates philosophical, methodological, and computational issues of granular computing as structured thinking, structured problem solving and structured information processing, respectively. A brief description of the theory is given in this section and more details can be found in other papers (Yao, 2005, 2006, 2007a, 2008a).

## 6.1. Granular Structures as Multiple Hierarchies

Granular computing emphasizes on structures. It seems that hierarchical granular structures is a good candidate for developing a theory of granular computing. By a *hierarchical structure* (i.e., *hierarchy*), I mean a loosely defined structure that is weaker than a tree or a lattice. The basic ingredients of a granular structure are a family of granules, a family of levels, and partial orderings on granules and levels.

Granules are used as an abstract and primitive notion whose physical meaning becomes clearer only when a particular application or concrete problem is considered. Intuitively speaking, granules are parts of a whole. They are the focal points of our current interest or the units we used to obtain a description or a representation. A granule serves dual roles: it is a single undividable unit when it is considered as a part of another granule; it is a whole consisting of interconnected and interacting granules when some other granules are viewed as its parts.

*Figure 2. The granular computing triangle*

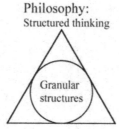

Philosophy:
Structured thinking

Granular structures

Methodology:
Structured problem solving

Computation:
Structured information processing

We need to characterize granules by a minimum set of three types of properties. The internal properties of a granule reflect its organizational structures and the relationships and interaction of its element granules. The external properties of a granule reveal its interaction with other granules. The contextual properties of a granule show its relative existence in a particular environment. The three types of properties together provide us a full understanding of the notion of granules.

We may collect a family of granules of a similar type together and study their collective properties. This leads to the notion of levels. While each granule provides a local view, a level provides a global view. An important property of granules and levels is their granularity, which enables us to order partially granules and levels. Such an ordering results in a hierarchical view. In building a hierarchical structure, we explore a vertical separation of levels and a horizontal separation of granules at the same hierarchical level (Simon, 1963). Usually, the two separations must ignore information that is irrelevant to the current interest or does not greatly affect our solution. Furthermore, a single hierarchy only represents one view. As illustrated by Figure 1, granular structures studied in granular computing may be more accurately described as a multilevel view given by a single hierarchy and a multiview understanding given by many hierarchies.

## 6.2. The Granular Computing Triangle

The core of the triarchic theory can be simply described by the granular computing triangle of Figure 2. The three vertices of the triangle represent the philosophical, methodological and computational perspectives.

## Philosophy

The philosophy of granular computing offers a worldview characterized by different sized, interacting and hierarchically organized granules. This view of the world in terms of structures as represented by multiple levels leads to a way of structured thinking, which is applicable to many branches of natural and social sciences. In fact, multilevel structures have been widely used, including levels of abstraction in almost every branch of sciences, levels of understanding in education, levels of interpretation in history and language understanding, levels of organization in ecology and social sciences, levels of complexity in computer science and systems theory, levels of processing in modeling human memory, levels of details in programming languages, and many others.

Broadly speaking, granular computing draws results from two complementary philosophical views about the complexity of real-world problems, namely, the traditional reductionist thinking and the more recent systems thinking. It combines analytical thinking for decomposing a whole into parts and synthetic thinking for integrating parts into a whole.

## Methodology

As a general method of structured problem solving, granular computing promotes systematic approaches, effective principles, and practical heuristics and strategies that have been used effectively by humans for solving real-world problems. A central issue is the exploration of granular structures. This involves three basic tasks: constructing granular structures, working within a particular level of the structure, and switching between levels. We can formulate a set of principles to highlight the methodology of granular computing.

Several such principles are considered here. The principle of *multilevel granularity* emphasizes the effective use of a hierarchical structure. According to this principle, we must consider multiple representations at different levels of granularity. The principle of *multiview* stresses the consideration of diversity in modeling. We need to look at the same problem from many angles and perspectives. Once granular structures are obtained, we can apply other principles to work based on such structures. For example, the principle of *focused efforts* calls for attention on the focal point at a particular stage of problem solving; the principle of *granularity conversion* links the different stages in this process. The principle of *view switching* allows us to change views and to compare different views. Those principles of granular computing have, in fact, been used extensively in different disciplines under different names and notations. Many principles of structured programming can be readily adopted for granular computing.

## Computation

As a new paradigm of structured information processing, granular computing focuses on computing methods based on the granular structures. The term computing needs to be understood in its broad meaning to include information processing in the abstract, in the brain and in machines. While information processing in the abstract deals with theories of computing without direct reference to their implementations, information processing in the brain and in machines represent the biological (natural) and the physical (artificial) implementations, respectively.

Two related basic issues of computation are representations and processes (operations). Representation covers the formal and precise description of granules and granular structures. Processes may be broadly divided into the two classes: granulation and computation with granules. Granulation processes involve the construction of the building blocks and structures, namely, granules, levels, and hierarchies. Computation processes explore the granular structures. This involves two-way communications up and down in a hierarchy, as well as switching between levels.

The three perspectives of granular computing are connected and mutually support each other. Their integration puts granular computing research on a firm basis. In addition, the granular computing triangle recommends a research direction towards an interdisciplinary wholeness approach. That is, researchers in different disciplines may investigate different perspectives of granular computing and at the same time integrate their individual results.

## 7. CONCLUDING REMARKS

In the chapter, I examine a view of granular computing as a human-inspired paradigm of problem solving and information processing. It covers two types of studies, namely, human-oriented studies and machine-oriented studies, and two goals, namely, granular computing for humans and granular computing for machines. The main stream of research focuses on machine-oriented studies with the goal of granular computing for machines. Human-oriented studies are a prerequisite of machine oriented-studies. As human-inspired structured approaches, granular computing is both for humans and for machines.

I outline a triarachic theory of granular computing based on results from related fields and most recent development of granular computing. The theory is based on granular structures and three perspectives of granular computing. Granular computing emphasizes the use of good structures representing multiview and multilevel. On the one hand, as a philosophy and general methodology, granular computing empowers everyone in problem solving; as a paradigm of structured information processing, granular computing supports human-inspired machines and systems. The triarchic theory enables us to develop granular computing as a field of study, rather than another theory or methodology.

# REFERENCES

Bargiela, A., & Pedrycz, W. (Eds.). (2002). *Granular computing: an introduction*. Boston: Kluwer Academic Publishers.

Bargiela, A., & Pedrycz, W. (2008). Toward a theory of granular computing for human-centered information processing. *IEEE Transactions on Fuzzy Systems*, *16*, 320–330. doi:10.1109/TFUZZ.2007.905912

Baars, B. J. (2002). The conscious access hypothesis: origins and recent evidence. *Trends in Cognitive Sciences*, *6*(1), 47–52. doi:10.1016/S1364-6613(00)01819-2

Bateson, G. (1978). *Mind and nature: a necessity unity*. New York: E.P. Dutton.

Beveridge, W. I. B. (1967). *The art of scientific investigation*. New York: Vintage Books.

Chen, Y. H., & Yao, Y. Y. (2008). A multiview approach for intelligent data analysis based on data operators. *Information Sciences*, *178*(1), 1–20. doi:10.1016/j.ins.2007.08.011

Crane, D. (1972). *Invisible colleges, diffusion of knowledge in scientific communities*. Chicago: The University of Chicago Press.

Dijkstra, E. W. (EWD237). A preliminary investigation into computer assisted programming. Retrieved September 22, 2008, from http://www.cs.utexas.edu/users/EWD/ewd02xx/EWD237.pdf

Dijkstra, E. W. (EWD245). On useful structuring. Retrieved September 22, 2008, from http://www.cs.utexas.edu/users/EWD/ewd02xx/EWD245.pdf

Friske, M. (1985). Teaching proofs: a lesson from software engineering. *The American Mathematical Monthly*, *92*, 142–144. doi:10.2307/2322651

Gilhooly, K. J. (1989). Human and machine problem solving, toward a comparative cognitive science. In Gilhooly, K. J. (Ed.), *Human and Machine Problem Solving* (pp. 1–13). New York: Plenum Press.

Han, J. C., & Dong, J. (2007). Perspectives of granular computing in software engineering. In: Lin, T. Y., Hu, X. H., Han, J. C., Shen, X. J., & Li, Z. J. (Eds.), *Proceedings of 2007 IEEE International Conference on Granular Computing* (pp. 66-71). Los Alamitos, CA: IEEE Computer Society Press.

Hawkins, J., & Blakeslee, S. (2004). *On intelligence*. New York: Henry Holt & Company.

Hobbs, J. R. (1985). Granularity. In: Aravind, K. J. (Ed.), *Proceedings of the Ninth International Joint Conference on Artificial Intelligence* (pp. 432-435). New York: Academic Press.

Keet, C. M. (2006). A taxonomy of types of granularity. In: Zhang, Y.Q., & Lin, T.Y. (Eds.), *Proceeding of 2006 IEEE International Conference on Granular Computing* (pp. 106-111). Piscataway, NJ: Institute of Electrical and Electronics Engineers, Inc.

Keet, C. M. (2008). *A formal theory of granularity.* PhD Thesis, KRDB Research Centre, Faculty of Computer Science, Free University of Bozen-Bolzano, Italy. Retrieved June 8, 2008, from http://www.meteck.org/files/AFormalTheoryOfGranularity_ CMK08.pdf

Knuth, D. E. (1984). Literate programming. *The Computer Journal, 27*(2), 97–111. doi:10.1093/comjnl/27.2.97

Leron, U. (1983). Structuring mathematical proofs. *The American Mathematical Monthly, 90,* 174–185. doi:10.2307/2975544

Lin, T. Y., Yao, Y. Y., & Zadeh, L. A. (Eds.). (2002). *Data mining, rough sets and granular computing.* Heidelberg, Germany: Springer-Verlag.

Marr, D. (1982). *Vision, a computational investigation into human representation and processing of visual information.* San Francisco: W.H. Freeman & Company.

Martella, R. C., Nelson, R., & Marchard-Martella, N. E. (1999). *Research methods: learning to become a critical research consumer.* Boston: Allyn & Bacon.

Minsky, M. (2007). *The emotion machine: commonsense thinking, artificial intelligence, and the future of the human mind.* New York: Simon & Schuster Paperbacks.

Newell, A., & Simon, H. A. (1972). *Human problem solving.* New Jersey: Prentice-Hall, Inc.

Pawlak, Z. (1998). Granularity of knowledge, indiscernibility and rough sets. In: *Proceedings of 1998 IEEE International Conference on Fuzzy Systems* (pp. 106-110). Piscataway, NJ: Institute of Electrical and Electronics Engineers, Inc.

Pedrycz, W., Skowron, A., & Kreinovich, V. (Eds.). (2008). *Handbook of granular computing.* West Sussex, UK: John Wiley & Sons Ltd.doi:10.1002/9780470724163

Pinker, S. (1997). *How the mind works.* New York: W.W. Norton & Company.

Samuel, A. L. (1962). Artificial intelligence: a frontier of automation. *The Annals of the American Academy of Political and Social Science, 340*(1), 10–20. doi:10.1177/000271626234000103

Schank, R. C. (1987). What is AI, anyway? *AI Magazine, 8*(4), 59–65.

Simon, H. A. (1963). The organization of complex systems. In Pattee, H. H. (Ed.), *Hierarchy Theory, the Challenge of Complex Systems* (pp. 1–27). New York: George Braziller.

Sternberg, R. J., & Frensch, P. A. (Eds.). (1991). *Complex problem solving, principles and mechanisms.* Mahwah, NJ: Lawrence Erlbaum Associates.

The national academy of engineering (2008). *Grand challenges for engineering.* Retrieved September 19, 2008, from http://www.engineeringchallenges.org

Wing, J. M. (2006). Computational thinking. *Communications of the ACM, 49*(3), 33–35. doi:10.1145/1118178.1118215

Xie, Y., Katukuri, J., Raghavan, V. V., & Johnsten, T. (2008). Examining granular computing from a modeling perspective. In: *Proceedings of 2008 Annual Meeting of the North American Fuzzy Information Processing Society* (pp. 1-5). Piscataway, NJ: Institute of Electrical and Electronics Engineers, Inc.

Yao, J. T. (2007). A ten-year review of granular computing. In: Lin, T.Y., Hu, X.H., Han, J.C., Shen, X.J., & Li, Z.J. (Eds.), *Proceedings of 2007 IEEE International Conference on Granular Computing* (pp. 734-739). Los Alamitos, CA: IEEE Computer Society Press.

Yao, J. T. (2008). Recent developments in granular computing: a bibliometrics study. In: Lin, T.Y., Hu, X.H., Liu, Q., Shen, X., Xia J., He, T., and Cercone, N. (Eds.) *Proceedings of 2008 IEEE International Conference on Granular Computing* (pp. 74-79). Piscataway, NJ: Institute of Electrical and Electronics Engineers, Inc.

Yao, Y. Y. (2000). Granular computing: basic issues and possible solution. *Proceedings of the 5th Joint Conference on Information Sciences* (pp. 186-189). Durham, NC: Association for Intelligent Machinery, Inc.

Yao, Y. Y. (2004a). A partition model of granular computing. *LNCS Transactions on Rough Sets I, LNCS 3100*, 232-253.

Yao, Y. Y. (2004b). Granular computing. [Ji Suan Ji Ke Xue]. *Computer Science, 31*, 1–5.

Yao, Y. Y. (2005). Perspectives of granular computing. In: Hu, X.H., Liu, Q., Skowron, A., Lin, T.Y., Yager, R.R., & Zhang, B. (Eds.), *Proceedings of 2005 IEEE International Conference on Granular Computing* (pp. 85-90). Piscataway, NJ: Institute of Electrical and Electronics Engineers, Inc.

Yao, Y. Y. (2006). Three perspectives of granular computing. *Journal of Nanchang Institute of Technology, 25*, 16–21.

Yao, Y. Y. (2007a). The art of granular computing. In: Kryszkiewicz, M., Peters, J.F., Rybinski, H., & Skowron, A. (Eds.), *Proceeding of the International Conference on Rough Sets and Emerging Intelligent Systems Paradigms, LNAI 4585* (pp. 101-112). Berlin, Germany: Springer.

Yao, Y. Y. (2007b). Structured writing with granular computing strategies. In: Lin, T.Y., Hu, X.H., Han, J.C., Shen, X.J., & Li, Z.J. (Eds.), *Proceedings of 2007 IEEE International Conference on Granular Computing* (pp. 72-77). Los Alamitos, CA: IEEE Computer Society.

Yao, Y. Y. (2008a). Granular computing: past, present and future. In: Lin, T.Y., Hu, X.H., Han, J.C., Shen, X.J., & Li, Z.J. (Eds.), *Proceedings of 2008 IEEE International Conference on Granular Computing* (pp. 80-85). Piscataway, NJ: Institute of Electrical and Electronics Engineers, Inc.

Yao, Y. Y. (2008b). The rise of granular computing. [Natural Science Edition]. *Journal of Chongqing University of Posts and Telecommunications, 20*, 299–308.

Zadeh, L. A. (1997). Towards a theory of fuzzy information granulation and its centrality in human reasoning and fuzzy logic. *Fuzzy Sets and Systems, 90*, 111–127. doi:10.1016/S0165-0114(97)00077-8

Zhang, L., & Zhang, B. (Eds.). (2007). *Theory and application of problem solving – theory and application of granular computing in quotient spaces (in Chinese)* (2nd ed.). Beijing, China: Tsinghua University Press.

Zhu, H. B. (2008). Granular problem solving and software engineering. In: Lin, T.Y., Hu, X.H., Han, J.C., Shen, X.J., & Li, Z.J. (Eds.), *Proceedings of 2008 IEEE International Conference on Granular Computing* (pp. 859-864) Piscataway, NJ: Institute of Electrical and Electronics Engineers, Inc.

# Chapter 2
# Discovery of Process Models from Data and Domain Knowledge:
## A Rough–Granular Approach

**Hung Son Nguyen**
*Warsaw University, Poland*

**Andrzej Jankowski**
*Institute of Decision Processes Support and AdgaM Solutions Sp. z o.o., Poland*

**James F. Peters**
*University of Manitoba, Canada*

**Andrzej Skowron**
*Warsaw University, Poland*

**Jarosław Stepaniuk**
*Białystok University of Technology, Poland*

**Marcin Szczuka**
*Warsaw University, Poland*

## ABSTRACT

*The rapid expansion of the Internet has resulted not only in the ever-growing amount of data stored therein, but also in the burgeoning complexity of the concepts and phenomena pertaining to that data. This issue has been vividly compared by the renowned statistician J.F. Friedman (Friedman, 1997) of Stanford University to the advances in human mobility from the period of walking afoot to the era of jet travel. These essential changes in data have brought about new challenges in the discovery of new data mining methods, especially the treatment of these data that increasingly involves complex processes that elude classic modeling paradigms. "Hot" datasets like biomedical, financial or net user behavior data are just a few examples. Mining such temporal or stream data is a focal point in the agenda of many research centers and companies worldwide (see, e.g., (Roddick et al., 2001; Aggarwal, 2007)). In the data mining community, there is a rapidly growing interest in developing methods for process mining,*

DOI: 10.4018/978-1-60566-324-1.ch002

*e.g., for discovery of structures of temporal processes from observed sample data. Research on process mining (e.g., (Unnikrishnan et al., 2006; de Medeiros et al., 2007; Wu, 2007; Borrett et al., 2007)) have been undertaken by many renowned centers worldwide[1]. This research is also related to functional data analysis (see, e.g., (Ramsay & Silverman, 2002)), cognitive networks (see, e.g., (Papageorgiou & Stylios, 2008)), and dynamical system modeling, e.g., in biology (see, e.g., (Feng et al., 2007)). We outline an approach to the discovery of processes from data and domain knowledge. The proposed approach to discovery of process models is based on rough-granular computing. In particular, we discuss how changes along trajectories of such processes can be discovered from sample data and domain knowledge.*

## INTRODUCTION: WISDOM TECHNOLOGY (WISTECH)

In this section, we discuss a research direction for discovery of process models from sample data and domain knowledge within the *Wisdom technology* (wistech) system presented recently in (Jankowski & Skowron, 2007; Jankowski & Skowron, 2008a).

Wisdom commonly means *rightly judging* based on available knowledge and interactions. This common notion can be refined. By *wisdom*, we understand an adaptive ability to make judgments correctly (in particular, correct decisions) to a satisfactory degree, having in mind real-life constraints. The intuitive nature of wisdom understood in this way can be metaphorically expressed by the so-called *wisdom equation* as shown in (1).

$$wisdom = adaptive\ judgment + knowledge + interaction. \tag{1}$$

Wisdom can be treated as a special type of knowledge processing. To explain the specificity of this type of knowledge processing, let us assume that a control system of a given agent *Ag* consists of a society of agent control components interacting with the other agent *Ag* components and with the agent *Ag* environments. Moreover, there are special agent components called as the agent coordination control components which are responsible for the coordination of control components. Any agent coordination control component mainly searches for answers for the following question: *What to do next?* or, more precisely: *Which of the agent Ag control components should be activated now?* Of course, any agent control component has to process some kind of knowledge representation. In the context of agent perception, the agent *Ag* itself (by using, e.g., interactions, memory, and coordination among control components) is processing a very special type of knowledge reflecting the agent perception of the hierarchy of needs (objectives, plans, etc.) and the current agent or the environment constraints. This kind of knowledge processing mainly deals with complex vague concepts (such as risk or safety) from the point of view of the *selfish* agent needs. Usually, this kind of knowledge processing is not necessarily logical reasoning in terms of proving statements (i.e., labeling statements by truth values such as TRUE or FALSE). This knowledge processing is rather analogous to the judgment process in a court aiming at recognition of evidence which could be used as an argument *for* or *against*. Arguments *for* or *against* are used in order to make the final decision which one of the solutions is the best for the agent in the current situation (i.e., arguments are labeling statements by judgment values expressing the action priorities). The evaluation of currents needs by agent *Ag* is realized from the point of view of hierarchy of agent *Ag life* values/needs). Wisdom type of knowledge processing by the agent *Ag* is characterized by the ability to improve quality of the judgment process based on the agent *Ag* experiences. In order to emphasize the importance of this ability, we use the concept of *adaptive judgment* in the wisdom equation instead of just *judgment*. An agent who is able to perform adaptive judgment in the above sense, we simply call as a *judge*.

The adaptivity aspects are also crucial from the point of view of interactions (Goldin et al., 2006; Nguyen & Skowron, 2008). The need for adaptation follows, e.g., from the fact that complex vague concepts on the basis of which the judgment is performed by the agent *Ag* are approximated by classification algorithms (classifiers) which should drift in time following changes in data and represented knowledge.

Wistech is a collection of techniques aimed at the further advancement of technologies to acquire, represent, store, process, discover, communicate, and learn *wisdom* in designing and implementing intelligent systems. These techniques include approximate reasoning by agents or teams of agents about vague concepts concerning real-life, dynamically changing, usually distributed systems in which these agents are operating. Such systems consist of other autonomous agents operating in highly unpredictable environments and interacting with each others. Wistech can be treated as the successor of database technology, information management, and knowledge engineering technologies. Wistech is the combination of the technologies represented in Equation (1) and offers an intuitive starting point for a variety of approaches to designing and implementing computational models for wistech in intelligent systems.

- *Knowledge technology* in wistech is based on techniques for reasoning about knowledge, information, and data, techniques that enable to employ the current knowledge in problem solving. This includes, e.g., extracting relevant fragments of knowledge from knowledge networks for making decisions or reasoning by analogy.
- *Judgment technology* in wistech is covering the representation of agent perception and adaptive judgment strategies based on results of perception of real life scenes in environments and their representations in the agent mind. The role of judgment is crucial, e.g., in adaptive planning relative to the Maslow Hierarchy of agents' needs or goals. Judgment also includes techniques used for perception, learning, analysis of perceived facts, and adaptive refinement of approximations of vague complex concepts (from different levels of concept hierarchies in real-life problem solving) applied in modeling interactions in dynamically changing environments (in which cooperating, communicating, and competing agents exist) under uncertain and insufficient knowledge or resources.
- *Interaction technology* includes techniques for performing and monitoring actions by agents and environments. Techniques for planning and controlling actions are derived from a combination of judgment technology and interaction technology.

The wistech system is strongly related to the idea of Gottfried Wilhelm Leibniz, one of the greatest mathematicians. He has discussed, in a sense, calculi of thoughts. In particular, he has written

*If controversies were to arise, there would be no more need of disputation between two philosophers than between two accountants. For it would suffice to take their pencils in their hands, and say to each other: 'Let us calculate'.--Gottfried Wilhelm Leibniz, Dissertio de Arte Combinatoria (Leipzig, 1666)*

*Languages are the best mirror of the human mind, and that a precise analysis of the signification of words would tell us more than anything else about the operations of the understanding.--Gottfried Wilhelm*

*Leibniz, New Essays on Human Understanding (1705) (Translated and edited by Peter Remnant and Jonathan Bennett Cambridge: Cambridge UP, 1982)*

Only much later, it was possible to recognize that new tools are necessary for developing such calculi, e.g., due to the necessity of reasoning under uncertainty about objects and (vague) concepts. Fuzzy set theory (Lotfi A. Zadeh, 1965) and rough set theory (Zdzisław Pawlak, 1982) represent two complementary approaches to vagueness. Fuzzy set theory addresses gradualness of knowledge expressed by fuzzy membership, whereas rough set theory addresses granularity of knowledge manifest in the classes (knowledge granules) contained in the partition of each set of sample data defined by the indiscernibility relation. Granular computing (Zadeh, 1973, 1998) may be now regarded as a unified framework for theories, methodologies and techniques for modeling of calculi of thoughts based on objects called granules.

There are many ways to build foundations for wistech computational models. One of them is based on the *rough-granular computing* (RGC). Rough-granular computing (RGC) is an approach for constructive definition of computations over sets of objects called information granules, aiming at searching for solutions of problems that are specified using vague concepts. Granules are obtained during a process called granulation. Granulation can be viewed as a human way of achieving data compression and it plays a key role in implementing the divide-and-conquer strategy in human problem-solving (Zadeh, 2006) Definitely, one can also find many phenomena in the nature that are based on granulation.

The proposed approach combines rough set methods with other soft computing methods, and methods based on granular computing (GC). RGC is used for developing one of the possible wistech foundations based on approximate reasoning about vague concepts. For more readings on granular computing, the reader is referred to (Bargiela & Pedrycz, 2003; Pedrycz et al., 2008; Pedrycz, 2001; Pal et al., 2004; Peters, 2008b).

There are several substantial differences between wistech and the traditional AI (Jankowski & Skowron, 2008a). Let us mention only that the decision making in witech is often based on complex vague concepts (e.g., concepts related to the Maslov hierarchy (Jankowski & Skowron, 2008a)). Approximations of these concepts performed by agents are changing over time due to their interaction with dynamically changing environments and due to acquisition of new knowledge by experts. We propose to base adaptive learning of concept approximations on interactive computations on objects called granules. Such granules represent structures of varying complexity, e.g., indiscernibility or similarity classes, patterns, rules, sets of rules, approximation spaces, clusters, classifiers. Interactive computations on granules result in the discovery of relevant granules for vague concept approximation. Understanding of the nature of interactive computations is nowadays one of the most challenging problems (Goldin et al., 2006). Vague concepts are often of a spatio-temporal nature. For approximation of these vague concepts, complex structures and their properties on different levels of hierarchical modeling should be discovered. Some of these structures represent complex interacting (concurrent) processes. In discovering such structures and their properties, we propose to use experimental (historical) data and domain knowledge represented, e.g., by ontologies (Bazan et al., 2006a; Bazan et al., 2006b; Bazan et al., 2005; Bazan & Skowron, 2005a; Bazan & Skowron, 2005b; Bazan et al., 2006c; Nguyen et al., 2004; Nguyen, 2005; Nguyen, 2008; Nguyen et al., 2006) gradually approximated in hierarchical modeling and multi-context modeling[2]. On different levels of hierarchical modeling, information systems with structural objects and their features can be discovered using experimental data and domain knowledge. They are gradually making it possible to construct granules (patterns) used for approximation of target vague concepts. For approximation, classification, or prediction of complex spatio-temporal concepts it is necessary to discover relevant granules (patterns) representing structures of complex (concurrent) processes (corresponding to analyzed objects or phenomena) and changes of these structures over time.

In the following sections, we first discuss some of the basic issues for RGC such as the optimization in discovery of compound granules and some basic issues on strategies in searching for compound granules. Next, we present an introduction to process mining based on RGC.

## OPTIMIZATION IN DISCOVERY OF COMPOUND GRANULES

This section is based on the approach discussed in (Jankowski et al., 2008). The problem considered in this section is the evaluation of perception as a means of optimizing various tasks. The solution to this problem hearkens back to early research on rough set theory and approximation. For example, in 1982, Ewa Orłowska observed that approximation spaces serve as a formal counterpart of perception.

In this chapter, the evaluation of perception is at the level of approximation spaces. The quality of an approximation space relative to a given approximated set of objects is a function of the description length of an approximation of the set of objects and the approximation quality of this set. In granular computing (GC), the focus is on discovering granules satisfying selected criteria. These criteria take inspiration from the minimal description length (MDL) principle proposed by Jorma Rissanen in 1983. In this section, the role of approximation spaces in modeling compound granules satisfying such criteria is discussed. For example, in terms of approximation itself, this chapter introduces an approach to function approximation in the context of a reinterpretation of the rough integral originally proposed by Zdzisław Pawlak in 1993.

First, we recall the definition of an approximation space from (Skowron & Stepaniuk, 1996). Approximation spaces can be treated as granules used for concept approximation. They are examples of special parameterized relational structures. Tuning parameters makes it possible to search for relevant approximation spaces relative to given concepts.

### Definition 1

*A parameterized approximation space is a system* $AS_{\#,\$} = \left(U, I_{\#}, \nu_{\$}\right)$, where

- $U$ is a non-empty *set of objects,* $I_{\#} : U \to P\left(U\right)$ *is an uncertainty function, where* $P\left(U\right)$ denotes the power set of $U$,
- $\nu_{\$} : P\left(U\right) \times P\left(U\right) \to \left[0,1\right]$ is a rough in*clusion function,*

and $\#, \$$ denote vectors of parameters (the indexes $\#, \$$ will be omitted if it does not lead to misunderstanding).

The uncertainty function defines for every object $x$, a set of objects described similarly to $x$. The set $I(x)$ is called the neighborhood of $x$ (see, *e.g.*, (Pawlak, 1991; Skowron & Stepaniuk, 1996)). The rough inclusion function $\nu_{\$}:P\left(U\right) \times P\left(U\right) \to \left[0,1\right]$ defines the degree of inclusion of $X$ in $Y$, where $X, Y \subseteq U$.

In the simplest case it can be defined by (see, *e.g.*, (Pawlak, 1991; Skowron & Stepaniuk, 1996)):

$$\nu_{SRI}(X,Y) = \begin{cases} \dfrac{card(X \cap Y)}{card(X)}, & if \quad X \neq \varnothing, \\ 1, & if \quad X = \varnothing. \end{cases}$$

The lower and the upper approximations of subsets of $U$ are defined as follows.

## Definition 2

*For any approximation space* $AS_{\#,\$} = \left(U, I_{\#}, \nu_{\$}\right)$ *and any subset* $X \subseteq U$, the lower and upper approximations are defined by

$$LOW\left(AS_{\#,\$}, X\right) = \left\{ x \in U : \nu_{\$}\left(I_{\#}(x), X\right) = 1 \right\},$$

$$UPP\left(AS_{\#,\$}, X\right) = \left\{ x \in U : \nu_{\$}\left(I_{\#}(x), X\right) > 0 \right\}, \text{respectively.}$$

The lower approximation of a set $X$ with respect to the approximation space $AS_{\#,\$}$ is the set of all objects that can be classified with certainty as objects of $X$ with respect to $AS_{\#,\$}$. The upper approximation of a set $X$ with respect to the approximation space $AS_{\#,\$}$ is the set of all objects, which can be possibly classified as objects of $X$ with respect to $AS_{\#,\$}$.

Several known approaches to concept approximations can be covered using this approach to approximation spaces, *e.g.*, (see, *e.g.*, references in (Skowron & Stepaniuk, 1996)). For more details on approximation spaces, the reader is referred to, *e.g.*, (Pawlak & Skowron, 2007; Bazan et al., 2006c; Skowron et al., 2006; Peters, 2007a; Peters et al., 2007b).

A key task in granular computing is the information granulation process that leads to the formation of information aggregates (with inherent patterns) from a set of available objects. A methodological and algorithmic issue is the formation of transparent (understandable) information granules inasmuch as they should provide a clear and understandable description of patterns present in sample objects (Bargiela & Pedrycz, 2003; Pedrycz et al., 2008). Such a fundamental property can be formalized by a set of constraints that must be satisfied during the information granulation process. Usefulness of these constraints is measured by quality of an approximation space:

$$Quality_1 : Set\_AS \times P(U) \rightarrow [0,1],$$

where $U$ is a non-empty set of objects and $Set\_AS$ is a set of possible approximation spaces with the universe $U$.

## Example 1

If $UPP(AS, X)) \neq \varnothing$ for $AS \in Set\_AS$ and $X \subseteq U$ then

$$Quality_1(AS, X) = \nu_{SRI}(UPP(AS, X), LOW(AS, X))$$
$$= \frac{card(LOW(AS, X))}{card(UPP(AS, X))}.$$

The value $1 - Quality_1(AS, X)$ expresses the degree of completeness of our knowledge about $X$, given the approximation space $AS$.

## Example 2

In applications, we usually use another quality measure analogous to the minimal length principle (Rissanen, 1985; Ślęzak, 2002), where also the description length of approximation is included. Let us denote by $description(AS, X)$ the description length of approximation of $X$ in $AS$. The description length may be measured, *e.g.*, by the sum of description lengths of algorithms testing membership for neighborhoods used in construction of the lower approximation, the upper approximation, and the boundary region of the set $X$. Then the quality $Quality_2(AS, X)$ can be defined by

$$Quality_2(AS, X) = g(Quality_1(AS, X), description(AS, X)),$$

where $g$ is a relevant function used for fusion of values $Quality_1(AS, X)$ and $description(AS, X)$. This function $g$ can reflect weights given by experts relative to both criteria.

One can consider different optimization problems relative to a given class $Set\_AS$ of approximation spaces. For example, for a given $X \subseteq U$ and a threshold $t \in [0,1]$, one can search for an approximation space $AS$ satisfying the constraint $Quality_2(AS, X) \geq t$.

Another example can be related to searching for an approximation space satisfying additionally the constraint $Cost(AS) < c$ where $Cost(AS)$ denotes the cost of approximation space $AS$ (*e.g.*, measured by the number of attributes used to define neighborhoods in $AS$) and $c$ is a given threshold. In the following example, we consider also costs of searching for relevant approximation spaces in a given family defined by a parameterized approximation space (see Figure 1). Any parameterized approximation space $AS_{\#,\$} = (U, I_\#, \nu_\$)$ is a family of approximation spaces. The cost of searching in such a family for a relevant approximation space for a given concept $X$ approximation can be treated as a factor of the quality measure of approximation of $X$ in $AS_{\#,\$} = (U, I_\#, \nu_\$)$. Hence, such a quality measure of approximation of $X$ in $AS_{\#,\$}$ can be defined by

*Figure 1. Granulation of parameterized approximation spaces*

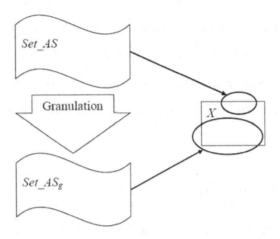

$$Quality_3(AS_{\#,\$}, X) = h(Quality_2(AS, X), Cost\_Search(AS_{\#,\$}, X)),$$

where $AS$ is the result of searching in $AS_{\#,\$}$, $Cost\_Search(AS_{\#,\$}, X)$ is the cost of searching in $AS_{\#,\$}$ for $AS$, and $h$ is a fusion function, *e.g.*, assuming that the values of $Quality_2(AS, X)$ and $Cost\_Search(AS_{\#,\$}, X)$ are normalized to interval $[0,1]$ $h$ could be defined by a linear combination of $Quality_2(AS, X)$ and $Cost\_Search(AS_{\#,\$}, X)$ of the form

$$\lambda Quality_2(AS, X) + (1 - \lambda) Cost\_Search(AS_{\#,\$}, X),$$

where $0 \leq \lambda \leq 1$ is a weight measuring an importance of quality and cost in their fusion.

We assume that the fusion functions $g, h$ in the definitions of quality are monotonic relative to each argument.

Let $AS \in Set\_AS$ be an approximation space relevant for approximation of $X \subseteq U$, *i.e.*, $AS$ is the optimal (or semi-optimal) relative to $Quality_2$. By $Granulation(AS_{\#,\$})$ we denote a new parameterized approximation space obtained by granulation of $AS_{\#,\$}$. For example, $Granulation(AS_{\#,\$})$ can be obtained by reducing the number of attributes or inclusion degrees (*i.e.*, possible values of the inclusion function). Let $AS'$ be an approximation space in $Granulation(AS_{\#,\$})$ obtained as the result of searching for optimal (semi-optimal) approximation space in $Granulation(AS_{\#,\$})$ for approximation of $X$.

We assume that three conditions are satisfied: after granulation of $AS_{\#,\$}$ to $Granulation(AS_{\#,\$})$ the following property holds: the cost $Cost\_Search(Granulation(AS_{\#,\$}), X)$, is much lower than the cost

$Cost\_Search(AS_{\#,\$}, X)$; $description(AS', X)$ is much shorter than $description(AS, X)$, *i.e.*, the description length of $X$ in the approximation space $AS'$ is much shorter than the description length of $X$ in the approximation space $AS$; $Quality_1(AS, X)$ and $Quality_1(AS', X)$ are sufficiently close.

The last two conditions should guarantee that the values $Quality_2(AS, X)$ and $Quality_2(AS', X)$ are comparable and this condition together with the first condition about the cost of searching should assure that:

$$Quality_3(Granulation(AS_{\#,\$}, X))$$
*is much better than* $Quality_3(AS_{\#,\$}, X)$.

Certainly, the phrases already mentioned such as *much lower, much shorter*, and *sufficiently close* should be further elaborated. The details will be discussed elsewhere.

Taking into account that parameterized approximation spaces are examples of parameterized granules, one can generalize the above example of parameterized approximation space granulation to the case of granulation of parameterized granules.

In the process of searching for {sub-}optimal approximation spaces, different strategies are used. Let us consider an example of such strategies (Skowron & Synak, 2004). In the example, $DT=(U, A, d)$ denotes a decision system (a given sample of data), where $U$ is a set of objects, $A$ is a set of attributes and $d$ is a decision. We assume that for any object $x$, there is accessible only partial information equal to the $A$-signature of $x$ (object signature, for short), *i.e.*, $Inf_A(x) = \{(a, a(x)) : a \in A\}$ and analogously for any concept there is only given a partial information about this concept by a sample of objects, *e.g.*, in the form of decision table. One can use object signatures as new objects in a new relational structure R. In this relational structure R are also modeled some relations between object signatures, *e.g.*, defined by the similarities of these object signatures. Discovery of relevant relations on object signatures is an important step in the searching process for relevant approximation spaces. In this way, a class of relational structures representing perception of objects and their parts is constructed. In the next step, we select a language L of formulas expressing properties over the defined relational structures and we search for relevant formulas in L. The semantics of formulas (*e.g.*, with one free variable) from L are subsets of object signatures. Observe that each object signature defines a neighborhood of objects from a given sample (*e.g.*, decision table $DT$) and another set on the whole universe of objects being an extension of $U$. In this way, each formula from L defines a family of sets of objects over the sample and also another family of sets over the universe of all objects. Such families can be used to define new neighborhoods of a new approximation space, *e.g.*, by taking unions of the above described families. In the searching process for relevant neighborhoods, we use information encoded in the given sample. More relevant neighborhoods make it possible to define relevant approximation spaces (from the point of view of the optimization criterion). It is worth to mention that often this searching process is even more compound. For example, one can discover several relational structures (not only one, *e.g.*, R as it was presented before) and formulas over such structures defining different families of neighborhoods from the original approximation space and next fuse them for obtaining one family of neighborhoods or one neighborhood in a new approximation space. This kind of modeling is typical for hierarchical modeling (Bazan et al., 2005), *e.g.*, when we search for a relevant approximation space for objects composed from parts for which some relevant approximation spaces have been already found.

## GRANULATION BY DECOMPOSITION AND CONTEXTUAL GRANULATION

In this section, we outline shortly two aspects of information granulation, namely (i) granulation by decomposition and (ii) granulation relative to a context.

Let us assume we would like to construct relevant patterns for a given concept $C$ approximation. By decomposition we mean the process of breaking the description of a complex object down into some smaller components.

Let $u=Inf_A(x)$ be an information vector, where $x \in U$ is an observed object, $U$ is a set of objects and $A$ is a set of attributes[3] and let $C \subseteq U$. Assuming that the object $x$ belongs to $C$, we would like to construct a more general pattern including $x$ which is also included into $C$ to a satisfactory degree.

In searching for relevant generalization of $u$, one can decompose the description vector $u$ into, *e.g.*, two information vectors $u_1$ and $u_2$. However, these components may not be relevant patterns for a given concept approximation because they are too general. Then one can try to fuse them using, *e.g.*, intersection or intersection with some constraints in searching for relevant patterns. If the results of decomposition are not general enough, one can try further to decompose them or one can use, *e.g.*, tolerance (similarity) relations for their generalization[4] (see Figure 2). This process may require several steps. In general, searching for relevant patterns has high computational complexity. For more compound concepts one can use a concept ontology to bound the search (Bazan et al., 2005; Skowron & Stepaniuk, 2003; Bazan et al., 2006a; Bazan, 2008). Evolutionary strategies are good candidates in searching for relevant patterns.

By a context of a given object $x$ we mean a relational structure over descriptions (or partial descriptions) of objects extracted from information system including the object $x$. The context of $x$ can be represented, *e.g.*, by a time window[5] ending at $Inf_A(x)$. The context of $x$ is used as an object on the

*Figure 2. Granulation through decomposition, clustering and intersection*

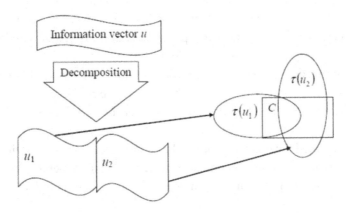

next level of hierarchical modeling where we construct an information (decision) system with features over contexts of objects. Any context can be treated as an information granule. The contexts can be granulated by means of, *e.g.*, similarities among them. In such hierarchical modeling we gradually construct new granules: models and features (attributes, properties) of more and more compound structural objects and finally we would like to discover relevant patterns for a given target concept $C$ approximation. These patterns describe sets of compound structural objects. The structural objects on the highest level of hierarchical modeling represent objects for the approximated concept $C$.

In the following illustrative example, we present one step of hierarchical modeling where a new information system with objects as time windows is constructed from information systems with objects observed in different time points.

## Example 3

Let us consider an intrusion detection system in a computer network. A given server is recording in a data base sequences of operations performed in the network. There is a given sample of (training) sequences such that each sequence is labelled by a *normal* or *abnormal* decision. The sequences recorded by a given server are decomposed into time windows and some relevant properties of time windows should be discovered in the process of constructing of classifier for the concepts *normal* or *abnormal*. Let us consider an example. Assume that the length of a time window is fixed. From sequences stored in the data base, a decision table is created with objects representing time windows. For example, for a sequence of twenty operations and windows with the width equal to five, we obtain sixteen objects. Every window is described by five attributes. First, we add to the new decision table windows by considering in the training sample sequences of operations labelled as *normal*. Next, we add to decision table windows using abnormal sequences of operations. We consider two cases in assigning the decision values to time windows:

- if the sequence of operations is labelled as *normal*, then all sixteen windows obtained from this sequence are labelled as *normal_window*;
- if the sequence of operations is labelled as *abnormal*, then we add to the decision table only windows which were not previously added with label *normal_window* and we label all these windows by *abnormal_window*.

From the above defined decision table, a new classifier can be induced for the decisions *normal_window*, *abnormal_window*. The characteristic function of this classifier can be used as a new feature for time windows. Note, that we have presented only one possible example of a time-window feature. Discovery of relevant features of windows is one of the challenging problems.

On the next level of modeling, objects are sequences of time windows and as features of such objects we consider some features of time windows together with some relations between time windows, *e.g.*, *before*, *after*. These features are used to induce the classifier for the concepts *normal*, *abnormal* related to sequences.

We have shortly described the main idea of two basic approaches to granulation, namely granulation by decomposition and granulation using context in which objects are perceived. The first one is based on decomposition of partial information about perceived objects and on inducing on the obtained parts some relevant relational structures. Properties of these structures are used to define relevant patterns. In this way we obtain information systems with objects represented by relational structures and conditional attributes represented by properties of such relational structures. The second approach is based on hierarchical synthesis of relational structures, representing structures of compound objects, on the basis of context in which such objects appear. In searching for a relevant context for objects we use information systems with objects represented by relational structures defined over the sets of values of given (*e.g.*, sensory) attributes or over relational structures over cartesian products of the value sets of conditional attributes and conditional attributes defining properties of such relational structures. In both cases, the searching process is aiming at discovery of relevant structures of objects and properties of objects represented by the discovered structures. Notice also that the descriptions of objects by means of conditional attributes are used in modeling of relational structures representing more compound objects on the next level of hierarchical modeling of structures of compound objects and their properties (see, e.g., (Bazan et al., 2005; Bazan et al., 2006a; Bazan, 2008)).

Finally, it is worthwhile mentioning that the process of searching for complex patterns and approximate reasoning in distributed systems is also strongly related to idea of information nets (Barwise and Seligman, 1997) and (Skowron et al., 2003). For example, the approach presented in (Skowron et al., 2003) makes it possible to construct information systems (or decision tables) on a given level of hierarchical modeling from information systems from a lower level of hierarchical modeling by using some constraints in joining objects from information systems. In this way, structural objects can be modeled and their properties can be represented in the construction of information systems by selecting relevant attributes. The attributes are defined over a language using attributes of systems from the lower hierarchical level as well as relations used to define constraints. Notice, that in a sense, the objects on the next level of hierarchical modeling are defined using the syntax from the level of the hierarchy. Domain knowledge is used to help to discover the relevant attributes (features) on each level of hierarchy. This domain knowledge can be provided, e.g., by concept ontology together with samples of objects for concepts from this ontology. Such knowledge makes it feasible searching for relevant attributes (features) on different levels of hierarchical modeling (Bazan et al., 2006a; Bazan et al., 2006b; Bazan et al., 2005; Bazan & Skowron, 2005a; Bazan & Skowron, 2005b; Bazan et al., 2006c; Nguyen et al., 2004; Nguyen, 2005; Nguyen, 2008; Nguyen et al., 2006).

## RGC IN PROCESS MINING

This section briefly introduces the rough granular computing approach to process mining.

## Introduction

As an opening point to the presentation of methods for the discovery of process models from data, we would like to mention the proposal by Zdzisław Pawlak. He proposed in 1992 (Pawlak, 1992) to use data tables (information systems) as specifications of concurrent systems. Any information system can be considered as a representation of a concurrent system: attributes are interpreted as local processes of the concurrent system, values of attributes -- as states of local processes, and objects -- as global states of the considered concurrent system. Several methods for synthesis of concurrent systems from data have been developed (see, e.g., (Peters, 1999; Skowron & Suraj, 1993; Skowron & Suraj, 1995; Suraj,

2000)). These methods are based on the following steps. In the first step, for a given information system $S$ is generated its theory $Th(S)$ consisting of a set of selected rules over descriptors defined by this system. These rules describe the coexistence constraints of local states in global states specified by $S$. In the next step, is defined a maximal extension $Ext(S)$ of $S$ consisting of all objects having descriptions consistent with all rules in $Th(S)$. Finally, a Petri net with the set of reachable markings equal to $Ext(S)$ is generated. There have been also developed methods for synthesis of Petri nets from information systems based on decomposition of information systems into the so called components defined by reducts.

Recently, it became apparent that rough set methods and information granulation established a promising perspective for the development of approximate reasoning methods in multi-agent systems. At the same time, it was shown that there exist significant limitations to prevalent methods of mining emerging very large datasets that involve complex vague concepts, phenomena or processes (see, e.g., (Breiman, 2001; Poggio and Smale, 2003; Vapnik, 1998)). One of the essential weaknesses of those methods is the lack of ability to effectively induce the approximation of complex concepts, the realization of which calls for the discovery of highly elaborated data patterns. Intuitively speaking, these complex target concepts are too far apart from available low-level sensor measurements. This results in huge dimensions of the search space for relevant patterns, which renders existing discovery methods and technologies virtually ineffective. In recent years, there emerged an increasingly popular view (see, e.g., (Domingos, 2007; Kriegel et al., 2007)) that one of the main challenges in data mining is to develop methods integrating the pattern and concept discovery with domain knowledge.

The dynamics of complex processes is often specified by means of vague concepts, expressed in natural languages, and of relations between those concepts. Approximation of such concepts requires a hierarchical modeling and approximation of concepts on subsequent levels in the hierarchy provided along with domain knowledge. Because of the complexity of the concepts and processes on top levels in the hierarchy, one can not assume that fully automatic construction of their models, or the discovery of data patterns required to approximate their components, would be straightforward. We propose to use in discovery of process models and their components through an interaction with domain experts. This interaction makes it possible to control the discovery process and make it computationally feasible. Thus, the proposed approach transforms a data mining system into an experimental laboratory, in which the software system, aided by human experts, will attempt to discover: (i) process models from data bounded by domain constraints, (ii) patterns relevant to user, e.g., required in the approximation of vague components of those processes. This research direction has been pursued by our team, in particular, toward the construction of classifiers for complex concepts (see, e.g., (Bazan et al., 2005; Bazan & Skowron, 2005b; Bazan & Skowron, 2005a; Bazan et al., 2006b; Bazan et al., 2006a; Bazan, 2008; Doherty et al., 2006; Nguyen et al., 2004; Nguyen, 2005; Nguyen, 2008; Nguyen et al., 2006)) aided by domain knowledge integration. Advances in recent years indicate a possible expansion of research into discovery of models for processes from temporal or spatio-temporal data involving complex objects.

The novelty of the proposed approach for the discovery of process models from data and domain knowledge as well as for reasoning about changes along trajectories of such processes lies in combining, on the one hand, a number of novel methods of granular computing for wistech developed using rough set methods and other known approaches to the approximation of vague, complex concepts (see, e.g., (Bazan et al., 2005; Bazan & Skowron, 2005b; Bazan & Skowron, 2005a; Bazan et al., 2006c; Bazan et al., 2006b; Bazan et al., 2006a; Bazan, 2008; Jankowski & Skowron, 2008b; Nguyen et al., 2004; Nguyen, 2005; Nguyen, 2008; Nguyen et al., 2006; Pawlak, 1982; Pawlak, 1991; Pawlak & Skowron, 2007; Pedrycz et al., 2008; Zadeh, 2001; Zadeh, 2006)), with, on the other hand, the discovery of process' structures from data through an interactive collaboration with domain experts(s) (see, e.g., (Bazan et al., 2005; Bazan & Skowron, 2005b; Bazan & Skowron, 2005a; Bazan et al., 2006c; Bazan et al., 2006b; Bazan et al., 2006a; Bazan, 2008; Jankowski & Skowron, 2008b; Nguyen et al., 2004; Nguyen, 2005; Nguyen, 2008; Nguyen et al., 2006; Pedrycz et al., 2008)). There are already promising results of real-life applications. In the current project we are working on development of RGC methods for application in areas such as prediction from temporal financial data, gene expression networks, web mining, identification of behavioral patterns, planning, learning interaction (e.g., cooperation protocols or coalition formation), autonomous prediction and control of autonomous robots, summarization of situation, or discovery of language for communication.

## Function Approximation and Rough Integral

Granulation plays an important role, in particular, in function approximation as well as in approximation of functionals[6] (*e.g.*, integrals). In this section, we introduce two basic concepts, function approximation and rough-integral. The approach to rough integration differs significantly from approach in (Pawlak, 1999; Pawlak et al., 2001). In particular, we propose to use a new concept of function approximation. Our approach is suitable for a number of applications where only sample function values are available, *e.g.*, sample radar signal values or seasonal temperatures in a particular geographic region. There are some relationships of our approach with functional data analysis (see, e.g., (Ramsay & Silverman, 2002)). However, in our approach, we are looking for high quality (in the rough set framework) of function approximation from available incomplete data rather than for its analytical model from the given class of function models. Our approach can be treated as a kind of rough clustering of functional data.

Let us consider an example of function approximation. We assume that a partial information is only available about a function, *i.e.*, some points from the graph of the function are known[7]. We would like to present a more formal description of function approximation and an application of this concept in defining a rough-integral over partially specified functions.

First, let us introduce some notation. Let us assume $X^\infty$ is the universe of objects and we assume that $\mu$ is a measure on a $\sigma$-field of subsets of $X^\infty$. By $X \subseteq X^\infty$, we denote a finite sample of objects from $X^\infty$. We assume that $\mu(X^\infty) < \infty$. By $R_+$, we denote the set of non-negative reals and by $\mu_0$ a measure on a $\sigma$-field of subsets of $R_+$. A function $f : X \to R_+$ will be called a sample of a function $f^* : X^\infty \to R_+$ if $f^*$ is an extension of $f$. For any $Z \subseteq X^\infty \times R_+$, let $\pi_1(Z)$ and $\pi_2(Z)$ denote the set $\{x \in X^\infty : \exists y \in R_+ \ (x, y) \in Z\}$ and $\{y \in R_+ : \exists x \in X^\infty (x, y) \in Z\}$, respectively.

If $C$ is a family of neighborhoods, *i.e.*, non-empty subsets of $X^\infty \times R_+$ (measurable relative to the product measure $\mu \times \mu_0$), then the lower approximation of $f$ relative to $C$ (see Figure 3) is defined by (2).

*Figure 3. Function approximation (neighborhoods marked by solid lines belong to the lower approximation and with dashed lines - to the upper approximation)*

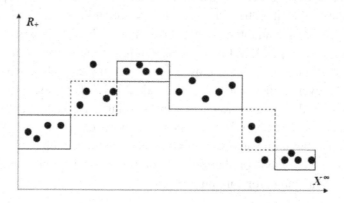

$$\underline{C}f{=}\bigcup\left\{c \in C{:}f\left(\pi_1(c) \cap X\right) \subseteq \pi_2(c)\right\}. \tag{2}$$

Observe that the definition in ((2)) is different from the standard definition of lower approximation (Pawlak, 1991; Pawlak & Skowron, 2007). This new definition makes it possible to express better the fact that the graph of $f$ is "well" matching a given neighborhood (Skowron et al., 2006). For expressing this, a classical set theoretical inclusion of neighborhood into the graph of $f$ is not satisfactory.

One can also define the upper approximation of $f$ relative to $C$ as shown in (3).

$$\overline{C}f{=}\bigcup\{c \in C{:}f(\pi_1(c) \cap X) \cap \pi_2(c) \neq \varnothing\}. \tag{3}$$

By $[\underline{C}f]$, we denote a family $\{c \in C{:}\ f(\pi_1(c) \cap X) \subseteq \pi_2(c)\}$. Hence, $\underline{C}f{=}\bigcup[\underline{C}f]$.

In applications, neighborhoods are defined constructively by semantics of some formulas. Let us assume that $F$ is a given set of formulas and for any formula $\alpha \in F$ there are defined two semantics:

$$\left\|\alpha\right\|_X \subseteq X \times R_+ \text{ and } \left\|\alpha\right\|_{X^\infty} \subseteq X^\infty \times R_+$$

*i.e.,* semantics on the sample $X$ and on the whole universe $X^\infty$. We obtain two families of neighborhoods $F_X{=}\{\left\|\alpha\right\|_X \subseteq X \times R_+ : \alpha \in F\}$ and $F_{X^\infty}{=}\{\left\|\alpha\right\|_{X^\infty} \subseteq X^\infty \times R_+ : \alpha \in F\}$. To this end, we consider (measurable) neighborhoods of the form $Z \times I$ where $Z \subseteq X^\infty$ and $I$ is an interval of reals. We also assume that $Z$ is defined by a formula $\alpha$ from a set $F'$, *i.e.,* $Z{=}\left\|\alpha\right\|_{X^\infty}$.

We know that $\left\|\alpha\right\|_X = \left\|\alpha\right\|_{X^\infty} \cap (X \times R_+)$ but having the sample we do not have information about the other objects from $X^\infty \setminus X$. Hence, for defining the lower approximation of $f$ over $X^\infty$ on the basis of the lower approximation over $X$ some estimation methods should be used.

## Example 4

We present an illustrative example showing an approximation of a function $f:X \to R_+$ where $X=\{1,2,4,5,7,8\}$. Let $f(1)=3, f(2)=2, f(4)=2, f(5)=5, f(7)=5, f(8)=2..$

We consider three indiscernibility classes $C_1=[0,3]\times[1.5,4]$, $C_2=[3,6]\times[1.7,4.5]$ and $C_3=[6,9]\times[3,4]$. We compute projections of indiscernibility classes:

$\pi_1(C_1)=[0,3]$, $\pi_2(C_1)=[1.5,4]$, $\pi_1(C_2)=[3,6]$, $\pi_2(C_2)=[1.7,4.5]$, $\pi_1(C_3)=[6,9]$ and $\pi_2(C_3)=[3,4]$.

Hence, we obtain

$$f(\pi_1(C_1)\cap X)=f(\{1,2\})=\{2,3\}\subseteq\pi_2(C_1),\ f(\pi_1(C_2)\cap X)=f(\{4,5\})=\{2,5\}\not\subseteq\pi_2(C_2)$$

but

$$f(\pi_1(C_2)\cap X)\cap\pi_2(C_2)=\{2,5\}\cap[1.7,4.5]\neq\varnothing,\ f(\pi_1(C_3)\cap X)=\varnothing.$$

We obtain the lower approximation $\underline{C}f=C_1$ and the upper approximation $\overline{C}f=C_1\cup C_2$

On can easily extend the discussed approach to function approximation for the case when instead of the partial graph of a function, it gives more general information consisting of many possible values for a given $x\in X$ due to repetitive measurements influenced by noise.

Let us consider now a family $Max[\underline{C}f]$ of all sub-families of $[\underline{C}f]$ such that after projection on $X^\infty$ a maximal (with respect to the measure $\mu$) family of pairwise disjoint sets is obtained. For any $P\in Max[\underline{C}f]$, we define the lower integral of $f$ over $P$ and the upper integral of $f$ over $P$ by

$$\underline{\int} f dP = \sum_{c\in P}(\mu\times\mu_0)(\pi_1(c)\times[0,min\pi_2(c)])$$
$$= \sum_{c\in P}\mu(\pi_1(c))\cdot min(\pi_2(c)),$$

and

$$\overline{\int} f dP = \sum_{c\in P}(\mu\times\mu_0)(\pi_1(c)\times[0,max\pi_2(c)])$$
$$= \sum_{c\in P}\mu(\pi_1(c))\cdot max(\pi_2(c)),$$

respectively, where $min\pi_2(c)=inf\{r\colon r\in\pi_2(c)\}$, $max\pi_2(c)=sup\{r\colon r\in\pi_2(c)\}$ and $\mu\times\mu_0$ is the product measure.

The pair $\left(\underline{\int} f dP, \overline{\int} f dP\right)$ is called the rough integral of $f$ relative to $P$.

One can search for the optimal family $P \in Max[\underline{C}f]$ taking into account the value $\left| \overline{\int} fdP - \underline{\int} fdP \right|$, the number of elements in $P$, and the coverage of $X^\infty$ is measured by

$$cover(f, P) = \frac{\mu\left( \cup \left\{ \pi_1(c) : c \in P \right\} \right)}{\mu(X^\infty)}.$$

Let us describe this in more detail. The size of the model for the rough integral of $f$ relative to $P$ can be defined by $Length(P)$, *i.e.*, the sum of the lengths of formulas defining elements from $P$. The quality $Quality(f, P)$ of the rough integral of $f$ relative to $P$ can be defined by a convex linear combination of the coverage of $X^\infty$ by projections on $X^\infty$ of neighborhoods from $P$ and the quality of the rough integral of $f$ relative to $P$

$$w_1 \left( \overline{\int} fdP - \underline{\int} fdP \right) + w_2 cover(X^\infty, P),$$

where $w_1, w_2$ are weights satisfying $w_1 + w_2 = 1, w_1, w_2 \in R_+$.

Now, one can define the quality of rough integral relative to $C$ by

$Quality(f, C)$
$= min\{C \in Max[\underline{C}f] : \lambda_1 Quality(f, C) + \lambda_2 Length(C)\}$,

where $\lambda_1 + \lambda_2 = 1$ and $\lambda_1, \lambda_2 \in R_+$. The optimization should be performed over the $Max[\underline{C}f]$. Usually, due to the computational complexity of this optimization, *i.e.*, searching for the optimal $P_{opt} \in Max[\underline{C}f]$ such that

$Quality(f, C) = Quality(f, P_{opt})$

one can obtain approximate solutions only (*i.e.*, a granule of numbers estimating the rough integral $\left( \underline{\int} fdP_{opt}, \overline{\int} fdP_{opt} \right)$ rather than a single number) by applying some heuristics.

It is worthwhile mentioning that in applications it is also necessary to discover the family $C$ of relevant neighborhoods for function approximation or for obtaining of rough integral of high quality. Moreover, the obtained approximation should be adaptively changed when new data are obtained or new family of neighborhoods is discovered. Such heuristics will be discussed elsewhere.

For constructive definition of neighborhoods from $C$, hierarchical modeling may be necessary. In the case of neighborhoods of the form $Z \times I$, where $Z \subseteq X^\infty$ and $I$ is an interval of reals it is enough to define a formula $\alpha$ such that $\|\alpha\|_{X^\infty} = Z$. Any such a formula $\alpha$ can be considered as a rule describing a region $Z \subseteq X^{\infty}$ in which the predicted deviation of approximated function $f$ is bounded by the height of the neighborhood, *i.e.*, the length of $I$.

## Interactions of Granules and Reasoning about Changes

Understanding interactions among different kinds of objects has become increasingly important for modeling and investigation of complex phenomena in different areas such as astronomy, biology, chemistry, geography, medicine, oceanography, philosophy, physics, psychology, sociology (see, *e.g.*, (Wikipedia; van Benthem, 2007; van Benthem, 2008) and (Feng et al., 2007; Goldin et al., 2006; Peters, 2005)). Investigations concerning interactions between objects were identified as crucial for understanding principles of modeling and for investigating properties of complex systems in such areas as multiagent systems, complex adaptive systems, and system engineering (see, e.g., (Luck et al., 2003; Mitchell, 2007; Sun, 2006; Peters, 2005; Peters et al., 2007a; Stevens et al., 1998)).

Figure 4 illustrates interactions between granules represented by agents and environments in which other agents may exist. We assume that the goal of multi-agent system is to preserve some invariants represented by some complex vague concepts and dependencies between them. These concepts may be relative to a particular agent, team of agents or the whole multi-agent system. In particular, constraints can have a global character and can represent, e.g., emergent patters of multi-agent systems.

By $s_0, s_1, \ldots$ are denoted states of environment. The results of perception of these states by agents are represented in Figure 4 by $Inf(s_0), Inf(s_1), \ldots$ where $Inf(s_i)$ represents the results of perception by sensors of the state $s_i$. $Inf(s_i)$ can include information about the environment state, existing agents, their states, messages sent by agents etc. Hence, perception is treated as a kind of interaction process leading to agent from the environment in which the agent is embedded.

The judgment engine is inducing a model $M_{s_i}$ of the current state $s_i$ using information about states and the knowledge network of agent. The model is represented by a special kind of granules such as relational structure or a cluster of relational structures on the relevant level of hierarchical modeling. Next, the judgment engine is extracting a relevant context of concepts (from the knowledge base network of this agent) for approximate reasoning about the induced model $M_{s_i}$. This approximate reasoning can

*Figure 4. Structure of granules*

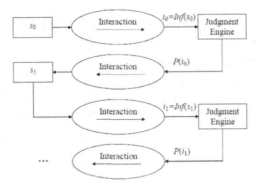

be described as matching the model against concepts from the context and is leading to degrees of satisfiability of the concepts from the context by $M_{s_i}$. These concepts labeled by degrees of their satisfiability by $M_{s_i}$ are used for predicting interaction with environment (leading from the agent to environment) represented by actions, plans or communication messages selected from the language of communication being at disposal of the agent. Observe that the messages sent by the agent can be related to cooperation or competition mechanisms, can be used for coalition formation etc. Coalitions are special granules important for approximate reasoning about properties of interactive computations performed on granules in distributed environments. Coalitions as a result of agent fusion are making it possible to look on computations performed by agents in a more abstract way. One can consider coalitions as meta-granules or meta-agents. Thanks to the hierarchical structure created by coalitions, coalitions of coalitions, etc., one can perform approximate reasoning about the computations performed by agents and finally prove that, e.g., the whole system is preserving invariants representing, e.g., emergent behavioral patterns. Moreover, the judgment engine is performing reasoning about changes for expressing differences between the current induced model and the model of the next state predicted in the previous step of computation. The results of such reasoning can be used, e.g., in the process of plan adaptation.

In Figure 4, interactions are assumed to be discrete. However, one can consider continuous interactions by assuming that interactions between agents and their environments are represented by continuous processes.

There is a need for the design of a unified approach for understanding interactions among compound objects with different compositions, modeling interactions among them, and approximate reasoning about them. The aim of such a theory is to develop tools for understanding interactions among granules and for approximate reasoning about interactions of granules that can be used in applications related to the different areas.

In the discussed approach, the reasoning about changes is important (see, *e.g.*, (Shoham, 1998; Gerbrandy and Groeneveld, 1997; Skowron & Synak, 2004)). Let us consider structural granules (Nguyen & Skowron, 2008), *i.e.*, granules having a structure defined by selector functions which are used for extracting from granules their parts representing some other granules[8]. We assume that any part of a given granule can be extracted by means of applying a proper composition of selector functions to the granule. By $\xi$ we denote a composition (path) of selectors representing, in a sense, a path used for selection of a part from a given granule. Under some assumptions, one can represent the structure of a given granule $G$ by a labeled tree in which paths are defined by compositions of selector functions leading to parts of $G$ labeling nodes in the tree (see Figure 5).

In particular, we assume that if two different paths defined by compositions of selector functions are pointing to some parts of a given granule $G$ then these parts are different and we consider only paths of selectors leading to some parts of $G$.[9]

Having a granule $G$ treated as a context[10] and a granule $G_0$ defined by the path $\xi$ applied to $G$ we define a $G$-neighborhood $N_G(G_0)$ of $G_0$ equal to a granule being a collection of granules defined by any, different from $\xi$, path applied to $G$ (more precisely we consider pairs with the first component denoting a path and with the second component equal to the granule pointed by this path in $G$).

*Figure 5. Structure of granules*

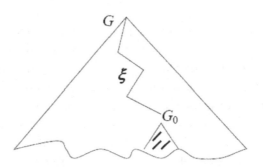

Let us consider granules changing in time. For a given moment of time $t$, a transient granule is denoted by $G(t)$ and by $G_0(t)$ is denoted its part defined by $\xi$ at time $t$. Let us assume that in a moment of time $t + \Delta t$ we observe the granule $G(t + \Delta t)$ and its part pointed by $\xi$ is equal to $G_0(t + \Delta t)$ (see Figure 6).

Now, the aim is to characterize changes between $G_0(t + \Delta t)$ and $G_0(t)$ in terms of features of $G_0(t)$ and features of $N_G(G_0)$. In searching for relevant features of $N_G(G_0)$ one should consider features of granules from $N_G(G_0)$ as well as different relations between them. Discovery of such relevant features from data and domain knowledge is a challenging problem. It is worthwhile mentioning that such relevant features cannot be, in general, defined by an *ad hoc* assumed linear combination of some measures computed on granules from $N_G(G_0)$ characterizing interactions of granules from $N_G(G_0)$ with $G_0(t)$ as it is often done when models are built using differential equations (see, e.g., (Feng et al., 2007)). Contrary to such an *ad hoc* approach, methods based on available data and domain knowledge should be developed for fusion of granules from $N_G(G_0)$, relations between these granules, and features of $G_0(t)$. The fusion is used for defining new higher level features describing interactions of granules from $N_G(G_0)$ and $G_0(t)$ which are next used for characterizing the degrees of changes $G_0(t)$ in time[11]. Finally, we obtain a decision system where decision values are characterizing the degrees of changes of $G_0(t)$ in time and conditional attributes are describing properties of $G_0(t)$ as well as properties of granules from $N_G(G_0)$

*Figure 6. Granule change*

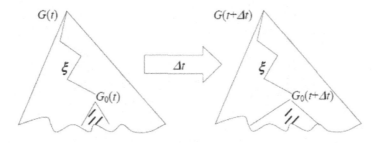

and some relationships between them. From the decision table it is necessary to induce the approximation of the decision function.

It is worthwhile noticing that for real-life problems the discovered models of processes are changing in time. Hence, it is necessary to discover temporal intervals in which the discovered models are valid as well as moments of time (granules of time) during which changes of models are occurring. Certainly, higher level laws are also relevant for analysis of the complex processes. For example, the discovered rules may describe the evolution of models in time. The other rules can help us to derive models of processes (or their properties) from the higher level of the hierarchical modeling by fusion of models of processes (or their properties) from the lower level of hierarchical modeling. In the fusion definition, the interactions between fused processes play a very important role.

A decision function approximation may be used for discovery from sample of objects and domain knowledge approximations of trajectories characterizing the dynamics of $G_0(t)$ considered in the context of $G(t)$. This is another challenging problem. We obtain only approximations of trajectories instead of exact trajectories generated, e.g., as solutions of differential equations. However, these approximations of trajectories may be more relevant for solutions of real-life problems than the exact trajectories. The latter trajectories represent exact solutions of differential equations but the models defined by differential equations may be *too far* from reality and in the consequence such exact solutions of differential equations may not be acceptable as the solutions of real-life problems. In Figure 7 is presented a general scheme for using function approximation in generation of the approximation of the next state from the currents state and trajectory approximation. We present some details on application of this idea at the end of the chapter. Interaction between granules representing objects (states) and components of classifiers (e.g., rules, in case of rule based classifiers together with their qualities relative to decision classes) should lead to compound patterns (called as approximate rules (see, e.g., (Bazan et al., 2005))) in the process analogous to fuzzyfication which are next fused to induce the approximation of the next trajectory state, in the process analogous to defuzzyfication (conflict resolution). In general, the above mentioned compound patterns should be discovered from data together with the relevant fusion or conflict resolution strategy.

*Figure 7. Trajectory approximation*

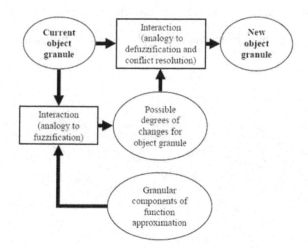

# Example 5

Let us consider some simple illustrative examples related to approximation of changes of attribute values. Let us consider an information system depicted in Table 1. In the example, we illustrate in a simple case how it is possible to induce classifiers for predicting changes of symbolic attribute values.

Using decomposition with respect to attribute $a_{current}$ we obtain two information systems: $IS_{a_{current}=0}$ and $IS_{a_{current}=1}$ (see Table 2 and 3, respectively).

The general scheme for generation of the next state approximation is depicted in Figure 7. Notice, that there are some analogies of this approach with the approach on action rules constructed for some other purpose (see, e.g., (Ras & Wyrzykowska, 2007)). One can observe some analogies of the discussed rules with action rules describing changes of some attribute values causing changes of some other attribute values. Our approach differs, e.g., in that the rules generated by using our approach describe how changes of some attributes coexist with changes of some other attributes.

From information systems presented in Table 1 and Table 2 we obtain:

- $Next(a=0)$ -- a rule based classifier built over decision rules:

**if** $a_{current}=0$ **then** $a_{next}=0$

**if** $a_{current}=1$ **and** $b_{current}=0$ **and** $c_{current}=0$ **then** $a_{next}=0$

- $Next(a=1)$ -- a rule based classifier built over decision rules:

**if** $a_{current}=1$ **and** $b_{current}=1$ **then** $a_{next}=1$

**if** $a_{current}=1$ **and** $c_{current}=1$ **then** $a_{next}=1$

Analogously, we obtain the following rule based classifiers:

*Table 1. Information system "current state"→ "next state"*

|  | $a_{current}$ | $b_{current}$ | $c_{current}$ | $a_{next}$ | $b_{next}$ | $c_{next}$ |
|---|---|---|---|---|---|---|
| $(x_1,y_1)$ | 0 | 0 | 0 | 0 | 0 | 1 |
| $(x_2,y_2)$ | 0 | 0 | 1 | 0 | 1 | 0 |
| $(x_3,y_3)$ | 0 | 1 | 0 | 0 | 0 | 1 |
| $(x_4,y_4)$ | 1 | 0 | 0 | 0 | 0 | 1 |
| $(x_5,y_5)$ | 1 | 0 | 1 | 1 | 1 | 0 |
| $(x_6,y_6)$ | 1 | 1 | 0 | 1 | 0 | 1 |

*Table 2. Information system $IS_{a_{current}=0}$*

|  | $b_{current}$ | $c_{current}$ | $a_{next}$ | $b_{next}$ | $c_{next}$ |
|---|---|---|---|---|---|
| $(x_1,y_1)$ | 0 | 0 | 0 | 0 | 1 |
| $(x_2,y_2)$ | 0 | 1 | 0 | 1 | 0 |
| $(x_3,y_3)$ | 1 | 0 | 0 | 0 | 1 |

*Table 3. Information system* $IS_{a_{current}=1}$

| | $b_{current}$ | $c_{current}$ | $a_{next}$ | $b_{next}$ | $c_{next}$ |
|---|---|---|---|---|---|
| $(x_4,y_4)$ | 0 | 0 | 0 | 0 | 1 |
| $(x_5,y_5)$ | 0 | 1 | 1 | 1 | 0 |
| $(x_6,y_6)$ | 1 | 0 | 1 | 0 | 1 |

*Table 4. Information system* $IS(c_{current}=0, c_{next}=1)$

| | $a_{current}$ | $b_{current}$ | $a_{next}$ | $b_{next}$ |
|---|---|---|---|---|
| $(x_1,y_1)$ | 0 | 0 | 0 | 0 |
| $(x_3,y_3)$ | 0 | 1 | 0 | 0 |
| $(x_4,y_4)$ | 1 | 0 | 0 | 0 |
| $(x_6,y_6)$ | 1 | 1 | 1 | 0 |

- $Next(b=0)$ -- a rule based classifier built over decision rule:

**if** $c_{current}=0$ **then** $b_{next}=0$

- $Next(b=1)$ -- a rule based classifier built over decision rule:

**if** $c_{current}=1$ **then** $b_{next}=1$

- $Next(c=0)$ -- a rule based classifier built over decision rule:

**if** $c_{current}=1$ **then** $c_{next}=0$

- $Next(c=1)$ -- a rule based classifier built over decision rule:

**if** $c_{current}=0$ **then** $c_{next}=1$.

Using generated classifiers we obtain the following trajectory

$(a=1, b=1, c=1; a=1, b=1, c=0)$,

$(a=1, b=0, c=1; a=1, b=1, c=0)$

generated by the transition relation induced from Table 1 with the initial state represented by $(a=1, b=1, c=1)$.

The example illustrates that instead of assuming analytical forms of changes (e.g., linear form of interactions of attributes influencing changes of a given attribute) as is often done in modeling by differential equations, one can try discover from data the approximation of these changes represented by means of induced classifiers. Observe that the decomposition of a given information systems makes it possible to extract from data rules describing changes of a given attribute values between current and next state using the value of the attribute on the current state and values of other attributes on this state reflecting interactions among attributes. Note, for more compound changes, it will be necessary to use also domain knowledge do induce relevant features for changes representation (by analogy to risk prediction or planning considered, e.g., in (Bazan et al., 2006b; Bazan et al., 2006a)).

In reasoning about changes, one should often discover dependencies between changes of different complexity (e.g., between or among compound parts of complex object). Let us consider a simple example illustrating this issue.

## Example 6: Rules about Changes

In this example, we consider decision rules for description of dependencies on changes of attribute values in transition from the current state to the next state.

Let $IS(c_{current}=0, c_{next}=1)$ be an information system obtained from $IS$ by selecting all objects satisfying the following conditions: $c_{current}=0$ and $c_{next}=1$ and next by deleting columns corresponding to attributes $c_{current}$ and $c_{next}$. We call the pair $(c_{current}=0, c_{next}=1)$ as a label of the constructed information system. We search for rules in this new information system.

For example, from information system presented in Table 1 we obtain information system presented in Table 4.

We denote by $i \rightarrow_a j$ a condition $a_{current}=i$ and $a_{next}=j$.

From information system $IS(c_{current}=0, c_{next}=1)$ (see Table 4) we obtain the following dependencies:

$0 \rightarrow_b 0$

$1 \rightarrow_b 0$

$0 \rightarrow_a 0$

**if** $b_{current}=0$ **then** $1 \rightarrow_a 0$

**if** $b_{current}=1$ **then** $1 \rightarrow_a 1$

We obtained examples of rules showing that the change $0 \rightarrow_a 1$ should coexists with other changes listed above. This is a first step to generalize the approach investigated in a number of papers (see, e.g., (Suraj, 2000)) where information systems were used as specifications of concurrent systems and methods for discovery of concurrent systems from information systems have been presented. The set of dependencies of the above form extracted from a given information system can be treated as a theory specifying constraints on dynamic transitions in the system. This is a new idea not explored so far even if some attempts for learning the transitions relation from examples were made (see, e.g., (Pancerz & Suraj, 2004)).

Certainly, more advanced methods are needed to extract rules about changes from real-life data. For example, one can consider instead of patterns defined by conjunction of descriptors, more general granules, the so called generalized patterns (i.e., conjunctions of generalized descriptors of the form $a \in V \subset V_a$) or clusters of known cases and search for evolutions of such patterns defined by the transition relation approximation characterizing changes. More precisely, one can study how images of patterns under the transition relation approximation are changing. Methods for inducing of rules of changes of patterns along trajectories defined by a partially specified transition relation will be presented in an extension of this chapter.

There are numerous examples of real-life problems of modeling of highly nonlinear complex phenomena where approximation of trajectories might be applicable (e.g., modeling of biological processes (Feng et al., 2007; Wu, 2007), identification and understanding of pathological processes in medicine as well as planning for therapy support (Bazan et al., 2006a; Bazan et al., 2005)). Another application can be related to discovery of unknown structure of complex objects or phenomena by means of relevant signal measurements (Guerrero, 2008. For example, in (Guerrero, 2008) two-way wave equations (differential equations as a function of space and time) describing seismic waves have been successfully used to generate 3D images of oil and natural gas reservoirs in the Gulf of Mexico. We propose to use together with exact mathematical models of changes defined by differential equations also approximate models of changes discovered from data and domain knowledge. The latter models can give better solutions for real-life problem because they can offer more relevant models of considered complex phenomena.

Let us now consider an example of reasoning about changes based on function approximation.

In the example, $s(t)$, $s(t + \Delta t)$ denote the state of the environment of a given agent $a$ at moment $t$ and $t + \Delta t$, respectively. By $a(t)$, $a(t + \Delta t)$ we denote the state of the agent $a$ at the moment $t$ and $t + \Delta t$, respectively. We assume that the changes of the environment state and agent state are described by the following system of equations

$$\Delta s\left(t\right) = F\left(\Delta t, s\left(t\right), a\left(t\right)\right); \tag{4}$$

$$\Delta a(t) = G(\Delta t, s(t), a(t)).$$

However, only a partial information $Inf(s(t)), Inf(s(t + \Delta t)), Inf(a(t)), Inf(a(t + \Delta t))$, is available on the states (see Figure 9), e.g., by the results of sensor measurements performed on the states. Moreover, we there is only a partial information about functions $F$ and $G$ given by a sample of values of these functions at some time points. Hence, it is necessary to approximate these functions. In Figure 8 the approximations of $F$ and $G$ are denoted by $Ap_F$ and $Ap_G$, respectively and $i_s = Inf(s(t))$, $i_a = Inf(a(t))$. These approximations of functions $F$ and $G$ are making it possible to compute information about changes of states $\Delta s(t)$ and $\Delta a(t)$ from partial information about states (see the Equations (4)). Next, this information together with components (e.g., rules in case of rule based classifiers) of function approximations and partial information about the state at time $t$ is sent to the judgment engine module (see Figures 7 and 9) for computing the approximation of the granules representing the image under the functions $F$ and $G$ of the set of objects satisfying patterns described by partial information

*Figure 8. From current to next state*     *Figure 9. Approximation of changes*

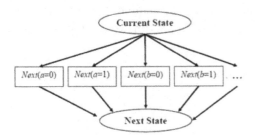     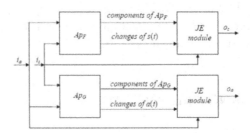

about states. In this way, granules approximating the next states $s(t + \Delta t)$, $s(t + \Delta t)$ can be obtained. In Figure 9, they are denoted by $o_s$ and $o_a$, respectively.

In the case of more complex phenomena, it may not be computationally feasible to approximate functions $F$, $G$ directly from partial information about global states $s(t)$ and $a(t)$. To overcome this difficulty one can use domain knowledge to decompose $F$, $G$ into simpler functions such that it becomes feasible to build approximations of $F,G$ from approximations of these simpler functions. Let us assume that $F$ ($G$) decomposes into simpler functions $F_1, F_2$ ($G_1, G_2$). Components of approximations of $F_1, F_2$ and $G_1, G_2$ used together with corresponding constraints allow us to specify components for approximation of $F$ and $G$.[12] To explain the role of constraints, let us assume that after decomposition of $F$ and $G$ we obtain the following new equations:

$$\Delta s_i(t) = F_i(\Delta t, s_i(t), a_i(t)) \tag{5}$$

$$\Delta a_i(t) = G_i(\Delta t, s_i(t), a_i(t)),$$

where $s_i(t), a_i(t)$ for $i=1,2$ denote parts of global states $s(t)$ and $a(t)$. These equations should be considered in conjunction with constraints that set conditions for the coexistence of parts in global states $s(t)$ and $a(t)$.

The constructions of more compound components from the less compound ones are analogous to those described by productions and approximate reasoning schemes investigated, e.g., in (Skowron & Stepaniuk, 2003). The decomposition process as described above is usually hierarchical, i.e., the decomposition is recursively repeated down to the level that already consists of functions which can be approximated directly from data.

## CONCLUSION

We discussed some issues of process mining from data and domain knowledge as well as approximate reasoning about changes along trajectories of approximated processes. We proposed the use of a rough-granular approach as the basic methodology for modeling the discovery process. We have emphasized the need for developing rough granular computing based on interactions among granules as well as learning strategies for approximation of functions characterizing changes, and approximation of trajectories of complex dynamical systems.

## ACKNOWLEDGMENT

The research has been partially supported by the grant N N516 368334 from Ministry of Science and Higher Education of the Republic of Poland. The research by James F. Peters is supported by Natural Sciences and Engineering Research Council of Canada (NSERC) Canada 185986 and Canadian Arthritis Network grant SRI-BIO-05. The research by Jaroslaw Stepaniuk is supported by the grant N N516 069235 from Ministry of Science and Higher Education of the Republic of Poland.

## REFERENCES

Aggarwal, C. (2007). *Data Streams: Models and Algorithms*. Berlin, Germany: Springer.

Bargiela, A., & Pedrycz, W. (2003). *Granular Computing: An Introduction*. Dordrecth, The Netherlands: Kluwer Academic Publishers.

Barwise, J., & Seligman, J. (1997). *Information Flow: The Logic of Distributed Systems*. Cambridge, UK: Cambridge University Press.

Bazan, J., Kruczek, P., Bazan-Socha, S., Skowron, A., & Pietrzyk, J. J. (2006, July 2-7). Risk pattern identification in the treatment of infants with respiratory failure through rough set modeling. In *Proceedings of Information Processing and Management under Uncertainty in Knowledge-Based Systems* (IPMU'2006), (no. 3, pp. 2650-2657). Paris, France

Bazan, J., Kruczek, P., Bazan-Socha, S., Skowron, A., & Pietrzyk, J. J. (2006a). Automatic planning of treatment of infants with respiratory failure through rough set modeling. In Greco, S., Hata, Y., Hirano, S., Inuiguchi, M., Miyamoto, S., Nguyen, H. S., and Słowiński, R. (eds.), *Fifth International Conference on Rough Sets and Current Trends in Computing (RSCTC 2006), Kobe, Japan, November 6-8, 2006*, volume 4259 of *Lecture Notes in Artificial Intelligence*, (pp. 418-427). Heidelberg, Germany: Springer.

Bazan, J., Peters, J. F., & Skowron, A. (2005, September 1-3). Behavioral pattern identification through rough set modelling. In Ślęzak, D., Szczuka, M., Duntsch, I., and Yao, Y., (eds.), *Proceedings of the Tenth International Conference on Rough Sets, Fuzzy Sets, Data Mining, and Granular Computing (RSFDGrC 2005), Regina, Canada* (volume 3642 of Lecture Notes in Artificial Intelligence, pp. 688-697). Berlin: Springer.

Bazan, J., & Skowron, A. (2005a). Classifiers based on approximate reasoning schemes. In Dunin-Kęplicz, B., Jankowski, A., Skowron, A., & Szczuka, M. (Eds.), *Monitoring, Security, and Rescue Techniques in Multiagent Systems, Advances in Soft Computing* (pp. 191–202). Heidelberg, Germany: Springer. doi:10.1007/3-540-32370-8_13

Bazan, J., Skowron, A., & Swiniarski, R. (2006b). Rough sets and vague concept approximation: From sample approximation to adaptive learning. *Transactions on Rough Sets V, LNCS 4100*(5), 39-62.

Borrett, S. R., & Bridewell, W., R., P. P. L. K., & Arrigo. (2007). A method for representing and developing process models. *Ecological Complexity, 4*(1-2), 1–12. doi:10.1016/j.ecocom.2007.02.017

Breiman, L. (2001). Statistical modeling: the two cultures. *Statistical Science, 16*(3), 199–231. doi:10.1214/ss/1009213726

Bronshtein, I., Semendyayev, K., Musiol, G., & Muehlig, H. (Eds.). (2003). *Handbook of Mathematics*. Berlin Heidelberg, Germany: Springer Verlag.

de Medeiros, A. K. A., Weijters, A. J. M. M., & van der Aalst, W. M. P. P. (2007). Genetic process mining: An experimental evaluation. *Data Mining and Knowledge Discovery, 14*, 245–304. doi:10.1007/s10618-006-0061-7

Doherty, P. ÃLukaszewicz, W., Skowron, A., & Szałas, A. (2006). Knowledge Representation Techniques: A Rough Set Approach, volume 202 of Studies in Fuzziness and Soft Computing. Berlin Heidelberg, Germany: Springer Verlag.

Domingos, P. P. (2007). Toward knowledge-rich data mining. *Data Mining and Knowledge Discovery, 15*, 21–28. doi:10.1007/s10618-007-0069-7

Feng, J., Jost, J., & Minping, Q. (2007). *Network: From Biology to Theory*. Berlin Heidelberg, Germany: Springer Verlag. doi:10.1007/978-1-84628-780-0

Friedman, J. H. (1997). Data mining and statistics. What's the connection? Keynote address. In *Proceedings of the 29th Symposium on the Interface: Computing Science and Statistics*, Houston, TX.

Gerbrandy, J., & Groeneveld, W. (1997). Reasoning about information change. *Journal of Logic Language and Information, 6*(2), 147–169. doi:10.1023/A:1008222603071

Goldin, D., Smolka, S., & Wegner, P. P. (2006). *Interactive Computation: The New Paradigm*. Berlin Heidelberg, Germany: Springer Verlag.

Guerrero, F. (2008). Solving the oil equation by a team of geophysicists and computer scientists. *IEEE Spectrum*, 33–36.

Jankowski, A., Peters, J., Skowron, A., & Stepaniuk, J. (2008). Optimization in discovery of compound granules. *Fundamenta Informaticae, 85*(1-4), 249–265.

Jankowski, A., & Skowron, A. (2007). A wistech paradigm for intelligent systems. *Transactions on Rough Sets VI, LNCS, 4374*(5), 94–132. doi:10.1007/978-3-540-71200-8_7

Jankowski, A., & Skowron, A. (2008a). Logic for artificial intelligence: The Rasiowa-Pawlak school perspective. In Ehrenfeucht, A., Marek, V., & Srebrny, M. (Eds.), *Andrzej Mostowski and Foundational Studies* (pp. 106–143). Amsterdam: IOS Press.

Kleinberg, J., Papadimitriou, C., & Raghavan, P. P. (1998). A microeconomic view of data mining. *Data Mining and Knowledge Discovery, 2*, 311–324. doi:10.1023/A:1009726428407

Kriegel, H.-P., Borgwardt, K. M., Kroger, P., Pryakhin, A., Schubert, M., & Zimek, A. (2007). Future trends in data mining. *Data Mining and Knowledge Discovery, 15*(1), 87–97. doi:10.1007/s10618-007-0067-9

Luck, M., McBurney, P., & Preist, C. (2003). *Agent technology. Enabling next generation computing: A roadmap for agent based computing*. Retrieved from AgentLink.org

Mitchell, M. (2007). Complex systems: Network thinking. *Artificial Intelligence, 170*(18), 1194–1212. doi:10.1016/j.artint.2006.10.002

Nguyen, H. S., & Skowron, A. (2008). A rough granular computing in discovery of process models from data and domain knowledge. *Journal of Chongqing University of Post and Telecommunications, 20*(3), 341–347.

Nguyen, S. H., Bazan, J., Skowron, A., & Nguyen, H. S. (2004). Layered learning for concept synthesis. *Transactions on Rough Sets I, LNCS 3100*(1), 187-208.

Nguyen, T. T., Paddon, C. P. P. W. D. J., & Nguyen, H. S. (2006). Learning sunspot classification. *Fundamenta Informaticae, 72*(1-3), 295–309.

Pal, S. K., Bandoyopadhay, S., & Biswas, S. (Eds.). (2005, December 18-22). *Proceedings of the First International Conference on Pattern Recognition and Machine Intelligence (PReMI'05), Indian Statistical Institute, volume 3776 of Lecture Notes in Computer Science*, Berlin Heidelberg, Germany. Springer Verlag.

Pal, S. K., Polkowski, L., & Skowron, A. (Eds.). (2004). *RoughNeural Computing: Techniques for Computing with Words*. Berlin: Cognitive Technologies. Springer.

Pancerz, K., & Suraj, Z. (2004). Discovering concurrent models from data tables with the ROSECON. *Fundamenta Informaticae, 60*(1-4), 251–268.

Pawlak, Z. (1981). *Classification of objects by means of attributes*. (Technical Report 429), Institute of Computer Science, Polish Academy of Sciences, Warsaw, Poland.

Pawlak, Z. (1982). Rough sets. *International Journal of Computer and Information Sciences, 11*, 341–356. doi:10.1007/BF01001956

Pawlak, Z. (1991). Rough Sets: Theoretical Aspects of Reasoning about Data: *Vol. 9. System Theory, Knowledge Engineering and Problem Solving*. Dordrecht, The Netherlands: Kluwer Academic Publishers.

Pawlak, Z. (1992). Concurrent versus sequential the rough sets perspective. *Bulletin of the EATCS, 48*, 178–190.

Pawlak, Z. (1999). Rough sets, rough functions and rough calculus. In Pal, S., & Skowron, A. (Eds.), *Rough Fuzzy Hybridization, A New Trend in Decision Making* (pp. 99–109). Berlin, Germany: Springer.

Pawlak, Z., Peters, J. F., Skowron, A., Suraj, Z., Ramanna, S., & Borkowski, M. (2001). Rough measures and integrals: A brief introduction. In Terano, T., Nishida, T., Namatame, A., Tsumoto, S., Ohsawa, Y., & Washio, T. (Eds.), *New Frontiers in Artificial Intelligence, Joint JSAI 2001 Workshop Post Proceedings, Lecture Notes in Artificial Intelligence* (*Vol. 2253*, pp. 374–379). Berlin, Germany: Springer.

Pawlak, Z., & Skowron, A. (2007). Rudiments of rough sets; Rough sets: Some extensions; Rough sets and boolean reasoning. *Information Sciences, 177*(1), 3–27, 28–40, 41–73. doi:10.1016/j.ins.2006.06.003

Pedrycz, W. (Ed.). (2001). *Granular Computing.* Berlin/Heidelberg, Germany: Springer/Verlag.

Pedrycz, W., Skowron, A., & Kreinovich, V. (Eds.). (2008). *Handbook of Granular Computing.* New York: John Wiley & Sons. doi:10.1002/9780470724163

Peters, J. F. (1998). Time and clock information systems: Concepts and roughly fuzzy petri net models. In *Rough Sets in Knowledge Discovery 2: Applications, Case Studies and Software Systems, of Studies in Fuzziness and Soft Computing* (*Vol. 19*, pp. 385–418). Berlin/Heidelberg, Germany: Springer/Verlag.

Peters, J. F. (2005). Rough ethology: Towards a biologically-inspired study of collective behavior in intelligent systems with approximation spaces. *Transactions on Rough Sets III, LNCS, 3100*(3), 153–174.

Peters, J. F. (2007a). Near sets: General theory about nearness of objects. *Applied Mathematical Sciences, 1*(53), 2609–2629.

Peters, J. F. (2007b). Near sets: Special theory about nearness of objects. *Fundamenta Informaticae, 75*(1-4), 407–433.

Peters, J. F. (2008a). Classification of perceptual objects by means of features. *International Journal of Information Technology and Intelligent Computing, 3*(2), 1–35.

Peters, J. F. (2008b). Discovery of perceptually near information granules. In Yao, J. (Ed.), *Novel Developments in Granular Computing: Applications for Advanced Human Reasoning and Soft Computation.* Hershey, PA: IGI Global.

Peters, J. F., Shahfar, S., Ramanna, S., & Szturm, T. (2007a). Biologically-inspired adaptive learning: A near set approach. In Proceedings of Frontiers in the Convergence of Bioscience and Information Technologies (FBIT07), (pp. 403-408). Washington, DC: SERSC, IEEE Computer Society.

Peters, J. F., & Skowron, A. (1999). Approximate realtime decision making: Concepts and rough fuzzy petri net models. *International Journal of Intelligent Systems, 14,* 805–839. doi:10.1002/(SICI)1098-111X(199908)14:8<805::AID-INT5>3.0.CO;2-R

Peters, J. F., Skowron, A., & Stepaniuk, J. (2007b). Nearness of objects: Extension of approximation space model. *Fundamenta Informaticae, 79*(3-4), 497–512.

Peters, J. F., & Wasilewski, P. P. (2008). (Manuscript submitted for publication). Foundations of near sets. [pending publication.]. *Information Sciences.*

Poggio, T., & Smale, S. (2003). The mathematics of learning: Dealing with data. *Notices of the AMS, 50*(5), 537–544.

Ramsay, J. O., & Silverman, B. W. (2002). *Applied Functional Data Analysis.* Berlin: Springer. doi:10.1007/b98886

Ras, Z. W., & Wyrzykowska, E. (2007). Extended action rule discovery based on single classification rules and reducts. In Hassanien, A., Suraj, Z., Slezak, D., & Lingras, P. (Eds.), *Rough Computing: Theories, Technologies and Applications* (pp. 175–184). Hershey, PA: IGI Global.

Rissanen, J. (1985). Minimum-description-length principle. In Kotz, S., & Johnson, N. (Eds.), *Encyclopedia of Statistical Sciences* (pp. 523–527). New York: John Wiley & Sons.

Roddick, J. F., Hornsby, K., & Spiliopoulou, M. (2001). An updated bibliography of temporal, spatial and spatio-temporal data mining research. In Roddick, J. F. and Hornsby, K., (eds.), *Post-Workshop Proceedings of the International Workshop on Temporal, Spatial and Spatio-Temporal Data Mining, Lecture Notes in Artificial Intelligence*, (volume 2007, pp. 147-163). Berlin, Germany: Springer.

Shoham, Y. (1998). *Reasoning about Change*. Cambridge, MA: MIT Press.

Skowron, A., & Stepaniuk, J. (1996). Tolerance approximation spaces. *Fundamenta Informaticae, 27*, 245–253.

Skowron, A., & Stepaniuk, J. (2003). Information granules and rough-neural computing. In Pal, S. K., Polkowski, L., & Skowron, A. (Eds.), *Rough-Neural Computing: Techniques for Computing with Words, Cognitive Technologies* (pp. 43–84). Berlin, Germany: Springer.

Skowron, A., Stepaniuk, J., Peters, J., & Swiniarski, R. (2006). Calculi of approximation spaces. *Fundamenta Informaticae, 72*(1-3), 363–378.

Skowron, A., Stepaniuk, J., & Peters, J. F. (2003). Rough sets and infomorphisms: Towards approximation of relations in distributed environments. *Fundamenta Informaticae, 54*(2-3), 263–277.

Skowron, A., & Suraj, Z. (1993). Rough sets and concurrency. *Bulletin of the Polish Academy of Sciences, 41*, 237–254.

Skowron, A., & Suraj, Z. (1995). Discovery of concurrent data models from experimental tables: A rough set approach. In *Proceedings of the First International Conference on Knowledge Discovery and Data Mining*, (pp. 288-293), Menlo Park, CA: AAAI Press.

Skowron, A., & Synak, P. P. (2004). Complex patterns. *Fundamenta Informaticae, 60*(1-4), 351–366.

Ślęzak, D. (2002). Approximate entropy reducts. *Fundamenta Informaticae, 53*(3-4), 365–387.

Stevens, R., Brook, P., Jacksona, K., & Arnold, S. (1998). *Systems Engineering. Coping with Complexity*. London: Prentice-Hall.

Sun, R. (Ed.). (2006). *Cognition and Multi-Agent Interaction. From Cognitive Modeling to Social Simulation*. Cambridge, UK: Cambridge University Press.

Suraj, Z. (2000). Rough set methods for the synthesis and analysis of concurrent processes. In Polkowski, L., Lin, T., & Tsumoto, S. (Eds.), *Rough Set Methods and Applications: New Developments in Knowledge Discovery in Information Systems, Studies in Fuzziness and Soft Computing* (*Vol. 56*, pp. 379–488). Heidelberg, Germany: Springer.

Unnikrishnan, K. P., & Ramakrishnan, N. S., Sastry, P., & Uthurusamy, R., (eds.) (2006). *Proceedings of 4th KDD Workshop on Temporal Data Mining: Network Reconstruction from Dynamic Data at KDD 2006 Conference*, Philadelphia. ACM SIGKDD.

van Benthem, J. (2007). Cognition as interaction. In Bouma, G., KrÄamer, I., and Zwarts, J., editors, Cognitive Foundations of Interpretation, (pp. 27-38). Amsterdam, KNAW.

van Benthem, J. (2008To appear). Logic games: From tools to models of interaction. In Gupta, A., Parikh, R., & van Benthem, J. (Eds.), *Logic at the Crossroads* (pp. 283–317). Mumbai, India: Allied Publishers.

Vapnik, V. (1998). *Statisctical Learning Theory*. New York: John Wiley & Sons.

Wikipedia (n.d.). *Wiki article on Interaction*. Retrieved from http://en.wikipedia.org/wiki/Interaction

Wu, F.-X. (2007). Inference of gene regulatory networks and its validation. *Current Bioinformatics*, *2*(2), 139–144. doi:10.2174/157489307780618240

Zadeh, L. A. (2001). A new direction in AI - toward a computational theory of perceptions. *AI Magazine*, *22*(1), 73–84.

Zadeh, L. A. (2006). Generalized theory of uncertainty (GTU)-principal concepts and ideas. *Computational Statistics & Data Analysis*, *51*, 15–46. doi:10.1016/j.csda.2006.04.029

## ENDNOTES

[1]   www.isle.org/126langley/, soc.web.cse.unsw.edu.au/bibliography/discovery/index.html

[2]   see http://mainesail.umcs.maine.edu/Context/context-conferences/

[3]   Each attribute of an object is represented by a function. Often, our knowledge about attribute functions is limited to the observed sample attribute values for each perceived object (see, e.g., (Peters, 2008a; Peters, 2007b; Peters, 2008b)). This fundamental insight about sample objects and sample attribute values comes from Zdzisław Pawlak (1981).

[4]   Let $\tau$ be a tolerance relation (reflexive and symmetric relation) defined on the set of information vectors. For any information vector $v$ we define $\tau(v) = \{w:(w,v) \in \tau\}$.

[5]   Rough set-based time windows were introduced in (Peters, 1998).

[6]   In general, a *functional* is a real number assigned to every function $f = f(t)$ from a given class of functions (Bronshtein et al., 2003).

[7]   A more general case, when only a partial information about points from the function graph is available will be discussed elsewhere.

[8]   Discovery of relevant selection functions and their composition for extracting parts of objects is strongly related to perception and is a challenging task for many problems (see, e.g., (Peters, 2008b; Peters, 2007a; Peters, 2008a; Peters and Wasilewski, 2008)).

[9]   Notice that some paths may be not applicable to $G$.

[10]  Observe that selection of a relevant context for a given granule is another challenging problem.

[11]  The analogous idea was formulated in (Kleinberg et al., 1998) for other kinds of fusion functions.

[12]  Let us recall that components for rule based classifiers can be interpreted as granules represented by decision rules together with their qualities relative to decision classes.

# Chapter 3
# Supervised and Unsupervised Information Granulation:
## A Study in Hyperbox Design

**Andrzej Bargiela**
*The University of Nottingham, UK*

**Witold Pedrycz**
*Polish Academy of Sciences, Poland*

## ABSTRACT

*In this study, we are concerned with information granulation realized both in supervised and unsupervised mode. Our focus is on the exploitation of the technology of hyperboxes and fuzzy sets as a fundamental conceptual vehicle of information granulation. In case of supervised learning (classification), each class is described by one or more fuzzy hyperboxes defined by their corresponding minimum and maximum vertices and the corresponding hyperbox membership function. Two types of hyperboxes are formed, namely inclusion hyperboxes that contain input patterns belonging to the same class, and exclusion hyperboxes that contain patterns belonging to two or more classes, thus representing contentious areas of the pattern space. With these two types of hyperboxes each class fuzzy set is represented as a union of inclusion hyperboxes of the same class minus a union of exclusion hyperboxes. The subtraction of sets provides for efficient representation of complex topologies of pattern classes without resorting to a large number of small hyperboxes to describe each class. The proposed fuzzy hyperbox classification is compared to the original Min-Max Neural Network and the General Fuzzy Min-Max Neural Network and the origins of the improved performance of the proposed classification are identified. When it comes to the unsupervised mode of learning, we revisit a well-known method of Fuzzy C-Means (FCM) by incorporating Tchebyschev distance using which we naturally form hyperbox-like prototypes. The design of hyperbox information granules is presented and the constructs formed in this manner are evaluated with respect to their abilities to capture the structure of data.*

DOI: 10.4018/978-1-60566-324-1.ch003

# 1. INTRODUCTION

Fuzzy hyperbox classification derives from the original idea of Zadeh (1965) of using fuzzy sets for representation of real-life data. Such data frequently is not *crisp* (has a binary inclusion relationship) but rather has a property of a *degree of membership*. In this case the use of traditional set theory introduces unrealistic constraint of forcing binary decisions where the graded response is more appropriate. An early application of fuzzy sets to the pattern classification problem (Bellman et al, 1966) proves the point that fuzzy sets represent an excellent tool simplifying the representation of complex boundaries between the pattern classes while retaining the full expressive power for the representation of the *core area* for each class. By having classes represented by fuzzy set membership functions it is possible to describe the degree to which a pattern belongs to one class or another.

Bearing in mind that the purpose of classification is the enhancement of interpretability of data or, in other words, derivation of a good abstraction of such data the use of hyperbox fuzzy sets as a description of pattern classes provides clear advantages. Each hyperbox can be interpreted as a fuzzy rule. However, the use of a single hyperbox fuzzy set for each pattern class is too limiting in that the topology of the original data is frequently quite complex (Zadeh, 1965) (and incompatible with the convex topology of the hyperbox). This limitation can be overcome by using a collection (union) of hyperboxes to cover each pattern class set (Simpson, 1992, 1993), (Gabrys, Bargiela, 2000). Clearly, the smaller the hyperboxes the more accurate cover of the class set can be obtained. Unfortunately, this comes at the expense of increasing the number of hyperboxes thus eroding the original objective of interpretability of the classification result. We have therefore a task of balancing the requirements of accuracy of coverage of the original data (which translates on the minimization of misclassifications) with the interpretability of class sets composed of many hyperboxes. These concerns are not unique to hyperboxes and they demonstrate themselves also in the context of other topologies of information granules, (Bargiela, 2001).

The tradeoff originally proposed by Simpson (1992) was the optimization of a single parameter defining the maximum hyperbox size as a function of misclassification rate. However, the use of a single maximum hyperbox size is somewhat restrictive. For class sets that are well separated from each other the use of large hyperboxes is quite adequate while for the closely spaced class sets, with a complex partition boundary, there is a need for small hyperboxes, so as to avoid high misclassification rates. One solution to this problem, proposed in (Gabrys, Bargiela, 2000), is the adaptation of the size of hyperboxes so that it is possible to generate larger hyperboxes in some areas of the pattern space while in the other areas the hyperboxes are constrained to be small to maintain low misclassification rates. The adaptation procedure requires however several presentations of data to arrive at the optimum sizes of hyperbox sizes for the individual classes.

In this paper we consider an alternative approach to achieving low misclassification rate while maintaining good interpretability of the classification results. Rather than trying to express the class sets as a union of fuzzy hyperbox sets (Gabrys, Bargiela, 2000), (Simpson, 1992), we represent them as a difference of two fuzzy sets. The first set is a union of hyperboxes produced in the standard way and the second set is a union of intersections of all hyperboxes that belong to different classes. We will refer to the first type of hyperboxes as inclusion hyperboxes and the second type as exclusion hyperboxes. By subtracting the exclusion hyperboxes from the inclusion ones it is possible to express complex topologies of the class set using fewer hyperboxes. Also, the three steps of the Min-Max clustering (Gabrys, Bargiela, 2000), (Simpson, 1992), namely *expansion*, *overlap test* and *contraction* can be reduced to two, namely *expansion* and *overlap* tests. Expansion step results in generating inclusion hyperboxes and the overlap test results in exclusion hyperboxes.

Clustering has been widely recognized as one of the dominant techniques of data analysis. The broad spectrum of the detailed algorithms and underlying technologies (fuzzy sets, neural networks, heuristic approaches) is impressive. In spite of this diversity, the key objective remains the same which is to understand the data. In this sense, clustering becomes an integral part of data mining (Cios, et al, 1998), (Zadeh, 1997). Data mining is aimed at making the findings that are inherently *transparent* to the end user. The transparency is accomplished through suitable knowledge representation mechanisms, namely a way in which generic data elements are formed, processed and presented to the user. The notion of information granularity becomes a cornerstone concept that needs to be discussed in this context, cf (Zadeh, 1997), (Maimon et al, 2001).

The underlying idea is that in any data set we can distinguish between a core part of a structure of the data that is easily describable and interpretable in a straightforward manner and a residual part, which does not carry any evident pattern of regularity. The core part can be described in a compact manner through several information granules while the residual part does not exhibit any visible geometry and requires some formal descriptors such as membership formulas. The scheme of unsupervised learning proposed in this study dwells on the augmentation of the standard FCM method which is now equipped with a Tchebyschev distance. This form of distance promotes hyperbox geometry of the information granules (hyperboxes). Starting from the results of clustering, our objective is to develop information granules forming a core structure in the data set, provide their characterization and discuss an interaction between the granules leading to their deformation.

The study is organized in the following fashion. Starting with the mode of supervised learning, we discuss the fuzzy min-max classification in Section 2. After discussing the inherent limitations of classes built as the union of hyperboxes, in Section 3, we proceed to introduce a novel approach to min-max classification by suggesting the coverage of complex class topologies by means of a set difference operator. This is discussed in Section 4 and is illustrated by some numerical examples in Section 5. We then look at the unsupervised learning mode in Section 6 where we emphasise the role of key parameters used in the information granulation process. A detailed clustering (unsupervised learning) algorithm together with a representative set of examples illustrating the topology of the resulting information granules is given in Section 7. The conclusions from our study are presented in Section 8.

## 2. FUZZY MIN-MAX CLASSIFICATION

The fuzzy Min-Max classification neural networks are built using hyperbox fuzzy sets. A hyperbox defines a region in $\mathbf{R}^n$, or more specifically in $[0\ 1]^n$ (since the data is normalized to $[0\ 1]$) and all patterns contained within the hyperbox have full class membership. A hyperbox $\mathbf{B}$ is fully defined by its minimum $\mathbf{V}$ and maximum $\mathbf{W}$ vertices. So that, $\mathbf{B}=[\mathbf{V},\ \mathbf{W}] \subset [0\ 1]^n$ with $\mathbf{V},\ \mathbf{W} \in [0\ 1]^n$.

Fuzzy hyperbox *B* is described by a membership function (in addition to its minimum and maximum vertices), which maps the universe of discourse ($\mathbf{X}$) into a unit interval.

$$B: \mathbf{X} \rightarrow [0,\ 1] \tag{1}$$

Formally, $\boldsymbol{B}(x)$ denotes a degree of membership that describes an extent to which x belongs to $\boldsymbol{B}$. If $\boldsymbol{B}(x) = 1$ then we say that x fully belongs to $\boldsymbol{B}$. If $\boldsymbol{B}(x)$ is equal to zero, x is fully excluded from $\boldsymbol{B}$. The values of the membership function that are in-between 0 and 1 represent a partial membership of x to $\boldsymbol{B}$. The higher the membership grade, the stronger is the association of the given element to $\boldsymbol{B}$. In this paper we will use an alternative notation for the hyperbox membership function $b(\boldsymbol{X}, \boldsymbol{V}, \boldsymbol{W})$ which gives an explicit indication of the min- and max- points of the hyperbox. The hyperbox fuzzy set will then be denoted as $B = \{\boldsymbol{X}, \boldsymbol{V}, \boldsymbol{W}, b(\boldsymbol{X}, \boldsymbol{V}, \boldsymbol{W})\}$. Note that $\boldsymbol{X}$ is an input pattern that in general represents a class-labelled hyperbox in $[0\ 1]^n$. To put it formally

$$X = \{[X^l X^u], d\} \tag{2}$$

where $X^l$ and $X^u$ represent min and max points of the input hyperbox $X$ and $d \in \{1, \ldots, p\}$ is the index of the classes that are present in the data set.

While it is possible to define various hyperbox membership functions that satisfy the boundary conditions with regard to full inclusion and full exclusion, it is quite intuitive to adopt a function that ensures monotonic (linear) change in-between these extremes. Following the suggestion in (Gabrys, Bargiela, 2000) we adopt here

$$b_j(X_h) = \min_{i=1,\ldots,n} (\min([1 - f(x_{hi}^u - w_{ji}, \gamma_i)], \ [1 - f(v_{ji} - x_{hi}^l, \gamma_i)])) \tag{3}$$

where $f(r, \gamma) = \begin{cases} 1 & if \quad r\gamma > 1 \\ r\gamma & if \quad 0 \le r\gamma \le 1 \\ 0 & if \quad r\gamma < 0 \end{cases}$ is a two parameter function in which $r$ represents the distance

of the test pattern $X_h$ from the hyperbox $[\boldsymbol{V}\,\boldsymbol{W}]$ and $\gamma = [\gamma_1, \gamma_2, \ldots, \gamma_n]$ represents the gradient of change of the fuzzy membership function. This is illustrated in Figure 1.

The fuzzy Min-Max algorithm is initiated with a single point hyperbox $[V_j W_j] = [\boldsymbol{0}\ \boldsymbol{0}]$. However, this hyperbox does not persist in the final solution. As the first input pattern $X_h = \{[X_h^l X_h^u], d\}$ is presented the initial hyperbox becomes $[V_j W_j] = [X_h^l X_h^u]$. Presentation of subsequent input patterns has an effect of creating new hyperboxes or modifying the size of the existing ones. A special case occurs when a new pattern falls inside an existing hyperbox in which case no modification to the hyperbox is needed.

## Hyperbox Expansion

When the input pattern $X_h$ is presented the fuzzy membership function for each hyperbox is evaluated. This creates a preference order for the inclusion of $X_h$ in the existing hyperboxes. However the inclusion of the pattern is subject to two conditions: (a) the new pattern can only be included in the hyperbox if the class label of the pattern and the hyperbox are the same and (b) the size of the expanded hyperbox that includes the new pattern must not be greater in any dimension than the maximum permitted size. To put it formally the expansion procedure involves the following

*Figure 1. One-dimensional (a) and two-dimensional (b) fuzzy membership function evaluated for a point input pattern $X_h$*

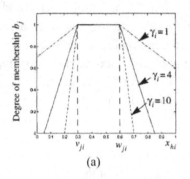

(a)

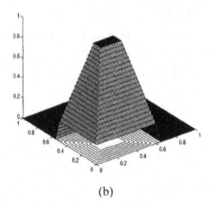

(b)

$$if \ class(B_j) = \begin{cases} d_h & \Rightarrow & test \ if \ B_j \ satisfies \ the \ \max imum \ size \ constra \ int \\ else & \Rightarrow & take \ another \ B_j \end{cases} \tag{4}$$

with the size constraint in (4) defined as

$$\underset{i=1,...,n}{\forall} (\max(w_{ji}, x_{hi}^u) - \min(v_{ji}, x_{hi}^l)) \leq \Theta \tag{5}$$

If expansion can be accomplished then the hyperbox min and max points are updated as

$$v_{ji} = \min(v_{ji}, x_{hi}^l), \quad for \ each \ i = 1, ..., n$$
$$w_{ji} = \max(w_{ji}, x_{hi}^u), \quad for \ each \ i = 1, ..., n$$

The parameter $\Theta$ can either be a scalar, as suggested in (Simpson, 1992), or a vector defining different maximum hyperbox sizes in different dimensions (Gabrys, Bargiela, 2000). It can be shown that the latter can result in fewer hyperboxes defining each pattern class but requires some a-priori knowledge about the topology of individual class sets or multiple presentations of data to facilitate adaptation.

## Overlap Test

The expansion of the hyperboxes can produce hyperbox overlap. The overlap of hyperboxes that have the same class labels does not present any problem but the overlap of hyperboxes with different class labels must be prevented since it would create ambiguous classification. The test adopted in (Gabrys, Bargiela, 2000) and (Simpson, 1992) uses the principle of minimal adjustment, where only the smallest overlap for one dimension is adjusted to resolve the overlap. This involves consideration of four cases for each dimension

**Case 1:** $v_{ji} < v_{ki} < w_{ji} < w_{ki}$

**Case 2:** $v_{ki} < v_{ji} < w_{ki} < w_{ji}$

**Case 3:** $v_{ji} < v_{ki} < w_{ki} < w_{ji}$

**Case 4:** $v_{ki} < v_{ji} < w_{ji} < w_{ki}$

The minimum value of overlap is remembered together with the index $i$ of the dimension, which is stored as variable $\Delta$. The procedure continues until no overlap is found for one of the dimensions (in which case there is no need for subsequent hyperbox contraction) or all dimensions have been tested.

## Hyperbox Contraction

The minimum overlap identified in the previous step provides basis for the implementation of the contraction procedure. Depending on which case has been identified the contraction is implemented as follows:

**Case 1:** $v_{k\Delta}^{new} = w_{j\Delta}^{new} = \dfrac{v_{k\Delta}^{old} + w_{j\Delta}^{old}}{2}$ or alternatively $(w_{j\Delta}^{new} = v_{k\Delta}^{old})$

**Case 2:** $v_{j\Delta}^{new} = w_{k\Delta}^{new} = \dfrac{v_{j\Delta}^{old} + w_{k\Delta}^{old}}{2}$ or alternatively $(v_{j\Delta}^{new} = w_{k\Delta}^{old})$

**Case 3:** if $w_{k\Delta} - v_{j\Delta} \le w_{j\Delta} - v_{k\Delta}$ then $v_{j\Delta}^{new} = w_{k\Delta}^{old}$ otherwise $w_{j\Delta}^{new} = v_{k\Delta}^{old}$

**Case 4:** if $w_{k\Delta} - v_{j\Delta} \le w_{j\Delta} - v_{k\Delta}$ then $w_{k\Delta}^{new} = v_{j\Delta}^{old}$ otherwise $v_{k\Delta}^{new} = w_{j\Delta}^{old}$

The above three steps of the fuzzy Min-Max classification can be expressed as training of a three-layer neural network. The network, represented in Figure 2, has a simple feed-forward structure and grows adaptively according to the demands of the classification problem. The input layer has $2*n$ processing elements, the first $n$ elements deal with the min point of the input hyperbox and the second $n$ elements deal with the max point of the input hyperbox $X_h = [X_h^l \ X_h^u]$. Each second-layer node represents a hyperbox fuzzy set where the connections of the first and second layers are the min-max points of the hyperbox including the given pattern and the transfer function is the hyperbox membership function. The connections are adjusted using the expansion, overlap test, contraction sequence described above.

Figure 2. *The three-layer neural network implementation of the GFMM algorithm*

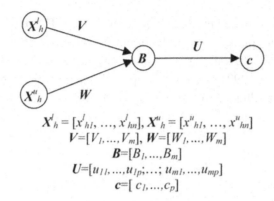

$$X^l_h = [x^l_{h1}, ..., x^l_{hn}], X^u_h = [x^u_{h1}, ..., x^u_{hn}]$$
$$V=[V_1, ..., V_m], W=[W_1, ..., W_m]$$
$$B=[B_1, ..., B_m]$$
$$U=[u_{11}, ..., u_{1p}; ...; u_{m1}, ..., u_{mp}]$$
$$c=[c_1, ..., c_p]$$

Note that the min points matrix $\mathbf{V}$ is modified only by the vector of lower bounds $X^l_h$ of the input pattern and the max points matrix $\mathbf{W}$ is adjusted in response to the vector of upper bounds $X^u_h$.

The connections between the second- and third-layer nodes are binary values. They are stored in matrix $\mathbf{U}$. The elements of $\mathbf{U}$ are defined as follows:

$$u_{jk} = \begin{cases} 1 & \text{if } B_j \text{ is a hyperbox for class } c_k \\ 0 & \text{otherwise} \end{cases} \tag{6}$$

where $B_j$ is the $j$th second-layer node and $c_k$ is the $k$th third-layer node. Each third-layer node represents a class. The output of the third-layer node represents the degree to which the input pattern $X_h$ fits within the class $k$. The transfer function for each of the third-layer nodes is defined as

$$c_k = \max_{j=1}^{m} B_j u_{jk} \tag{7}$$

for each of the $p$ third-layer nodes. The outputs of the class layer nodes can be fuzzy when calculated using expression (7), or crisp when a value of one is assigned to the node with the largest $c_k$ and zero to the other nodes.

## 3. INHERENT LIMITATIONS OF THE FUZZY MIN-MAX CLASSIFICATION

Training of the Min-Max neural network involves adaptive construction of hyperboxes guided by the class labels. The input patterns are presented in a sequential manner and are checked for a possible inclusion in the existing hyperboxes. If the pattern is fully included in one of the hyperboxes no adjustment of the min- and max-point of the hyperbox is necessary, otherwise a hyperbox *expansion* is initiated. However, after expansion is accomplished it is necessary to perform an *overlap test* since it is possible that the expansion resulted in some areas of the pattern space belonging simultaneously to two distinct classes,

*Figure 3. Training of the fuzzy min-max neural network (a) hyperboxes belonging to two different classes class($B_1$) ≠ class($B_2$);(b) inclusion of pattern {$X_h$, class($B_2$)} in $B_2$ implying overlap with $B_1$;(c) contraction of $B_1$ and $B_2$ with adjustment along two coordinates; (d) contraction of $B_1$ and $B_2$ with adjustment along one coordinate*

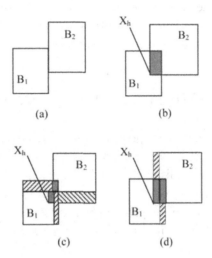

thus contradicting the classification itself. If the overlap test is negative, the expanded hyperbox does not require any further adjustment and the next input pattern is being considered. If, on the other hand, the overlap test is positive the hyperbox *contraction* procedure is initiated. This involves subdivision of the hyperboxes along one or several overlapping coordinates and the consequent adjustment of the min- and max-points of the overlapping hyperboxes. However, the contraction procedure has an inherent weakness in that it inadvertently eliminates from the two hyperboxes some part of the pattern space that was unambiguous while in the same time retaining some of the contentious part of the pattern space in each of the hyperboxes. This is illustrated in Figure 3.

By inspecting Figure 3 it is clear that the contraction step of the fuzzy Min-Max network training resolves only part of the problem created by the expansion of the hyperbox $B_2$. Although the hyperboxes $B_1$ and $B_2$ no longer overlap after the contraction has been completed (Figure 3(c) and 3(d)), some part of the original hyperbox $B_1$ remains included in $B_2$ and similarly some part of the hyperbox $B_2$ remains included in the contracted $B_1$. The degree of this residual inclusion depends on the contraction method that is chosen but it is never completely eliminated. Incidentally, it is worth noting that the intuitive approach proposed in (Simpson, 1992) of subdividing overlapping hyperboxes along a single coordinate with the smallest overlap does produce worse residual inclusion problem than the alternative subdivision along all overlapping coordinates (compare Figure 3(c) and 3(d)).

Another problem inherent to the contraction procedure is that it unnecessarily eliminates parts of the original hyperboxes. These eliminated portions are marked in Figure 3 with diagonal pattern lines. The elimination of these parts of hyperboxes implies that the contribution to the training of the Min-Max neural network of the data contained in these areas is nullified. If the neural networktraining involves only one pass through the data, then this is an irreversible loss that demonstrates itself in a degraded classification performance. The problem can be somewhat alleviated by allowing multiple presentations of data in the training process, as in (Gabrys, Bargiela, 2000), or reducing the maximum size of hyperboxes. In either case the result is that additional hyperboxes are created to cover the eliminated portions of the original hyperboxes. Unfortunately, the increased number of hyperboxes reduces the interpretability of classification so that there is a limit as to how far this problem can be resolved in the context of the standard Min-Max expansion/contraction procedure.

Finally, it is worth noting that the training pattern $\{X_h, class(B_2)\}$ continues to be misclassified in spite of the contraction of the hyperboxes. This means that a 100% correct classification rate is not always possible even with the multiple-pass Min-Max neural network training.

## 4. EXCLUSION/INCLUSION FUZZY CLASSIFICATION NETWORK (EFC)

The solution proposed here is the explicit representation of the contentious areas of the pattern space as *exclusion hyperboxes*. This is illustrated in Figure 4. The original hyperbox *b1* and the expanded hyperbox *b2* do not lose any of the undisputed area of the pattern space but the patterns contained in the exclusion hyperbox are eliminated from the relevant classes in the $\{c_1, ..., c_p\}$ set and are instead assigned to class $c_{p+1}$ (contentious area of the pattern space class). This overruling implements in effect the subtraction of hyperbox sets which allows for the representation of non-convex topologies with a relatively few hyperboxes.

The additional second-layer nodes *e* are formed adaptively in a similar fashion as for nodes *b*. The min-point and the max-point of the exclusion hyperbox are identified when the overlap test is positive for two hyperboxes representing different classes. These values are stored as new entries in matrix *S* and matrix *T* respectively. If the new exclusion hyperbox contains any of the previously identified exclusion hyperboxes, the included hyperboxes are eliminated from the set *e*. The connections between the nodes *e* and nodes *c* are binary values stored in matrix *R*. The elements of *R* are defined as follows:

$$r_{lk} = \begin{cases} 1 & \textit{if } e_l \textit{ overlapped hyperbox of class } c_k \textit{ and } 1 < k < p \\ 1 & \textit{if } k = p+1 \\ 0 & \textit{otherwise} \end{cases} \tag{8}$$

*Figure 4. The concept of the exclusion/inclusion fuzzy hyperboxes (a) hyperboxes belonging to two different classes class($B_1$) $\neq$ class($B_2$); (b) inclusion of pattern $\{X_h, class(B_2)\}$ in $B_2$ implying overlap with $B_1$ and consequent identification of the exclusion hyperbox*

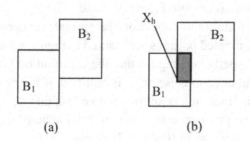

(a)          (b)

Note that the third layer has $p+1$ nodes $[c_1, ..., c_p, c_{p+1}]$ with the node $c_{p+1}$ representing the new exclusion hyperbox class. The output of the third-layer is now moderated by the output from the exclusion hyperbox nodes $e$ and the values of matrix $R$. The transfer function for the third-layer nodes is defined as:

$$c_k = \max_{k=1}^{p+1}(\max_{j=1}^{m} b_j u_{jk} - \max_{i=1}^{q} e_i r_{ik})$$

(9)

The second component in (9) cancels out the contribution from the overlapping hyperboxes that belonged to different classes.

## 5. NUMERICAL EXAMPLE

The EFC was applied to a number of synthetic data sets and demonstrated improvement over the GFMM and the original FMM (Simpson, 1992). As a representative example, we illustrate the performance of the network using the IRIS data-set from the Machine Learning Repository (http://www.ics.uci.edu/~mlearn/ MLRepository.html). It is important to emphasise however that the use of a single specific data set does not detract from the essence of the topological argument that we are making in this paper; that is, that the pattern classes are covered more efficiently by the difference of fuzzy sets compared to the usual covering with the union of fuzzy sets.

Using the IRIS data set we have trained the network on the first 75 patterns and the EFC performance was checked using the remaining 75 patterns. The results for FMM have been obtained using our implementation of the FMM algorithm, which produced results consistent with those reported in (Simpson, 1992). The results are summarized in Table 1.

The results reported in Table 1 deserve some additional commentary. First we need to point out that the EFC algorithm would normally start without any constraint on the hyperbox size, i.e. $\Theta=1$. This is in contrast to the two other algorithms that do require precise control of the maximum hyperbox size. So, in the interest of comparability of the results we have run the EFC algorithm with $\Theta$ equal to 0.03, 0.06, 0.2 and 0.4.

*Figure 5. Exclusion/inclusion fuzzy classification network*

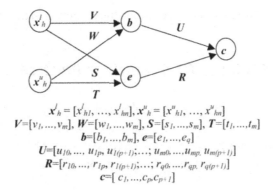

$$x^l_h = [x^l_{h1}, ..., x^l_{hn}], x^u_h = [x^u_{h1}, ..., x^u_{hn}]$$
$$V=[v_1,...,v_m], W=[w_1,...,w_m], S=[s_1,...,s_m], T=[t_1,...,t_m]$$
$$b=[b_1,...,b_m], e=[e_1,...,e_q]$$
$$U=[u_{10}, ..., u_{1p}, u_{1(p+1)};...; u_{m0}, ...,u_{mp}, u_{m(p+1)}]$$
$$R=[r_{10}, ..., r_{1p}, r_{1(p+1)};...; r_{q0}, ...,r_{qp}, r_{q(p+1)}]$$
$$c=[c_1,...,c_p,c_{p+1}]$$

*Table 1. Comparison of performance of FMM, GFMM and EFC*

| Performance criterion | FMM [14] | GFMM [8] | EFC |
|---|---|---|---|
| **Correct classification rate (range)** | **97.33-92%** | **100-92%** | **100-97%** |
| Number of hyperboxes (max. size 0.03) | 56 | 49 | 34 |
| Number of hyperboxes (max. size 0.06) | 32 | 29 | 18 |
| Number of hyperboxes (max. size 0.20) | 16 | 12 | 7 |
| Number of hyperboxes (max. size 0.40) | 16 | 12 | 4* |

\* The smallest number of classes; the number is not affected by the increase of the maximum size of hyperbox $\Theta$

The detailed results obtained with EFC for other values of the parameter $\Theta$ (0.1, 0.25, 0.35 and 0.45) are illustrated in Figures 6-10. Figure 6 shows the projection of the IRIS data onto a two-dimensional space of petal-length/petal-width. Subsequent figures show the effect of the gradual increase of the value of the maximum hyperbox size parameter $\Theta$. Although it is clear that for $\Theta=0.10$ (Figure 7) the covering of the data with hyperboxes is more accurate than for $\Theta=0.45$ (Figure 10), we argue that this is achieved at a too great expense of reduced interpretability of the classification. The large number of rules, implied by the individual hyperboxes, is clearly counterproductive. From the viewpoint of the interpretability of classification the result illustrated in Figure 10, is much preferred. Also, by comparing Figures 9 and 10, we note that for large $\Theta$ the result of classification is no longer dependent on the value of the parameter but is exclusively defined by the data itself. This in itself is a very desirable feature of the proposed algorithm.

Another point worth emphasizing is that the number of classes identified by the EFC is $p+1$ where $p$ is the number of classes identified by the FMM and GFMM. This implies that the calculation of the "classification rate" is not identical in all three cases. We have taken the view that the exclusion hyperbox(es) offer a positive identification of the patterns that are ambiguous. In this sense the fact of having some test data fall into the exclusion hyperbox is not considered a misclassification. Clearly, this has an effect of improving the classification rate of the EFC with respect to the other two methods. However, to do otherwise and to report all data falling into the exclusion hyperboxes as misclassified would be also misleading since we already have a knowledge about the nature of the exclusion hyperbox and it would effectively make no use of the "$p+1^{st}$" pattern class.

Of course we do need to balance the assessment of the EFC algorithm by highlighting the importance of the ratio of the volumes of the exclusion and inclusion hyperbox sets. If this ratio is small (e.g. 1/35 in the case of the IRIS dataset) the classification results are very good. However, if the ratio increases significantly, the classification is likely to return a large proportion of patterns as belonging to the "exclusion" class. This in itself offers a constructive advice on the reduction of the maximum size of hyperboxes.

## 6. FROM FUZZY CLUSTERING TO HYPERBOX INFORMATION GRANULES

Let us briefly recall the basic notions and terminology of unsupervised learning. As before the set of data (patterns) is denoted by X, where $X = \{x_1, x_2, ..., x_N\}$ while each pattern is an element in the n-dimensional unit hypercube, that is $[0,1]^n$. The objective is to cluster X into "c" clusters and the problem is cast as an optimization task (objective function based optimization)

*Figure 6. IRIS data projected onto petal-length/ petal-width two-dimensional space*

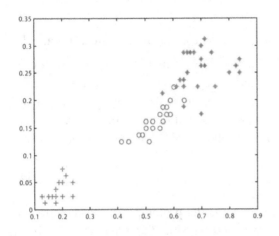

*Figure 7. Exclusion/inclusion hyperboxes evaluated for θ=0.10*

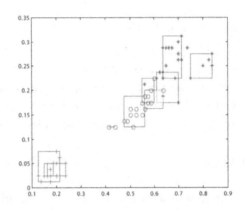

*Figure 8. Exclusion/inclusion hyperboxes evaluated for θ=0.25*

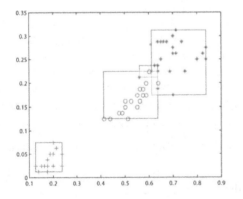

*Figure 9. Exclusion/inclusion hyperboxes evaluated for θ=0.35*

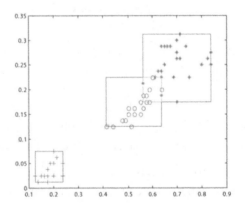

*Figure 10. Exclusion/inclusion hyperboxes evaluated for θ=0.45*

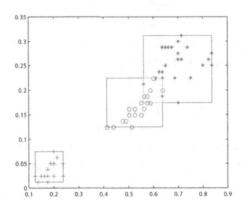

$$Q = \sum_{i=1}^{c} \sum_{k=1}^{N} u_{ik}^2 d_{ik} \qquad (10)$$

where $U = [u_{ik}]$, $u_{ik} \geq 0$, i=1,2,..,c, k=1, 2, ...,N is a partition matrix describing clusters in data. The distance function (metric) between the k-th pattern and i-th prototype is denoted by $d_{ik}$. $d_{ik} = \text{dist}(\mathbf{x}_k, \mathbf{v}_i)$ while $\mathbf{v}_1, \mathbf{v}_2, ..., \mathbf{v}_c$ are the prototypes characterizing the clusters. The type of the distance implies certain geometry of the clusters one is interested in exploiting when analyzing the data. For instance, it is well known that a commonly used Euclidean distance promotes an ellipsoidal shape of the clusters.

Emphasizing the role of the parameters to be optimized, the above objective function reads now as

Min Q with respect to $\mathbf{v}_1, \mathbf{v}_2, ...,\mathbf{v}_c$ and U $\qquad (11)$

Its minimization carried out for the partition matrix as well as the prototypes. With regard to the prototypes (centroids), we end up with a constraint-free optimization while the other one calls for the constrained optimization. The constraints assure that U is a partition matrix meaning that the following well-known conditions are met

$$\sum_{i=1}^{c} u_{ik} = 1 \quad \text{for all k} = 1,2,..,N \qquad (12)$$

$$0 < \sum_{k=1}^{N} u_{ik} < N \quad \text{for all i} = 1,2,..,c \qquad (13)$$

The choice of the distance function is critical to our primary objective of achieving the transparency of the findings. We are interested in such distances whose equidistant contours are "boxes" with the sides parallel to the coordinates. The Tchebyschev distance ($l_\infty$ distance) is a distance satisfying this property. The boxes are decomposable that is the region within a given equidistant contour of the distance can be treated as a decomposable relation R in the feature space, viz.

$$R = A \times B \qquad (14)$$

where A and B are sets (or more generally information granules) in the corresponding feature spaces. It is worth noting that the Euclidean distance does not lead to the decomposable relations in the above sense (as the equidistant regions in such construct are spheres or ellipsoides). The illustration of the decomposability property is illustrated in Figure 11.

The above clustering problem known in the literature as an $l_\infty$ FCM was introduced and discussed by Bobrowski and Bezdek (1991) more than 15 years ago. Some recent generalizations can be found in (Groenen, Jajuga, 2001). This motivation behind the introduction of this type of distance was the one about handling data structures with "sharp" boundaries (clearly the Tchebyschev distance is more suitable with this regard than the Euclidean distance). The solution proposed in (Bobrowski, Bezdek, 1991) was obtained by applying a basis exchange algorithm.

*Figure 11. Decomposability property provided by the Tchebyschev distance; the region of equidistant points is represented as a Cartesian product of two sets in the corresponding feature spaces*

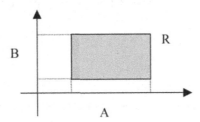

In this study, as already highlighted, the motivation behind the use of the Tchebyschev distance is different. We are after the description of data structure and the related interpretability of the results of clustering so that the clusters can be viewed as basic models of associations existing in the data. Here, we derive a gradient-based FCM technique enhanced with some additional convergence mechanism.

## 7. THE CLUSTERING ALGORITHM: DETAILED CONSIDERATIONS

The FCM optimization procedure is standard to a high extent (Bezdek, 1981) and consists of two steps: a determination of the partition matrix and calculations of the prototypes. The use of the Lagrange multipliers converts the constrained problem into its constraint-free version. The original objective function (10) is transformed to the form

$$V = \sum_{i=1}^{c} \sum_{k=1}^{N} u_{ik}^2 d_{ik} + \sum_{k=1}^{N} \lambda_k \left( \sum_{i=1}^{c} u_{ik} - 1 \right) \tag{15}$$

with $\lambda = [\lambda_1, \lambda_2, ..., \lambda_N]$ being a vector of Lagrange multipliers. The problem is then solved with respect to each pattern separately, that is, we consider the relationship below for each data point (t=1, 2, ...,N)

$$\frac{\partial V}{\partial u_{st}} = 0 \text{ and } \frac{\partial V}{\partial \lambda_t} = 0 \tag{16}$$

s=1,2, ..., c, t=1,2, ..., N. Straightforward calculations lead to the expression

$$u_{st} = \frac{1}{\sum_{j=1}^{c} \frac{d_{st}}{d_{jt}}} \tag{17}$$

The determination of the prototypes is more complicated as the Tchebyschev distance does not lead to a closed-type expression (unlike the standard FCM with the Euclidean distance). Let us start with the objective in which the distance function is spelled out in an explicit manner

$$Q = \sum_{i=1}^{c} \sum_{k=1}^{N} u_{ik}^2 \max_{j=1,2,\ldots,n} | x_{kj} - v_{ij} | \tag{18}$$

The minimization of Q carried out with respect to the prototype (more specifically its t-th coordinate) follows a gradient-based scheme

$$v_{st}(iter+1) = v_{st}(iter) - \alpha \frac{\partial Q}{\partial v_{st}} \tag{19}$$

where $\alpha$ is an adjustment rate (learning rate) assuming positive values. This update expression is iterative; we start from some initial values of the prototypes and keep modifying them following the gradient of the objective function. The detailed calculations of the gradient lead to the expression

$$\frac{\partial Q}{\partial v_{st}} = \sum_{k=1}^{N} u_{sk}^2 \frac{\partial}{\partial v_{st}} \{ \max_{j=1,2,\ldots,n} | x_{kj} - v_{sj} | \} \tag{20}$$

Let us introduce the following shorthand notation

$$A_{kst} = \max_{\substack{j=1,2,\ldots,n \\ j \neq t}} | x_{kj} - v_{sj} | \tag{21}$$

Evidently, $A_{kst}$ does not depend on $v_{st}$. This allows us to concentrate on the term that affects the gradient. We rewrite the above expression for the gradient as follows

$$\frac{\partial Q}{\partial v_{st}} = \sum_{k=1}^{N} u_{sk}^2 \frac{\partial}{\partial v_{st}} \{ \max(A_{kst}, | x_{kt} - v_{st} |) \} \tag{22}$$

The derivative is nonzero if $A_{kst}$ is less or equal to the second term standing in the expression,

$$A_{kst} \leq | x_{kt} - v_{st} | \tag{23}$$

Next, if this condition holds we infer that the derivative is equal to either 1 or $-1$ depending on the relationship between $x_{kt}$ and $v_{st}$, that is $-1$ if $x_{kt} > v_{st}$ and 1 otherwise.
Putting these conditions together, we get

$$\frac{\partial Q}{\partial v_{st}} = \sum_{k=1}^{N} u_{sk}^2 \begin{cases} -1 & \text{if } A_{kst} \leq |x_{kt} - v_{st}| \text{ and } x_{kt} > v_{st} \\ +1 & \text{if } A_{kst} \leq |x_{kt} - v_{st}| \text{ and } x_{kt} \leq v_{st} \\ 0 & \text{otherwise} \end{cases} \tag{24}$$

The primary concern that arises about this learning scheme is not the one about a piecewise character of the modulus (absolute value) function (a concern that can be raised from the formal standpoint but that is easily remedied by the appropriate selection of α in (19)) but a fact that the derivative zeroes for a significant number of situations. This may result in a poor performance of the optimization method as it could be trapped when the overall gradient becomes equal to zero. To enhance the method, we relax the binary character of the predicates (less or greater than) standing in (24). These predicates are Boolean (two-valued) as they return values equal to 0 or 1 (which translates into an expression "predicate is satisfied or it does not hold). The modification comes in the form of a degree of satisfaction of this predicate, meaning that we compute a multivalued predicate degree (a is included in b) (25) that returns 1 if a is less or equal to b. Lower values of the degree arise when this predicate is not fully satisfied. This form of augmentation of the basic concept was introduced in (Dubois, Prade, 1995), (Gottwald, 1995), (Pedrycz, 1989), (Pedrycz, Gomide, 1998) in conjunction to studies in fuzzy neural networks and relational structures (fuzzy relational equations).

The degree of satisfaction of the inclusion relation is equal to

$$Degree(a \text{ is included in } b) = a \to b \tag{26}$$

where a and b are in the unit interval. The implication operation $\to$ is a residuation operation, cf. (Pedrycz, 1989), (Pedrycz, Gomide, 1998). Here we consider a certain implementation of such operation where the implication is implied by the product t-norm, namely

$$a \to b = \begin{cases} 1 & \text{if } a \leq b \\ b/a & \text{otherwise} \end{cases} \tag{27}$$

Using this construct, we rewrite (24) as follows

$$\frac{\partial Q}{\partial v_{st}} = \sum_{k=1}^{N} u_{sk}^2 \begin{cases} -(A_{kst} \to |x_{kt} - v_{st}|) & \text{if } x_{kt} > v_{st} \\ (A_{kst} \to |x_{kt} - v_{st}|) & \text{if } x_{kt} \leq v_{st} \end{cases} \tag{28}$$

In the overall scheme, this expression will be used to update the prototypes of the clusters (28). Summarizing, the clustering algorithm arises as a sequence of the following steps:

- *Repeat*
   - Compute partition matrix using (17);
   - Compute prototypes using the partition matrix obtained in the first phase. (It should be noted that the partition matrix does not change at this stage and all updates of the prototypes work with this matrix. This phase is more time consuming in comparison with the FCM method equipped with the Euclidean distance)
- *Until* a termination criterion satisfied

Both the termination criterion and the initialization of the method are standard. The termination

*Figure 12. Two-dimensional synthetic data with four visible clusters of unequal size*

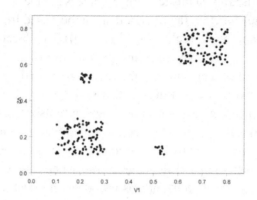

takes into account changes in the partition matrices at two successive iterations that should not exceed a certain threshold level. The initialization of the partition matrix is random.

As an illustrative example, we consider a synthetic data involving 4 clusters, see Figure 12. The two larger data groupings consist of 100 data-points and the two smaller ones have 20 and 10 data-points respectively.

Table 2 gives a representative set of clustering results for 2 to 8 clusters. As expected, the two larger data groupings exercise dominant influence on the outcome of the FCM algorithms. Both Euclidean and Tchebyschev distance based FCM exhibit robust performance in that they find approximately the same clusters in their successive runs (within the limits of the optimization convergence criterion). While most of the identified prototypes fall within the large data groupings, the Tchebyschev distance based FCM consistently manages to associate a prototype with one of the smaller data grouping (underlined in the table). This is clearly a very advantageous feature of our modified FCM algorithm and confirms our assertion that the objective of enhancing the interpretability of data through the identification of decomposable relations is enhanced with Tchebyschev distance based FCM.

The above results are better understood if we examine the cluster membership function over the entire pattern space. The visualization of the membership function for one of the two clusters, positioned in the vicinity of (0.2, 0.2), (c=2) is given in Figure 13.

It is easily noticed that for higher values of the membership grades (e.g. 0.9), the shape of contours is rectangular. This changes for lower values of the membership grades when we witness a gradual departure from this geometry of the clusters. This is an effect of interaction between the clusters that manifests itself in a deformation of the original rectangles. The deformation depends on the distribution of the clusters, their number and a specific threshold $\beta$ being selected. The lower is the value of this threshold, the more profound departure from the rectangular shape. For higher values of $\beta$ such deformation is quite limited. This suggests that when using high values of the threshold level the rectangular (or hyperbox) form of the core part of the clusters is fully legitimate.

Let us contrast these results with the geometry of the clusters constructed when using a Euclidean distance. Again, we consider two prototypes, as identified by the Euclidean distance based FCM, see Figure 14. The results are significantly different: the clusters are close to the Gaussian-like form and do not approximate well by rectangular shapes.

The above effect is even more pronounced when there are more clusters interacting with each other. We consider 8 prototypes identified by the two FCM algorithms, see Figure 15. In the case of Chebyschev

*Table 2. Prototypes identified by two FCM algorithms, with Euclidean and Tchebyschev distance measure respectively, for the varying number of clusters (the underlined prototypes correspond to the smaller data groupings)*

*Figure 13. Visualization of the first cluster (membership function) centered around (0.2088 0.1998): (a) 3D space and (b) contour plots*

| Number of clusters | Prototypes for FCM with Euclidean distance | Prototypes for FCM with Tchebyschev distance |
|---|---|---|
| 2 | 0.6707 0.6706<br>0.2240 0.2236 | 0.2088 0.1998<br>0.6924 0.6831 |
| 3 | 0.2700 0.3011<br>0.6875 0.6841<br>0.2302 0.2127 | 0.7000 0.6847<br><u>0.2440 0.4914</u><br>0.2124 0.1852 |
| 4 | 0.2255 0.2035<br>0.2323 0.2479<br>0.6872 0.6814<br>0.6533 0.6588 | 0.7261 0.7377<br><u>0.2278 0.5178</u><br>0.2092 0.1846<br>0.6523 0.6498 |
| 5 | 0.2525 0.2784<br>0.2282 0.2014<br>0.6721 0.6757<br>0.2343 0.2389<br>0.6919 0.6841 | 0.2189 0.1451<br><u>0.2272 0.5188</u><br>0.1960 0.2258<br>0.6568 0.6868<br>0.7268 0.6593 |
| 6 | 0.2329 0.2562<br>0.6809 0.6777<br>0.6857 0.6830<br>0.2272 0.2206<br>0.2261 0.2008<br>0.6447 0.6500 | 0.7469 0.6650<br>0.2151 0.1364<br><u>0.2278 0.5208</u><br>0.6570 0.6840<br>0.2619 0.2648<br>0.1945 0.2239 |
| 7 | 0.6646 0.6697<br>0.7036 0.6619<br>0.6993 0.7100<br>0.2395 0.5019<br>0.2382 0.1935<br>0.2164 0.1955<br>0.2271 0.2018 | 0.1967 0.2255<br>0.2200 0.1450<br>0.7278 0.6594<br><u>0.2277 0.5183</u><br>0.3976 0.4051<br>0.6099 0.6117<br>0.6588 0.6923 |
| 8 | 0.6962 0.6892<br><u>0.2398 0.5088</u><br>0.2360 0.1980<br>0.2441 0.2203<br>0.6962 0.6882<br>0.6850 0.6756<br>0.2385 0.1942<br>0.2166 0.1965 | 0.6607 0.7615<br>0.2122 0.1327<br>0.3209 0.3097<br>0.6565 0.6830<br>0.7267 0.6590<br>0.6460 0.6492<br><u>0.2277 0.5191</u><br>0.2108 0.2249 |

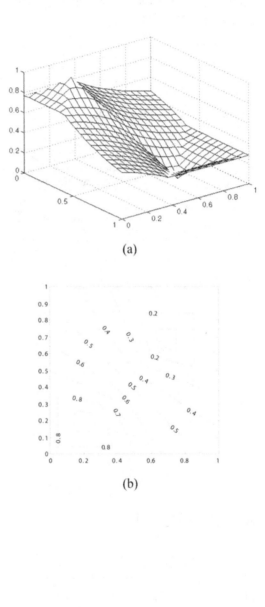

(a)

(b)

FCM, it is clear that despite strong interactions between the clusters, the rectangular shape of the cluster membership function is preserved for a range of values of this function. These undistorted rectangles cover a good proportion of the original data, which is represented by the selected prototype. On the other hand, the Euclidean FCM results in contours of the membership function that are undistorted circles only in the very close proximity of the prototype itself. Thus the task of linking the original data with the prototype representing an association existing in the data is quite difficult for most of the data points.

*Figure 14. Visualization of the first cluster (membership function) centered around (0.2240 0.2236): (a) 3D space and (b) contour plots. The Euclidean distance function was used in the clustering algorithm*

*Figure 15. Contour plots for one of the 8 clusters (membership function) centered around (0.2108 0.2248) for the Tchebyschev distance (a); and (0.2441 0.2203) for the Euclidean distance (b)*

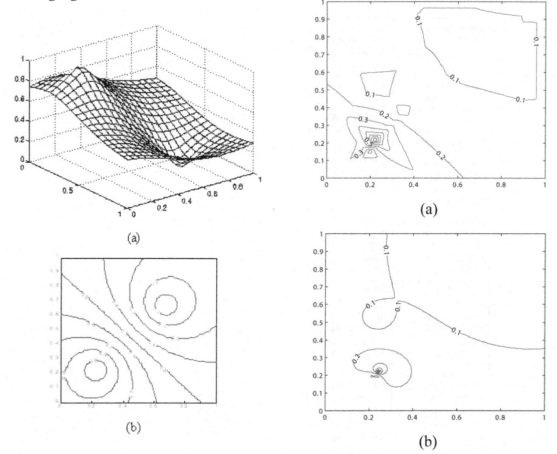

## 8. CONCLUSION

In this chapter we discuss a new algorithm for pattern classification that is based on novel representation of class sets as a difference of two types of fuzzy sets (the union of hyperboxes belonging to the given class and the union of hyperboxes belonging to different classes). It has been shown that, compared to the standard hyperbox paving approaches, the proposed algorithm results in a more efficient genera-tion of complex topologies that are necessary to describe the pattern classes. The consequence of the adoption of the exclusion/inclusion framework is a greater interpretability of the classification results (smaller number of hyperboxes needed to cover the data). It has been shown that in the proposed ap-proach the size of the hyperboxes does not need to be pre-determined and is indeed defined by the data itself. This is a very beneficial feature as it frees the analyst from making arbitrary choices with regard to the parameters of the algorithm. The low misclassification rate and good interpretability of the results of the proposed algorithm is achieved at the expense of rejecting a proportion of patterns that fall into the exclusion hyperbox set. If this proportion is small the algorithm provides an optimum mix of good classifier features. However, if the exclusion set becomes comparable in size to the inclusion set the maximum size of hyperboxes needs to be reduced. This is analogous to the standard hyperbox paving approaches but unlike in the standard approaches we do not use the misclassifications rate (that is dependent on the test data set) but instead use the ratio of exclusion to inclusion hyperbox sets (evaluated with training data only) as an indicator of how small hyperboxes need to be.

A general point raised by this investigation is that of a benefit of a richer vocabulary of topological constructs in describing data sets in multi-dimensional pattern spaces.

## ACKNOWLEDGMENT

Support from the Engineering and Physical Sciences Research Council (UK) and the Natural Sciences and Engineering Research Council of Canada (NSERC) is gratefully acknowledged.

## REFERENCES

Bargiela, A. (2001). Interval and Ellipsoidal Uncertainty Models. In Pedrycz, W. (Ed.), *Granular Computing*. Berlin Heidelberg, Germany: Springer Verlag.

Bargiela, A., & Pedrycz, W. (2001, June 113-120). Granular clustering with partial supervision. In *Proceedings of the European Simulation Multiconference,* (ESM2001). Prague, Czech Republic.

Bellman, R. E., Kalaba, R., & Zadeh, L. (1966). Abstraction and pattern classification. *Journal of Mathematical Analysis and Applications, 13*, 1–7. doi:10.1016/0022-247X(66)90071-0

Bezdek, J. C. (1981). *Pattern Recognition with Fuzzy Objective Function Algorithms*. New York: Plenum Press.

Bobrowski, L., & Bezdek, J. C. (1991). C-Means clustering with the $l_1$ and $l_\infty$ norms. *IEEE Transactions on Systems, Man, and Cybernetics, 21*, 545–554. doi:10.1109/21.97475

Cios, K., Pedrycz, W., & Swiniarski, R. (1998). *Data Mining Techniques*. Boston: Kluwer Academic Publishers.

Dubois, D., & Prade, H. (1995). Fuzzy relation equations and causal reasoning. *Fuzzy Sets and Systems, 75*, 119–134. doi:10.1016/0165-0114(95)00105-T

Gabrys, B., & Bargiela, A. (2000). General fuzzy min-max neural network for clustering and classification. *IEEE Transactions on Neural Networks, 11*, 769–783. doi:10.1109/72.846747

Gottwald, S. (1995). Approximate solutions of fuzzy relational equations and a characterization of t-norms that define metrics for fuzzy sets. *Fuzzy Sets and Systems, 75*, 189–201. doi:10.1016/0165-0114(95)00011-9

Groenen, P. J. F., & Jajuga, K. (2001). Fuzzy clustering with squared Minkowski distances. *Fuzzy Sets and Systems, 120*, 227–237. doi:10.1016/S0165-0114(98)00403-5

Maimon, O., Kandel, A., & Last, M. (2001). Information-theoretic fuzzy approach to data reliability and data mining. *Fuzzy Sets and Systems, 117*, 183–194. doi:10.1016/S0165-0114(98)00294-2

Pedrycz, W. (1989). *Fuzzy Control and Fuzzy Systems*. New York: Wiley.

Pedrycz, W., & Gomide, F. (1998). *An Introduction to Fuzzy Sets*. Cambridge, MA: MIT Press.

Simpson, P. K. (1992). Fuzzy min-max neural networks-Part1: Classification. *IEEE Transactions on Neural Networks, 3*(5), 776–786. doi:10.1109/72.159066

Simpson, P. K. (1993). Fuzzy min-max neural networks – Part 2: Clustering. *IEEE Transactions on Neural Networks, 4*(1), 32–45.

Zadeh, L. A. (1965). Fuzzy sets. *Information and Control, 8*, 189–200. doi:10.1016/S0019-9958(65)90241-X

Zadeh, L. A. (1997). Toward a theory of fuzzy information granulation and its centrality in human reasoning and fuzzy logic [FSS]. *Fuzzy Sets and Systems, 90*, 111–117. doi:10.1016/S0165-0114(97)00077-8

# Chapter 4
# On Characterization of Relation Based Rough Set Algebras

**Wei-Zhi Wu**
*Zhejiang Ocean University, P. R. China*

**Wen-Xiu Zhang**
*Xi'an Jiaotong University, P. R. China*

## ABSTRACT

*Rough set theory is one of the most advanced areas popularizing GrC. The basic notions in rough set theory are the lower and upper approximation operators. A rough set algebra is a set algebra with two additional lower and upper approximation operators. In this chapter, we analyze relation based rough set algebras in both crisp and fuzzy environments. We first review the constructive definitions of generalized crisp rough approximation operators, rough fuzzy approximation operators, and fuzzy rough approximation operators. We then present the essential properties of the corresponding lower and upper approximation operators. We also characterize the approximation operators by using the axiomatic approach. Finally, the connection between fuzzy rough set algebras and fuzzy topological spaces is established.*

## 1. INTRODUCTION

Granulation of a universe of discourse is one of the important aspects whose solution has significant bearing on Granular Computing (GrC). Many models and methods of GrC concentrating on concrete models in special contexts have been proposed and studied over the years. Rough set theory is one of the most advanced areas popularizing GrC. The concept of a rough set was originally proposed by Pawlak (1982) as a formal tool for modeling and processing intelligent systems characterized by insufficient and incomplete information. Using the concepts of lower and upper approximations in rough set theory, knowledge hidden in information systems may be unravelled and expressed in the form of decision rules (Pawlak, 1991; Zhang et al, 2003).

DOI: 10.4018/978-1-60566-324-1.ch004

The basic operators in rough set theory are approximations. There are at least two approaches to the development of rough set theory, namely the constructive and axiomatic approaches. In the constructive approach, binary relations on a universe of discourse, partitions of the universe of discourse, neighborhood systems, and Boolean algebras are all primitive notions. The lower and upper approximation operators are constructed by means of these notions (Boixader et al., 2000; Dubois & Prade, 1990; Mi et al., 2005; Nanda & Majumda, 1992; Pei, 2005; Pei & Xu, 2004; Pomykala, 1987; Skowron et al., 2003; Slowinski & Vanderpooten, 2000; Wu & Zhang, 2002, 2004; Yao, 1998a, b, c; Yeung et al., 2005; Zhu & Wang, 2007). The constructive approach is suitable for practical applications of rough sets. On the other hand, the axiomatic approach, which is appropriate for studying the structures of rough set algebras, takes the lower and upper approximation operators as primitive notions. In this approach, a set of axioms is used to characterize approximation operators that are the same as the ones produced by using the constructive approach (Lin & Liu, 1994; Liu, 2008); Mi et al., 2008; Mi & Zhang, 2004; Morsi & Yakout, 1998; Radzikowska & Kerre, 2002; Thiele, 2000a, b, 2001a, b; Wu et al., 2003, 2005; Wu & Zhang, 2004; Yang, 2007; Yang & Li, 2006; Yao, 1996, 1998a, b; Yeung et al., 2005). Under this point of view, rough set theory may be interpreted as an extension theory with two additional unary operators. The lower and upper approximation operators are related to the necessity (box) and possibility (diamond) operators in modal logic, the interior and closure operators in topological spaces, and the belief and plausibility functions in Dempster-Shafer theory of evidence (Chuchro, 1993, 1994; Qin & Pei, 2005; Skowron, 1989; Wu et al., 2002; Yao & Lingras, 1998).

The majority of studies on rough sets have been concentrated on the constructive approach. In Pawlak's rough set model (Pawlak, 1991), an equivalence relation is a key and primitive notion. This equivalence relation, however, seems to be a very stringent condition that may limit the application domain of the rough set model. To solve this problem, many authors have generalized the notion of approximation operators by using nonequivalence binary relations (Slowinski & Vanderpooten, 2000; Wu & Zhang, 2002; Yao, 1998a, b, c; Yao & Lin, 1996; Zhang et al., 2003). The These extensions of rough set model may be used in reasoning and knowledge acquisition in incomplete information systems and incomplete decision tables. Moreover, rough sets can also be generalized to the fuzzy environment and the results are called rough fuzzy sets (fuzzy sets approximated by a crisp approximation space) and fuzzy rough sets (fuzzy or crisp sets approximated by a fuzzy approximation space) (Boixader et al., 2000; Dubois & Prade, 1990; Mi et al., 2005; Mi & Zhang, 2004; Morsi & Yakout, 1998; Radzikowska & Kerre, 2002; Wu & Zhang, 2004; Wu et al., 2005; Yao, 1997; Yeung et al., 2005), these models have been employed to handle fuzzy and quantitative data (Hu et al., 2006, 2007; Jensen & Shen, 2007; Kuncheva, 1992). For example, the rough fuzzy set model can be used to in reasoning and knowledge acquisition in complete or incomplete information systems with fuzzy decisions and the fuzzy rough set model can be employed to apply to knowledge discovery in fuzzy information systems or fuzzy decision tables.

Compared with the constructive approach, lesser effort has been made on the axiomatic approach. Zakowski (1982) studied a set of axioms on approximation operators. Comer (1991, 19993) investigated axioms on approximation operators in relation to cylindric algebras. Within the framework of topological spaces, Lin and Liu (1994) suggested six axioms on a pair of abstract operators on the power set of a universe of discourse. Under these axioms, there exists an equivalence relation such that the derived lower and upper approximations are the same as the abstract operators. Similar result was also stated earlier by Wiweger (1989). A problem arisen is that all of these studies are restricted to Pawlak rough set algebra defined by equivalence relations. Wybraniec-Skardowska (1989) examined many axioms on various classes of approximation operators. Different constructive methods were suggested to produce such approximation operators. Thiele (2001b) explored axiomatic characterizations of approximation operators within modal logic for a crisp diamond and box operator represented by an arbitrary binary crisp relation. The most important axiomatic studies for crisp rough sets were made by Yao (1996, 1998a, 1998b), and Yao and Lin (1996), in which various classes of crisp rough set algebras are characterized by different sets of axioms. As to the fuzzy cases, Morsi and Yakout (1998) studied a set of axioms on fuzzy rough sets based on a triangular norm and a residual implicator, but their studies were restricted to fuzzy T-rough sets defined by fuzzy T-similarity relations which were equivalence crisp relations in the degenerated case. Thiele (2000a, b, 2001a) investigated axiomatic characterizations of fuzzy rough approximation operators and rough fuzzy approximation operators within modal logic for fuzzy diamond and box operators. Nevertheless, he did not solve the problem under which the minimal axiom set is necessary and sufficient for the existence of a fuzzy relation (and a crisp relation, respectively) producing the same fuzzy rough (and rough fuzzy, respectively) approximation operators. Wu et al. (2003), Wu and Zhang (2004), examined many axioms on various classes of rough fuzzy and fuzzy rough approximation operators when $T = \min$. Mi and Zhang (2004) discussed axiomatic characterization of a pair of dual lower and upper fuzzy approximation operators based on a residual implication. Based on a fuzzy similarity relation, Radzikowska and Kerre (2002) defined a broad family of the so-called $(I, T)$-fuzzy rough sets which is determined by an implicator $I$ and a triangular norm $T$.

Wu et al. (2005) gave a general framework for the study of $(I, T)$-fuzzy rough sets corresponding to an arbitrary fuzzy relation.

In this chapter, we focus mainly on rough set algebras characterized by a dual pair of lower and upper approximation operators in both of crisp and fuzzy environments. We will review the definitions of generalized crisp rough sets, rough fuzzy sets and fuzzy rough sets, and we will present the essential properties of the corresponding lower and upper approximation operators. We then characterize the approximation operators by axioms, and as an example, the connection between fuzzy rough set algebras and fuzzy topological spaces are established.

## 2. GENERALIZED CRISP ROUGH SET MODELS

### 2.1. Construction of Crisp Approximation Operators

Throughout this chapter the class of all subsets of a set $X$ will be denoted by $P(X)$. For $A \in P(X)$, we will denote by $\sim A$ the complement of $A$, i.e., $\sim A = X - A$.

Let $U$ be a finite and nonempty universe of discourse and $R \subseteq U \times U$ an equivalence binary relation on $U$, then the pair $(U, R)$ is called a Pawlak approximation space. The equivalence relation $R$ partitions the universe $U$ into disjoint subsets. The class of such subsets is a quotient space which we denote as $U / R$. Elements of $U / R$ are called the elementary sets which reflect the granules of the available information: the knowledge basis under consideration induced by the approximation space $(U, R)$. The empty set $\varnothing$ and the union of one or more elementary sets are called definable, observable, measurable, or composed sets. The family of all definable sets, denoted by $\sigma(U / R)$, is a $\sigma$-algebra of subsets of $U$

generated by the quotient set $U / R$. Given an arbitrary set $X \subseteq U$, it may be impossible to describe $X$ precisely using the equivalence classes of $R$. In this case, one may characterize $X$ by a pair of lower and upper approximations:

$$\underline{R}(X) = \left\{ x \in U : [x]_R \subseteq X \right\} = \bigcup \{ [x]_R : [x]_R \subseteq X \} \tag{1}$$

$$\overline{R}(X) = \left\{ x \in U : [x]_R \cap X \neq \varnothing \right\} = \bigcup \left\{ [x]_R : [x]_R \cap X \neq \varnothing \right\} \tag{2}$$

where $[x]_R = \{ y \in U : (x, y) \in R \}$ is the $R$-equivalence class containing $x$. The lower approximation $\underline{R}(X)$ is the union of all the elementary sets which are subsets of $X$, and the upper approximation $\overline{R}(X)$ is the union of all the elementary sets which have a nonempty intersection with $X$. It is natural to say that an element of $U$ necessarily belongs to $X$ if all its equivalent elements belong to $X$ whereas it possibly belongs to $X$ if at least one of its equivalent elements belongs to $X$. The pair $\left( \underline{R}(X), \overline{R}(X) \right)$ is the representation of $X$ in the approximation space $(U, R)$, or simply the Pawlak rough set of $X$ with respect to $(U, R)$. And $\underline{R}, \overline{R} : P(U) \rightarrow P(U)$ are respectively called the lower and upper approximation operators, and the system $(P(U), \cap, \cup, \sim, \underline{R}, \overline{R})$ is called a Pawlak rough set algebra (Yao, 1996) which is an extension of the set algebra $(P(U), \cap, \cup, \sim)$. It can be observed that $\underline{R}(X)$ is the greatest definable set contained in $X$, and $\overline{R}(X)$ is the least definable set containing $X$, i.e.,

$$\underline{R}(X) = \bigcup \{ Y : Y \in \sigma(U / R), Y \subseteq X \}, \tag{3}$$

$$\overline{R}(X) = \bigcap \{ Y : Y \in \sigma(U / R), Y \supseteq X \}. \tag{4}$$

The Pawlak approximation operators satisfy the following properties (Pawlak, 1991): for $X, Y \in P(U)$,

- **(P1)** $\underline{R}(X) = \sim \overline{R}(\sim X)$, $\overline{R}(X) = \sim \underline{R}(\sim X)$,

- **(P2)** $\underline{R}(U) = \overline{R}(U) = U$, $\underline{R}(\varnothing) = \overline{R}(\varnothing) = \varnothing$,

- **(P3)** $\underline{R}(X \cap Y) = \underline{R}(X) \cap \underline{R}(Y)$, $\overline{R}(X \cup Y) = \overline{R}(X) \cup \overline{R}(Y)$,

- **(P4)** $X \subseteq Y \Rightarrow \underline{R}(X) \subseteq \underline{R}(Y)$, $\overline{R}(X) \subseteq \overline{R}(Y)$,

- **(P5)** $\underline{R}(X \cup Y) \supseteq \underline{R}(X) \cup \underline{R}(Y)$, $\overline{R}(X \cap Y) \subseteq \overline{R}(X) \cap \overline{R}(Y)$,

- **(P6)** $\underline{R}(X) \subseteq X \subseteq \overline{R}(X)$,

- **(P7)** $\overline{R}\left(\underline{R}(X)\right) \subseteq X \subseteq \underline{R}\left(\overline{R}(X)\right)$,

- **(P8)** $\underline{R}(X) = \underline{R}\left(\underline{R}(X)\right)$, $\overline{R}\left(\overline{R}(X)\right) = \overline{R}(X)$,

- **(P9)** $\overline{R}\left(\underline{R}(X)\right) = \underline{R}(X)$, $\overline{R}(X) = \underline{R}\left(\overline{R}(X)\right)$.

The Pawlak rough set model can be used to discover knowledge hidden in complete information tables in the sense of decision rules (Pawlak, 1991). However, the equivalence relation in the Pawlak rough set model is a very stringent condition that may limit the application domain of the rough set model. The notion of approximation operators can be generalized by considering an arbitrary binary relation, even in two universes. The non-equivalence relation-based rough set models have been used in reasoning and knowledge acquisition in data set presented as incomplete information tables.

Let $U$ and $W$ be two nonempty and finite universes, $R \in P(U \times W)$ a binary relation from $U$ to $W$, the triple $(U,\ W,\ R)$ is called a generalized approximation space. For $x \in U$, denote $R_s(x) = \{y \in W : xRy\}$; it is called the successor neighborhood of $x$. For any $X \subseteq W$, we define a pair of lower and upper approximations of $X$ with respect to $(U,W,R)$ by replacing the equivalence class $[x]_R$ with the successor neighborhood $R_s(x)$:

$$\underline{R}(X) = \left\{x \in U : R_s(x) \subseteq X\right\}, \tag{5}$$

$$\overline{R}(X) = \left\{x \in U : R_s(x) \cap X \neq \varnothing\right\}. \tag{6}$$

The pair $\left(\underline{R}(X), \overline{R}(X)\right)$ is called the generalized crisp rough set of $X$ with respect to $(U,\ W,\ R)$, $\underline{R}$, $\overline{R} : P(W) \to P(U)$ are called the generalized lower and upper approximation operators, and the system $(P(W), P(U), \cap, \cup, \sim, \underline{R}, \overline{R})$ is called a generalized rough set algebra.

The generalized rough set approximation operators satisfy the following properties (Yao, 1998b, c): for $X, Y \in P(W)$,

- **(LD)** $\underline{R}(X) = \sim \overline{R}(\sim X)$,

- **(UD)** $\overline{R}(X) = \sim \underline{R}(\sim X)$,

- **(L1)** $\underline{R}(W) = U$,

- **(U1)** $\overline{R}(\varnothing) = \varnothing$,

- **(L2)** $\underline{R}(X \cap Y) = \underline{R}(X) \cap \underline{R}(Y)$,

- **(U2)** $\overline{R}(X \cup Y) = \overline{R}(X) \cup \overline{R}(Y)$,

- **(L3)** $X \subseteq Y \Rightarrow \underline{R}(X) \subseteq \underline{R}(Y)$,

- **(U3)** $X \subseteq Y \Rightarrow \overline{R}(X) \subseteq \overline{R}(Y)$,

- **(L4)** $\underline{R}(X \cup Y) \supseteq \underline{R}(X) \cup \underline{R}(Y)$,

- **(U4)** $\overline{R}(X \cap Y) \subseteq \overline{R}(X) \cap \overline{R}(Y)$.

Properties (LD) and (UD) show that the approximation operators $\underline{R}$ and $\overline{R}$ are dual to each other. Properties with the same number (e.g., (L1) and (U1)) may be regarded as dual properties. Properties (L1) and (L2) are independent, dually, (U1) and (U2) are independent. Property (L2) implies (L3) and (L4), likewise, (U2) implies (U3) and (U4).

We can also generalize rough set models constructed from special types of binary relations. A binary relation $R$ from $U$ to $W$ is referred to as serial if $R_s(x) \neq \varnothing$ for all $x \in U$. If $W = U$ and $R \in P(U \times U)$ is binary relation on $U$, then $R$ is referred to as reflexive if $x \in R_s(x)$ for all $x \in U$ ; $R$ is referred to as symmetric if $x \in R_s(y)$ implies $y \in R_s(x)$ for all $x, y \in U$ ; $R$ is referred to as transitive if $x \in R_s(y)$ and $y \in R_s(z)$ imply $x \in R_s(z)$ for all $x, y, z \in U$.

With respect to a serial relation from $U$ to $W$ we have

$R$ is serial $\Leftrightarrow$ (L0) $\underline{R}(\varnothing) = \varnothing$,

$\Leftrightarrow$ (U0) $\overline{R}(W) = U$,

$\Leftrightarrow$ (LU0) $\underline{R}(X) \subseteq \overline{R}(X),\ \forall X \in P(W)$.

If $R \in P(U \times U)$ is binary relation on $U$, the properties of special types of binary relations can be characterized by the properties of approximation operators (Yao, 1998a, b, c):

$R$ is reflexive $\Leftrightarrow$ (L5) $\underline{R}(X) \subseteq X,\ \forall X \in P(U)$,

$\Leftrightarrow$ (U5) $X \subseteq \overline{R}(X),\ \forall X \in P(U)$.

$R$ is symmetric $\Leftrightarrow$ (L6) $\overline{R}(\underline{R}(X)) \subseteq X, \forall X \in P(U)$,

$\Leftrightarrow$ (U6) $X \subseteq \underline{R}(\overline{R}(X)), \forall X \in P(U)$.

$R$ is transitive $\Leftrightarrow$ (L7) $\underline{R}(X) \subseteq \underline{R}(\underline{R}(X)), \forall X \in P(U)$,

$\Leftrightarrow$ (U7) $\overline{R}(\overline{R}(X)) \subseteq \overline{R}(X), \forall X \in P(U)$.

## 2.2. Axiomatic Characterization of Generalized Approximation Operators

In an axiomatic approach, rough sets are axiomatized by abstract operators. The primitive notion is a system $\left( P(W), P\left(U\right), \cap, \cup, \sim, L, H \right)$, where $L, H : P\left(W\right) \rightarrow P\left(U\right)$ are operators from $P(W)$ to $P(U)$. Now we employ the abstract set-theoretic operators $L, H : P\left(W\right) \rightarrow P\left(U\right)$ to characterize the generalized approximation operators. It should be pointed out that Yao (1996, 1998) obtained the main results for characterizing generalized crisp rough set approximation operators and Yang and Li (2006) further improved Yao's results.

### Definition 1

A mapping $L : P\left(W\right) \rightarrow P\left(U\right)$ is called a lower approximation operator if it satisfies two axioms:

- **(1L)** $L\left(W\right) = U$,

- **(2L)** $L\left(X \cap Y\right) = L\left(X\right) \cap L\left(Y\right), \forall X, Y \in P(W)$.

A mapping $H : P\left(W\right) \rightarrow P\left(U\right)$ is called an upper approximation operator if it satisfies two axioms:

- **(1U)** $H\left(\varnothing\right) = \varnothing$,

- **(2U)** $H\left(X \cup Y\right) = H\left(X\right) \cup H\left(Y\right), \forall X, Y \in P(W)$.

### Definition 2

Let $L, H : P\left(W\right) \rightarrow P\left(U\right)$ be two operators. They are referred to as dual operators if

- **(DL)** $L\left(X\right) = \sim H\left(\sim X\right), \forall X \in P(W)$.

- **(DU)** $H\left(X\right) = \sim L\left(\sim X\right), \forall X \in P(W)$.

Given an upper approximation operator $H : P\left(W\right) \rightarrow P\left(U\right)$, by defining a binary relation $R$ from $U$ to $W$ : for $(x, y) \in U \times W$,

$$(x, y) \in R \Leftrightarrow x \in H(1_y), \tag{7}$$

similar to the proof of Theorem 3 in Yao (1996), we can obtain axiomatic characterization of dual approximation operators:

## Theorem 1

Suppose that $L, H : P(W) \to P(U)$ are two dual operators. Then there exists a binary relation $R$ from $U$ to $W$ such that

$$L(X) = \underline{R}(X) \text{ and } H(X) = \overline{R}(X) \text{ for all} \qquad X \in P(W) \tag{8}$$

iff $L$ satisfies the axioms (1L) and (2L), or equivalently, $H$ satisfies axioms (1U) and (2U).

## Definition 3

A system $(P(W), P(U), \cap, \cup, \sim, L, H)$ is called a rough set algebra if $L$ satisfies the axiom set {(DL), (1L), (2L)} or $H$ satisfies axiom set {(DU), (1U), (2U)}. If there exists a serial relation $R$ from $U$ to $W$ such that Equation (8) holds, then we call $(P(W), P(U), \cap, \cup, \sim, L, H)$ a serial rough set algebra. If $W = U$ we will write $(P(U), \cap, \cup, \sim, L, H)$ instead of

$(P(W), P(U), \cap, \cup, \sim, L, H)$,

in such a case, if there exists a reflexive (respectively, a symmetric, a transitive) relation on $U$ such that Equation (8) holds, we then called $(P(U), \cap, \cup, \sim, L, H)$ a reflexive (respectively, a symmetric, a transitive) rough set algebra.

Theorems 2-5 below show that a special type of rough set algebra can be characterized by axioms, the proofs of these theorems are similar to or can be found in Yao (1998a).

## Theorem 2

Let $(P(W), P(U), \cap, \cup, \sim, L, H)$ be a rough set algebra. Then $(P(W), P(U), \cap, \cup, \sim, L, H)$ is a serial rough set algebra iff $L$ and $H$ satisfy one in the axiom set {(0L), (0U), (0LH)}:

- **(0L)** $L(\varnothing) = \varnothing$,

- **(0U)** $H(W) = U$,

- **(0LU)** $L(X) \subseteq H(X), \forall X \in P(W)$.

**Remarks:** It should be pointed out that under the axioms {(DL), (1L), (2L)}, axioms (0L), (0U), and (0LU) are equivalent, and axioms (DL), (1L), (2L), and (0L) are independent (Yang & Li, 2006), thus {(DL), (0L), (1L), (2L)} is an independent complete axiom set to characterize a serial rough set algebra.

## Theorem 3. (Yao, 1998a)

Let $(P(U), \cap, \cup, \sim, L, H)$ be a rough set algebra. Then $(P(U), \cap, \cup, \sim, L, H)$ is a reflexive rough set algebra iff $L$ satisfies axiom (5L), or equivalently, $H$ satisfies axiom (5U):

- **(5L)** $L(X) \subseteq X$, $\forall X \in P(U)$,

- **(5U)** $X \subseteq H(X)$, $\forall X \in P(U)$.

   **Remarks:** Axioms (1L), (2L), and (5L) are independent (Yang & Li, 2006), thus {(DL), (1L), (2L), (5L)} is an independent complete axiom set to characterize a reflexive rough set algebra.

## Theorem 4. (Yao, 1998a)

Let $(P(U), \cap, \cup, \sim, L, H)$ be a rough set algebra. Then $(P(U), \cap, \cup, \sim, L, H)$ is a symmetric rough set algebra iff $L$ satisfies axiom (6L), or equivalently, $H$ satisfies axiom (6U):

- **(6L)** $H(L(X)) \subseteq X, \forall X \in P(U)$,

- **(6U)** $X \subseteq L(H(X)), \forall X \in P(U)$.

   **Remarks:** Axioms (1L), (2L), and (6L) are dependent (Yang & Li, 2006), in fact, axioms (2L) and (6L) imply axiom (1L), thus {(DL), (2L), (6L)} is an independent complete axiom set to characterize a symmetric rough set algebra.

## Theorem 5. (Yao, 1998a)

Let $(P(U), \cap, \cup, \sim, L, H)$ be a rough set algebra. Then $(P(U), \cap, \cup, \sim, L, H)$ is a transitive rough set algebra iff $L$ satisfies axiom (7L), or equivalently, $H$ satisfies axiom (7U):

- **(7L)** $L(X) \subseteq L(L(X)), \forall X \in P(U)$,

- **(7U)** $H(H(X)) \subseteq H(X), \forall X \in P(U)$.

   **Remarks:** Axioms (1L), (2L), and (7L) are independent (Yang & Li, 2006), thus {(DL), (1L), (2L), (7L)} is an independent complete axioms to characterize a transitive rough set algebra.

## 3. ROUGH FUZZY SET MODELS

A rough fuzzy set results from the approximation of a fuzzy set with respect to a crisp approximation space. In this section, we will investigate rough fuzzy approximation operators within both constructive and axiomatic approaches.

## 3.1. Construction of Rough Fuzzy Approximation Operators

For a finite and nonempty set $U$, the class of all fuzzy subsets of $U$ will be denoted by $F(U)$. For any $\alpha \in [0,1]$, $\underline{\alpha}$ will be denoted by the constant fuzzy set of $U$, i.e., $\underline{\alpha}(x) = \alpha$ for all $x \in U$. For $A \in F(U)$, we denote by $\sim A$ the complement of $A$.

Let $(U, W, R)$ be a generalized approximation space. $\forall A \in F(W)$, the lower and upper approximations of $A$, $\underline{RF}(A)$ and $\overline{RF}(A)$, with respect to the approximation space $(U, W, R)$ are fuzzy sets of $U$ whose membership functions are as follows:

$$\overline{RF}(A)(x) = \bigvee_{y \in R_s(x)} A(y), \; x \in U, \tag{9}$$

$$\underline{RF}(A)(x) = \bigwedge_{y \in R_s(x)} A(y), \; x \in U. \tag{10}$$

The pair $\left( \underline{RF}(A), \overline{RF}(A) \right)$ is referred to as the rough fuzzy set of $A$ with respect to $(U, W, R)$ and $\underline{RF}, \overline{RF} : F(W) \to F(U)$ are referred to as lower and upper rough fuzzy approximation operators respectively, and the system $(F(W), F(U), \cap, \cup, \sim, \underline{RF}, \overline{RF})$ is called a generalized rough fuzzy set algebra.

The generalized rough fuzzy approximation operators satisfy the following properties: $\forall A, B \in F(W)$, $\forall \alpha \in [0,1]$,

- **(FLD)** $\underline{RF}(A) = \sim \overline{RF}(\sim A)$

- **(FUD)** $\overline{RF}(A) = \sim \underline{RF}(\sim A)$

- **(RFL1)** $\underline{RF}(A \cup \underline{\alpha}) = \underline{RF}(A) \cup \underline{\alpha}$

- **(RFU1)** $\overline{RF}(A \cap \underline{\alpha}) = \overline{RF}(A) \cap \underline{\alpha}$

- **(RFL2)** $\underline{RF}(A \cap B) = \underline{RF}(A) \cap \underline{RF}(B)$

- **(RFU2)** $\overline{RF}(A \cup B) = \overline{RF}(A) \cup \overline{RF}(B)$

- **(RFL3)** $A \subseteq B \Rightarrow \underline{RF}(A) \subseteq \underline{RF}(B)$

- **(RFU3)** $A \subseteq B \Rightarrow \overline{RF}(A) \subseteq \overline{RF}(B)$

- **(RFL4)** $\underline{RF}(A \cup B) \supseteq \underline{RF}(A) \cup \underline{RF}(B)$

- **(RFU4)** $\overline{RF}\left(A \cap B\right) \subseteq \overline{RF}\left(A\right) \cap \overline{RF}\left(B\right)$

If the generalize rough set models constructed from special types of crisp binary relations, then (Wu & Zhang, 2004)

$R$ is serial $\Leftrightarrow$ (RFL0) $\underline{RF}\left(\underline{\underline{\alpha}}\right) = \underline{\underline{\alpha}}$, $\forall \alpha \in [0,1]$,

$\Leftrightarrow$ (RFU0) $\overline{RF}\left(\underline{\underline{\alpha}}\right) = \underline{\underline{\alpha}}$, $\forall \alpha \in [0,1]$,

$\Leftrightarrow$ (RFL0)' $\underline{RF}\left(\varnothing\right) = \varnothing$,

$\Leftrightarrow$ (RFU0)' $\overline{RF}\left(W\right) = U$,

$\Leftrightarrow$ (RFLU) $\underline{RF}\left(A\right) \subseteq \overline{RF}\left(A\right)$, $\forall A \in F\left(W\right)$.

If $R \in P(U \times U)$ is binary relation on $U$, the properties of special types of binary relations can be characterized by the properties of rough fuzzy approximation operators (Wu, 2004):

Moreover, if

$R$ is reflexive $\Leftrightarrow$ (RFL5) $\underline{RF}\left(A\right) \subseteq A$, $\forall A \in F\left(U\right)$,

$\Leftrightarrow$ (RFU5) $A \subseteq \overline{RF}\left(A\right)$, $\forall A \in F\left(U\right)$.

$R$ is symmetric $\Leftrightarrow$ (RFL6) $A \subseteq \underline{RF}\left(\overline{RF}\left(A\right)\right)$, $\forall A \in F\left(U\right)$,

$\Leftrightarrow$ (RFU6) $\overline{RF}\left(\underline{RF}\left(A\right)\right) \subseteq A$, $\forall A \in F\left(U\right)$,

$\Leftrightarrow$ (RFL6)' $\underline{RF}\left(1_{U-\{x\}}\right)\left(y\right) = \underline{RF}\left(1_{U-\{y\}}\right)\left(x\right)$, $\forall\left(x,y\right) \in U \times U$,

$\Leftrightarrow$ (RFU6)' $\overline{RF}\left(1_{x}\right)\left(y\right) = \overline{RF}\left(1_{y}\right)\left(x\right)$, $\forall\left(x,y\right) \in U \times U$.

$R$ is transitive $\Leftrightarrow$ (RFL7) $\underline{RF}\left(A\right) \subseteq \underline{RF}\left(\underline{RF}\left(A\right)\right)$, $\forall A \in F\left(U\right)$,

$\Leftrightarrow$ (RFU7) $\overline{RF}\left(\overline{RF}\left(A\right)\right) \subseteq \overline{RF}\left(A\right)$, $\forall A \in F\left(U\right)$.

where $1_{x}$ denotes the fuzzy singleton with value 1 at $x$ and 0 elsewhere.

## 3.2. Axiomatic Characterization of Rough Fuzzy Approximation Operators

### Definition 4

Let $L, H : F(W) \to F(U)$ be two operators. They are called dual operators if

- **(DFL)** $L(A) = \sim H(\sim A)$, $\forall A \in F(W)$,

- **(DFU)** $H(A) = \sim L(\sim A)$, $\forall A \in F(W)$.

### Theorem 6. (Wu and Zhang, 2004)

Let $L, H : F(W) \to F(U)$ be two dual operators. Then there exists a crisp binary relation $R$ from $U$ to $W$ such that

$$L(A) = \underline{RF}(A) \text{ and } H(A) = \overline{RF}(A) \text{ for all } \quad A \in F(W) \tag{11}$$

iff $L$ satisfies axioms (RFL), (1RFL), (2RFL), or equivalently, $H$ satisfies axioms (RFU), (1RFU), (2RFU):

- **(RFL)** $L\left(1_{W-\{y\}}\right) \in P(U)$, $\forall y \in W$,

- **(RFU)** $H\left(1_y\right) \in P(U)$, $\forall y \in W$,

- **(1RFL)** $L(A \cup \underline{\underline{\alpha}}) = L(A) \cup \underline{\underline{a}}$, $\forall A \in F(U)$, $\forall \alpha \in [0,1]$,

- **(1RFU)** $H(A \cap \underline{\underline{\alpha}}) = H(A) \cap \underline{\underline{\alpha}}$, $\forall A \in F(U)$, $\forall \alpha \in [0,1]$,

- **(2RFL)** $L(A \cap B) = L(A) \cap L(B)$, $\forall A, B \in F(U)$,

- **(2RFU)** $H(A \cup B) = H(A) \cup H(B)$, $\forall A, B \in F(U)$.

   **Remarks:** Axioms (RFL), (1RFL), and (2RFL) are independent, and axioms (RFU), (1RFU), and (2RFU) are independent.

### Definition 5

A system $(F(W), F(U), \cap, \cup, \sim, L, H)$ is called a rough fuzzy set algebra if $L$ satisfies the axiom set $\{(RFL), (DFL), (1RFL), (2RFL)\}$ or $H$ satisfies axiom set $\{(RFU), (DFU), (1RFU), (3RFU)\}$. If there exists a serial relation $R$ from $U$ to $W$ such that Equation (11) holds, then we call $(F(W), F(U), \cap, \cup, \sim, L, H)$ a serial rough fuzzy set algebra. If $W = U$ we will write $(F(U), \cap, \cup, \sim, L, H)$ instead of

$(F(W), F(U), \cap, \cup, \sim, L, H)$,

in such a case, if there exists a reflexive (respectively, a symmetric, a transitive) relation on $U$ such that Equation (11) holds, we then called $(F(U), \cap, \cup, \sim, L, H)$ a reflexive (respectively, a symmetric, a transitive) rough fuzzy set algebra.

## Theorem 7. (Wu and Zhang, 2004)

Let $(F(W), F(U), \cap, \cup, \sim, L, H)$ be a rough fuzzy set algebra. Then $(F(W), F(U), \cap, \cup, \sim, L, H)$ is a serial rough fuzzy set algebra iff $L$ and $H$ satisfy one in the axiom set $\{(0RFL), (0RFU), (0RFL)\,', (0RFU)\,', (0RFLH)\}$:

- **(0RFL)** $L\left(\underset{=}{\alpha}\right) = \underset{=}{\alpha}$, $\forall \alpha \in [0,1]$,

- **(0RFU)** $H\left(\underset{=}{\alpha}\right) = \underset{=}{\alpha}$, $\forall \alpha \in [0,1]$,

- **(0RFL)** ' $L\left(\varnothing\right) = \varnothing$,

- **(0RFU)** ' $H\left(W\right) = U$,

- **(0RFLU)** $L\left(X\right) \subseteq H\left(X\right)$, $\forall X \in F\left(W\right)$.

**Remarks:** Axioms (RFL), (DFL), (1RFL), (2RFL), and (0RFL) are independent, and axioms (RFU), (DFU), (1RFU), (2RFU), and (0RFU) are independent, thus {(RFL), (DFL), (1RFL), (2RFL), (0RFL)} is an independent complete axiom set to characterize a serial rough fuzzy set algebra.

## Theorem 8. (Wu and Zhang, 2004)

Let $(F(U), \cap, \cup, \sim, L, H)$ be a rough fuzzy set algebra. Then $(F(U), \cap, \cup, \sim, L, H)$ is a reflexive rough fuzzy set algebra (that is, there exists a reflexive binary relation $R$ on $U$ such that

$$L\left(A\right) = \underline{RF}\left(A\right) \text{ and } H\left(A\right) = \overline{RF}\left(A\right), \ \forall A \in \ F\left(U\right) \tag{12}$$

hold) iff $L$ satisfies axiom (5RFL), or equivalently, $H$ satisfies axiom (5RFU):

- **(5RFL)** $L\left(X\right) \subseteq X$, $\forall X \in F\left(U\right)$,

- **(5RFU)** $X \subseteq H\left(X\right)$, $\forall X \in F\left(U\right)$.

**Remarks:** Axioms (RFL), (DFL), (1RFL), (2RFL), and (5RFL) are independent, and axioms (RFU), (DFU), (1RFU), (2RFU), and (5RFU) are independent, thus {(RFL), (DFL), (1RFL), (2RFL), (5RFL)} is an independent complete axiom set to characterize a reflexive rough fuzzy set algebra (Yang, 2007).

## Theorem 9. (Wu and Zhang, 2004)

Let $(F(U), \cap, \cup, \sim, L, H)$ be a rough fuzzy set algebra. Then $(F(U), \cap, \cup, \sim, L, H)$ is a symmetric rough fuzzy set algebra iff $L$ satisfies axiom (6RFL), or equivalently, $H$ satisfies axiom (6RFU):

- **(6RFL)** $A \subseteq L(H(A))$, $\forall A \in F(U)$,

- **(6RFU)** $H(L(A)) \subseteq A$, $\forall A \in F(U)$.

**Remarks:** Axioms (RFL), (DFL), (1RFL), (2RFL), and (6RFL) are dependent, and axioms (RFU), (DFU), (1RFU), (2RFU), and (6RFU) are independent, in fact, axiom (6RFL) implies axiom (RFL) (Wu, 2004), thus {(DFL), (1RFL), (2RFL), (6RFL)} is an independent complete axiom set to characterize a reflexive rough fuzzy set algebra.

## Theorem 10. (Wu and Zhang, 2004)

Let $(F(U), \cap, \cup, \sim, L, H)$ be a rough fuzzy set algebra. Then $(F(U), \cap, \cup, \sim, L, H)$ is a transitive rough fuzzy set algebra iff $L$ satisfies axiom (7RFL), or equivalently, $H$ satisfies axiom (7RFU):

- **(7RFL)** $L(A) \subseteq L(L(A))$, $\forall A \in F(U)$,

- **(7RFU)** $H(H(A)) \subseteq H(A)$, $\forall A \in F(U)$.

**Remarks:** Axioms (RFL), (DFL), (1RFL), (2RFL), and (7RFL) are independent, and axioms (RFU), (DFU), (1RFU), (2RFU), and (7RFU) are independent (Yang, 2007), thus {(RFL), (DFL), (1RFL), (2RFL), (7RFL)} is an independent complete axiom set to characterize a transitive rough fuzzy set algebra.

## 4. FUZZY ROUGH SET MODELS DETERMINED BY A TRIANGULAR NORM

When a fuzzy/crisp set is approximated by a fuzzy approximation space, we can obtain a fuzzy rough set. In this section, we characterize fuzzy rough approximation operators determined by a triangular norm.

### 4.1. Construction of Fuzzy Rough Approximation Operators

A triangular norm, or *t*-norm in short, is an increasing, associative and commutative mapping $T : [0,1] \times [0,1] \to [0,1]$ that satisfies the boundary condition: for all $a \in [0,1]$, $T(a,1) = a$.

A triangular conorm (*t*-conorm in short) is an increasing, associative and commutative mapping $S : [0,1] \times [0,1] \to [0,1]$ that satisfies the boundary condition: for all $a \in [0,1]$, $T(a,0) = a$. A *t*-norm $T$ and a *t*-conorm $S$ are said to be dual with each other if for all $a, b \in [0,1]$,

$$S(1-a, 1-b) = 1 - T(a,b), \quad T(1-a, 1-b) = 1 - S(a,b). \tag{13}$$

Let $U$ and $W$ be two non-empty universes of discourse and $R$ a fuzzy relation from $U$ to $W$ The triple $(U, W, R)$ is called a fuzzy approximation space. Let $T$ and $S$ be a $t$-norm and a $t$-conorm which are dual to each other. For any set $A \in F(W)$, the lower and upper T- fuzzy rough approximations of $A$, $\underline{TR}(A)$ and $\overline{TR}(A)$, with respect to the fuzzy approximation space $(U, W, R)$ are fuzzy sets of $U$ whose membership functions, for each $x \in U$, are defined, respectively, by

$$\underline{TR}(A)(x) = \underset{y \in W}{\wedge} S(1 - R(x, y), A(y)), \tag{14}$$

$$\overline{TR}(A)(x) = \underset{y \in U}{\vee} T(R(x, y), A(y)). \tag{15}$$

The pair $\left(\underline{TR}(A), \overline{TR}(A)\right)$ is referred to as a fuzzy rough set, and $\underline{TR}$ and $\overline{TR} : F(W) \rightarrow F(U)$ are referred to as lower and upper T-fuzzy rough approximation operators, respectively.

The lower and upper T-fuzzy rough approximation operators $\underline{TR}$ and $\overline{TR}$ satisfy the properties: $\forall A, B \in F(W)$, $\forall \alpha \in [0, 1]$,

- **(FLD)** $\underline{TR}(A) = \sim \overline{TR}(\sim A)$,

- **(FUD)** $\overline{TR}(A) = \sim \underline{TR}(\sim A)$,

- **(FRL1)** $\underline{TR}(A \cup \underline{\underline{\alpha}}) = \underline{TR}(A) \cup \underline{\underline{\alpha}}$,

- **(FRU1)** $\overline{TR}(A \cap \underline{\underline{\alpha}}) = \overline{TR}(A) \cap \underline{\underline{\alpha}}$,

- **(FRL2)** $\underline{TR}(A \cap B) = \underline{TR}(A) \cap \underline{TR}(B)$,

- **(FRU2)** $\overline{TR}(A \cup B) = \overline{TR}(A) \cup \overline{TR}(B)$,

- **(FRL3)** $A \subseteq B \Rightarrow \underline{TR}(A) \subseteq \underline{TR}(B)$,

- **(FRU3)** $A \subseteq B \Rightarrow \overline{TR}(A) \subseteq \overline{TR}(B)$,

- **(FRL4)** $\underline{TR}(A \cup B) \supseteq \underline{TR}(A) \cup \underline{TR}(B)$

- **(FRU4)** $\overline{TR}(A \cap B) \subseteq \overline{TR}(A) \cap \overline{TR}(B)$.

If the generalize fuzzy rough set models constructed from special types of fuzzy binary relations, then

$R$ is serial $\Leftrightarrow$ (FRL0) $\underline{TR}(\underline{\underline{\alpha}}) = \underline{\underline{\alpha}}$, $\forall \alpha \in [0, 1]$,

$\Leftrightarrow$ (FRU0) $\overline{TR}\left(\underset{=}{\alpha}\right) = \underset{=}{\alpha}$, $\forall \alpha \in [0,1]$,

$\Leftrightarrow$ (FRL0)' $\underline{TR}\left(\varnothing\right) = \varnothing$,

$\Leftrightarrow$ (FRU0)' $\overline{TR}\left(W\right) = U$,

$\Leftrightarrow$ (FRLU) $\underline{TR}\left(A\right) \subseteq \overline{TR}\left(A\right)$, $\forall A \in F\left(W\right)$.

If $R \in F(U \times U)$ is binary relation on $U$, the properties of special types of fuzzy binary relations can be characterized by the properties of fuzzy rough approximation operators:

$R$ is reflexive $\Leftrightarrow$ (FRL5) $\underline{TR}\left(A\right) \subseteq A$, $\forall A \in F\left(U\right)$,

$\Leftrightarrow$ (FRU5) $A \subseteq \overline{TR}\left(A\right)$, $\forall A \in F\left(U\right)$.

$R$ is symmetric $\Leftrightarrow$ (FRL6) $\underline{TR}\left(1_{U-\{x\}}\right)\left(y\right) = \underline{TR}\left(1_{U-\{y\}}\right)\left(x\right)$, $\forall \left(x,y\right) \in U \times U$,

$\Leftrightarrow$ (FRU6) $\overline{TR}\left(1_{x}\right)\left(y\right) = \overline{TR}\left(1_{y}\right)\left(x\right)$, $\forall \left(x,y\right) \in U \times U$.

$R$ is transitive $\Leftrightarrow$ (FRL7) $\underline{TR}(A) \subseteq \underline{TR}(\underline{TR}(A))$, $\forall A \in F\left(U\right)$,

$\Leftrightarrow$ (FRU7) $\overline{TR}(\overline{TR}(A)) \subseteq \overline{TF}(A)$, $\forall A \in F\left(U\right)$.

## 4.2. Axiomatic Characterization of Fuzzy Rough Approximation Operators

Theorem 11. (Wu et al., 2005)

Let $L, H : F\left(W\right) \to F\left(U\right)$ be two dual operators. Then there exists a fuzzy binary relation $R$ on $U$ such that

$$L\left(A\right) = \underline{TR}\left(A\right) \text{ and } H\left(A\right) = \overline{TR}\left(A\right) \text{ for all } A \in F\left(W\right) \tag{16}$$

iff $L$ satisfies axioms (1FRL), (2FRL), or equivalently, $H$ satisfies axioms (1FRU), (2FRU):

- **(1FRL)** $L\left(A \cup \underset{=}{\alpha}\right) = L\left(A\right) \cup \underset{=}{\alpha}$, $\forall A \in F\left(U\right)$, $\forall \alpha \in [0,1]$,
- **(1FRU)** $H\left(A \cap \underset{=}{\alpha}\right) = H\left(A\right) \cap \underset{=}{\alpha}$, $\forall A \in F\left(U\right)$, $\forall \alpha \in [0,1]$,
- **(2FRL)** $L\left(A \cap B\right) = L\left(A\right) \cap L\left(B\right)$, $\forall A, B \in F\left(U\right)$,

- **(2FRU)** $H\left(A \cup B\right) = H\left(A\right) \cup H\left(B\right),\ \forall A, B \in F\left(U\right).$

**Remarks:** Axioms (1FRL) and (2FRL) are independent, and, similarly, axioms (1FRU) and (2FRU) are independent too (Mi et al., 2008).

## Definition 6

A system $(F(W), F(U), \cap, \cup, \sim, L, H)$ is called a fuzzy rough set algebra if $L$ satisfies the axiom set {(DFL), (1FRL), (2FRL)} or $H$ satisfies axiom set {(DFU), (1FRU), (2FRU)}. If there exists a serial fuzzy relation $R$ from $U$ to $W$ such that Equation (16) holds, then we call $(F(W), F(U), \cap, \cup, \sim, L, H)$ a serial fuzzy rough set algebra. If $W = U$ we will write $(F(U), \cap, \cup, \sim, L, H)$ instead of

$(F(W), F(U), \cap, \cup, \sim, L, H),$

in such a case, if there exists a reflexive (respectively, a symmetric, a transitive) fuzzy relation on $U$ such that Equation (11) holds, we then called $(F(U), \cap, \cup, \sim, L, H)$ a reflexive (respectively, a symmetric, a transitive) fuzzy rough set algebra.

## Theorem 12. (Wu et al., 2005)

Let $(F(W), F(U), \cap, \cup, \sim, L, H)$ be a fuzzy rough set algebra. Then $(F(W), F(U), \cap, \cup, \sim, L, H)$ is a serial fuzzy rough set algebra iff $L$ and $H$ satisfy one in the axiom set {(0FRL), (0FRU), (0FRL) ', (0FRU) ', (0FRLH)}:

- **(0FRL)** $L\left(\underline{\underline{\alpha}}\right) = \underline{\underline{\alpha}},\ \forall \alpha \in [0,1],$

- **(0FRU)** $H\left(\underline{\underline{\alpha}}\right) = \underline{\underline{\alpha}},\ \forall \alpha \in [0,1],$

- **(0FRL)** ' $L\left(\varnothing\right) = \varnothing,$

- **(0FRU)** ' $H\left(W\right) = U,$

- **(0RFLU)** $L\left(X\right) \subseteq H\left(X\right), \forall X \in F\left(W\right).$

## Theorem 13. (Wu et al., 2005)

Let $(F(U), \cap, \cup, \sim, L, H)$ be a fuzzy rough set algebra. Then $(F(U), \cap, \cup, \sim, L, H)$ is a reflexive fuzzy rough set algebra (that is, there exists a reflexive fuzzy binary relation $R$ on $U$ such that

$$L\left(A\right) = \underline{RF}\left(A\right) \text{ and } H\left(A\right) = \overline{RF}\left(A\right) \text{ for all } A \in F\left(U\right) \tag{17}$$

hold) iff $L$ satisfies axiom (5FRL), or equivalently, $H$ satisfies axiom (5FRU):

- **(5FRL)** $L(X) \subseteq X$, $\forall X \in F(U)$,

- **(5FRU)** $X \subseteq H(X)$, $\forall X \in F(U)$.

**Remarks:** Axioms (DFL), (1FRL), (2FRL), and (5FRL) are independent, and axioms (DFU), (1FRU), (2FRU), and (5FRU) are independent, thus {(DFL), (1FRL), (2FRL), (5FRL)} is an independent complete axiom set to characterize a reflexive fuzzy rough set algebra.

## Theorem 14. (Wu et al., 2005)

Let $(F(U), \cap, \cup, \sim, L, H)$ be a fuzzy rough set algebra. Then $(F(U), \cap, \cup, \sim, L, H)$ is a symmetric fuzzy rough set algebra iff $L$ satisfies axiom (6FRL), or equivalently, $H$ satisfies axiom (6FRU):

- **(6FRL)** $L\left(1_{U-\{x\}}\right)(y) = L\left(1_{U-\{y\}}\right)(x)$, $\forall (x, y) \in U \times U$,

- **(6FRU)** $H\left(1_x\right)(y) = H\left(1_y\right)(x)$, $\forall (x, y) \in U \times U$.

**Remarks:** Axioms (DFL), (1FRL), (2FRL), and (6FRL) are independent, and axioms (DFU), (1FRU), (2FRU), and (6FRU) are independent, thus {(DFL), (1RFL), (2RFL), (6RFL)} is an independent complete axiom set to characterize a transitive fuzzy rough set algebra.

## Theorem 15. (Wu et al., 2005)

Let $(F(U), \cap, \cup, \sim, L, H)$ be a fuzzy rough set algebra. Then $(F(U), \cap, \cup, \sim, L, H)$ is a transitive fuzzy rough set algebra iff $L$ satisfies axiom (7FRL), or equivalently, $H$ satisfies axiom (7FRU):

- **(7FRL)** $L(A) \subseteq L(L(A))$, $\forall A \in F(U)$,

- **(7FRU)** $H(H(A)) \subseteq H(A)$, $\forall A \in F(U)$.

**Remarks:** Axioms (DFL), (1FRL), (2FRL), and (7FRL) are independent, and axioms (DFU), (1FRU), (2FRU), and (7FRU) are independent, thus {(DFL), (1FRL), (2FRL), (7FRL)} is an independent complete axiom set to characterize a transitive fuzzy rough set algebra.

## 4.3. Relationship Between Fuzzy Rough Set Algebras and Fuzzy Topological Spaces

Let $U$ be a nonempty set, a family of fuzzy subset $\tau \subseteq F(U)$ is referred to as a fuzzy topology on $U$, if

- **(FT1)** $\underline{\underline{\alpha}} \in \tau$, $\forall \alpha \in [0,1]$,

- **(FT2)** $A, B \in \tau \Rightarrow A \cap B \in \tau$,

- **(FT3)** $\{A_j : j \in J\} \subseteq \tau$, $J$ is an index set $\Rightarrow \bigcup_{j \in J} A_j \in \tau$.

The pair $(U, \tau)$ is called a fuzzy topological space, and the elements of the fuzzy topology $\tau$ are referred to as open fuzzy sets.

A map $\Psi : F(U) \to F(U)$ is referred to as a fuzzy interior operator iff

(1)  $\Psi(A) \subseteq A$, $\forall A \in F(U)$,

(2)  $\Psi(A \cap B) = \Psi(A) \cap \Psi(B)$, $\forall A, B \in F(U)$

(3)  $\Psi(\Psi(A)) = \Psi(A)$, $\forall A \in F(U)$,

(4)  $\Psi(\underline{\underline{\alpha}}) = \underline{\underline{\alpha}}$, $\forall \alpha \in [0,1]$.

A map $\Phi : F(U) \to F(U)$ is referred to as a fuzzy closure operator iff

(1)  $A \subseteq \Phi(A)$, $\forall A \in F(U)$,

(2)  $\Phi(A \cup B) = \Phi(A) \cup \Phi(B)$, $\forall A, B \in F(U)$,

(3)  $\Phi(\Phi(A)) = \Phi(A)$, $\forall A \in F(U)$,

(4)  $\Phi(\underline{\underline{\alpha}}) = \underline{\underline{\alpha}}$, $\forall \alpha \in [0,1]$.

It is easy to show that if $\Psi : F(U) \to F(U)$ is an interior operator, then

$$\tau_\Psi = \{A \in F(U) : \Psi(A) = A\} \tag{18}$$

is a fuzzy topology. So the open fuzzy sets are the fixed points of $\Psi$.

Given a reflexive and transitive fuzzy rough set algebra $K = \left( F(U), \cap, \cup, \sim, L, H \right)$, by defining a fuzzy topology $\tau_K$ on $U$ as follows:

$$\tau_K = \left\{ A \in F(U) : L(A) = A \right\}. \tag{19}$$

We can conclude following.

## Theorem 16

Let $K = \left( F(U), \cap, \cup, \sim, L, H \right)$ be a fuzzy rough set algebra. Then there exists a fuzzy topology $\tau_K$ such that $L$ and $H$ are respectively the fuzzy interior operator and fuzzy closure operator induced by $\tau_K$ iff

$K = \left( F\left(U\right), \cap, \cup, \sim, L, H \right)$ is a reflexive and transitive fuzzy rough set algebra.

Combining Theorems 13 and 15, we can obtain following theorem which presents the conditions that a fuzzy topological space can be derived from a fuzzy rough set algebra.

## Theorem 17

Assume that $\tau$ is a fuzzy topology on $U$, and $\Psi$ and $\Phi$ are respectively the fuzzy interior operator and fuzzy closure operator of $\tau$, then there exists a fuzzy rough set algebra

$$K_{\tau} = \left( F\left(U\right), \cap, \cup, \sim, L, H \right)$$

on $U$ such that

$$L\left(A\right) = \Psi\left(A\right) \text{ and } H(A) = \Phi(A), \forall A \in F(U) \tag{20}$$

Iff $\Psi$ satisfies axioms (1FRL) and (2FRL), and $\Phi$ satisfies axioms (1FRU) and (2FRU).

## 5. CONCLUSION

The theory of rough sets is studied based on the notion of an approximation space and its inducing lower and upper approximation operators. A binary relation in the approximation space forms the granules of knowledge of the available information. Using the concepts of lower and upper approximations in rough set theory, knowledge hidden in a decision table may be unraveled in the form of decision rules. With reference to various requirements, generalized rough set models in both of crisp and fuzzy environment can be formulated and studied from constructive and algebraic points of view. In the constructive approach, lower and upper approximation operators are defined by binary relations, this approach is useful for practical applications of rough set theory. In the algebraic approach, approximation operators are characterized by abstract axioms, that is, a set of axioms is used to characterize approximation operators that are the same as the ones produced by using the constructive approach. The algebraic approach will help us to gain much more insights into the mathematical structures of the approximation operators. In this approach, rough set theory may be regarded as an extension of set theory.

## ACKNOWLEDGMENT

This work was supported by grants from the National Natural Science Foundation of China (Nos. 60673096 and 60773174) and the Natural Science Foundation of Zhejiang Province in China (No. Y107262).

## REFERENCES

Boixader, D., Jacas, J., & Recasens, J. (2000). Upper and lower approximations of fuzzy sets. *International Journal of General Systems*, 29, 555–568. doi:10.1080/03081070008960961

Chuchro, M. (1993). A certain conception of rough sets in topological Boolean algebras. *Bulletin of the Section of Logic, 22*, 9–12.

Chuchro, M. (1994). On rough sets in topological Boolean algebras. In Ziarko, W. (Ed.), *Rough Sets, Fuzzy Sets and Knowledge Discovery* (pp. 157–160). Berlin, Germany: Springer-Verlag.

Comer, S. (1991). An algebraic approach to the approximation of information. *Fundamenta Informaticae, 14*, 492–502.

Comer, S. (1993). On connections between information systems, rough sets, and algebraic logic. In C. Rauszer (Ed.), Algebraic Methods in Logic and Computer Science (vol. 28, pp. 117–127). Polish Academy of Sciences: Banach Center Publisher.

Dubois, D., & Prade, H. (1990). Rough fuzzy sets and fuzzy rough sets. *International Journal of General Systems, 17*, 191–208. doi:10.1080/03081079008935107

Hu, Q. H., Xie, Z. X., & Yu, D. R. (2007). Hybrid attribute reduction based on a novel fuzzy rough model and information granulation. *Pattern Recognition, 40*, 3509–3521. doi:10.1016/j.patcog.2007.03.017

Hu, Q. H., Yu, D. R., & Xie, Z. X. (2006). Information-preserving hybrid data reduction based on fuzzy rough techniques. *Pattern Recognition Letters, 27*, 414–423. doi:10.1016/j.patrec.2005.09.004

Jensen, R., & Shen, Q. (2007). Fuzzy-rough sets assisted attribute selection. *IEEE Transactions on Fuzzy Systems, 15*, 73–89. doi:10.1109/TFUZZ.2006.889761

Kuncheva, L. I. (1992). Fuzzy rough sets: application to feature selection. *Fuzzy Sets and Systems, 51*, 147–153. doi:10.1016/0165-0114(92)90187-9

Lin, T. Y., & Liu, Q. (1994). Rough approximate operators: axiomatic rough set theory. In Ziarko, W. (Ed.), *Rough Sets, Fuzzy Sets and Knowledge Discovery* (pp. 256–260). Berlin, Germany: Springer.

Liu, G. L. (2008). Axiomatic systems for rough sets and fuzzy rough sets. *International Journal of Approximate Reasoning, 48*, 857–867. doi:10.1016/j.ijar.2008.02.001

Mi, J.-S., Leung, Y., & Wu, W.-Z. (2005). An uncertainty measure in partition-based fuzzy rough sets. *International Journal of General Systems, 34*, 77–90. doi:10.1080/03081070512331318329

Mi, J.-S., Leung, Y., Zhao, H.-Y., & Feng, T. (2008). Generalized fuzzy rough sets determined by a triangular norm. *Information Sciences, 178*, 3203–3213. doi:10.1016/j.ins.2008.03.013

Mi, J.-S., & Zhang, W.-X. (2004). An axiomatic characterization of a fuzzy generalization of rough sets. *Information Sciences, 160*, 235–249. doi:10.1016/j.ins.2003.08.017

Morsi, N. N., & Yakout, M. M. (1998). Axiomatics for fuzzy rough sets. *Fuzzy Sets and Systems, 100*, 327–342. doi:10.1016/S0165-0114(97)00104-8

Nanda, S., & Majumda, S. (1992). Fuzzy rough sets. *Fuzzy Sets and Systems, 45*, 157–160. doi:10.1016/0165-0114(92)90114-J

Pawlak, Z. (1982). Rough sets. *International Journal of Computer and Information Science, 11*, 341–356. doi:10.1007/BF01001956

Pawlak, Z. (1991). *Rough Sets: Theoretical Aspects of Reasoning about Data*. Boston: Kluwer Academic Publishers.

Pei, D. W. (2005). A generalized model of fuzzy rough sets. *International Journal of General Systems, 34*, 603–613. doi:10.1080/03081070500096010

Pei, D. W., & Xu, Z. B. (2004). Rough set models on two universes. *International Journal of General Systems, 33*, 569–581. doi:10.1080/0308107042000193561

Pomykala, J. A. (1987). Approximation operations in approximation space. *Bulletin of the Polish Academy of Sciences: Mathematics, 35*, 653–662.

Qin, K. Y., & Pei, Z. (2005). On the topological properties of fuzzy rough sets. *Fuzzy Sets and Systems, 151*, 601–613. doi:10.1016/j.fss.2004.08.017

Radzikowska, A. M., & Kerre, E. E. (2002). A comparative study of fuzzy rough sets. *Fuzzy Sets and Systems, 126*, 137–155. doi:10.1016/S0165-0114(01)00032-X

Skowron, A. (1989). The relationship between the rough set theory and evidence theory. *Bulletin of Polish Academy of Science: Mathematics, 37*, 87–90.

Skowron, A., Stepaniuk, J., & Peters, J. F. (2003). Rough sets and infomorphisms: Towards approximation of relations in distributed environments. *Fundamenta Informaticae, 54*, 263–277.

Slowinski, R., & Vanderpooten, D. (2000). A Generalized definition of rough approximations based on similarity. *IEEE Transactions on Knowledge and Data Engineering, 12*, 331–336. doi:10.1109/69.842271

Thiele, H. (2000a). On axiomatic characterisations of crisp approximation operators. *Information Sciences, 129*, 221–226. doi:10.1016/S0020-0255(00)00019-0

Thiele, H. (2000b, October 19). On axiomatic characterisation of fuzzy approximation operators I, the fuzzy rough set based case. In [Banff Park Lodge, Bariff, Canada.]. *Proceedings of RSCTC, 2000*, 239–247.

Thiele, H. (2001a). On axiomatic characterisation of fuzzy approximation operators II, the rough fuzzy set based case. In *Proceedings of the 31st IEEE International Symposium on Multiple-Valued Logi* (pp. 330–335).

Thiele, H. (2001b). On axiomatic characterization of fuzzy approximation operators III the fuzzy diamond and fuzzy box cases. In *The 10th IEEE International Conference on Fuzzy Systems* (vol. 2, pp. 1148–1151).

Wiweger, R. (1989). On topological rough sets. *Bulletin of Polish Academy of Sciences: Mathematics, 37*, 89–93.

Wu, W.-Z., Leung, Y., & Mi, J.-S. (2005). On characterizations of (I, T)-fuzzy rough approximation operators. *Fuzzy Sets and Systems, 154*(1), 76–102. doi:10.1016/j.fss.2005.02.011

Wu, W.-Z., Leung, Y., & Zhang, W.-X. (2002). Connections between rough set theory and Dempster-Shafer theory of evidence. *International Journal of General Systems, 31*, 405–430. doi:10.1080/0308107021000013626

Wu, W.-Z., Mi, J.-S., & Zhang, W.-X. (2003). Generalized fuzzy rough sets. *Information Sciences, 151*, 263–282. doi:10.1016/S0020-0255(02)00379-1

Wu, W.-Z., & Zhang, W.-X. (2002). Neighborhood operator systems and approximations. *Information Sciences, 144*, 201–217. doi:10.1016/S0020-0255(02)00180-9

Wu, W.-Z., & Zhang, W.-X. (2004). Constructive and axiomatic approaches of fuzzy approximation operators. *Information Sciences, 159*, 233–254. doi:10.1016/j.ins.2003.08.005

Wybraniec-Skardowska, U. (1989). On a generalization of approximation space. *Bulletin of the Polish Academy of Sciences: Mathematics, 37*, 51–61.

Yang, X.-P. (2007). Minimization of axiom sets on fuzzy approximation operators. *Information Sciences, 177*, 3840–3854. doi:10.1016/j.ins.2007.03.008

Yang, X.-P., & Li, T.-J. (2006). The minimization of axiom sets characterizing generalized approximation operators. *Information Sciences, 176*, 887–899. doi:10.1016/j.ins.2005.01.012

Yao, Y. Y. (1996). Two views of the theory of rough sets in finite universes. *International Journal of Approximate Reasoning, 15*, 291–317. doi:10.1016/S0888-613X(96)00071-0

Yao, Y. Y. (1997). Combination of rough and fuzzy sets based on alpha-level sets. In Lin, T. Y., & Cercone, N. (Eds.), *Rough Sets and Data Mining: Analysis for Imprecise Data* (pp. 301–321). Boston: Kluwer Academic Publishers.

Yao, Y. Y. (1998a). Constructive and algebraic methods of the theory of rough sets. *Journal of Information Science, 109*, 21–47. doi:10.1016/S0020-0255(98)00012-7

Yao, Y. Y. (1998b). Generalized rough set model. In Polkowski, L., & Skowron, A. (Eds.), *Rough Sets in Knowledge Discovery 1. Methodology and Applications* (pp. 286–318). Berlin Heidelberg, Germany: Springer Verlag.

Yao, Y. Y. (1998c). Relational interpretations of neighborhood operators and rough set approximation operators. *Information Sciences, 111*, 239–259. doi:10.1016/S0020-0255(98)10006-3

Yao, Y. Y., & Lin, T. Y. (1996). Generalization of rough sets using modal logic. *Intelligent Automation and Soft Computing, 2*, 103–120.

Yao, Y. Y., & Lingras, P. J. (1998). Interpretations of belief functions in the theory of rough sets. *Information Sciences, 104*, 81–106. doi:10.1016/S0020-0255(97)00076-5

Yeung, D. S., Chen, D. G., & Tsang, E. C. C. (2005). On the generalization of fuzzy rough sets. *IEEE Transactions on Fuzzy Systems, 13*(3), 343–361. doi:10.1109/TFUZZ.2004.841734

Zakowski, W. (1982). On a concept of rough sets. *Demonstratio Mathematica, 15*, 1129–1133.

Zhang, W.-X., Leung, Y., & Wu, W.-Z. (2003). *Information Systems and Knowledge Discovery*. Beijing, China: Science Press.

Zhu, W., & Wang, F.-Y. (2007). On three types of covering rough sets. *IEEE Transactions on Knowledge and Data Engineering, 19*, 1131–1144. doi:10.1109/TKDE.2007.1044

# Chapter 5
# A Top–Level Categorization of Types of Granularity

**C. Maria Keet**
*Free University of Bozen-Bolzano, Italy*

## ABSTRACT

*Multiple different understandings and uses exist of what granularity is and how to implement it, where the former influences success of the latter with regards to storing granular data and using granularity for automated reasoning over the data or information, such as granular querying for information retrieval. We propose taxonomy of types of granularity and discuss for each leaf type how the entities or instances relate within its granular level and between levels. Such distinctions give guidelines to a modeller to better distinguish between the types of granularity in the design phase and the software developer to improve on implementations of granularity. Moreover, these foundational semantics of granularity provide a basis from which to develop a comprehensive theory of granularity.*

## INTRODUCTION

Granularity deals with articulating something (hierarchically) according to certain criteria, the granular perspective, where a lower level within a perspective contains information or knowledge (*i.e.*, entities, concepts, relations, constraints) or data (measurements, laboratory experiments etc.) that is more detailed than contents in the adjacent higher level. Conversely, a higher level 'abstracts away'—simplifies or makes indistinguishable—finer-grained details. A granular level, or level of granularity, contains one or more entity types and/or instances. What granularity comprises can differ between research disciplines that tend to emphasize one aspect or the other. It combines efforts from philosophy, AI, machine learning, database theory and data mining, (applied) mathematics with fuzzy sets, fuzzy logic, and rough sets Yao (2005, 2007), for example (Peters *et al.*, 2002; Yao, 2004; Zadeh, 1997; Zhang *et al.*, 2002). Several

DOI: 10.4018/978-1-60566-324-1.ch005

usages of granularity capture subtle, but essential, differences in interpretation, representation, and/or emphasis. For example, data clustering fuzzyness or roughness can be desired for *allocating* entities to their appropriate level. Reasoning over granulated data and information and *retrieving* granulated information requires clearer distinctions that utilize precise and finer-grained semantics of granularity to obtain correct behaviour of the application software, due in part because it emphasizes a *qualitative* component of granularity, albeit not ignoring the quantitative aspects. For instance, reasoning with a partonomy (hierarchy based on the part-of relation) requires different functions compared to aggregating—calculating—precisely 60 seconds into a minute, 60 minutes in to an hour and so forth.

The aim of this chapter is to elucidate foundational semantics of granularity, that is, identifying the different *kinds* of granulation hierarchies and, hence, *ways of granulation* of a subject domain. The outcome of this analysis is a top-level *taxonomy of types of granularity* that has a first main branching between scale-based and not scale-based granularity—or, roughly, quantitative and qualitative granularity—and has subsequent more detailed distinctions up to the current eight leaf types in the taxonomy. Each of these types of granularity has its own set of constraints, requirements for representation, and consequences for implementation. These differences can be used to model granulation hierarchies (also called granular perspectives) that are based on the *mechanism of granulation*; hence, the types of granularity are reusable both within a particular subject domain and across domains. This, in turn, simplifies reuse of program code or query formulation—as opposed to repetitive hard-coding—through enabling one to recognise and deal in a consistent way with different kinds of recurring granularity structures.

The remainder of this chapter is organised as follows. I first consider related works and analyse four different viewpoints on granularity. The taxonomy of types of granularity is introduced and elaborated on in the section after that, which also contains examples for usage in modeling and implementation. Last, we look at future trends and close with conclusions.

## BACKGROUND

To provide an overview of the state of the art, we have to take a two-pronged approach. First, we briefly consider the scope of disciplines where granularity has played an important role, which reveals implicitly the various approaches toward granularity and differences in emphases of aspects of granularity. Second, these approaches will be thoroughly analysed and illustrated with examples in the second subsection.

## Related Works

This section contains a summary of existing approaches and solutions to deal with granularity, which range from informal usage of granularity without software support to formal partial theories for either qualitative or quantitative aspects of granularity. The literature can be assessed along three dimensions, being (i) Formal characterisations of granularity and ontological approaches, (ii) Engineering solutions that mainly emphasise the quantitative aspects of granularity, and (iii) Informal approaches to (biological) granularity. The first two items can be grouped as granular computing with the aim of *structured thinking* and *structured problem solving*, respectively, where the latter can be divided into methodologies and processes (Yao, 2005, 2007). When the former is clear, the latter ought to fall in place with ease to, in turn, solve the methodologies and processes. Conversely, the former has to match reality sufficiently to be applicable, thereby closing the loop. Such informal considerations will have to be taken into account when developing a generic theory of granularity.

## Modelling: Subject Domain Semantics and Ontology

All contributions have implicit or partially explicit assumptions about the basic entities and relations that have to do or are needed for handling granularity, be it for modelling of a particular subject domain or ontological and formal investigations into the nature of such entities. These are depicted in Figure 1 with indicative labels, such as the underspecified `precedes` relation (be it ≺ or ≼) between adjacent levels of granularity or granules, and the `links` relation to somehow relate the different hierarchies. In anticipation of the next section, we have added an appropriate place for where the taxonomy of `TypesOfGranularity` can fit.

Looking first at informal approaches, Tange *et al.* (1998) constructed granular perspectives and levels for medical practice based on term usage in literature that was intended for text mining and categorisation of scientific literature. Hierarchies, such as `Physical examination - Lungs - Auscultation` that informally combines a process, structural part of the human body and "type of observation", have to be organised more clearly and preferably in an ontologically consistent manner. Other examples of informal approaches in biology and medicine are (Elmasri *et al.*, 2007; Grizzi & Chiriva-Internati, 2005; Hunter & Borg, 2003; Ribba *et al.*, 2006; Salthe, 1985).

On the border of biomedicine and formal approaches is Kumar *et al.*'s granularity for human structural anatomy and relatively simple *gran* function (Kumar *et al.*, 2005; Keet & Kumar, 2005). They have *GR* as the ordered set of levels of granularity applicable to a domain and *U* denoting the set of biological universals, so that *gran*(*x*) returns the level of granularity where the universal of interest resides. It assumes that granulated domain knowledge already exists and it requires patchwork in the logic, design, and implementation, as demonstrated with the 9 granular perspectives (granulation hierarchies) for

*Figure 1. Graphical depiction of the main entity types for granularity: a 'granular perspective' (granulation hierarchy) must contain at least two 'granular levels' and for each such related instances, both have, or adhere to, the same 'type of granularity' (mechanism for how to granulate) and a perspective can be identified by its type of granularity and its 'criterion' for granulation*

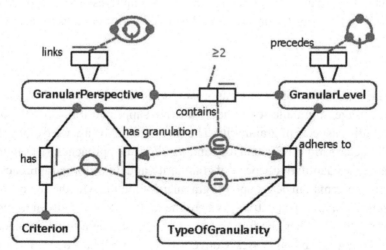

infectious diseases (Keet & Kumar, 2005). This can be addressed using contextual information, that is, proper management of granular perspectives, thereby avoiding inconsistencies in the software system. A separate issue is its bottom-updevelopment of granular levels limited to human beings, which are not reusable in an expanded subject domain such as all eukaryotes instead of only humans. For computational implementations, however, an underlying domain-independent logically consistent theory of granularity is an imperative to meet requirements such as reusability, flexibility, and interoperability. Similar issues can be observed for conceptual data modelling for multi-representation geo-spatial databases in geographical information systems (Fent *et al.*, 2005; Fonseca *et al.*, 2002; Parent *et al.*, 2006a). An interesting addition for geographic information systems was made explicit by Camossi *et al.* (2003). They elaborated on the requirement for cross-hierarchy conditional information retrieval; for instance, where one has two granular perspectives, one for administrative regions and one for rive sizes, then a realistic query is "if one makes a map with granularity at the `Province`-level then only rivers with a flow ≥ 10 000 litres/min should be included in the map". One easily can imagine a similar example in the medical domain—though, to the best of my knowledge not raised yet—as, for example, "if the medical doctor needs a day-by-day view of the growth of the cancer in patient1, then deliver the tissue samples" as opposed to delivering cell cultures (`Cell`-level in a anatomy granular perspective with the `Hour`-level using time granularity) or microarrays (genes linked to the `Minute`-level).

Formal approaches motivated by engineering usefulness are restricted to a partial account of granularity and incorporate modelling decisions suitable for the engineering scope, such as data warehouse design (Kamble, 2004; Luján-Mora *et al.*, 2006; Malinowski & Zimányi, 2006), UML (Abelló *et al.*, 2006), and databases as linguistic corpus (Fagin *et al.*, 2005), and therefore are not easily transportable to other implementation scenarios such as Geographic Information Systems (GIS) and ontologies. Also, they have specified a large set of one-off functions and data manipulation operators only at the design or implementation layer, requiring a re-coding of functions, such as for calendar hierarchies and products sold; compare for example, GMD, MSD, MADS, and MultiDimER (Kamble, 2004; Fagin *et al.*, 2005; Parent *et al.*, 2006a; Malinowski & Zimányi, 2006), or see Euzenat & Montanari (2005) for an overview on theories of and functions for time granularity and Ning *et al.* (2002) for a particular example.

Hobbs (1985) has introduced several core components of granularity and Bittner & Smith (2003) have developed an ontologically-motivated formal "theory of granular partitions" (TGP) based on mereology. The TGP is relatively comprehensive and useful for granular levels, but it is limited to mereology, does not address the types of aggregation commonly used with data mining and conceptual data modelling, has no functions, no mechanism to deal with multiple granulation hierarchies for different perspectives, and does not allow for the kind of granularity and abstraction commonly used in biology or Mani's (1998) folding operations in linguistics. There are few contributions on granularity from philosophy, which is addressed mostly within themes such as hierarchical systems and emergent properties in biology (Cariani, 1997; Edmonds, 2000; Salthe, 1985; Wimsatt, 1995; Yao, 2005) where the main emphasis is on use of levels of detail to demarcate models to achieve better scientific explanations of natural phenomena and to address the limitations of those models with different theories for different levels of detail. Thus, it does not focus specifically on the ontological status or nature of what granularity is.

## Granular Computing

Other types of implementations exist in different research disciplines, such as data mining and clustering techniques, which are grouped recently under the term Granular Computing, which focuses primarily on computational problem solving aspects. It combines efforts primarily from machine learning, data mining, and (applied) mathematics with fuzzy logic and rough sets. Lin (2006) summarises several example usages and Bargiela & Pedrycz (2006) and Yao (2007) describe background and trends. In this context, the comprehensive description of granule and granulation by Zadeh (1997) is useful for grouping together several notions about granular computing: "Informally, granulation of an object A results in a collection of granules of *A*, with a granule being a clump of objects (or points) which are drawn together by indistinguishability, similarity, proximity or functionality... In general, granulation is hierarchical in nature.". The notions of similarity, equivalence, and indistinguishability relations have been well investigated with set-based approaches (Bittner & Stell, 2003; Chen & Yao, 2006; Hata & Mukaidono, 1999; Keet, 2007a; Mencar *et al.*, 2007; Peters *et al.*, 2002; Skowron & Peters, 2003; Yao, 2004). However, this set-based approach has issues that can be better addressed with mereology proper (Abelló *et al.*, 2006; Bittner & Smith, 2003; Keet, 2008a). The research programme of rough mereology (see, e.g., Polkowski (2006); Polkowski & Semeniuk-Polkowska (2008) for recent results) has, from an ontological (Varzi, 2004; Keet & Artale, 2008) and logical (Pontow & Schubert, 2006) perspective, a comparatively weak mereology component, because it is tightly coupled with the set-based approach and remains close to Lesniewski's pioneering work without considering newer mereological theories. For instance, modifying General Extensional Mereology, or a mereotopological version (Varzi, 2007), with the orthogonal roughness dimension would be an interesting and useful avenue to investigate.

Characteristic for these Granular Computing approaches is the applied mathematics, data-centric view, and quantitative aspects of data for problem-solving tasks, although the notion of "computing with words" (Zadeh, 1997, 2002; Broekhoven *et al.*, 2007; Mendel and Wu, 2007) clearly moves in the direction of subject domain semantics. The notion of a granularity *framework* with formally defined perspectives and levels is absent, but there are notable steps in that direction. Skowron & Peters (2003) have granule g as primitive, although they use it only for attaching lower and upper approximation bound to it. Yao's (2004) comprehensive partition model based on rough sets[1] has been discussed before (Keet, 2008a). It is mainly quantitative, but recognises the need for qualitative aspects and seeks to accommodate a criterion for granulation although it does not have proper levels and only a lattice of sets. Rough sets' approximation spaces can be lifted up to the ontological layer by, first, to conceptualise the various possibilities to augment any crisp theory admitting normal sets. We have drawn three options for such an *orthogonally positioned* extension to Figure 1 in Figure 2. Observe that each option admits to a different ontological commitment, with the top two most different from the bottom one: the former assumes roughness (or, in analogy, fuzzyness) to be an *optional* property for granulation whereas the latter imposes that roughness is in some sense at least *mandatory*, if not *essential*, to any granular level; in the current paper, we do not commit to such a strong ontological commitment because one can identify granularity also for non-rough crisp data, information, and knowledge. In later work, Chen & Yao (2006) put more emphasis on granular perspectives, called "multiviews", and a lattice as flexible granulation hierarchy. Qiu *et al.* (2007) make steps from set extension to concept, name a granular level a "granular world" that denotes a set of "concept granules", have a mapping function to go from the finer-to the coarser level, and the union of such levels is a "full granular space", which corresponds to what we refer to here as granular perspective where one always must have *is a* as relation between entities. This clearly moves in the direction of the TOG (Keet, 2008a), although it is limited to taxonomies only, and, most notably, misses a granulation criterion, a specification of the relation between the levels, and quantitative granularity.

The principal other formal approaches with a computational scope for granularity are (rough and/or fuzzy) clustering, fuzzy sets, and to a lesser extent the combination of rough sets and fuzzy sets into fuzzy rough sets. The latter considers, among others, a fuzzy similarity relation to add another dimension with *degree* of similarity, and attribute reduction of fuzzy attributes using rough sets (refer to Chen *et al.* (2007) for recent results). Within the scope of fuzzy sets, one can distinguish the purely quantitative focus from the computing with words with, for example, linguistic fuzzy models for classification in the context of macroinvertebrate habitat suitability in aquatic ecosystems (Broekhoven *et al.*, 2007), which involves manual adjustment by domain experts of the numerical membership functions associated to the "linguistic values". The named sets in the linguistic fuzzy model, however, do not yet deal with levels of granularity among the sets. Hierarchical and fuzzy clustering (Dawyndt *et al.*, 2006; Kaplan *et al.*, 2005; Vernieuwe *et al.*, 2007), among many, have quantitative granularity implicit in the mathematical models, which, ideally, should be made explicit to benefit transparency and to improve reusability. Limitations of such parameter-adjustable generated hierarchies are discussed by Zhou *et al.* (2005). They developed an algorithm to generate just that hierarchy whose data points group together into set extensions of the universals in the Gene Ontology. This, as well as Tsumoto's (2007) mining with a diagnostic taxonomy for headaches, could be interesting in conjunction with classification in logic-based ontologies and bottom-up generation or validation of the granular levels in a granular perspective. None of them, however, addresses that there are different kinds of granulation hierarchies and how and why they come about from a subject domain perspective.

Hata & Mukaidono (1999) explore granulation with fuzzy logic, where three classes of fuzzy information granulation are distinguished. First, their example for fuzzy Kleene classes uses informal granulation through mixing granulation criteria: first a transformation function from a colour gradient to a x-y plot with the usual range [0,1] and then to select parts of the line. Second, their fuzzy probabilistic classes formalise the informal usage of more detailed attributes to calculate an overall probability for an event, which needs further investigation to take a structured approach to 'component-probabilities' of aggregated 'whole probabilities'. The third fuzzy information granulation is based on fuzzy Lukasiewicz classes, which, for the given example, amounts to fuzzy mereology (detecting anatomical parts in images of the whole brain), that, when worked out in greater detail, could be an interesting combination of qualitative with quantitative granularity and traditional bio-ontologies in the Semantic Web with fuzzy OWL-DL (Straccia, 2006); put differently: adding the orthogonal dimension for fuzziness alike depicted for roughness in Figure 2.

Thus, major themes addressed for computational problem solving are quantitative granularity and—like with DWHs and GIS—it takes a data-centric or ontologically poor linguistic approach toward granularity, whereas for conceptual data modelling, ontologies, and the Semantic Web, there is also the need to deal with both qualitative aspects of granularity and with the conceptual modelling and ontological analysis layers. In addition, while the mathematics-rich Granular Computing is good for mathematical foundations, it is relatively poor in incorporating subject domain semantics and lacks mechanisms for *how* the levels and hierarchies come about for a particular domain, such as administrative boundaries or human anatomy. Practically, many granulation hierarchies have been described in the above-cited literature across disciplines. For instance, we have cartographic maps that represent cities, provinces, regions, and countries, and a simple time granularity may start from second, to minute, hour, and day. With the latter hierarchy we can move from the chosen lowest level to the minute level by aggregating 60 seconds—that is, one uses a mathematical function—which cannot be devised consistently for administrative areas (e.g., 'each province must be an aggregate of 15 cities' or 'exactly 5 provinces must comprise a region' does not hold in any country). By analysing hierarchies and, moreover, differences

*Figure 2. Three options for adding the orthogonal notion of roughness with approximation values for the levels (or, in analogy, fuzzyness) to granular levels. The top figure requires a bounded space when one specifies one of the values, the middle one permits specifying either one or both bounds, and the bottom one adds further mandatory constraints to impose approximation spaces with both lower and upper bounds for each granular level*

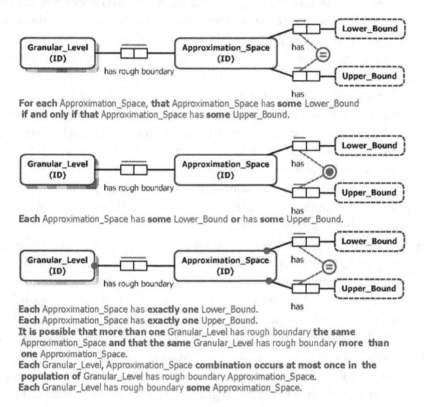

in emphases when modelling a hierarchy, common and differentiating characteristics can be uncovered. This analysis is the topic of the next subsection.

## ANALYSIS OF DIFFERENT EMPHASES REGARDING GRANULARITY

Granularity deals with organising data, information, and knowledge in greater or lesser detail that resides in a *granular level* or *level of granularity* and is granulated according to certain *criteria*, which thereby give a perspective—also called view, context, or dimension—on the subject domain, henceforth called *granular perspective*. A lower level within a perspective contains knowledge, information, or data that is more detailed than the adjacent higher level. Conversely, a higher level 'abstracts away', simplifies, or makes indistinguishable, finer-grained details. A granular level contains one or more entities, that is, representations of entity types or their instances; note that granular level is sometimes called granule, but we reserve *granule* to denote a cell or 'part of the pie'. Several interpretations of granularity and diagrammatical representations are shown in Figure 3, capturing subtle, but essential, differences in interpretation, representation, and/or emphasis. These differences in viewpoints are discussed in the remainder of this section. Successively, the emphasis will be on entity types & instances, the relation between levels and their contents, the perspective & criteria for granulation, and on consequences of choosing a particular formal representation. The main distinctions are summarised at the end of this section.

## Emphasis on Entity Types and Their Instances

We first consider Figure 3: *A1-A5*. The circles A1-A4 in Figure 3 are examples where the circles can represent the subject domain or a granular level. This gives four possible interpretations.

i.  If it represents a subject domain, then the four respectively five parts in A1 (A2) are finer grained than the circle, that is, each one provides more detail about the domain than a plain circle (C1). With $\prec$ denoting a strict order, then A1 $\prec$ C1 and A2 $\prec$ C1 hold.

ii. If it represents a granular level, it shows the four (A1) respectively five (A2) granules resulting from granulating the contents of a level where each level is disjoint exhaustively granulated (fully divided). Without further clarification, it cannot be excluded that one of the granules denotes `Everything else`, or, if there is always one entity (/type) (A6) or possibly more (A7) entities in each granule (see also below on A6 and A7).

iii. If the circles A1 and A2 are the same domain or granular level, then a different grid corresponds to granulation according to different perspectives or criteria on the same domain.

iv. If A3 (resp. A4) is at a lower level of granularity compared to A1 (A2), then A3 $\prec$ A1 (A4 $\prec$ A2, respectively) and the granules of A1 (A2) are fully divided into more granules in A3 (A4), thereby representing finer-grained divisions that can be made when more details are taken into account, but which are indistinguishable at the level of A1 (A2).

*Figure 3. Several graphical representations of granularity. A1/A5: (i) is the domain or a level with (ii) a partition and (iii) possible non-included rest depending on the interpretation. B1-B4 may be alternative representations of A1-A4. See text for explanation*

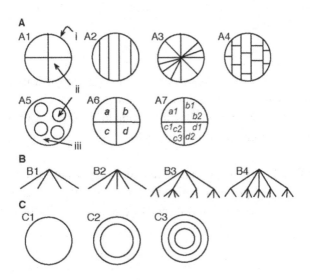

From the possible interpretations assigned to A1-A4, A5 suggests that it contains four granules and empty space that falls outside the four nested smaller circles. However, it equally may be an inappropriately used ER diagram or Venn diagram requiring additional clarification to disambiguate its exact meaning regarding levels and granulation, such as if the four circles are disjoint exhaustive or not. Important to realise is that Figure 3-A has *implicit* the granular perspective with its criterion how to granulate: there is some criterion $x$ why A1 has four parts and another criterion $y$ such that A2 has five, but $x$ and $y$ are assumed in the representation and the criterion for granulation—hence also the granular perspective—is omitted.

In Figure 3: A6 and A7 the two circles containing $a,...,d$ can represent a fundamental distinction on how to model granularity. Both A6 and A7 represent a populated A1, but depending on the interpretation of the figure, $a,...,d$ in A6 can denote entity types or instances, and the indexed $a_1,...,d_2$ in A7 then denote instances:

i.  If $a$, $b$, $c$, and $d$ are entity types, then
    1.  *without* granulation as in C1, $\{a, b, c, d\}$ is an unordered set of entities of the domain of interest, thus $a, b, c, d \in D$ although in C1 they are indistinguishable;
    2.  *with* granulation, as in A6, $\{a, b, c, d\}$ are distinguishable and found to be distinct. Moreover, there is *exactly one* entity type in each granule, which can be either by design—one granule, one entity—or accidental in that there may be an e that also fits in the granule where, for example, a resides but is not included due to either unintended omission or known incomplete coverage of the domain.

ii. If $a$, $b$, $c$ and $d$ in A6 are instances, then either
    1.  the current 4 granules are accidental in the sense that at a time $t_1 > t_{present}$ there may be more or less than 4 granules because at least one of the objects may have ceased to exist or a new one added, or
    2.  at $t_1$ where an object has ceased to exist, there is an empty granule; hence, one commits to the original granulation for a set of instances. Thus, it can be that at time $t_2$, where $t_2 > t_1$, that granule is not empty anymore.

In both options, the outcome of granulation is dependent on the instances present at the time of identifying or creating the granules.

iii. If it is the case of i-2, then either
    1.  A7 shows the corresponding instances of the entity types in A6, or
    2.  there was an unordered set of instances $\{a_1,..., d_2\}$ that were grouped according to some criterion. Based on their similarity, they are grouped into their corresponding classes as in A6 that may or may not correspond to universals.

iii-1 and iii-2 are different only in the starting point, one being the entity types and the other instance-motivated. Some of the points in this and the previous paragraph will be illustrated with an example; the new topic it introduces about measurement scales will be discussed afterwards.

## Example 1

Let the circles A1 and A2 each represent a human population, where its parts (granules) are labelled with, respectively:

- **a1:** (Single, Married, Divorced, Widowed)
- **a2:** (Newborn, Child, Adolescent, Adult, Elderly)

Hence, A1's criterion is Marital status and A2's criterion can be Life stage. Considering A7, let $a_1,..., d_2$ be (not necessarily exhaustive) instances of months, then each granule could represent the quarters:

- **a7:** (Quarter1, Quarter2, Quarter3, Quarter4)

This indicates that the domain or coarser-grained level C1 is Year; if there were semesters, then an intermediate level $x$ would have to be added, such that A7 $\prec x \prec$ C1 and $x$ having two granules for Semester1 and Semester2. More importantly, this granulation uses a 'smallest element': in this closed-world assumption, Month is chosen as the arbitrary atom (or *Urelement*) that is aggregated in such a way that each aggregate denotes a set extension of a class. Another example of this concerns phone points, where the phone point instances are granulated into Cell, Land line, Direct line, and PABX where a class was created from sets of phone points (Kamble, 2004). Thus, this relies on set theory for representing granularity, where each set neither necessarily must be the set-extension of a universal nor a defined class.

Another aspect of the figures in A is, for example, granulating temperature using a measurement scale in a lower grain size of integer degrees 19, 20, 21, for isotherms and moving up to a higher level where Isotherm20 suffices with coarser-grained rounding off (see also Example *3*). In both cases, the *same* thing is granulated with more or less detail. This interpretation is prevalent in GIS for making a grid over land plots. Analogous is the case with spatial and time scales that for, for example, humans cover factor differences of $10^{15}$ for spatial and $10^9$ for time, ranging from proteins (in nm) to height of humans (in m) and from $\mu$s for Brownian motion to decades for lifespan of a human, respectively (Hunter & Borg, 2003).

It is essential to note that when granulating according to a *scale*, one defines a *smallest unit* or a *standard unit* from which other levels are generated using a mathematical formula, according to which the domain is to be granulated. This is another, less problematic, granulation compared to trying to figure out the relation between Tissue and Cell or Cell and Organelle, if and how developmental stages of an organism have granularity, or characterising the type(s) of components of the Second messenger system that comprise distinct objects, its parts, processes, events etc. The second section of Example *1* above deals with larger or smaller parts of arbitrary scales, but each level still concerns values according to the same arbitrary scale. Non-scale-dependent finer levels involve *other* types of entities, as, for instance, a biological cell is not equal to a tissue slice of 0.05mm thin. The latter puts a higher emphasis on the criterion for granulation and its levels than on the entities and instances one may find at a certain level of detail. This is especially useful for biological granularity, because of the incomplete knowledge of the domain that prevents disjoint exhaustive categorisations of its contents and its emphasis on qualitative information and knowledge as opposed to quantitative data. Granularity comprises both methods, but they involve fundamentally different granularity between coarser and finer levels.

In addition, while a1 and a7 in Example *1* may seem alike, they are not: members of a population are different from elements in a set. With the latter, granularity *depends* on its instances: with another set of instances, the levels of granularity, ordering of the elements in a level, and perspectives may turn out to be different, and therefore can be time-inconsistent. In contradistinction, granulation involving an entity type identified with a collective noun like (human) population and how one can group the *members* of the population: from time $t_0$ to a later time $t_1$ the instances (members of the human population) have changed, but this does neither affect the principle/criterion nor the levels.

## Emphasis on Relation between Entities and Levels

Continuing with the possible interpretations, we proceed to Figure 3: *B1-B4*. Two first basic observations are that

i.    B1-B4 correspond to A1-A4, where the top equals the circle and each edge leads to a node (cell) at the end of each line. The tree structure is favourable when depicting multiple granular levels, because it is more concise than the figures in A (compare A3 and A4 to B3 and B4, respectively).

ii.   The lines in B emphasise the relation between levels of granularity, or at least between its entities (/types) residing in coarser-and finer-grained levels.

Point ii highlights the point of departure or focus—the relations involved—but is ignorant about which types of relations are relevant for granularity, both regarding the relation between the entities in different levels and how granular levels relate to each other. Committing to one type of relation or the other can imply an ontological commitment how one formally represents granularity (see below); in particular, partonomic versus taxonomic (generalisation/specialisation) granulation that are used or considered regarding informal biological granularity (a.o., Degtyarenko & Contrino, 2004; Fonseca *et al.*, 2002; Zhang *et al.*, 2002; Pandurang Nayak & Levy, 1995; Kiriyama & Tomiyama, 1993). Such deliberations for one type of relation or the other is a distinct issue from using arbitrary scales and puts in the background the entities (/types) in each level and how the contents is allocated to a level. In addition, it may be that there is a taxonomic division for contents within a level, as depicted in Figure 7. Using the *is_a* relation for granulation means that each layer in the tree with the same depth should correspond to a granular level. However, this does not necessarily hold for granularity as perceived by domain experts. For instance, 'folding' deals with polysemy and underspecification in language and the so-called black-box usage in biology, which is illustrated for cell physiology and book ordering in Example *2*.

> **Example 2.** Combining different types of entities and relations between granular levels may be useful in particular for abstracting biological complex types like `Second messenger system` or `MAPK cascade`. With the former, its processes such as `Activation`, `GTP-GDP exchange`, `α-subunit release`, states like `Activated`, and components such as `Hormone receptor`, `G_s protein`, and `cAMP`, collapse together into one entity type `Second messenger system`. `MAPK cascade` is already used as a module in systems biology that at a higher level of abstraction is treated as a black box, containing (sub-)processes, inputs/outputs, parameters and their values, etc. (Sontag, 2004).

A variant not uncommon in hierarchical modeling of conceptual data models is to have, for example, an entity type `Book order`, where the ordering consists of several procedural processes and entities involving, among others, `Billing`, `Paying`, `Supplier`, and `Shipment`.

As the example shows, that what is a type of endurant at the higher level of granularity, is composed of a combination of endurant parts, processes, and states. For an implementation, it is possible to separate the different types of components into different granular perspectives and levels, but this does not capture what is meant with the higher-level entity type like `Second messenger system`. Put differently: if separated in a granular perspective of structural components and another one for processes, the "Second messenger system" at the higher level in each perspective is only a *partial* representation of the entity type. If one allows relating levels of granularity by folding with type shifting (Mani, 1998), then this complicates what the parts are and how they relate to the whole, but on the other hand, saves integrating or linking granular perspectives. Either way, the relation-view between levels and between the entities (/types) is there; which granulation relations can be used and how will be summarised further below.

## Emphasis on the Perspective and Criteria for Granulation

Last, Figure 3: *C1-C4* show three levels of granularity where a smaller circle denotes a finer-grained level. This is unlike the Russian dolls analogy, where a similar smaller doll is contained in the larger one, but alike dissecting an organism to see what organs are inside, zooming in on parts of the organ, the tissue, cells and so forth. Thus, the parts are different types of entities and one uses, for example, human structural anatomy to identify finer-and coarser-grained levels that contain, respectively, all types of organs, tissues, and cells. In addition, each level has its distinguishing characteristic, that is, the property of a level is emphasised. In contrast with the first approach, one looks first at the property or properties, decides on the levels, and only possibly subsequently allocates entities to the levels based on the pre-selected properties.

Less explicit is how these properties relate to each other, except that it must relate in some way to both the finer-and coarser-grained level. I call the unifying rationale that links these properties the *criterion*. For instance, within the domain of human anatomy, one can granulate according to different criteria, such as structural anatomy, functional anatomy, or the processes they are involved in. Subsequently, one can identify granular levels according to certain properties that have to do with structural aspects or with containment and so forth. Observe that this entails a commitment to a granulation relation.

Because of the property-focus, C1-C3 do not bear any information if the cascaded granulation of the contents in each level is disjoint or complete. It does suggest that each level of granularity has one *type* of entity, such the outer circle representing the `Cell`-level containing cell types, with a smaller circle the `Organelle`-level containing entities such as `Endoplasmatic reticulum` and `Lysosome`. Although these examples may indicate the physical size is a criterion, this is not necessarily the case. For example, if one were to represent the phylogenetic tree in the diagrammatic representation of B or C, a `Mammal`-level has no physical size associated with its definition. More generally, with the emphasis on the perspective and criteria for granulation, this approach is more useful for non-scale dependent granularity.

## Emphasis on Formal Representation

The difference between scale and non-scale dependency mentioned in the previous sections roughly fits with Sowa's (2000) epistemic and intentional granularity. Sowa bases his three types of granularity on Peirce's three categories of Firstness, Secondness and Thirdness. Firstness then maps to actual granularities with axioms for discrete, continuous or lumpy aggregates (Sowa (2000) and below) and concerns the entities that populate a level. Secondness for granularity uses epistemic logics involving measurements, including error ranges, or axioms & measurements (Sowa, 2000) and corresponds to the scale-dependent granularity with fuzzyness and roughness in allocating objects to their level of granularity. The Thirdness for granularity, corresponds to intentional, which requires a three-place predicate relating "an agent *a* to an entity *x* for a reason *r*" (Sowa, 2000), where a reason r depends on the perspective on takes. However, depending on how one uses granularity in a subject domain, devising *levels* does not require asking oneself questions if entity *x* has at least one atom as part, if there is an infinite regress of parts that is cut at the lowest level defined, or if the entity is lumpy, but the allocation of entities to a given level does use aggregates and entities. More precisely, in mereology an *Atom* is an entity that has no proper parts (1).

$$Atom(x) \triangleq \neg \exists y (y < x) \tag{1}$$

Then, there are three kinds of aggregates (with "$\leq$" as part-of and "$<$" as proper-part-of). First, *Discrete*: everything has at least one atom as part (2); thus, that things can be subdivided up to the point where nothing is left but atoms.

$$\forall x \exists y (Atom(y) \wedge y \leq x) \tag{2}$$

Second, *Continuous*: everything has at least one proper part (3), which permits indefinite sub-division, implying that there are no atoms,

$$\forall x \exists y (y < x) \tag{3}$$

Third, *Lumpy*: some things are atoms, some are continuous (4). (Sowa, 2000).

$$\exists x Atom(x) \wedge \exists y \forall z (z \leq y \rightarrow \exists w (w < z)) \tag{4}$$

Thus, representing granularity using mereology may have *but does not require* atoms as 'ultimate part' or Urelement that is used for set theory-based granularity. Observe also that Urelement can, in fact, be defined in terms of atoms, where Urelement is the "atom at the finest-grained level in a granulation hierarchy", provided that 'granular level' and 'granulation hierarchy' are defined (e.g., as in the TOG by Keet, 2008a). Both set theory and mereology have their advantages and disadvantages for representing granularity that better approximates reality. Ease, difficulty, or even impossibility, to identify an Urelement is illustrated in the following example.

**Example 3.** Let us take calendar entities and set-theory based granularity. Entity types such as Week, Month, Quarter, and Year can be defined based on a chosen Urelement Day and then can be represented by distinct sets of days. However, if we take isotherms, then what has to be chosen as Urelement? If one uses `Degree` as smallest element to build coarser-grained isotherms, then with a set as the extension of `Isotherm20`, like {15, 16, 17, 18, 19, 20, 21, 22, 23, 24}, and where `Isotherm20` is a subtype of `Isotherm` that has other subtypes (such as `Isotherm30`), there are two problems: the extension is not the entity type and the numbers are not degrees but integers (see also Johansson, 2004b). Within the subject domain of biology, identifying or choosing a smallest element is more challenging. In one scenario, a general practitioner who is not interested in smaller entity types than tissue will make `Tissue` the Urelement (atom) to populate the lowest level, but this would also mean that all higher-level entities are composed of tissue *only*: we *know* this is biologically incorrect and thereby not a good representation of reality. Moreover, if one takes the lowest level of the Foundational Model of Anatomy (FMA) (Rosse & Mejino, 2003)—that is, `Biological macromolecule`, which does not include other molecules without which a human body cannot survive, such as $H_2O$—and deem that all coarser-grained levels up to `Body` are varying sets of macromolecules, then a body changes identity each time a molecule is synthesised/metabolised, which happens continuously, resulting in the situation that a body has no enduring identity but is in flux[2]. In a similar fashion, entomologists study the same ant colony over time, even though ants were born and have died. More generally, regardless if a set-theoretic logical theory or model is logically valid and corresponding knowledge base in a legal state, basing reasoning on represented knowledge that is not adequately grounded in the reality it aims to represent can lead to undesirable outcomes for patients, ecosystems and the like.

Both ways of representing granularity, through *is_a* with set theory and mereological *part_of,* are from a logical viewpoint mostly interchangeable (Pontow & Schubert, 2006), but not from an ontological viewpoint as the intended meaning captured in a formalisation is distinct. This difference has been recognised earlier by Salthe (2001) and are not considered to be *competing* interpretations of granularity, but *both* considered as distinct, valid ways of understanding granularity. One does not have to force one type of granularity in the straightjacket of the other; doing so anyway always will deprive another type of granularity from representing nature as accurate as possible.

Moving to the notion of 'thirdness', reason *r* might be useful for granular perspectives in non-scale dependent granularity: although it is not necessarily modelled as a triadic predicate, separating and re-using the reason, or criterion, benefits scaling up the granularity framework. Such differences in types of granularity have, at the meta-level, a major effect on granulation relation between entities (/types) residing in different granular levels, because scale-dependent levels are identified and ordered according to a combination of a property and an arbitrary scale whereas non-scale-dependent levels are ordered according to a combination of properties where level identification is less straightforward. Properties will be analysed in detail in the next chapter.

## MAIN DIFFERENCES CONCERNING APPROACHES TOWARD GRANULARITY

An attempt to merge the graphical representations depicted in Figure 3 is shown in Figure 4 for two granular perspectives, where the top ellipses are coarse-grained granular levels with less detail in larger cells—that is, conceptually more encompassing entities—than the two finer-grained granular levels.

*Figure 4. Merging emphases on aspects of granularity (A-C of Figure 3): top ellipse (i) is a coarse-grained granular level granulated with less detail in larger cells or coarser-grained entities (ii) than in the finer-grained granular level (iii)*

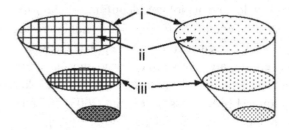

*Figure 5. Top-level taxonomy of types of granularity*

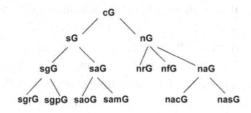

Summarizing, one can identify the 4 principal dimensions for types of granularity and the perception thereof:

1.  Arbitrary scale versus non-scale-dependent granularity;
2.  How levels, and its contents, in a perspective relate to each other;
3.  Difference in emphases, being entity-, relation-, or criterion-focused;
4.  The perception and (mathematical) representation, such as based on set theory versus mereology.

These differences do not imply one cannot switch from one to the other, represent one way into another, or let them work together orthogonally. When analysing of some subject domain, one apparently seamlessly shifts perspectives and alternately emphasises the criterion used for granularity and the partitioning within a level itself, or taking a type versus instance-inspired approach. Teaching a computer program to do so, however, requires a formal approach to implement it in a consistent manner that can be used and reused across different types of software applications.

## TAXONOMY OF TYPES OF GRANULARITY

Given the types of granularity informally introduced in the previous paragraphs, they will be structured into a taxonomy of types of granularity in this section. Hereby it is emphasised that there is not one granularity, but several types—mechanisms of granulation—that have additional constraints extending the **core** Granularity, **cG**, as root. Figure 5 shows the top-level taxonomy, where the meaning behind the labels of the types are important, and Table 1 summarizes the distinguishing characteristic at each branching point. This will be elaborated on in the next two sections by first showing a general bird's eye view and then providing a description of the characteristics in detail in the second subsection. We consider several typical examples more comprehensively in the third subsection and also give an outline where and how the taxonomy of types of granularity can simplify implementations.

*Table 1. Distinguishing characteristics at the branching points in the taxonomy of types of granularity depicted in Figure 5*

| Branching point | Distinguishing feature |
|---|---|
| sG – nG | scale – non-scale (or, roughly: quantitative – qualitative) |
| sgG – saG | grain size – aggregation (or: scale *on* entity – scale *of* entity) |
| sgrG – sgpG | resolution – size of the entity |
| saoG – samG | overlay aggregated – entities aggregated according to scale |
| naG – nrG – nfG | semantic aggregation – one type of relation between entities in different levels – different type of relation between entities in levels and relations among entities in level |
| nacG – nasG | parent-child not taxonomic and relative independence of contents of higher/lower level – parent-child with taxonomic inheritance |

## Overview of the Top-Level Taxonomy

In this section, the types of granularity and the distinguishing characteristic at each branching point in the taxonomy are briefly described to give a general idea.

- **cG**: **c**ore Granularity, consisting of the basic characteristic common to all considered types of granularity and basic constraints.
- **nG**: **n**on-scale-dependent Granularity, where other types of entities reside in each finer-grained level; subtypes have additional constraints and granulation relations.
- **nrG**: levels of **n**on-scale dependent Granularity are ordered according to one type of **r**elation in a perspective; for example, (structural-)*part_of,* (spatially-)*contained_in*. The primary types of granulation relations were identified and formally defined (Keet, 2008a; Keet & Artale, 2008) and include, at least, *is_a, participates_in, member_of,* and *proper_part_of* with its subtypes *contained_in* and *involved_in*.
- **nfG**: levels of **n**on-scale dependent Granularity are ordered by simultaneous **f**olding ≥ 2 different (types of) entities, such as folding events and states, and consequently folding relations between those entities, upon going to a coarser-grained level; for example, the 'black boxes' in biology such as the Second messenger system, the Abstraction Hierarchy, ER clustering.
- **naG**: **n**on-scale-dependency with some form of **a**ggregation.
- **nasG**: **n**on-scale-dependency using **a**ggregation of the **s**ame collection of instances of one type that subsequently can be granulated using semantic criteria. The class at a lower level is a subtype of the class at the coarser-grained level; for example, a collection of phone points and at the finer-grained level we have land-line and mobile phone points.
- **nacG**: **n**on-scale dependency using **a**ggregation attributed to the notion of an entity generally labelled with a **c**ollective noun, has an existing semantics, the instances of the aggregate are different from instances of its members, and a change in its members does not affect the meaning of the whole; for example, `Population` with `Organisms of type x`, or `Team` as aggregate of its `Players`.
- **sG**: **s**cale-dependent Granularity where the contents is structured according to a more or less obvious arbitrary scale; for **c**G and additional constraints. For instance, calendar hierarchy, rounding off of altitude lines on a cartographic map.

- **sgG**: **s**cale dependency with relation to **g**rain size, or resolution, scale-based zooming.
- **sgrG**: **s**cale dependency, taking into account **g**rain size with respect to **r**esolution; for example, `Cell wall` represented as line, as lipid bi-layer, and as three-dimensional structure, or a building on cartographic maps as polygon or as point depending on the resolution of the map.
- **sgpG**: **s**cale dependency, with **g**rain size and **p**hysical size of the entities; for example, sieves with different pore sizes that retains the entities or lets them through, a Euro coins separator, or two objects touching each other (e.g., wallpaper and the wall).
- **saG**: **s**cale dependency with some form of **a**ggregation and its immediate parts are of one type.
- **samG**: **s**cale dependency and using **a**ggregation of the same collection of instances of the same top type or Urelement that subsequently can be granulated in various ways at lower levels of detail using a **m**athematical function; for example, `Second`, `Minute`, and `Hour`, where 60 seconds go in a minute.
- **saoG**: **s**cale-dependency the carving up of the same entity at each level according to a coarser or finer grid of which the cells can be **a**ggregated and lay **o**ver the representation of a material entity[3]. For instance, the earth with its isotherms, where the isotherms are in steps of 10 degrees, 5 degrees, 1 degree detail[4].

The current version of the taxonomy of types of granularity roughly fits the distinction between quantitative and qualitative features and added versus inherent granularity. At some branching point in the taxonomic structure, more than one desideratum is used to distinguish between the subtypes, which can be remedied by introducing 'fillers' to ensure only one desideratum at a time is added. However, these fillers are not used anyway and unnecessarily enlarge the top-level structure, and therefore have been omitted. Other categorisations of types of granularity are conceivable, but these are much less consistent and structured. For instance, aggregation versus 'granularity by other means', instead of the (non) scale dependency because one has both **saG** and **naG** each with their subtypes. However, using aggregation emphasises the internal structure of a level, how entities and instances relate, or is implementation-driven, but it does not take into account the properties *how* to make the distinction between types because having a remainder group of types of granularity does not capture the semantics adequately and then the same desiderata would re-appear in both branches thereby creating redundancy. In addition, using aggregation as distinguishing criterion *implicitly* makes a distinction between set theory and mereology, but this should be a representational issue only. Last, aggregation is underspecified, both with respect to its ontological nature and variants in implementations. There are two other options to categorise the types, being entity-focussed and human-centred, which might aid understanding of the types. However, because several types can be categorised twice, it does not serve to devise an unambiguous classification[5]. In contrast, the proposed taxonomy takes a purely *semantic*, ontological, approach, thereby also separating restrictions of (formal) representation and implementation from the intended meaning.

## Characteristics in Detail

A consequence of different types of granularity is the influence on the structure of the contents of each level, independent of the actual data source. For instance, completeness and disjointness: a grid is automatically disjoint and, depending on the level and implementation decisions, complete, which does not necessarily hold for contents of levels that has a **nG**-type of granulation. It also affects the allocation of contents into the levels and reasoning over it, which will be illustrated below. A first formalization of the structural aspects of the contents of a level for each leaf type was presented in (Keet, 2006a). The drawback of that formalization is that it requires many primitives and, as it turns out, we can avail of the theory of granularity, TOG (Keet, 2008a), to provide a more elegant formal characterization. However, it is outside the current scope to introduce the TOG. Put differently, (i) The TOG—or any other theory of granularity—does not have as prerequisite a comprehensive formalization of the taxonomy of types of granularity; (ii) A precise characterisation of the types of granularity is very useful to grasp several modeling decisions for development of a theory of granularity, but not mandatory; (iii) Only an implementation of comprehensive granular reasoning needs both. Therefore, in this chapter, we only formalise aspects where possible and clearly indicate which kind of predicates one would need in a theory of granularity. To be precise about the formalisation in this chapter, we need a few preliminaries about first order logic, such as described in (Hedman, 2004), classes, universals and particulars (e.g., Earl (2005); MacLeod & Rubenstein (2005); Smith (2004))[6] , and have to introduce several basic granularity functions and relations. For the present purpose, it suffices to let *GL* denote *granularlevel*, which is a unary predicate, *U* as universal and *PT* a particular, DL denotes the set of levels in the domain granularity framework ($D^f$, which contains all granular perspectives and their levels), and $D^s$ denotes the subject domain (not to be confused with a specific data source, such as an instance of the FMA database). Given these preliminaries, (5) says there is a relation between an entity (/type) *x* and the level it resides in and with the *grain* function (6) we retrieve level *y* where *x* resides; an alternative notation for (6) is $\forall x(grain(x) = y \rightarrow D^s(x) \land GL(y))$. The *assignGL(x, y)* function assigns an entity (/type) *x* to a granular level *y*, where *U(x)* or *PT (x)* and *GL(y)* (7, 8).

$$\forall x, y(in\_level(x, y) \triangleq ((PT (x) \underline{\lor} U(x)) \land GL(y) \land grain(x) = y)) \tag{5}$$

$$\text{grain: } D^s \mapsto GL \tag{6}$$

$$\text{assignGL: } D^s \times GL \tag{7}$$

$$\forall x, y(assignGL(x, y) \rightarrow GL(y) \land (PT(x) \underline{\lor} U(x)) \land in\_level(x, y)) \tag{8}$$

Further, one can enforce that each entity must reside in a granular level with (9).

$$\forall x(D^s(x) \rightarrow \exists y(grain(x) = y \land GL(y))) \tag{9}$$

Put differently, it represents an ontological commitment that the world—or at least the subject domain under consideration—is granular, which may or may not be truthful to reality. Moreover, this constraint may be too restrictive for deployed information systems where for some part of the $D^s$ either the granulation is not known or beyond the interest of the domain experts and software developers.

## Characteristics of the Eight Leaf Types

The 8 leaf types inherit characteristics from their parent type of granularity. There are several general conditions that the structure of the entities (/types)[7] within a level must satisfy, which all types inherit from **cG**. Based on the previous section, one can draw a preliminary list of general characteristics for the entities (/types) that are granulated according to any of the subtypes of **cG**.

i.      The contents of a level can be either entity types or instances, but not both.

ii.     The entities (/types) in a particular level have at least one property (value) in common.

iii.    The entities (/types) are disjoint, but not necessarily exhaustive due to our gaps in knowledge of nature. Within a closed world assumption, they are disjoint exhaustive.

iv.     Provided an entity (/type) is not an orphan and the subject domain is covered fully with granular perspectives, it must reside in at least one granular level.

v.      An entity (/type) never can reside in more than one granular level within the same perspective and that entity (/type) is classified as the same (instance of) universal.

vi.     The entity (/type) in a granular level may reside also in $\geq 1$ other levels, provided that each level the entity (/type) resides in is contained in a distinct granular perspective.

In addition, only lists of ingredients are given to formally characterise the eight leaf types, whereas an elegant, comprehensive formalization that relies on both the TOG and a generic foundational ontology, such as DOLCE (Masolo *et al.*, 2003), is a topic of current work. For instance, the underspecified "$<$" over levels can be defined (called *RL* in the TOG), several of its properties proven, and a clear distinction can be made between the relation between levels and the granulation relation between entities (/types) residing in the levels. Further, notions such as endurant, *ED*, physical region, *PR*, how they relate, and so forth have precisely defined meaning with constraints in DOLCE, whereas the intuitive primitives that will be suggested for several types of granularity may be cast in terms of DOLCE categories and constraints, too, after closer investigation. The respective characteristics for the eight leaf types of granularity are then as follows.

## saoG

All instances in the ordered set belonging to a particular level are instances of the same type. The amount of whole instances is not necessarily determined by the size of the entity that is granulated (see section 1 for an example with granulating a lake). The instances are automatically disjoint because the granulation results in a grid. In addition, the instances within the same level make up the set-extension of its corresponding universal, such as a set of plots of $km^2$ where the amount of plots depends on both the entity that is granulated and on the decisions to include or discard 'partial' plots where a cell of the grid covers a larger area than the part of the entity. Combining these constraints, we need to represent, at least:

- a notion of region to represent the cells of the grid (e.g., DOLCE's region *R*) and that these cells are of the same type, so that if we denote the granulation region with, say, *granR*, then $\forall x(granR(x) \rightarrow R(x))$ and for a particular grid where the shapes are squares (with squares defined the usual way), then we have also that for that particular granular perspective $\forall x(granR(x) \rightarrow Square(x))$ holds;
- a way to relate the boundary of one cell to another and to state these cells are disjoint;
- the entity (/type) to which the grid is applied (e.g., DOLCE's endurant *ED*);
- that the endurant can be associated to each level in the granular perspective, but granulation regions of certain size are in one level of granularity only and those of a larger measure must be in a coarser-grained level than those of a smaller measure.

## samG

All instances in the ordered set belonging to a particular level are instances of the same type and they are whole instances at that level. Further, there is an exact, known, number of instances that can be in that level. In addition, the entities and instances at the higher levels are ultimately composed of the chosen Urelement at the lowest granular level. In contradistinction with **saoG**, the set is grouped into particular amounts, like {Hour 1,..., Hour 24} at the Hour-level $y_i$, which are ultimately built up from the same Urelement, such as Second at level $y_{i+2}$. Combining these constraints, we need to represent, at least:

- Urelement defined as the arbitrarily chosen atom at the most fine-grained level in the granular perspective, which may or may not be Atom *sensu* (1);
- a function to calculate the amount of elements that have to be aggregated and to relate that function to the level;
- the granulation relation between the aggregates in different levels versus the relation between granular levels;
- that the aggregates in different levels are the set extensions of different universals (as opposed to arbitrary aggregates).

## sgpG

This involves a 'zooming in' and 'zooming out' factor, where at a coarser-grained level, for example, the wall and wallpaper touch each other, but at a greater magnification, there is wall-gluewallpaper, and again in smaller detail, one looks at the molecules in the paper, glue, and wall. The zooming factor is like a grain size when relating levels of granularity, where *within one* level one can distinguish instances of, for example, ≥1mm but instances <1mm, metaphorically, fall through the sieve and are indistinguishable from each other, but are distinguishable at lower levels of granularity. In practice, this is used, for example, when filtering substances with filters having different pore sizes and dialysis tubes. With **sgpG**, differences in physical size of the entities (/types) is *the* property for granulation. To characterise the content, we need a function, for example, *size_of*, which returns a value in, say, length, square or cubic size, which can be categorised as physical regions alike DOLCE's *PR*. Thus, the instances of an entity type $\varphi$, *inst*($x$, $\varphi$) recorded at some instance of *GL*, say, level $gl_j$, are physically smaller than the instances at a higher level ($gl_i$), with $gl_j \prec gl_i$, and thereby are related to each other at least or possibly only by the relation that they fall within the same physical size range. Combining these constraints, we need to represent, at least:

- access to the measurement of the physical size of the objects, for example, with a function *size_of*: $PT \mapsto PR$ for the measured region (*PR*) of an object (*PT*), and comparison of measured regions so that, in rudimentary form, *size_of*($x$) < *size_of*($y$) provided we have *in_level*($x$, $gl_j$), *in_level*($y$, $gl_i$), and $gl_j \prec gli$;
- that this measurement is taken by using a direct or indirect measurement property of the entities (/types);
- a value range for each level in the granular perspective and to ensure that those ranges of coarser levels are larger than those of finer-grained levels;

- that, consequently, the (type of) entities in different levels are different—following the first item, then $\forall x, y(inst(x, \varphi) \rightarrow \neg inst(y, \psi))$—and can also be different within the same level.

## sgrG

The entities in reality associated with the levels are the same in the coarse-and finer-grained levels, but their representations change according to pre-defined resolutions. That is, the real world entity is the same universal or its instance, but one chooses to represent them as if they were instantiating different universals; for example, `Cell wall` as circle, lipid bi-layer, three-dimensional structure, or also considering the movements of the lipids and proteins. In this case, the resolution-motivated representation is a figurine where that at a coarser-grained level is, in fact, a proper part of the figurine at the finer-grained level, as, for example, a point is a proper part of a polygon and circle a proper part of a sphere. This is common in cartography and GIS in general, where at a greater resolution, a street is represented as a single line, two parallel lines, or even more detail. Thus, there are several mappings from the same entity to different figurines, resulting in the situation where ordering the figurines with respect to the resolution (hence, also their attributes) are more important than the actual entity. To capture this multi-representation, we could introduce a primitive $rep\_of(x, y)$ to denote the relation between the real-world entity and its coarser-or finer-grained representation $Rep(y)$. Combining these constraints, we need to represent, at least:

- associate a value to the granular level to represent the resolution applicable to the level;
- the entity (/type) that has a multi-representation (e.g., DOLCE's endurant $ED$) and thereby that the endurant can be associated to each level in the granular perspective;
- the figurines with, say, $Rep(x)$ (but preferably a more detailed characterisation);
- the association of the entity (/type) with the figurines with, say, $rep\_of(x, y)$ where $ED(x)$ and $Rep(y)$;
- that given any $rep\_of(x, y_i)$ and $rep\_of(x, y_j)$, then they must be in different levels;
- that given the previous item, if $in\_level(y_i, gl_i)$ and $in\_level(y_j, gl_j)$ and $gl_j \prec gl_i$, then $Rep(y_i)$ is a proper part of $Rep(y_j)$.

## nrG

The entities in a level are of a different type, but all are of the same category, such as all being non-agentive physical objects (*NAPO*) or processes (*PRO*) and so forth. For instance, at the `Cell-level`, there are many *types* of cells, but they are all of the category *NAPO* structural component (`Hemal cell`, `Leukocyte`,...), or function (`Hormone excretor`, `Insulin excretor`,...), and so forth, or a `Protein unit structure`-level with items such as $\alpha$-helices and $\beta$-sheets. Thus, the entities are structured in a hierarchy where the direct children are in a lower level of granularity than its supertype. The characteristic of the **nrG** type is the type of relation between entities, which is of the same type throughout; the currently suggested types of relation were given in section 1, which is denoted here with granulation relation *GR*. In the level, without further specification, the entities can be in an unordered set. It may be, however, that the content has some other additional structure within the level alike a **nasG**, or another **nrG** structure, as illustrated in Example 4 and Figure 7. Alternatively, one can group the unordered set such that it takes into account the additional tree (or other) structure in the level, where each granule correspond to a different branch. Either way, the entities are disjoint thanks to the underlying structure in the data source. Combining these constraints, we need to represent, at least:

- the granulation relation *GR* between the entities (/types) that relate these entities (/types) residing in adjacent levels;
- that for each granular perspective only one granulation relation is used;
- the permitted granulation relations by which one can granulate the data.

## nfG

The entities in a level can be of different kinds, such as folding *NAPOs* with their processes and states, combining types of entities into *one* entity residing in an adjacent higher level. It is not the case that the entities contained in the lower granular level is an (un)ordered set, but the entities (/types) are always related to at least one other entity (/type) within that level. For instance, the hierarchical modeling to improve comprehension of large conceptual data models that was illustrated in Example *2* and different folding operations—that is, what is folded and how—can be identified, concerning perdurants and endurants and some of their subtypes (this has been elaborated on in (Keet, 2008a, 2007b)). Combining these constraints, we need to represent, at least:

- the assertion that the entities (/types) in a level are related to each other;
- the granulation relations between the entities (/types) and their relations in the finer-grained level as the domain of the relations on the one hand and the single entity (/type) they are are folded into in the coarse-grained level as the range on the other hand;
- the permitted granulation relations between the coarse-grained entity (/type) and the finer-grained entities (/types) and relations it expands into.

## nacG

Like **samG**, all instances in the set belonging to a particular level are all of the same type and at that level they are whole instances. It is not necessarily the case that the amount of instances in a particular level is known and can be computed. For instance, `Sports team` does have a predefined amount of instances of `Player` per team, but sales department members of a company do not have to have always the same amount of members. The instances that are member of such populations change over time but the entity (/type), generally labelled with a collective noun, and its meaning endures. Thus, looking at the structure of the data in a level, it is at least an unordered set but can be an ordered set of instances, and the instances populating the set can vary over time, although the entity (/type) keeps its identity. It might be possible, to have not an (un)ordered set but a taxonomy or other additional aggregation within the level alike a **nasG** or **nrG** structure, such as an employee hierarchy (with `Junior sales person`, `Senior sales person`, `Trainee`, `Manager`, etc), or aggregated by the organisational unit (`teamA1`, `teamA2`, etc). Combining these constraints, we need to represent, at least:

- that the instances in the level instantiate the same type, that is, $\forall x(inst(x, \varphi))$ for a particular level, or, at the type-level, that they are subsumed by a root entity type;

- that this type is, at least, a subtype of endurant *ED*, such as a social object and not defined by its extension;
- a notion of 'membership' of the entities (/types) in the finer-grained level as members of the entity (/type) in the adjacent coarser-grained level, such as through the meronymic *member_of* as granulation relation.

## nasG

The structure of the data is like **samG**, but if one combines the subsets at each level, then the amount of unique instances residing in *eac*h level is always the same amount as they are instances of the chosen counting element. For instance, at level $gl_1$ there are 100 phone points and in a $gl_2$, such that $gl_2 \prec gl_1$, the 100 phone points may be divided into three subsets `Land line`, `Mobile`, `Phone over IP` each with, say, 2, 35, 63 elements of the original set, respectively, hence, `Mobile ⊂ Phone point`. There may be a $gl_3$ with `Classic cell phone` and `Skype mobile phone` that granulates `Mobile` phone points and that each have 20 and 15 elements in the set, respectively, which adds up to the 35 elements for `Mobile` of the higher level $gl_2$ (assuming that `Classic cell phone ∩ Skype mobile phone` = Ø, although in certain cases there may be a 'rest group'). Thus, at each level there are subsets with instances as elements of the set that, depending on the granulation criterion, are disjoint. Combining these constraints, we need to represent, at least:

- define the counting element as the arbitrarily chosen atom at the most coarse-grained level in the granular perspective, which serves to count the number of instances in all levels;
- that the number of instances at a given time are the same for each level in the granular perspective, hence, are fully partitioned at each level;
- for all instances that are member of a class φ in a finer-grained level, their coarser-grained representations are instances of ψ residing in a coarser-grained level, that is, $\forall x(inst(x, \varphi) \rightarrow inst(x, \psi))$ so that taxonomic subsumption (*is_a*) may be a relation by which to granulate the data;
- following from the previous point and proper taxonomy development, then the instances at some level $gl_2$ have in their representation either at least one more attribute or more constrained attribute values than their respective representation in the coarser grained-level $gl_1$.

One may opt for the design decision to demand from the chosen criterion that the sets never overlap, or, for 'just in case', create two subtypes of **nasG** where one does allow overlapping sets and the other subtype does not. It does not merit a subtyping because the core ontological aspect is the same, but it may be useful for software systems to distinguish between these two cases.

Some types of relation between the entities or instances within a level can be combined, because one does not have to take into account that some are granulated according to arbitrary scale and others are not. (The (non-)arbitrary scale division is relevant for the relations between levels, but do not always act out on the relation between entity types or instances contained within a level.) **nasG**, **nacG**, **nrG**, and **sgG** may be unordered sets, **samG** and **saoG** may be ordered sets, and **nfG**, **nrG**, **sgG**, and **nacG** can have a more complex additional orthogonal structure of the data inside the level that itself may be subject to a granular structure. This, among other topics, will be illustrated in the next section.

# SAMPLE USAGE OF THE TYPES OF GRANULARITY IN MODELING AND IMPLEMENTATION

We return to several typical examples that passed the revue in previous sections, which now can be cast in the light of a type of granularity so as to both be more precise about the way of granulation and to hint toward finer-grained as well as orthogonal properties that can facilitate implementations and stimulate further analysis toward extending the top-level taxonomy of types of granularity in the scale-dependent branch in particular. After analysis typical examples, we sketch a simplification for implementing granularity thanks to the reusability of the types of granularity.

## Granular Perspectives and Their Type of Granularity

In this section we take a closer look at examples for, primarily, **saoG**, **samG**, and **nrG**, and their modeling options and novel inferences in particular.

### Content of a Level with Arbitrary Scales

For granularity type **saoG**, each level is granulated alike a grid with cells that may or may not be exhaustive for its contents. In the remainder of this paragraph we take a closer look at consequences of constraining granulation to be exhaustive versus permitting non-exhaustiveness that was briefly mentioned for the **cG** type at the start of the previous section. Consider a GIS application used for, for example, laying a grid on a lake as depicted in Figure 6-A for a coarser-grained level, which ensures each part of the lake is covered by the grid. Alternatively, one might want to apply a rule alike "when > 50% of a cell is occupied it must be covered by a grid cell", shown in Figure 6-A′ that consequently discards parts of the lake that occupy < 50% of a cell. This leads to a second question and a consequence: if the

*Figure 6. Grid with cells partitioning a 'lake' according to different rules*

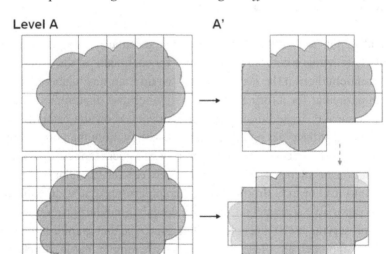

discarded cells in Figure 6-A' should be taken into account at a lower level. If one does, then one arrives at a granulation as depicted in Figure 6-B, if one does not (Figure 6-B'), then the parts at the lower level do not make the whole at the coarser-grained level as can be observed from the difference between moving from A' to B' instead of from A to B to B' (the seven shaded squares would have been absent moving from A' to B'). The discarding rule means that granulation is not exhaustive for we have thrown out a remainder. This type of impreciseness is characteristic for any coarse-grained level and applies to scales for features such as surfaces, volumes, isotherms, and isobars. Developments in rough set theory, rough mereology, and fuzzy logic might serve as an appealing implementation method, and is further elaborated on in (Chen *et al.*, 2007; Hata & Mukaidono, 1999; Keet, 2007a; Klawonn & Kruse, 2004; Peters *et al.*, 2002; Yao, 2004; Zadeh, 1997). Yet differently, instead of including part of the shore of the lake, one can divide the lake by making the grid *inside* the coloured area only, but then one would have to deal with incomplete cells, that is, cells of different size within one granular level, which complicates computation and would not solve the aforementioned boundary problems. Clearly, this is straightforward for **samG**, thanks to the measurement scale and the explicit requirement for a function to move between entities residing in different levels.

Another type of (non) exhaustiveness occurs with less obvious scales, which was briefly illustrated in Example *1*. For instance, if it had only (Baby, Child, Adolescent, Adult) based on age, then Elderly is omitted, hence, that the granulation is either non-exhaustive or assumed to be included in Adult and thereby meeting the exhaustiveness criterion. Because we have created the scale, we can easily decide one way or the other. Alternatively, we could have two levels, one coarse-grained with (Young person, Old person) that partitions a population between persons ≤ 40 year and > 40 years old and a finer-grained one with (Baby, Child, Adolescent, Young adult, Mature adult, Senior, Elderly) using the age brackets 0-5 years, 5-10, 10-20, 20-40, 40-55, 55-70 and > 70 years, respectively. Moreover, bringing the requirement to decide on such issue to the fore, which can be done thanks to the types of granularity, this can be made explicit during the software design phase so as to enhance possibilities for transparent use, reusability, and interoperability of granulated information systems.

## Non-Scale-Dependent Content of a Level

One might conceptualise non-scale-dependent, qualitative granularity as squeezing in a grid-structure in a level—one entity type, with or without its instances for each 'cell' in the grid—but this ignores the relations between parent/children in the hierarchy and would then be a changeable grid and no (pairwise) disjoint tree, in particular for information in biology because disjointness and exhaustiveness is aimed for but rarely achieved[8]. In addition, disjointness depends on the categorisation one is accustomed to, where it may be that the types and their instance satisfy more than one category; for example, LAB streptococci are types of lactic acid bacteria and types of cocci (sphere-shaped) that aggregate in grape-like bunches. Of greater interest is the interaction between the granulation relations and levels of granularity that adhere to **nfG** or **nrG**. In this setting, granularity provides an additional layer to infer more knowledge than is possible separately. Loading a domain granularity framework with data is—or should be—structure-preserving with respect to the data source so that granularity *enhances* the domain data. Advantages of this approach are illustrated in the next example that uses **nrG**-granulated human anatomy by the parthood relation throughout whilst at the same time exploiting a taxonomic structure within in the granular levels.

## Example 4

The Foundational Model of Anatomy (Rosse & Mejino, 2003) uses both *is_a* and *part_of* relations between anatomical entities. Let us take parthood for granulation, then the taxonomic structure can be preserved in the levels, as depicted in Figure 7-B for cells. The FMA lists that `Blood` has as parts: `Plasma, Erythrocyte, Neutrophil, Eosinophil, Basophil, Lymphocyte, Mono-cyte, Platelet, B lymphocyte, T lymphocyte, Natural killer cell, Granular leukocyte,` and `Leukocyte`. Relying on this unordered set alone, one cannot know if it is exhaustive: 1) the list was created manually and some entity type may have been omitted by accident, 2) an ontology adheres to the open-world assumption, and 3) the development tool, FMA-Protégé, does not include axioms for disjoint exhaustive. Combining the taxonomy subsumed by `Cell` and intersecting it with the parts of `Blood`, it is immediately evident that both the parent and child types of `Non-granular leukocyte` are part of blood, but not `Non-granular leukocyte` itself, even though logically it should be. In addition, two cell types that are directly subsumed by `Non-granular leukocyte` are `Peripheral blood mononuclear cell` and `Lymphoblast`, but they are not listed as parts of blood. Monocytes are definitely part of blood, whereas lymphoblasts are "immature lymphocytes" and either not non-granular leukocytes or should be subsumed by `Lymphocyte`. Either way, the structure-preserving loading of granular levels brings afore such areas for improvements. Obviously, one would want to take advantage of the already encoded structure of the taxonomy and have returned something alike Figure 7-B instead of *A*.

This example can be automated at least in part, from which the need has arisen to have a set of usable and reusable types of granular queries (Keet, 2008a). An important advantage of this structure-preserving approach—in particular in conjunction with automation—is that when presenting the combination of taxonomy with granularity demarcations, one gets for free the detection of inconsistent or incomplete

*Figure 7. Two levels with examples of their contents, unordered as in the FMA versus structure-preserving; entities subsumed by Hemal cell present a section of the FMA where terms in bold-face are listed (as in A) as part of blood*

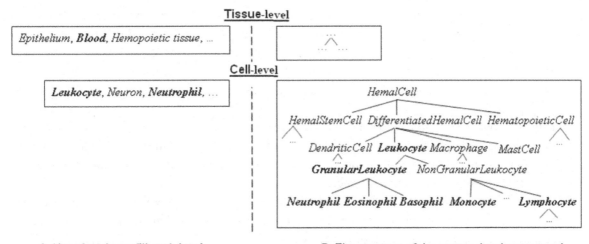

knowledge in either the taxonomy or in the partonomy. Thus, conflicting information is highlighted, can be used for formulating research questions, and be investigated.

Example *4*, however, implicitly illustrated another issue. Lower levels may contain many more entities—1 human body, 12 organ systems, 300+ cell types, 100000+ proteins (Hunter & Borg, 2003)—which is difficult to understand if these entity types (let alone their instances) were represented as an unordered set for each level. This can be pruned through conditional selections and intersections as done in the example (see also the follow-up examples, below). For instance, if one searches the contents at the Cell-level combined with a particular selection of, say, Blood at the Tissue-level, then the types returned contain only the entity types in the selected levels & type, indicated in bold face in Figure 7-B.

A related facet of utilising the structure of the contents compared to an unordered set for each level concerns the 'size' aspect, where it is crucial that the relations between the entities at different levels are not destroyed when applying non-scale-dependent granularity to the subject domain. The typical problem it otherwise raises is that of chicken anatomy where the chicken egg at the Cell-level is physically larger than some of the chicken's organs and body parts, such as Head. Without the parthood relations between the anatomical entities, one might erroneously assume that cells are part of body parts, hence the chicken egg part of head. Conversely, when one maintains the parthood relation and using **nrG**-granulation, then such inferences cannot be drawn because there is explicitly no path from chicken egg to chicken head. Aside from preventing incorrect inferences, one can obtain more benefits from using the underlying structure, in addition to those already illustrated in Example *4*, which are demonstrated in the following example that also takes into account more than one granular perspective with corresponding type of granularity.

> **Example 5.** Whereas Example *4* looked at the finer-grained levels, here we also consider coarse-grained levels of Blood. (1) Represents three levels in the mode of transmission perspective for infectious diseases (Keet & Kumar, 2005), and (2) is taken from the FMA partonomy; thus, Blood is positioned at the intersection of two levels in distinct perspectives, being Mode of transmission and Anatomy, and one can derive (3) from (1) and (2) by traversing the levels 'up.' (4) Is another branch in the FMA: one branch descends to Blood and another one to Skin-associated lymphoid tissue (SALT), and both are ultimately part of the Hemolymphoid system.
>
> 1. Blood involved_in Person-to-person involved_in Direct contact
> 2. Blood part_of Hematopoietic system part_of Hemolymphoid system
> 3. Hemolymphoid system involved_in Direct contact
> 4. Hemolymphoid system has_part Lymphoid System has_part Non-lymphatic lymphoid system has_part Skin-associated lymphoid tissue

However, one cannot conclude that SALT is involved in transmission via Direct contact, but it does pose hypotheses on involvement. In fact, SALT *prevents* infectious agents to enter the vascular system (hence, blood). Although the involvement is different, new combinations may be identified and suggest directions for new research.

Traversing the partonomy downwards, one can infer that at least one of Blood's 13 parts must be involved in transmission of infectious agents because blood is. This is already supported by scientific evidence: transmission of hepatitis C virus via Erythrocytes (Widell *et al.*, 1996) and West Nile Virus via blood `Plasma` (Hollinger & Kleinman, 2003). Consequently, one may wonder if it is the whole cell or if one can isolate parts of cells that are involved. The latter has been established manually with, for example, *Listeria* infections at the `Organelle`-level (subcellular) and nucleation of actin filament polymerization (Rodal *et al.*, 2005).

Note that the assumption in the above example implies a reductionist viewpoint, and philosophically encounters the problem of infinite regress; however, the finest-grained level that is defined for the subject domain demarcates a *finite* regress. It is possible that when the implementation predicts involvement of a lower level it either is not known, hence an epistemological issue where the system generates new research questions, or for good scientific reasons involvement of a lower level is not possible due to a systems-level complex combination of events and substances. Either way, using biological granularity in combination with ontologies can speed up the discovery process because it combines existing information—and gaps therein—in a novel way, thereby offering a new view on the same information.

## Simplifying Implementation by Using the Types of Granularity

In addition to allocation of entities in the appropriate level(s) of granularity, *retrieving* granulated information—just that part of the user's interest—is important. Of the various types of queries (Keet, 2008a,b), we will take a closer look at one of the requirements: retrieving the contents of a granular level with the *getC* function. This is conceptually straightforward, but hides many details, in particular the need to use the structure of the contents given the different types of granularity to ensure correct behaviour. Let us first define the function as follows. Let $gl_i$ be a particular granular level such that $gl_i \in L$, with $i \leq n_{max}$, $n_{max}$ the total amount of levels declared, hence, corresponding to the amount of elements in the set L, and $y_1,..., y_n$ are the entity types or instances residing in that particular level, *i.e.* $y_j \in U$ or $y_j \in PT$ with $U$ the set of universals and *PT* the set of particulars in the granulated information system, and E denotes the collection of universals or particulars that reside in a single granular level.

*Goal*: *retrieve the contents E, entities (/types), of a selected granular level $gl_i$; input is the selected level, where $gl_i \in L$ (and L the set of levels) and output is a set of entities (/types), $E \in E$, that takes into account the structure of the contents in the level.*
*Specification*: *getC*: $L \mapsto E$.

For instance, $getC(gl_2)= \{y_1,..., y_n\}$. *getC* takes a particular granular level as argument and returns the contents of that granular level, *irrespective of how the contents themselves may be structured*. Figure 8 depicts this graphically for two levels, reflecting that the structure of the levels' contents varies according to the type of granularity they adhere to. The current characterisation of *getC*, however, does not guarantee preserving the structure of the source data like conveniently depicted in Figure 8. Although this could be ignored here and deferred to the implementation stage, it can be solved relatively easily by nesting other functions specific for each type of granularity. Before we resolve this, salient problems are illustrated if it were ignored.

**Example 6.** Consider the domain granularity framework for infectious diseases (Keet & Kumar, 2005), we have nine granular perspectives where we focus first on $gp_9 = $ `Predisposing factors` that has two levels. Retrieving contents of both (1 and 2) [9] below, one has to note that (2) is

*Figure 8. Left: selection of levels, with the contents of gp₃gl₂ depicted; Right: selection of levels, with the contents of gp₁gl₂ depicted; Left: selection of levels, with the contents of gp₈gl₂ depicted. The black dot indicates that the entity type labelled with C is selected and contained in the hierarchy in gp₃gl₂ and in an ordered list in gp₁gl₂*

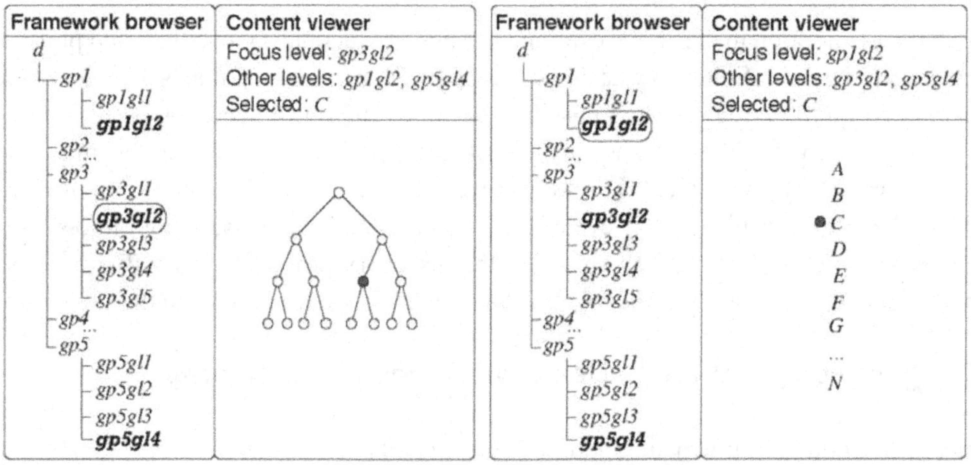

now merely an unordered set without further structure among the entity types in the level, but its simple approach ignores that in the data source the environmental factors are in a different branch of the taxonomy than the four types of living habit predisposing factors; that is, there is not one top type in $gp_9gl_2$. Its coarser-grained level $gp_9gl_1$ contains the entity type Environment that in the subject domain subsumes SocEnv, PolEnv, EcoEnv, and BioEnv, whereas Living habits subsumes Diet, Stress, Smoking, and PersHyg.

1.  getC(gp₉gl₁) = {LivingHabits, Hereditary, Environment, Age}
2.  getC(gp9gl2) = {SocEnv, PolEnv, EcoEnv, BioEnv, Diet, Stress, Smoking, PersHyg}
3.  getC(gp8gl2) = {Congestion, Red hepatization, Grey hepatization, Resolution}

If, on the other hand, we would have selected $gp_8$ = Pathological process, one of its levels ($gp_8gl_2$), and retrieve the contents (3), then there is an internal structure among the entities within the level and not only between the types in adjacent levels, for they are successive sub-processes of the Inflammatory process of pneumococcal pneumonia. However, neither (2) nor (3) reveals that the former is part of a taxonomy and the latter represent successive processes.

The problems illustrated in Example *6* are caused by inadequate usage of the original data. To solve this, we first need to look at the types of granularity and their influence on *getC*. Having recorded the type of granularity used for each granular perspective—in the TOG, this is achieved with the *has_granulation* and *adheres_to* relations—and the structure of the contents of each type of granularity, we can obtain both the type of granularity and the content structure upon using *getC*. Therefore, the specifics for retrieving the contents of each type of granularity can be solved automatically and has to be defined only *once* for each leaf type of granularity used in the application. Let us use a function, *tgL* (an abbreviation of *type of granularity* that the *level* adheres to), which is constrained as *tgL*: L $\mapsto$ *TG*, where *TG* is one of the types of granularity, and L as before. Given the types of granularity and their corresponding content structure, their impact on nested functions for *getC* are as follows.

- For **saoG** we have a grid at each level, hence *getC* typically will retrieve this grid, which is a 2D representation fixed according to its coordinates. Typically, one wants to retrieve the associated representation of the material entity or its cartographic map, too; hence retrieval with *getC* will contain at least two sub-functions to handle this.
- **samG** has its instances within a level as an ordered set, and does not need further processing for retrieval.
- **sgpG**: entities with additional data about their size, which can be retrieved, for example, as a two-column table.
- **sgrG**: textual representation and corresponding figurines, which can be retrieved as with sgpG but with two attributes—label of the entity and figurine—for each object.
- **nasG** types have unordered sets and do not need further processing for retrieval.
- Depending on the implementation, **nacG** can be an unordered set that is aggregated or have additional 'subgroups' in a level. Members at the lower level can be a) aggregated as an unordered set, b) ordered taxonomically, or c) another representation, like a graph with the positions of sports team players on the field. Consequently, finer-grained behaviour of the sub-procedures of *getC* depends on the data source.
- **nfG**: incluentities within a level, which is useful together with the *getC* to retrieve all the entities and its relations. (This works only if those entities do not have relations with other entities beyond the level they reside in, else an additional verification is needed that checks that the candidate entity to retrieve is not in another level within the same perspective.) The minimal structure of the representation of the contents are triples with $\langle$*entity, relation, entity*$\rangle$, which can be listed as unordered set, or rendered in some graphical representation.
- Using *getC* with a level adhering to **nrG**-type granulated entities: one may want to take into account their respective supertypes at the adjacent coarser-grained level, and then aggregate the subsumees in the branch into a granule in the focal level. An example of this is the query to retrieve the cells from the `Cell`-level that are part of blood, thereby omitting the other types of cells residing in the `Cell`-level. Hence, *getC* uses at least a recursive query to retrieve hierarchically organised content and may use entity selection to retrieve a subset of the contents.

Once the content is retrieved, it can be used for further processing, such as intersecting contents of two levels. Regarding Example *6*, we can ensure retrieval of the sequential processes for hepatization thanks to **nfG**-type of granularity where the procedure requires retrieval of the within-level relations as well, and thanks to **nrG**-type for the predisposing factors granular perspective, use the recursive query with its auxiliary functions, illustrated in Example *7*.

> **Example 7.** The predisposing factors are of the granularity type **nrG** and the goal is to answer queries such as "given the predisposing factor `Environment` at level $gp_9gl_1$, retrieve the contents at level $gp_9gl_2$"; for example, condensed in (1). If the supertype is unknown beforehand, the query needs a preliminary step to retrieve the parent type of the selected entity; for example, "retrieve the granule of `Stress`" where `Stress` is subsumed by `Living habit` (2).

*Figure 9.*

---

**Algorithm 1** Retrieving a level's contents by taking into account the content structure

---

**Require:** $x \Leftarrow selectL(x)$

**procedure** $getC(x)$

1:  $\phi \Leftarrow tgL(x)$
2:  **switch**
3:      **case** $\phi = \text{samG}$ : $\ll$ see text for details $\gg$
4:          RESULT $\Leftarrow$ query and sort the set

5:      $\vdots$
6:      **case** $\phi = \text{nrG}$ : $\ll$ see text for details $\gg$
7:          RESULT $\Leftarrow$ recursive query over granulation relation $GR$
8:  **end switch**
9:  **return** RESULT

---

1.  if grain(Environment) = $gp_9gl_1$ and grain(x) = $gp_9gl_2$
    then getContent($gp_9gl_2$) = {SocEnv, PolEnv, EcoEnv, BioEnv}and is_a(x, Environment)
2.  if grain(Stress) = $gp_9gl_2$ and is_a(Stress, x) and grain(x) = $gp_9gl_1$
    and grain(y) = $gp_9gl_2$
    then getContent($gp_9gl_2$) = {Diet, Stress, Smoking, PersHyg} and subsumes(x,y)

    More examples can be found in (Keet, 2008a).

A suggested procedure that demonstrates the nesting of this function in *getC* is included as Figure 9. *Algorithm 1* (*selectL* is an auxiliary level-selection function). The goal of each **case**-option—*what* to do to retrieve it—is the same but actual operations depend on the software implementation, such as using a recursive query in STRUQL or a method in a C++ program; that is, its practical realisation depends on how the data, information or knowledge is organised in the type of application. Thus, to achieve the *purpose* of *getC*, one has to *use the type of granularity to which a level adheres* and the finer-grained application-specific procedures it requires to retrieve the content. Clearly, once one has defined the procedure for retrieval, such as the need for recursive query for **nrG**-granulation, one can re-apply this to a different granular perspective that uses the same granulation, thereby avoiding re-analysis and promoting transparency of the software.

## FUTURE TRENDS

The top-level taxonomy of types of granularity as proposed in this chapter makes explicit the main distinctions between the different ways how people granulate data, information, and knowledge, and, tentatively, how it may exist in reality. This is, however, only a first step in characterising the foundational semantics of granularity, for which there are two principle directions of further research concerning the topic. First, upon closer inspection, there may be uncovered more detailed distinctions between the types so as to refine the taxonomy with a fourth or even fifth layer. This in particular for the scale-dependent branch, because more theoretical and practical results are known compared to the non-scale-dependent branch (e.g., with an ontology of measurement, usage of attribute values in clustering, rough and fuzzy sets and fuzzy logic). In addition, the interplay between and concurrent use of quantitative with qualitative granularity (Bender & Glen, 2004; Keet, 2007a; Zhou *et al.*, 2005) may reveal additional insights in dependencies between the two principal ways of granulation. Second, there is the need to formalise the taxonomy elegantly with as few primitives as necessary and to result in a logically consistent theory. To this end, it is necessary to have a theory of granularity that adequately addresses, among others, what a granular level is, what the nature of the relation between levels is, and what constitutes a granular perspective (granulation hierarchy). To the best of my knowledge, the most comprehensive proposal that lays bare premises and their (logical) consequences to define a theory of granularity has been proposed by Keet (2008a), which could be used in the endeavour to formalise the taxonomy, although a comparatively 'lightweight' theory might also suffice for scalable information systems.

Both directions, however, focus on more theoretical development as opposed to "*Applications* for Advanced Human Reasoning" as the book title indicates. Clearly, the taxonomy already can be used to better represent granular perspectives *manually*, hence it contributes to *human* reasoning for we have obtained a better understanding of granularity. However, efficient *computational* applications that use the types of granularity—be it *de novo* or as enhancements to existing granulated information systems—have yet to be developed. The latter may be seen as a shortcoming by engineers on the short-term, but a sound theoretical basis is a necessity for each field of study, which has been a noted point for improvement for granular computing already[10]. Moreover, the manual examples unambiguously demonstrated several of the benefits one can harvest by first identifying the type of granularity, in particular for granular information retrieval. This may provide an incentive to commence novel usage of the types of granularity or to use it to verify existing granular perspectives in, for example, geographic information systems (Keet, 2009) so as to facilitate information system integration.

## CONCLUSION

The aim of this chapter was to elucidate foundational semantics of granularity. Ontological distinctions between different types of granularity were identified based on differences in (i) scale-and non-scale-dependent types of granularity; (ii) How levels, and its contents, in a granular perspective relate to each other; (iii) Difference in emphases, being entity-, relation-, or criterion-focused; and (iv) its representation (mathematical or otherwise). Based on the differences uncovered, a top-level taxonomy of types of granularity was developed and it was characterised for each of the eight leaf types of granularity how content (entity types, object, and their relations) residing within levels adhering to a particular type of granularity relate to each other within and across adjacent levels. These types of granularity can guide a conceptual data modeler to better distinguish between the different hierarchies and the software developer to improve on implementations of granularity, in particular when used for reasoning over the data or information. For instance, one can discover implied relations between entities/instances by positioning orthogonally a taxonomy and a partonomy, and make valid inferences with relation to (spatial) inclusion of ecological and/or GIS data. Last, sample contents of a level of granularity were illustrated with examples from several subject domains and advantages of use and reuse of the taxonomy for granular information retrieval was demonstrated.

Current research is focused on a formalisation of the taxonomy and a case study in the subject domain of agriculture for defining granular perspectives using the types of granularity.

# REFERENCES

Abelló, A., Samos, J., & Saltor, F. (2006). YAM²: a multidimensional conceptual model extending UML. *Information Systems, 31*(6), 541–567. doi:10.1016/j.is.2004.12.002

Bargiela, A., & Pedrycz, W. (2006, May 10-12). The roots of granular computing. *IEEE International Conference on Granular Computing 2006* (GrC06), (vol. 1, pp. 806-809). Atlanta, GA.

Bender, A., & Glen, R. C. (2004). Molecular similarity: a key technique in molecular informatics. *Organic & Biomolecular Chemistry, 2*, 3204–3218. doi:10.1039/b409813g

Bittner, T., & Smith, B. (2003). A Theory of Granular Partitions. In Duckham, M., Goodchild, M. F., & Worboys, M. F. (Eds.), *Foundations of Geographic Information Science* (pp. 117–151). London: Taylor & Francis Books. doi:10.1201/9780203009543.ch7

Bittner, T., & Stell, J. (2003). Stratified rough sets and vagueness, In Kuhn, W., Worboys, M., Timpf, S. (eds.), *Spatial Information Theory. Cognitive and Computational Foundations of Geographic Information Science. International Conference* (COSIT'03), (pp. 286-303).

Broekhoven, E., van, Adriaenssens, V., & De Baets, B. (2007). Interpretability-preserving genetic optimization of linguistic terms in fuzzy models for fuzzy ordered classification: an ecological case study. *International Journal of Approximate Reasoning, 44*, 65–90. doi:10.1016/j.ijar.2006.03.003

Camossi, E., Bertolotto, M., Bertino, E., & Guerrini, G. (2003, September 23). Issues on Modelling Spatial Granularity. In *Proceedings of the Workshop on fundamental issues in spatial and geographic ontologies*. Ittingen, Switzerland.

Cariani, P. (1997). Emergence of new signal-primitives in neural systems. *Intellectica, 25*, 95–143.

Chen, D., Wang, X., & Zhao, S. (2007). Attribute Reduction Based on Fuzzy Rough Sets. In Kryszkiewicz, M., Peters, J.F., Rybinski, H., Skowron, A. (Eds.), *Proceedings of the International Conference Rough Sets and Intelligent Systems Paradigms* (RSEISP 2007), (Lecture Notes in Artificial Intelligence vol. *4585*, pp. 381-390). Berlin, Germany: Springer.

Chen, Y. H., & Yao, Y. Y. (2006). Multiview intelligent data analysis based on granular computing. *IEEE International Conference on Granular Computing* (GrC'06), (pp. 281-286). Washington, DC: IEEE Computer Society.

Dawyndt, P., De Meyer, H., & De Baets, B. (2006). UPGMA clustering revisited: A weight-driven approach to transitive approximation. *International Journal of Approximate Reasoning, 42*(3), 174–191. doi:10.1016/j.ijar.2005.11.001

de Fent, I., Gubiani, D., & Montanari, A. (2005). Granular GeoGraph: a multi-granular conceptual model for spatial data. In Calì, A., Calvanese, D., Franconi, E., Lenzerini, M., Tanca, L. (eds), *Proceedings of the 13th Italian Symposium on Advanced Databases* (SEBD'05), (pp368-379). Rome: Aracne editrice.

Degtyarenko, K., & Contrino, S. (2004). COMe: the ontology of bioinorganic proteins. *BMC Structural Biology, 4*(3).

Dongrui, M. J., & Wu, D. (2007, November 2-4). Perceptual Reasoning: A New Computing With Words Engine. *IEEE International Conference on Granular Computing* (GrC2007), (pp. 446-451). San Francisco: IEEE Computer Society.

Earl, D. (2005). The classical theory of concepts. *Internet Encyclopedia of Philosophy*. Retrieved from http://www.iep.utm.edu/c/concepts.htm

Edmonds, B. (2000). Complexity and scientific modelling. *Foundations of Science, 5*(3), 379–390. doi:10.1023/A:1011383422394

Elmasri, R., Fu, J., & Ji, F. (2007, June 20-22). Multi-level conceptual modeling for biomedical data and ontologies integration. *20th IEEE International Symposium on Computer-Based Medical System*s (CBMS'07), (pp. 589-594). Maribor, Slovenia.

Euzenat, J., & Montanari, A. (2005). Time granularity. In Fisher, M., Gabbay, D., & Vila, L. (Eds.), *Handbook of temporal reasoning in artificial intelligence* (pp. 59–118). Amsterdam: Elsevier. doi:10.1016/S1574-6526(05)80005-7

Fagin, R., Guha, R., Kumar, R., Novak, J., Sivakumar, D., & Tomkins, A. (2005, June 13-16). Multi-Structural Databases. In *Proceedings of PODS 2005*. Baltimore, MD.

Fonseca, F., Egenhofer, M., Davis, C., & Camara, G. (2002). Semantic granularity in ontology-driven geographic information systems. *Annals of Mathematics and Artificial Intelligence, 36*(1-2), 121–151. doi:10.1023/A:1015808104769

Grizzi, F., & Chiriva-Internati, M. (2005). The complexity of anatomical systems. *Theoretical Biology & Medical Modelling, 2*(26).

Hata, Y., & Mukaidono, M. (1999, May 20-22). On Some Classes of Fuzzy Information Granularity and Their Representations. In *Proceedings of the Twenty Ninth IEEE International Symposium on Multiple-Valued Logic*, (pp. 288-293). Freiburg im Breisgau, Germany.

Hedman, S. (2004). *A first course in logic—an introduction to model theory, proof theory, computability, and complexity*. Oxford, UK: Oxford University Press.

Hobbs, J. R. (1985). Granularity. *International Joint Conference on Artificial Intelligence (IJCAI85)*, 432-435.

Hollinger, F. B., & Kleinman, S. (2003). Transfusion transmission of West Nile virus: a merging of historical and contemporary perspectives. *Transfusion, 43*(8), 992–997. doi:10.1046/j.1537-2995.2003.00501.x

Hunter, P. J., & Borg, T. (2003). Integration from proteins to organs: The physiome project. *Nature, 4*(3), 237–243.

Johansson, I. (2004b). The Ontology of temperature. *Philosophical Communications, 32*, 115–124.

Kamble, A. S. (2004). *A Data Warehouse Conceptual Data Model for Multidimensional Information*. (PhD thesis), University of Manchester, UK.

Kaplan, N., Sasson, O., Inbar, U., Friedlich, M., Fromer, M., & Fleischer, H. (2005). ProtoNet 4.0: A hierarchical classification of one million protein sequences. *Nucleic Acids Research, 33*, 216–218. doi:10.1093/nar/gki007

Keet, C. M. (2006, May 10-12). A taxonomy of types of granularity. *IEEE Conference in Granular Computing* (GrC2006), (vol. 1, pp. 106-111). Atlanta, GA: IEEE Computer Society.

Keet, C. M. (2007, November 2-4). Granulation with indistinguishability, equivalence or similarity. *IEEE International Conference on Granular Computing* (GrC2007), (pp. 11-16). San Francisco: IEEE Computer Society.

Keet, C. M. (2007, September 10-13). Enhancing comprehension of ontologies and conceptual models through abstractions. In Basili, R., Pazienza, M.T. (Eds.), *10th Congress of the Italian Association for Artificial Intelligence* (AIIA 2007), (Lecture Notes in Artificial Intelligence vol. 4733, pp. 814-822). Berlin Heidelberg, Germany: Springer-Verlag

Keet, C. M. (2008, June 2). Toward cross-granular querying over modularized ontologies. *International Workshop on Ontologies: Reasoning and Modularity* (WORM'08), (CEUR-WS Vol-348, pp. 6-17). Tenerife, Spain.

Keet, C. M. (2008a). *A Formal Theory of Granularity*. (PhD Thesis), KRDB Research Centre, Faculty of Computer Science, Free University of Bozen-Bolzano, Italy.

Keet, C. M. (2009, February 10-12). Structuring GIS information with types of granularity: a case study. In *Proceedings of the 6th International Conference on Geomatics*. La Habana, Cuba

Keet, C. M., & Artale, A. (2008). Representing and reasoning over a taxonomy of part-whole relations. *Applied Ontology, 3*(1-2), 91–110.

Keet, C. M., & Kumar, A. (2005, August 28-31). Applying partitions to infectious diseases. In Engelbrecht, R., Geissbuhler, A., Lovis, C. Mihalas, G. (eds.), *XIX International Congress of the European Federation for Medical Informatics* (MIE2005), Geneva, Switzerland.

Kiriyama, T., & Tomiyama, T. (1993, May 16-20). Reasoning about Models across Multiple Ontologies. In *Proceedings of the International Qualitative Reasoning Workshop*. Washington, DC.

Klawonn, F., & Kruse, R. (2004). The Inherent Indistinguishability in Fuzzy Systems. In Lenski, W. (ed.), Logic versus Approximation: Essays Dedicated to Michael M. Richter on the Occasion of his 65th Birthday, (Lecture Notes in Computer Science, vol. 3075, pp. 6-17). Berlin Heidelberg, Germany: Springer Verlag.

Kumar, A., Smith, B., & Novotny, D. D. (2005). Biomedical informatics and granularity. *Comparative and Functional Genomics, 5*(6-7), 501–508. doi:10.1002/cfg.429

Lin, T. Y. (2006, May 10-12). Toward a Theory of Granular Computing. *IEEE International Conference on Granular Computing* (GrC06). Atlanta, GA: IEEE Computer Society.

Luján-Mora, S., Trujillo, J., & Song, I. (2006). A UML profile for multidimensional modeling in data warehouses. *Data & Knowledge Engineering, 59*(3), 725–769. doi:10.1016/j.datak.2005.11.004

MacLeod, M. C., & Rubenstein, E. M. (2005). Universals. *The Internet Encyclopedia of Philosophy.* Retrieved from http://www.iep.utm.edu/u/universa.htm

Malinowski, E., & Zimányi, E. (2006). Hierarchies in a multidimensional model: From conceptual modeling to logical representation. *Data & Knowledge Engineering, 59*(2), 348–377. doi:10.1016/j. datak.2005.08.003

Mani, I. (1998). A theory of granularity and its application to problems of polysemy and underspecification of meaning. In A.G. Cohn, L.K. Schubert, and S.C. Shapiro (eds.), *Principles of Knowledge Representation and Reasoning: Proceedings of the Sixth International Conference,* (KR98), (pp. 245-255). San Francisco: Morgan Kaufmann.

Masolo, C., Borgo, S., Gangemi, A., Guarino, N., & Oltramari, A. (2003). *Ontology Library.* WonderWeb Deliverable D18 (ver. 1.0, 31-12-2003). Retrieved from http://wonderweb.semanticweb.org

Mencar, C., Castellanoa, G., & Fanellia, A. M. (2007). Distinguishability quantification of fuzzy sets. *Information Sciences, 177*(1), 130–149. doi:10.1016/j.ins.2006.04.008

Ning, P., Wang, X. S., & Jajodia, S. (2002). An algebraic representation of calendars. *Annals of Mathematics and Artificial Intelligence, 63*(1-2), 5–38. doi:10.1023/A:1015835418881

Pandurang, N. P., & Levy, A. Y. (1995). A semantic theory of abstractions. In Mellish, C. (ed.), *Proceedings of the International Joint Conference on Artificial Intelligence,* (pp.196-203). San Francisco: Morgan Kaufmann.

Parent, C., Spaccapietra, S., & Zimányi, E. (2006a). *Conceptual modeling for traditional and spatio-temporal applications—the MADS approach.* Berlin Heidelberg, Germany: Springer Verlag.

Pawlak, Z., & Skowron, A. (2007a). Rudiments of rough sets. *Information Sciences, 177*(1), 3–27. doi:10.1016/j.ins.2006.06.003

Pawlak, Z., & Skowron, A. (2007b). Rough sets: Some extensions. *Information Sciences, 177*(1), 28–40. doi:10.1016/j.ins.2006.06.006

Peters, J. F., Skowron, A., Ramanna, S., & Synak, P. (2002). Rough sets and information granulation. In: T.B. Bilgic, D. Baets, and O. Kaynak (eds.), *Proceedings of 10th International Fuzzy Systems Association World Congress,* (Lecture Notes in Artificial Intelligence vol. *2715*, pp. 370-377). Berlin Heidelberg, Germany: Springer-Verlag.

Polkowski, L. (2006). Rough Mereological Reasoning in Rough Set Theory: Recent Results and Problems. In *Proceedings of Rough Sets and Knowledge Technology* (RSKT 2006), (LNCS vol. 4062, pp. 79-92). Berlin, Germany: Springer

Polkowski, L., & Semeniuk-Polkowska, M. (2008). Reasoning about Concepts by Rough Mereological Logics. In *Proceedings of Rough Sets and Knowledge Technology* (RSKT 2008), (Springer LNCS vol. 5009, pp. 205-212).

Pontow, C., & Schubert, R. (2006). A mathematical analysis of theories of parthood. *Data & Knowledge Engineering, 59,* 107–138. doi:10.1016/j.datak.2005.07.010

Qiu, T., Chen, X., Liu, Q., & Huang, H. (2007, November 2-4). A Granular Space Model for Ontology Learning. *IEEE International Conference on Granular Computing* (GrC2007), (pp. 61-65). San Francisco: IEEE Computer Society.

Ribba, B., Colin, T., & Schnell, S. (2006). A multiscale mathematical model of cancer, and its use in analyzing irradiation therapies. *Theoretical Biology & Medical Modelling, 3*(7).

Rodal, A. A., Sokolova, O., Robins, D. B., Daugherty, K. M., Hippenmeyer, S., & Riezman, H. (2005). Conformational changes in the Arp2/3 complex leading to actin nucleation. *Nature Structural & Molecular Biology, 12*, 26–31. doi:10.1038/nsmb870

Rosse, C., & Mejino, J. L. V. (2003). A reference ontology for biomedical informatics: the foundational model of anatomy. *Journal of Biomedical Informatics, 36*, 478–500. doi:10.1016/j.jbi.2003.11.007

Salthe, S. N. (1985). *Evolving hierarchical systems—their structure and representation*. New York: Columbia University Press.

Salthe, S. N. (2001, Novomber). Summary of the Principles of Hierarchy Theory. Retrieved on October 10, 2005, from http://www.nbi.dk/~natphil/salthe/hierarchy th.html

Skowron, A., & Peters, J. F. (2003). Rough sets: Trends and challenges -plenary paper. In Wang, G., Liu, Q., Yao, Y., Skowron, A. (eds.), *Proceedings of RSFDGrC 2003: Rough Sets, Fuzzy Sets, Data Mining, and Granular Computing.* (Lecture Notes in Artificial Intelligence vol. *2639*, pp. 25-34). Berlin Heidelberg, Germany: Springer-Verlag

Smith, B. (2004). Beyond Concepts, or Ontology as Reality Representation. In Varzi, A., Vieu, L. (eds.), *Formal Ontology and Information Systems. Proceedings of the Third International Conference* (FOIS 2004), (pp. 73-84). Amsterdam: IOS Press.

Sontag, E. D. (2004). Some new directions in control theory inspired by systems biology. *Systems Biology, 1*(1), 9–18. doi:10.1049/sb:20045006

Sowa, J. F. (2000). *Knowledge representation: logical, philosophical, and computational foundations*. Beijing, China: China Machine Press.

Straccia, U. (2006). A Fuzzy Description Logic for the Semantic Web. In Sanchez, E. (Ed.), *Capturing Intelligence: Fuzzy Logic and the Semantic Web*. Amsterdam: Elsevier.

Tange, H. J., Schouten, H. C., Kester, A. D. M., & Hasman, A. (1998). The granularity of medical narratives and its effect on the speed and completeness of information retrieval. *Journal of the American Medical Informatics Association, 5*(6), 571–582.

Tsumoto, S. (2007). Mining Diagnostic Taxonomy and Diagnostic Rules for Multi-Stage Medical Diagnosis from Hospital Clinical Data. *IEEE International Conference on Granular Computing* (GrC2007), (pp. 611-616). Washington, DC: IEEE Computer Society.

Varzi, A. C. (2004). Mereology. In Zalta, E.N. (ed.), *The Stanford Encyclopedia of Philosophy*. Retrieved from http://plato.stanford.edu/archives/fall2004/entries/mereology/

Varzi, A. C. (2007). Spatial reasoning and ontology: parts, wholes, and locations. In Aiello, M., Pratt-Hartmann, I., & van Benthem, J. (Eds.), *Handbook of Spatial Logics* (pp. 945–1038). Berlin, Germany: Springer. doi:10.1007/978-1-4020-5587-4_15

Vernieuwe, H., Verhoest, N. E. C., De Baets, B., Hoeben, R., & De Troch, F. P. (2007). Cluster-based fuzzy models of groundwater transport. *Advances in Water Resources*, *30*(4), 701–714. doi:10.1016/j.advwatres.2006.06.012

Widell, A., Elmud, H., Persson, M. H., & Jonsson, M. (1996). Transmission of hepatitis C via both erythrocyte and platelet transfusions from a single donor in serological window-phase of hepatitis C. *Vox Sanguinis*, *71*(1), 55–57. doi:10.1046/j.1423-0410.1996.7110055.x

Wimsatt, W. C. (1995). The ontology of complex systems: Levels of organization, perspectives, and causal thickets. *Canadian Journal of Philosophy*, *20*, 207–274.

Yao, J. T. (2007). A ten-year review of granular computing. *IEEE International Conference on Granular Computing 2007* (GrC'07), (pp. 734-739). IEEE Computer Society.

Yao, Y. Y. (2004). A partition model of granular computing. *Lecture Notes in Computer Science Transactions on Rough Sets*, *1*, 232–253.

Yao, Y. Y. (2005). Perspectives of Granular Computing. *IEEE Conference on Granular Computing* (GrC2005), (vol. *1*, pp. 85-90).

Yao, Y. Y. (2007). The art of granular computing. In *Proceedings of the International Conference on Rough Sets and Emerging Intelligent Systems Paradigms*.

Yao, Y. Y. (2008, August). (in press). Granular computing: Past, present, and future. *IEEE Conference on Granular Computing 2008,* (GrC'08). Beijing, China: IEEE. *Computers & Society*.

Zadeh, L. A. (1997). Toward a theory of fuzzy information granulation and its centrality in human reasoning and fuzzy logic. *Fuzzy Sets and Systems*, *90*(2), 111–127. doi:10.1016/S0165-0114(97)00077-8

Zadeh, L. A. (2002). From computing with numbers to computing with words—from manipulations of measurements to manipulation of perceptions. *International Journal of applied mathematics and computer science, 12*(3), 307-324.

Zhang, J., Silvescu, A., & Honavar, V. (2002). *Ontology-Driven Induction of Decision Trees at Multiple Levels of Abstraction.* (Technical Report ISU-CS-TR 02-13), Computer Science, Iowa State University. Retrieved from http://archives.cs.iastate.edu/documents/disk0/00/00/02/91/

Zhou, Y., Young, J. A., Santrosyan, A., Chen, K., Yan, S. F., & Winzeler, E. A. (2005). In silico gene function prediction using ontology-based pattern identification. *Bioinformatics (Oxford, England)*, *21*(7), 1237–1245. doi:10.1093/bioinformatics/bti111

## ENDNOTES

[1]   For an excellent recent review paper on rough sets and several extensions, consult Pawlak & Skowron (2007a,b), where the latter also contains an overview of approximation spaces conceptualized by Pawlak in a series of papers from the early 1980s onwards.

[2]   Four-dimensionalism of perdurantists is outside the scope.

[3]   The grid is over the representation of a *material* entity, because one cannot put a grid over the representation of a non-material entity like an organisation, but one can do this with, for example, a lake—that is, with GIS objects such as representations of entities on cartographic maps.

[4]   This does not consider roughness or fuzziness of the measurement, which is an orthogonal issue.

[5]   For instance, entity-focussed: i) Different real-world entities in different levels with **sgpG**, **nrG**, **nfG**, **nacG**, ii) The same real-world entities in different levels, reordered/restructured with **sgrG**, **samG**, **saoG**, **nasG**, **nrG**. Human-centred: i) Human-imposed granularity with **sgrG**, **sgpG**, **samG**, **saoG**, **nacG**, **nasG**, and ii) Not necessarily human-imposed granularity with **sgpG**, **nrG**, **nfG**, **nacG**, **nasG**.

[6]   "Universals are a class of mind independent entities, usually contrasted with individuals, postulated to ground and explain relations of qualitative identity and resemblance among individuals. Individuals are said to be similar in virtue of sharing universals." (MacLeod & Rubenstein, 2005). Philosophically, universals are not always considered to be distinct from concepts (Earl, 2005), but, in practice, the term *concept* tends to refer to mind-dependent entities (Smith, 2004). A *class* is a set, which may correspond to a universal or a concept in its intension.

[7]   The use of the word "structure" in the context of contents in granular levels refers to its organisation of the entities (/types), such as an ordered list or grid, which can coincide with structure *sensu* model theory if the TOG is applied to instance data but its underlying idea will also be used where the contents is type-level knowledge.

[8]   This is primarily due to epistemological reasons: there are many things of nature we just do not know enough about, accumulation of knowledge about nature is in flux, and discoveries are not made following a balanced binary tree representation but as they come and where most funding is.

[9]   The retrieved entity types are abbreviated here for brevity; see (Keet & Kumar, 2005) for the full terms like `Social environment` and `Personal hygiene`.

[10]  It has been a noted shortcoming for Granular Computing numerous times by leading researchers like T.Y. Lin in his GrC'06 keynote speech and Yao (2005, 2007, 2008).

# Chapter 6
# From Interval Computations to Constraint–Related Set Computations:
## Towards Faster Estimation of Statistics and ODEs under Interval, p–Box, and Fuzzy Uncertainty

**Martine Ceberio**
*University of Texas at El Paso, USA*

**Vladik Kreinovich**
*University of Texas at El Paso, USA*

**Andrzej Pownuk**
*University of Texas at El Paso, USA*

**Barnabás Bede**
*University of Texas - Pan American, USA*

## ABSTRACT

*One of the important components of granular computing is interval computations. In interval computations, at each intermediate stage of the computation, we have intervals of possible values of the corresponding quantities. In our previous papers, we proposed an extension of this technique to set computations, where on each stage, in addition to intervals of possible values of the quantities, we also keep sets of possible values of pairs (triples, etc.). In this paper, we show that in several practical problems, such as estimating statistics (variance, correlation, etc.) and solutions to ordinary differential equations (ODEs) with given accuracy, this new formalism enables us to find estimates in feasible (polynomial) time.*

DOI: 10.4018/978-1-60566-324-1.ch006

# 1. FORMULATION OF THE PROBLEM

## 1.1. Need for Data Processing

In many real-life situations, we are interested in the value of a physical quantity $y$ that is difficult or impossible to measure directly. Examples of such quantities are the distance to a star and the amount of oil in a given well. Since we cannot measure $y$ directly, a natural idea is to measure $y$ *indirectly*. Specifically, we find some easier-to-measure quantities $x_1, \ldots, x_n$ which are related to $y$ by a known relation $y = f(x_1, \ldots, x_n)$; this relation may be a simple functional transformation, or complex algorithm (e.g., for the amount of oil, numerical solution to a partial differential equation). Then, to estimate $y$, we first measure or estimate the values of the quantities $x_1, \ldots, x_n$ and then we use the results $\tilde{x}_1, \ldots, \tilde{x}_n$ of these measurements (estimations) to compute an estimate $\tilde{y}$ for $y$ as $\tilde{y} = f(\tilde{x}_1, \ldots, \tilde{x}_n)$

Computing an estimate for $y$ based on the results of direct measurements is called *data processing*; data processing is the main reason why computers were invented in the first place, and data processing is still one of the main uses of computers as number crunching devices.

## 1.2. Measurement Uncertainty: From Probabilities to Intervals

Measurement are never 100% accurate, so in reality, the actual value $x_i$ of $i$-th measured quantity can differ from the measurement result $\tilde{x}_i$. Because of these *measurement errors* $\Delta x_i \stackrel{def}{=} \tilde{x}_i - x_i$, the result $\tilde{y} = f(\tilde{x}_1, \ldots, \tilde{x}_n)$ of data processing is, in general, different from the actual value $y = f(x_1, \ldots, x_n)$ of the desired quantity $y$.

It is desirable to describe the error $\Delta y \stackrel{def}{=} \tilde{y} - y$ of the result of data processing. To do that, we must have some information about the errors of direct measurements.

*Figure 2.*

*Figure 1.*

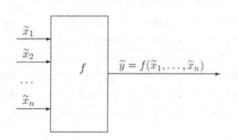

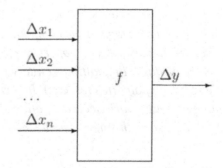

What do we know about the errors $\Delta x_i$ of direct measurements? First, the manufacturer of the measuring instrument must supply us with an upper bound $\Delta_i$ on the measurement error. If no such upper bound is supplied, this means that no accuracy is guaranteed, and the corresponding "measuring instrument" is practically useless. In this case, once we performed a measurement and got a measurement result $\tilde{x}_i$, we know that the actual (unknown) value $x_i$ of the measured quantity belongs to the interval $\mathbf{x}_i = [\underline{x}_i, \overline{x}_i]$, where $\underline{x}_i = \tilde{x}_i - \Delta_i$ and $\overline{x}_i = \tilde{x}_i + \Delta_i$.

In many practical situations, we not only know the interval $[-\Delta_i, \Delta_i]$ of possible values of the measurement error; we also know the probability of different values $\Delta x_i$ within this interval. This knowledge underlies the traditional engineering approach to estimating the error of indirect measurement, in which we assume that we know the probability distributions for measurement errors $\Delta x_i$.

In practice, we can determine the desired probabilities of different values of $\Delta x_i$ by comparing the results of measuring with this instrument with the results of measuring the same quantity by a standard (much more accurate) measuring instrument. Since the standard measuring instrument is much more accurate than the one use, the difference between these two measurement results is practically equal to the measurement error; thus, the empirical distribution of this difference is close to the desired probability distribution for measurement error. There are two cases, however, when this determination is not done:

- First is the case of cutting-edge measurements, for example, measurements in fundamental science. When we use the largest particle accelerator to measure the properties of elementary particles, there is no "standard" (much more accurate) located nearby that we can use for calibration: our accelerator is the best we have.
- The second case is the case of measurements in manufacturing. In principle, every sensor can be thoroughly calibrated, but sensor calibration is so costly–usually costing ten times more than the sensor itself–that manufacturers rarely do it.

In both cases, we have no information about the probabilities of $\Delta x_i$; the only information we have is the upper bound on the measurement error.

In this case, after we performed a measurement and got a measurement result $\tilde{x}_i$, the only information that we have about the actual value $x_i$ of the measured quantity is that it belongs to the interval $\mathbf{x}_i = [\tilde{x}_i - \Delta_i, \tilde{x}_i + \Delta_i]$. In such situations, the only information that we have about the (unknown) actual value of $y = f(x_1, \ldots, x_n)$ is that $y$ belongs to the range $\mathbf{y} = [\underline{y}, \overline{y}]$ of the function $f$ over the box $\mathbf{x}_1 \times \ldots \times \mathbf{x}_n$:

$$\mathbf{y} = [\underline{y}, \overline{y}] = f(\mathbf{x}_1, \ldots, \mathbf{x}_n) \overset{def}{=} \left\{ f(x_1, \ldots, x_n) \mid x_1 \in \mathbf{x}_1, \ldots, x_n \in \mathbf{x}_n \right\}.$$

*Figure 3.*

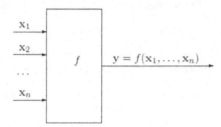

The process of computing this interval range based on the input intervals $\mathbf{x}_i$ is called *interval computations*; see, for example, Jaulin et al. (2001).

## 1.3. Case of Fuzzy Uncertainty and Its Reduction to Interval Uncertainty

An expert usually describes his/her uncertainty by using words from the natural language, like "most probably, the value of the quantity is between 3 and 4". To formalize this knowledge, it is natural to use *fuzzy set theory*, a formalism specifically designed for describing this type of informal ("fuzzy") knowledge; see, for example, Klir and Yuan (1995).

In fuzzy set theory, the expert's uncertainty about $x_i$ is described by a fuzzy set, that is, by a function $\mu_i(x_i)$ which assign, to each possible value $x_i$ of the $i$-th quantity, the expert's degree of certainty that $x_i$ is a possible value. A fuzzy set can also be described as a nested family of $\alpha$-cuts

$$\mathbf{x}_i(\alpha) \stackrel{def}{=} \{x_i \mid \mu(x_i) > \alpha\} \ .$$

Zadeh's extension principle can be used to transform the fuzzy sets for $x_i$ into a fuzzy set for $y$. It is known that for continuous functions $f$ on a bounded domain, this principle is equivalent to saying that for every $\alpha$,

$$\mathbf{y}(\alpha) = f(\mathbf{x}_1(\alpha), \ldots, \mathbf{x}_n(\alpha)).$$

In other words, fuzzy data processing can be implemented as layer-by-layer interval computations. In view of this reduction, in the following text, we will mainly concentrate on interval computations.

## 1.4. Outline

We start by recalling the basic techniques of interval computations and their drawbacks, then we will describe the new set computation techniques and describe a class of problems for which these techniques are efficient. Finally, we talk about how we can extend these techniques to other types of uncertainty (e.g., classes of probability distributions).

## 2. INTERVAL COMPUTATIONS: BRIEF REMINDER

### 2.1. Interval Computations: Main Idea

Historically the first method for computing the enclosure for the range is the method which is sometimes called "straightforward" interval computations. This method is based on the fact that inside the computer, every algorithm consists of elementary operations (arithmetic operations, $\min$, $\max$, etc.). For each elementary operation $f(a,b)$, if we know the intervals $\mathbf{a}$ and $\mathbf{b}$ for $a$ and $b$, we can compute the exact range $f(\mathbf{a},\mathbf{b})$. The corresponding formulas form the so-called *interval arithmetic*:

$$[\underline{a},\overline{a}]+[\underline{b},\overline{b}]=[\underline{a}+\underline{b},\overline{a}+\overline{b}]; \quad [\underline{a},\overline{a}]-[\underline{b},\overline{b}]=[\underline{a}-\overline{b},\overline{a}-\underline{b}];$$

$$[\underline{a},\overline{a}]\cdot[\underline{b},\overline{b}]=[\min(\underline{a}\cdot\underline{b},\underline{a}\cdot\overline{b},\overline{a}\cdot\underline{b},\overline{a}\cdot\overline{b}),\max(\underline{a}\cdot\underline{b},\underline{a}\cdot\overline{b},\overline{a}\cdot\underline{b},\overline{a}\cdot\overline{b})];$$

$$1/[\underline{a},\overline{a}]=[1/\overline{a},1/\underline{a}] \text{ if } 0\notin[\underline{a},\overline{a}]; [\underline{a},\overline{a}]/[\underline{b},\overline{b}]=[\underline{a},\overline{a}]\cdot(1/[\underline{b},\overline{b}]).$$

In straightforward interval computations, we repeat the computations forming the program $f$ step-by-step, replacing each operation with real numbers by the corresponding operation of interval arithmetic. It is known that, as a result, we get an enclosure $\mathbf{Y}\supseteq\mathbf{y}$ for the desired range.

### 2.2. From Main Idea to Actual Computer Implementation

Not every real number can be exactly implemented in a computer; thus, for example, after implementing an operation of interval arithmetic, we must enclose the result $[r^-,r^+]$ in a computer-representable interval: namely, we must round-off $r^-$ to a smaller computer-representable value $\underline{r}$, and round-off $r^+$ to a larger computer-representable value $\overline{r}$.

### 2.3. Sometimes, We Get Excess Width

In some cases, the resulting enclosure is exact; in other cases, the enclosure has excess width. The excess width is inevitable since straightforward interval computations increase the computation time by at most a factor of 4, while computing the exact range is, in general, NP-hard (see, e.g., Kreinovich et al. (1997)), even for computing the population variance $V=\dfrac{1}{n}\cdot\sum_{i=1}^{n}(x_i-\overline{x}_i)^2$, where $\overline{x}=\dfrac{1}{n}\cdot\sum_{i=1}^{n}x_i$ (see Ferson et al. (2002)). If we get excess width, then we can use more sophisticated techniques to get a better estimate, such as centered form, bisection, etc.; see, for example, Jaulin et al. (2001).

## 2.4. Reason for Excess Width

The main reason for excess width is that intermediate results are dependent on each other, and straight-forward interval computations ignore this dependence. For example, the actual range of $f(x_1) = x_1 - x_1^2$ over $\mathbf{x}_1 = [0, 1]$ is $\mathbf{y} = [0, 0.25]$ Computing this $f$ means that we first compute $x_2 := x_1^2$ and then subtract $x_2$ from $x_1$. According to straightforward interval computations, we compute $\mathbf{r} = [0, 1]^2 = [0, 1]$ and then $\mathbf{x}_1 - \mathbf{x}_2 = [0, 1] - [0, 1] = [-1, 1]$. This excess width comes from the fact that the formula for interval subtraction implicitly assumes that both $a$ and $b$ can take arbitrary values within the corresponding intervals $\mathbf{a}$ and $\mathbf{b}$, while in this case, the values of $x_1$ and $x_2$ are clearly not independent: $x_2$ is uniquely determined by $x_1$, as $x_2 = x_1^2$

## 3. CONSTRAINT-BASED SET COMPUTATIONS

## 3.1. Main Idea

The main idea behind constraint-based set computations (see, e.g., Ceberio et al. (2006)) is to remedy the above reason why interval computations lead to excess width. Specifically, at every stage of the computations, in addition to keeping the *intervals* $\mathbf{x}_i$ of possible values of all intermediate quantities $x_i$, we also keep several *sets*:

sets $\mathbf{x}_{ij}$ of possible values of pairs $(x_i, x_j)$;

if needed, sets $\mathbf{x}_{ijk}$ of possible values of triples $(x_i, x_j, x_k)$; etc.

In the above example, instead of just keeping two intervals $\mathbf{x}_1 = \mathbf{x}_2 = [0, 1]$, we would then also generate and keep the set $\mathbf{x}_{12} = \{(x_1, x_1^2) | x_1 \in [0, 1]\}$. Then, the desired range is computed as the range of $x_1 - x_2$ over this set–which is exactly $[0, 0.25]$.

To the best of our knowledge, in interval computations context, the idea of representing dependence in terms of sets of possible values of tuples was first described by Shary; see, for example, Shary (2003, 2004) and references therein.

How can we propagate this set uncertainty via arithmetic operations? Let us describe this on the example of addition, when, in the computation of $f$, we use two previously computed values $x_i$ and $x_j$ to compute a new value $x_k := x_i + x_j$. In this case, we set

$$\mathbf{x}_{ik} = \{(x_i, x_i + x_j) | (x_i, x_j) \in \mathbf{x}_{ij}\}, \qquad \mathbf{x}_{jk} = \{(x_j, x_i + x_j) | (x_i, x_j) \in \mathbf{x}_{ij}\},$$

and for every $l \neq i, j$, we take

$$\mathbf{x}_{kl} = \{(x_i + x_j, x_l) \,|\, (x_i, x_j) \in \mathbf{x}_{ij}, (x_i, x_l) \in \mathbf{x}_{il}, (x_j, x_l) \in \mathbf{x}_{jl}\}.$$

## 3.2. From Main Idea to Actual Computer Implementation

In interval computations, we cannot represent an arbitrary interval inside the computer, we need an enclosure. Similarly, we cannot represent an arbitrary set inside a computer, we need an enclosure.

To describe such enclosures, we fix the number $C$ of granules (e.g., $C = 10$). We divide each interval $\mathbf{x}_i$ into $C$ equal parts $\mathbf{X}_i$; thus each box $\mathbf{x}_i \times \mathbf{x}_j$ is divided into $C^2$ subboxes $\mathbf{X}_i \times \mathbf{X}_j$. We then describe each set $\mathbf{x}_{ij}$ by listing all subboxes $\mathbf{X}_i \times \mathbf{X}_j$ which have common elements with $\mathbf{x}_{ij}$; the union of such subboxes is an enclosure for the desired set $\mathbf{x}_{ij}$.

This implementation enables us to implement all above arithmetic operations. For example, to implement $\mathbf{x}_{ik} = \{(x_i, x_i + x_j) \,|\, (x_i, x_j) \in \mathbf{x}_{ij}\}$, we take all the subboxes $\mathbf{X}_i \times \mathbf{X}_j$ that form the set $\mathbf{x}_{ij}$; for each of these subboxes, we enclosure the corresponding set of pairs

$$\{(x_i, x_i + x_j) \,|\, (x_i, x_j) \in \mathbf{X}_i \times \mathbf{X}_j\}$$

into a set $\mathbf{X}_i \times (\mathbf{X}_i + \mathbf{X}_j)$. This set may have non-empty intersection with several subboxes $\mathbf{X}_i \times \mathbf{X}_k$; all these subboxes are added to the computed enclosure for $\mathbf{x}_{ik}$. Once can easily see if we start with the exact range $\mathbf{x}_{ij}$, then the resulting enclosure for $\mathbf{x}_{ik}$ is an $(1/C)$-approximation to the actual set–and so when $C$ increases, we get more and more accurate representations of the desired set.

Similarly, to find an enclosure for

$$\mathbf{x}_{kl} = \{(x_i + x_j, x_l) \,|\, (x_i, x_j) \in \mathbf{x}_{ij}, (x_i, x_l) \in \mathbf{x}_{il}, (x_j, x_l) \in \mathbf{x}_{jl}\},$$

we consider all the triples of subintervals $(\mathbf{X}_i, \mathbf{X}_j, \mathbf{X}_l)$ for which $\mathbf{X}_i \times \mathbf{X}_j \subseteq \mathbf{x}_{ij}$, $\mathbf{X}_i \times \mathbf{X}_l \subseteq \mathbf{x}_{il}$, and $\mathbf{X}_j \times \mathbf{X}_l \subseteq \mathbf{x}_{jl}$; for each such triple, we compute the box $(\mathbf{X}_i + \mathbf{X}_j) \times \mathbf{X}_l$; then, we add subboxes $\mathbf{X}_k \times \mathbf{X}_l$ which intersect with this box to the enclosure for $\mathbf{x}_{kl}$.

## 3.3. First Example: Computing the Range of $x - x$

For $f(x) = x - x$ on $[0,1]$, the actual range is $[0,0]$, but straightforward interval computations lead to an enclosure $[0,1] - [0,1] = [-1,1]$. In straightforward interval computations, we have $r_1 = x$ with the exact interval range $\mathbf{r}_1 = [0,1]$, and we have $r_2 = x$ with the exact interval range $\mathbf{x}_2 = [0,1]$. The variables $r_1$ and $r_2$ are dependent, but we ignore this dependence.

In the new approach: we have $\mathbf{r}_1 = \mathbf{r}_2 = [0,1]$ and we also have $\mathbf{r}_{12}$:

For each small box, we have $[-0.2, 0.2]$, so the union is $[-0.2, 0.2]$.

If we divide into more pieces, we get an interval closer to 0.

## 3.4 Second Example: Computing the Range of $x - x^2$

In straightforward interval computations, we have $r_1 = x$ with the exact interval range interval $\mathbf{r}_1 = [0,1]$, and we have $r_2 = x^2$ with the exact interval range $\mathbf{x}_2 = [0,1]$. The variables $r_1$ and $r_2$ are dependent, but we ignore this dependence and estimate $\mathbf{r}_3$ as $[0,1] - [0,1] = [-1,1]$.

In the new approach: we have $\mathbf{r}_1 = \mathbf{r}_2 = [0,1]$ and we also have $\mathbf{r}_{12}$. First, we divide the range $[0,1]$ into 5 equal subintervals $\mathbf{R}_1$. The union of the ranges $\mathbf{R}_1^2$ corresponding to these 5 subintervals $\mathbf{R}_1$ is $[0,1]$, so $\mathbf{r}_2 = [0,1]$. We divide this interval $\mathbf{r}_2$ into 5 equal sub-intervals $[0,0.2]$, $[0.2,0.4]$, etc. We now compute the set $\mathbf{r}_{12}$ as follows:

for $\mathbf{R}_1 = [0,0.2]$, we have $\mathbf{R}_1^2 = [0,0.04]$, so only sub-interval $[0,0.2]$ of the interval $\mathbf{r}_2$ is affected;

for $\mathbf{R}_1 = [0.2,0.4]$, we have $\mathbf{R}_1^2 = [0.04,0.16]$, so also only sub-interval $[0,0.2]$ is affected;

for $\mathbf{R}_1 = [0.4,0.6]$, we have $\mathbf{R}_1^2 = [0.16,0.36]$ so two sub-intervals $[0,0.2]$ and $[0.2,0.4]$ are affected, etc.

For each possible pair of small boxes $\mathbf{R}_1 \times \mathbf{R}_2$ we have $\mathbf{R}_1 - \mathbf{R}_2 = [-0.2,0.2]$, $[0,0.4]$, or $[0.2, 0.6]$, so the union of $\mathbf{R}_1 - \mathbf{R}_2$ is $\mathbf{r}_3 = [-0.2,0.6]$.

If we divide into more and more pieces, we get the enclosure which is closer and closer to the exact range $[0,0.25]$.

*Figure 4.*                 *Figure 5.*

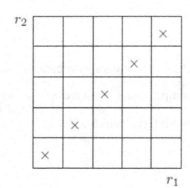

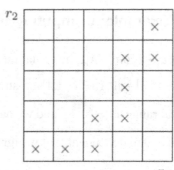

## 3.5. How to Compute $r_{ik}$

The above example is a good case to illustrate how we compute the range $r_{13}$ for $r_3 = r_1 - r_2$. Indeed, since $r_3 = [-0.2, 0.6]$, we divide this range into 5 subintervals $[-0.2, -0.04]$, $[-0.04, 0.12]$, $[0.12, 0.28]$, $[0.28, 0.44]$, $[0.44, 0.6]$.

For $\mathbf{R}_1 = [0, 0.2]$, the only possible $\mathbf{R}_2$ is $[0, 0.2]$ so $\mathbf{R}_1 - \mathbf{R}_2 = [-0.2, 0.2]$. This covers $[-0.2, -0.04]$, $[-0.04, 0.12]$, and $[0.12, 0.28]$.

For $\mathbf{R}_1 = [0.2, 0.4]$, the only possible $\mathbf{R}_2$ is $[0, 0.2]$, so $\mathbf{R}_1 - \mathbf{R}_2 = [0, 0.4]$. This interval covers $[-0.04, 0.12]$, $[0.12, 0.28]$, and $[0.28, 0.44]$.

For $\mathbf{R}_1 = [0.4, 0.6]$, we have two possible $\mathbf{R}_2$: for $\mathbf{R}_2 = [0, 0.2]$, we have $\mathbf{R}_1 - \mathbf{R}_2 = [0.2, 0.6]$ this covers $[0.12, 0.28]$, $[0.28, 0.44]$, and $[0.44, 0.6]$; for $\mathbf{R}_2 = [0.2, 0.4]$, we have $\mathbf{R}_1 - \mathbf{R}_2 = [0, 0.4]$ this covers $[-0.04, 0.12]$, $[0.12, 0.28]$, and $[0.28, 0.44]$.

For $\mathbf{R}_1 = [0.6, 0.8]$, we have $\mathbf{R}_1^2 = [0.36, 0.64]$ so three possible $\mathbf{R}_2$: $[0.2, 0.4]$, $[0.4, 0.6]$, and $[0.6, 0.8]$, to the total of $[0.2, 0.8]$. Here, $[0.6, 0.8] - [0.2, 0.8] = [-0.2, 0.6]$, so all 5 subintervals are affected.

Finally, for $\mathbf{R}_1 = [0.8, 1.0]$, we have $\mathbf{R}_1^2 = [0.64, 1.0]$, so two possible $\mathbf{R}_2$: $[0.6, 0.8]$ and $[0.8, 1.0]$, to the total of $[0.6, 1.0]$. Here, $[0.8, 1.0] - [0.6, 1.0] = [-0.2, 0.4]$, so the first 4 subintervals are affected.

## 3.6. Limitations of This Approach

The main limitation of this approach is that when we need an accuracy $\varepsilon$, we must use $\sim 1 / \varepsilon$ granules; so, if we want to compute the result with $k$ digits of accuracy, that is, with accuracy $\varepsilon = 10^{-k}$, we must consider exponentially many boxes ($\sim 10^k$). In plain words, this method is only applicable when we want to know the desired quantity with a given accuracy (e.g., 10%).

*Figure 6.*

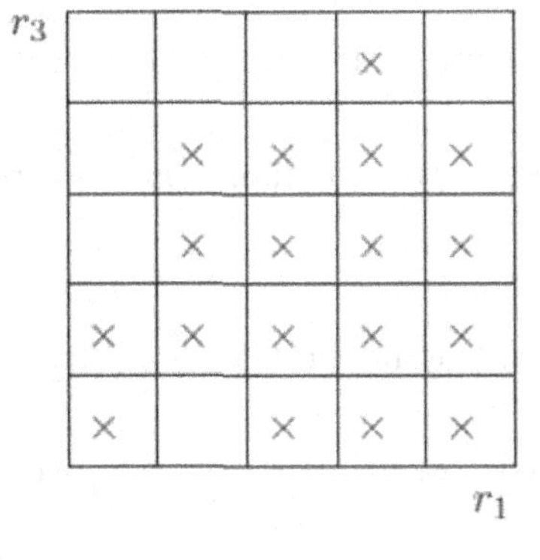

## 3.7. Cases When This Approach is Applicable

In practice, there are many problems when it is sufficient to compute a quantity with a given accuracy: for example, when we detect an outlier, we usually do not need to know the variance with a high accuracy, an accuracy of 10% is more than enough.

Let us describe the case when interval computations do not lead to the exact range, but set computations do–of course, the range is "exact" modulo accuracy of the actual computer implementations of these sets.

## 3.8. Example: Estimating Variance under Interval Uncertainty

Suppose that we know the intervals $\mathbf{x}_1, \ldots, \mathbf{x}_n$ of possible values of $x_1, \ldots, x_n$, and we need to compute

the range of the variance $V = \dfrac{1}{n} \cdot M - \dfrac{1}{n^2} \cdot E^2$, where $M \overset{def}{=} \sum_{i=1}^{n} x_i^2$ and $E \overset{def}{=} \sum_{i=1}^{n} x_i$.

This problem is important, for example, in detecting outliers. Outliers are useful in many application areas. For example, in medicine, to detect possible illnesses, we analyze the healthy population, compute the averages $E[x]$ and the standard deviations $\sigma[x]$ of different characteristics $x$, and if for some person, the value of a blood pressure, weight, body temperature, etc., is outside the corresponding 2- or 3-sigma interval $[E[x] - k_0 \cdot \sigma[x], E[x] + k_0 \cdot \sigma[x]]$, then we perform additional tests to see if there is any hidden problem with this person's health. Similarly, in geophysics, when we look for rare minerals, we know the typical values for a given area, and if at some location, the values of the geophysical characteristics are outliers (i.e., they are outside the corresponding interval), then these area are probably the most promising.

Traditional algorithms for detecting outliers assume that we know the exact values $x_i$ of the corresponding characteristics but in practice, these values often come from estimates or crude measurements. For example, most routine blood pressure measurements performed at health fairs, in drugstores, at the dentist office, etc., are very approximate, with accuracy 10 or more; their objective is not to find the exact values of the corresponding characteristics but to make sure that we do not miss a dangerous anomaly. When we estimate the mean and the standard deviations based on these approximate measurements, we need to take into account that these values are very approximate, that is, that, in effect, instead of the exact value $x_i$ (such as 110), we only know that the actual (unknown) value of the blood pressure is somewhere within the interval

$$[\tilde{x}_i - \Delta_i, \tilde{x}_i + \Delta_i] = [110 - 10, 110 + 10] = [100, 120]$$

In all these situations, we need to compute the range on the variance $V$ under the interval uncertainty on $x_i$.

A natural way to compute $V$ is to compute the intermediate sums $M_k \overset{def}{=} \sum_{i=1}^{k} x_i^2$ and $E_k \overset{def}{=} \sum_{i=1}^{k} x_i$.

We start with $M_0 = E_0 = 0$; once we know the pair $(M_k, E_k)$, we compute

$$(M_{k+1}, E_{k+1}) = (M_k + x_{k+1}^2, E_k + x_{k+1}).$$

Since the values of $M_k$ and $E_k$ only depend on $x_1, \ldots, x_k$ and do not depend on $x_{k+1}$, we can conclude that if $(M_k, E_k)$ is a possible value of the pair and $x_{k+1}$ is a possible value of this variable, then $(M_k + x_{k+1}^2, E_k + x_{k+1})$ is a possible value of $(M_{k+1}, E_{k+1})$. So, the set $\mathbf{p}_0$ of possible values of $(M_0, E_0)$ is the single point $(0, 0)$; once we know the set $\mathbf{p}_k$ of possible values of $(M_k, E_k)$, we can compute $\mathbf{p}_{k+1}$ as

$$\{(M_k + x^2, E_k + x) | (M_k, E_k) \in \mathbf{p}_k, x \in \mathbf{x}_{k+1}\}$$

For $k = n$, we will get the set $\mathbf{p}_n$ of possible values of $(M, E)$; based on this set, we can then find the exact range of the variance $V = \dfrac{1}{n} \cdot M - \dfrac{1}{n^2} \cdot E^2$.

What $C$ should we choose to get the results with an accuracy $\varepsilon \cdot \overline{V}$? On each step, we add the uncertainty of $1/C$; to, after $n$ steps, we add the inaccuracy of $n/C$. Thus, to get the accuracy $n/C \approx \varepsilon$, we must choose $C = n/\varepsilon$.

What is the running time of the resulting algorithm? We have $n$ steps; on each step, we need to analyze $C^3$ combinations of subintervals for $E_k$, $M_k$, and $x_{k+1}$. Thus, overall, we need $n \cdot C^3$ steps, that is, $n^4/\varepsilon^3$ steps. For fixed accuracy $C \sim n$, so we need $O(n^4)$ steps–a polynomial time, and for $\varepsilon = 1/10$, the coefficient at $n^4$ is still $10^3$–quite feasible.

For example, for $n = 10$ values and for the desired accuracy $\varepsilon = 0.1$, we need $10^3 \cdot n^4 \approx 10^7$ computational steps–"nothing" for a Gigaherz ($10^9$ operations per second) processor on a usual PC. For $n = 100$ values and the same desired accuracy, we need $10^4 \cdot n^4 \approx 10^{12}$ computational steps, that is, $10^3$ seconds (15 minutes) on a Gigaherz processor. For $n = 1000$, we need $10^{15}$ steps, that is, $10^6$ computational steps–12 days on a single processor or a few hours on a multi-processor machine.

In comparison, the exponential time $2^n$ needed in the worst case for the exact computation of the variance under interval uncertainty, is doable ($2^{10} \approx 10^3$ step) for $n = 10$, but becomes unrealistically astronomical ($2^{100} \approx 10^{30}$ steps) already for $n = 100$.

## Comment

When the accuracy increases $\varepsilon = 10^{-k}$, we get an exponential increase in running time–but this is OK since, as we have mentioned, the problem of computing variance under interval uncertainty is, in general, NP-hard.

## 3.9. Other Statistical Characteristics

Similar algorithms can be presented for computing many other statistical characteristics. For example, for every integer $d > 2$, the corresponding higher-order central moment $C_d = \frac{1}{n} \cdot \sum_{i=1}^{n} (x_i - \bar{x})^d$ is a linear combination of $d$ moments $M^{(j)} \stackrel{def}{=} \sum_{i=1}^{n} x_i^j$ for $j = 1, \ldots, d$; thus, to find the exact range for $C_d$, we can keep, for each $k$, the set of possible values of $d$-dimensional tuples $(M_k^{(1)}, \ldots, M_k^{(d)})$, where $M_k^{(j)} \stackrel{def}{=} \sum_{i=1}^{k} x_i^j$ For these computations, we need $n \cdot C^{d+1} \sim n^{d+2}$ steps–still a polynomial time.

Another example is covariance $\mathrm{Cov} = \frac{1}{n} \cdot \sum_{i=1}^{n} x_i \cdot y_i - \frac{1}{n^2} \cdot \sum_{i=1}^{n} x_i \cdot \sum_{i=1}^{n} y_i$. To compute covariance, we need to keep the values of the triples $(\mathrm{Cov}_k, X_k, Y_k)$, where $\mathrm{Cov}_k \stackrel{def}{=} \sum_{i=1}^{k} x_i \cdot y_i$, $X_k \stackrel{def}{=} \sum_{i=1}^{k} x_i$, and $Y_k \stackrel{def}{=} \sum_{i=1}^{k} y_i$. At each step, to compute the range of

$(\mathrm{Cov}_{k+1}, X_{k+1}, Y_{k+1}) = (\mathrm{Cov}_k + x_{k+1} \cdot y_{k+1}, X_k + x_{k+1}, Y_k + y_{k+1})$, we must consider all possible combinations of subintervals for $\mathrm{Cov}_k$, $X_k$, $Y_k$, $x_{k+1}$, and $y_{k+1}$–to the total of $C^5$. Thus, we can compute covariance in time $n \cdot C^5 \sim n^6$.

Similarly, to compute correlation $\rho = \mathrm{Cov} / \sqrt{V_x \cdot V_y}$, we can update, for each $k$, the values of $(C_k, X_k, Y_k, X_k^{(2)}, Y_k^{(2)})$, where $X_k^{(2)} = \sum_{i=1}^{k} x_i^2$ and $Y_k^{(2)} = \sum_{i=1}^{k} y_i^2$ are needed to compute the variances $V_x$ and $V_y$. These computations require time $n \cdot C^7 \sim n^8$.

## 3.10. Systems of Ordinary Differential Equations (ODEs) under Interval Uncertainty

A general system of ODEs has the form $\dot{x}_i = f_i(x_1, \ldots, x_m, t)$, $1 \leq i \leq m$. Interval uncertainty usually means that the exact functions $f_i$ are unknown, we only know the expressions of $f_i$ in terms of parameters, and we have interval bounds on these parameters.

There are two types of interval uncertainty: we may have global parameters whose values are the same for all moments $t$, and we may have noise-like parameters whose values may different at different moments of time–but always within given intervals. In general, we have a system of the type $\dot{x}_i = f_i(x_1, \ldots, x_m, t, a_1, \ldots, a_k, b_1(t), \ldots, b_l(t))$, where $f_i$ is a known function, and we know the intervals $\mathbf{a}_j$ and $\mathbf{b}_j(t)$ of possible values of $a_i$ and $b_j(t)$.

## 3.11 Example

For example, the case of a differential inequality when we only know the bounds $\underline{f}_i(x_1,\ldots,x_n,t)$ and $\overline{f}_i(x_1,\ldots,x_n,t)$ on $f_i(x_1,\ldots,x_n,t)$ can be described as $\tilde{f}_i(x_1,\ldots,x_n,t) + b_1(t) \cdot \Delta(x_1,\ldots,x_n,t)$, where

$$\tilde{f}_i(x_1,\ldots,x_n,t) \stackrel{def}{=} (\underline{f}_i(x_1,\ldots,x_n,t) + \overline{f}_i(x_1,\ldots,x_n,t))/2$$

$$\Delta(x_1,\ldots,x_n,t) \stackrel{def}{=} (\overline{f}_i(x_1,\ldots,x_n,t) - \underline{f}_i(x_1,\ldots,x_n,t))/2 \text{ and } \mathbf{b}_1(t) = [-1,1].$$

## 3.12. Solving Systems of Ordinary Differential Equations (ODEs) under Interval Uncertainty

For the general system of ODEs, Euler's equations take the form

$$x_i(t + \Delta t) = x_i(t) + \Delta t \cdot f_i(x_1(t),\ldots,x_m(t),t,a_1,\ldots,a_k,b_1(t),\ldots,b_l(t)).$$
Thus, if for every $t$, we keep the set of all possible values of a tuple $(x_1(t),\ldots,x_m(t),a_1,\ldots,a_k)$ then we can use the Euler's equations to get the exact set of possible values of this tuple at the next moment of time.

The reason for exactness is that the values $x_i(t)$ depend only on the previous values $b_j(t - \Delta t)$, $b_j(t - 2\Delta t)$, etc., and not on the current values $b_j(t)$.

To predict the values $x_i(T)$ at a moment $T$, we need $n = T / \Delta t$ iterations.

To update the values, we need to consider all possible combinations of $m + k + l$ variables $x_1(t),\ldots,x_m(t),a_1,\ldots,a_k,b_1(t),\ldots,b_l(t)$; so, to predict the values at moment $T = n \cdot \Delta t$ in the future for a given accuracy $\varepsilon > 0$, we need the running time $n \cdot C^{m+k+l} \sim n^{k+l+m+1}$. This is still polynomial in $n$.

## 3.13. Other Possible Cases When Our Approach Is Efficient

Similar computations can be performed in other cases when we have an iterative process where a fixed finite number of variables is constantly updated.

In such problems, there is an additional factor which speeds up computations. Indeed, in the modern computers, fetching a value from the memory, in general, takes much longer than performing an arithmetic operation. To decrease this time, computers have a hierarchy of memories–from registers from which the access is the fastest, to cash memory (second fastest), etc. Thus, to take full use of the speed of modern processors, we must try our best to keep all the intermediate results in the registers. In the problems in which, at each moment of time, we can only keep (and update) a small current values of the values, we can store all these values in the registers–and thus, get very fast computations (only the input values $x_1, \ldots, x_n$ need to be fetched from slower-to-access memory locations).

## Comment

The discrete version of the class of problems when we have an iterative process where a fixed finite number of variables is constantly updated is described in Suvorov (1976), where efficient algorithms are proposed for solving these discrete problems–such as propositional satisfiability. The use of this idea for interval computations was first described in Chapter 12 of Kreinovich et al. (1997).

## 3.14. Additional Advantage of Our Technique: Possibility to Take Constraints into Account

Traditional formulations of the interval computation problems assume that we can have arbitrary tuples $(x_1, \ldots, x_n)$ as long as $x_i \in \mathbf{x}_i$ for all $i$. In practice, we may have additional constraints on $x_i$. For example, we may know that $x_i$ are observations of a smoothly changing signal at consequent moments of time; in this case, we know that $|x_i - x_{i+1}| \leq \varepsilon$ for some small known $\varepsilon > 0$. Such constraints are easy to take into account in our approach.

For example, if know that $\mathbf{x}_i = [-1, 1]$ for all $i$ and we want to estimate the value of a high-frequency Fourier coefficient $f = x_1 - x_2 + x_3 - x_4 + \ldots - x_{2n}$, then usual interval computations lead to an enclosure $[-2n, 2n]$, while, for small $\varepsilon$, the actual range for the sum $(x_1 - x_2) + (x_3 - x_4) + \ldots$ where each of $n$ differences is bounded by $\varepsilon$, is much narrower: $[-n \cdot \varepsilon, n \cdot \varepsilon]$ (and for $x_i = i \cdot \varepsilon$, these bounds are actually attained).

Computation of $f$ means computing the values $f_k = x_1 - x_2 + \ldots + (-1)^{k+1} \cdot x_k$ for $k = 1, \ldots$ At each stage, we keep the set $\mathbf{s}_k$ of possible values of $(f_k, x_k)$, and use this set to find

$$\mathbf{s}_{k+1} = \{(f_k + (-1)^k \cdot x_{k+1}, x_{k+1}) | (f_k, x_k) \in \mathbf{s}_k \ \& \ | x_k - x_{k+1} | \leq \varepsilon\}.$$

In this approach, when computing $f_{2k}$, we take into account that the value $x_{2k}$ must be $\varepsilon$-close to the value $x_k$ and thus, that we only add $\leq \varepsilon$. Thus, our approach leads to almost exact bounds–modulo implementation accuracy $1 / C$.

In this simplified example, the problem is linear, so we could use linear programming to get the exact range, but set computations work for similar non-linear problems as well.

## 3.15. Toy Example with a Constraint

The problem is to find the range of $r_1 - r_2$ when $\mathbf{r}_1 = [0,1]$, $\mathbf{r}_2 = [0,1]$, and $|r_1 - r_2| \le 0.1$. Here, the actual range is $[-0.1, 0.1]$, but straightforward interval computations return $[0,1] - [0,1] = [-1,1]$

In the new approach, first, we describe the constraint in terms of subboxes (see Figure 7). Next, we compute $\mathbf{R}_1 - \mathbf{R}_2$ for all possible pairs and take the union. The result is $[-0.6, 0.6]$.

If we divide into more pieces, we get the enclosure closer to $[-0.1, 0.1]$.

# 4. POSSIBLE EXTENSION TO P-BOXES AND CLASSES OF PROBABILITY DISTRIBUTIONS

## 4.1. Classes of Probability Distributions and p-Boxes: A Reminder

Often, in addition to the interval $\mathbf{x}_i$ of possible values of the inputs $x_i$, we also have partial information about the probabilities of different values $x_i \in \mathbf{x}_i$. An exact probability distribution can be described, for example, by its cumulative distribution function $F_i(z) = \text{Prob}(x_i \le z)$. In these terms, a partial information means that instead of a single cdf, we have a *class* F of possible cdfs.

A practically important particular case of this partial information is when, for each $z$, instead of the exact value $F(z)$, we know an interval $\mathbf{F}(z) = [\underline{F}(z), \overline{F}(z)]$ of possible values of $F(z)$; such an "interval-valued" cdf is called a *probability box*, or a *p-box*, for short; see, for example, Ferson (2002).

*Figure 7.*

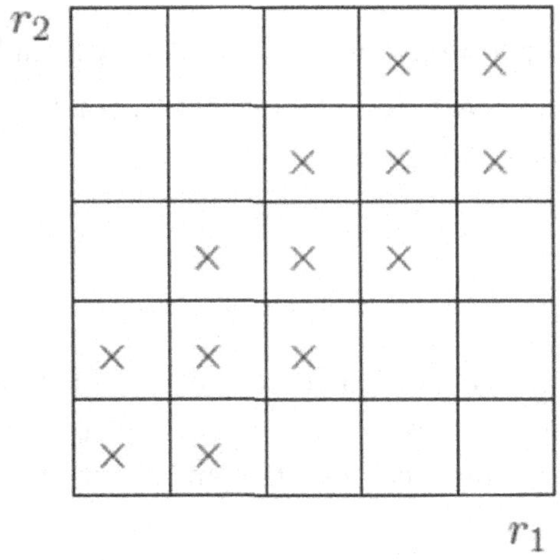

## 4.2. Propagating p-Box Uncertainty via Computations: A Problem

Once we know the classes $F_i$ of possible distributions for $x_i$, and a data processing algorithms $f(x_1, \ldots, x_n)$, we would like to know the class F of possible resulting distributions for $y = f(x_1, \ldots, x_n)$.

## 4.3. Idea

For problems like systems of ODES, it is sufficient to keep, and update, for all $t$, the set of possible joint distributions for the tuple $(x_1(t), \ldots, a_1, \ldots)$.

## 4.4. From Idea to Computer Implementation

We would like to estimate the values with some accuracy $\varepsilon \sim 1 / C$ and the probabilities with the similar accuracy $1 / C$. To describe a distribution with this uncertainty, we divide both the $x$-range and the probability ($p$-) range into $C$ granules, and then describe, for each $x$-granule, which $p$-granules are covered. Thus, we enclose this set into a finite union of p-boxes which assign, to each of $x$-granules, a finite union of $p$-granule intervals.

A general class of distributions can be enclosed in the union of such p-boxes. There are finitely many such assignments, so, for a fixed $C$, we get a finite number of possible elements in the enclosure.

We know how to propagate uncertainty via simple operations with a finite amount of p-boxes (see, e.g., Ferson (2002)), so for ODEs we get a polynomial-time algorithm for computing the resulting p-box for $y$.

## 4.5. For p-Boxes, We Need Further Improvements to Make This Method Practical

Formally, the above method is polynomial-time. However, it is not yet practical beyond very small values of $C$. Indeed, in the case of interval uncertainty, we needed $C^2$ or $C^3$ subboxes. This amount is quite feasible even for $C = 10$.

To describe a p-subbox, we need to attach one of $C$ probability granules to each of $C$ $x$-granules; these are $\sim C^C$ such attachments, so we need $\sim C^C$ subboxes. For $C = 10$, we already get an unrealistic $10^{10}$ increase in computation time.

## ACKNOWLEDGMENT

This work was supported in part by NSF grants HRD-0734825, EAR-0225670, and EIA-0080940, by Texas Department of Transportation Research Project No. 0-5453, by the Japan Advanced Institute of Science and Technology (JAIST) International Joint Research Grant 2006-08, and by the Max Planck

Institut für Mathematik. Many thanks to Sergey P. Shary for valuable suggestions, and to the anonymous referees for their help.

## REFERENCES

Ceberio, M., Ferson, S., Kreinovich, V., Chopra, S., Xiang, G., Murguia, A., & Santillan, J. (2006, February 22-24). How To Take Into Account Dependence Between the Inputs: From Interval Computations to Constraint-Related Set Computations. In *Proceedings of the 2nd Int'l Workshop on Reliable Engineering Computing*. Savannah, Georgia, (pp. 127–154), *Journal of Uncertain Systems, 1*(1), 11–34.

Ferson, S. (2002). *RAMAS Risk Calc 4.0*. Boca Raton, FL: CRC Press.

Ferson, S., Ginzburg, L., Kreinovich, V., Longpré, L., & Aviles, M. (2002). Computing variance for interval data is NP-hard. *ACM SIGACT News, 33*(2), 108–118. doi:10.1145/564585.564604

Jaulin, L., Kieffer, M., Didrit, O., & Walter, E. (2001). *Applied Interval Analysis*. London: Springer.

Klir, G., & Yuan, B. (1995). *Fuzzy sets and fuzzy logic: theory and applications*. Upper Saddle River, NJ: Prentice Hall.

Kreinovich, V., & Lakeyev, A. Rohn, & J., Kahl, P. (1997). Computational complexity and feasibility of data processing and interval computations. Dordrecht, The Netherlands: Kluwer.

Shary, S. P. (2003, July 8-9). Parameter partitioning scheme for interval linear systems with constraints In *Proceedings of the International Workshop on Interval Mathematics and Constraint Propagation Methods* (ICMP'03), (pp. 1–12). Novosibirsk, Akademgorodok, Russia. (in Russian).

Shary, S. P. (2004). Solving tied interval linear systems. [in Russian]. *Siberian Journal of Numerical Mathematics, 7*(4), 363–376.

Suvorov, P. Yu. (1980). On the recognition of the tautological nature of propositional formulas. *J. Sov. Math., 14*, 1556–1562. doi:10.1007/BF01693987

# Chapter 7
# Granular Computing Based Data Mining in the Views of Rough Set and Fuzzy Set

**Guoyin Wang**
*Chongqing University of Posts and Telecommunications, P.R. China*

**Jun Hu**
*Chongqing University of Posts and Telecommunications, P.R. China*

**Qinghua Zhang**
*Chongqing University of Posts and Telecommunications, P.R. China*

**Xianquan Liu**
*Chongqing University of Posts and Telecommunications, P.R. China*

**Jiaqing Zhou**
*Southwest Jiaotong University, P.R. China*

## ABSTRACT

*Granular computing (GRC) is a label of theories, methodologies, techniques, and tools that make use of granules in the process of problem solving. The philosophy of granular computing has appeared in many fields, and it is likely playing a more and more important role in data mining. Rough set theory and fuzzy set theory, as two very important paradigms of granular computing, are often used to process vague information in data mining. In this chapter, based on the opinion of data is also a format for knowledge representation, a new understanding for data mining, domain-oriented data-driven data mining (3DM), is introduced at first. Its key idea is that data mining is a process of knowledge transformation. Then, the relationship of 3DM and GrC, especially from the view of rough set and fuzzy set, is discussed. Finally, some examples are used to illustrate how to solve real problems in data mining using granular computing. Combining rough set theory and fuzzy set theory, a flexible way for processing incomplete information systems is introduced firstly. Then, the uncertainty measure of*

DOI: 10.4018/978-1-60566-324-1.ch007

*covering based rough set is studied by converting a covering into a partition using an equivalence domain relation. Thirdly, a high efficient attribute reduction algorithm is developed by translating set operation of granules into logical operation of bit strings with bitmap technology. Finally, two rule generation algorithms are introduced, and experiment results show that the rule sets generated by these two algorithms are simpler than other similar algorithms.*

## 1. INTRODUCTION

Across a wide variety of fields, data are being collected and accumulated at a dramatic pace. It is necessary to acquire useful knowledge from large quantity of data. Traditionally, data mining is considered as the nontrivial extraction of implicit, previously unknown, and potentially useful information from data. That is to say, knowledge is generated from data. But in our opinion, knowledge is originally existed in the data, but just not understandable for human. In a data mining process, knowledge existed in a database is transformed from data format into another human understandable format like rule.

Granular computing is a label of theories, methodologies, techniques, and tools that make use of granules in the process of problem solving. The philosophy of granular computing has appeared in many fields, and it is likely playing a more and more important role in data mining. Rough set theory and fuzzy set theory are two very important paradigms in granular computing.

In this chapter, a new understanding for data mining, domain-oriented data-driven data mining (3DM), will be proposed. Moreover, we will introduce basic concepts of granular computing and analyze the relationship of granular computing and 3DM. We will also discuss the granular computing based data mining in the views of rough set and fuzzy set, and introduce some applications of granular computing in data mining. In the end, some conclusions are drawn.

## 2. BASIC CONCEPTS OF RELATED THEORIES

### Domain-Oriented Data-Driven Data Mining (3DM)

Data mining (also known as Knowledge Discovery in Databases - KDD) is the nontrivial extraction of implicit, previously unknown, and potentially useful information from data (Frawley, Piatetsky-Shapiro, & Matheus, 1991). It uses machine learning, statistical and visualization techniques to discover knowledge from data and represent it in a form that is easily comprehensible for humans. There are many commonly used techniques in data mining like artificial neural networks, fuzzy sets, rough sets, decision trees, genetic algorithms, nearest neighbor method, statistics based rule induction, linear regression and linear predictive coding, et al.

Unfortunately, most data mining researchers pay much attention to technique problems for developing data mining models and methods, while little to basic issues of data mining. What is data mining? Our answer would be "data mining is a process of knowledge transformation". It is consistent with the process of human knowledge understanding. In our opinion, data is also a format for knowledge representation. The knowledge we mined from data was originally stored in data. Unfortunately, we cannot read, understand, or use it, since we cannot understand data. In a data mining process, we are transforming knowledge from a data format, which is not understandable for human, into another understandable symbolic format like rule, formula, theorem, etc. No new knowledge will be generated in a data mining process. That is, we are transforming knowledge from one format into another format while not producing new knowledge. Based on this understanding for data mining, we could have the knowledge transformation framework for data mining as shown in Figure 1.

From Figure 1, one can find that knowledge could be encoded into natural format, data format, symbolic format, and neural link format. That is, knowledge could be stored in a natural world system, a data system, a symbol system, or a biological neural network system. The knowledge expressed in each form should have some properties, that is, $P_i$'s. There should be some relationship between the knowledge in different formats. In order to keep the knowledge unchanged in a data mining process, properties of the knowledge should remain unchanged during the knowledge transformation process. Otherwise, there should be some mistake in the knowledge transformation process. This information could provide some guideline for designing data mining algorithms. It would also be helpful for us to keep the knowledge in the data format unchanged in a data mining process. Thus, in order to keep the knowledge unchanged in a data mining process, we need to know some properties of the knowledge in data format, and use it to control the data mining process and keep it unchanged. This is the key idea of data-driven data mining.

Many real world data mining tasks, for instance financial data mining in capital markets, are highly constraint-based and domain-oriented. Thus, it targets actionable knowledge discovery, which can afford important grounds for performing appropriate actions. Many data mining researchers proposed domain-driven or user-driven data mining methods for such tasks (Cao, Schurmann, & Zhang, 2005; Dorado, Pedrycz, & Izquierdo, 2005; Kuntz, Guillet, Lehn, & Briand, 2000; Patrick, Palko, Munro, & Zappavigna, 2002; Zhang & Cao, 2006; Zhao & Yao, 2005).

Does data-driven data mining conflicts with user-driven data mining? Our answer is No. Different users could access different data of a database from their own view. If we take data as a format of knowledge representation, a database (data set) could also be taken as a knowledge base. So, different user could find and use different subset of the whole knowledge base for his/her own task. That is, through his/her view, a user could access a subset of knowledge in the data format and transform it from data format into the format he/she required. The knowledge transformation process for each user could still be done in a data-driven manner.

In a domain-driven data mining process, user's interesting, constraint, and prior domain knowledge are very important. An interaction between user and machine is needed. The data mining process might

*Figure 1. Knowledge transformation framework for data mining*

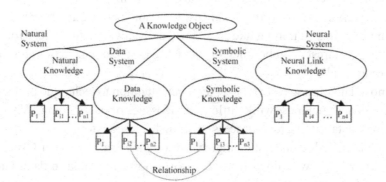

be controlled by a user. In this case, the knowledge source of this mining process includes data and the user, while not just data. So, the domain prior knowledge is also a source for the data mining process. The control of a user to the data mining process could also be taken as a kind of dynamic input of the data mining process. Thus, a data mining process is not only mining knowledge from data, but also from human. Data is not the only source of knowledge. This is so called domain-oriented data-driven data mining (3DM) (Wang, 2006, 2007).

## Granular Computing

Human problem solving involves the perception, abstraction, representation and understanding of real world problems, as well as their solutions. Granular computing (GrC) is an emerging conceptual and computing paradigm of information processing at different levels of granularity. It has been motivated by the increasingly urgent need for intelligent processing for large quantities heterogeneous data (Lin, 1997; Skowron, 2001; Skowron & Stepaniuk, 2001; Yao, 2000; Zadeh, 1997). By taking human knowledge generation as a basic reference, granular computing offers a landmark change from the current machine-centric to human-centric approach for information and knowledge.

The basic ingredients of granular computing are granules such as subsets, classes, objects, clusters, and elements of a universe. The basic notions and principles of granular computing, though under different names, have appeared in many related fields, such as programming, artificial intelligence, divide and conquer, interval computing, quantization, data compression, chunking, cluster analysis, rough set theory, quotient space theory, belief functions, machine learning, databases, and many others (Hu et al., 2005; Zadeh, 1998; Zhang & Lin, 2006). In recent years, granular computing played an important role in bioinformatics, e-Business, security, machine learning, data mining, high-performance computing and wireless mobile computing in terms of efficiency, effectiveness, robustness and structured representation of uncertainty (Bargiela & Pedrycz, 2006; Yao & Yao, 2002, 2002).

Although extensive work has been done on granular computing, different researchers have various understanding on granular computing. Zadeh considers granular computing as a basis for computing with words, i.e., computation with information described in natural language (Zadeh, 1997, 1998, 2006). Yao views granular computing as a triangle: structured thinking in the philosophical perspective, structured problem solving in the methodological perspective and structured information processing in the computational perspective (Yao, 2005, 2007). Bargiella and Pedrycz emphasize essential features of granular computing: the semantical transformation of data in the process of granulation and the non-computational verification of information abstractions (Bargiela & Pedrycz, 2005, 2006; Bargiela, Pedrycz, & Hirota, 2004; Bargiela, Pedrycz, & Tanaka, 2004).

In our opinion, granular computing is a conceptual framework for data mining (Wang, 2006, 2007). The process of data mining is a transformation of knowledge in different granularities. In general, the original data is not understandable for human. That is because data is a representation of knowledge in the finest granularity. However, human is often sensitive with knowledge in a coarser granularity. So, the process of data mining is to transform the knowledge from a finer granularity to a coarser granularity. Moreover, it is variable to different problems how coarse a granularity is suitable. That is to say, the granularity is not the coarser the better, and it relies on the given domain. In addition, the uncertainty of knowledge hiding in data cannot be changed in the process of transformation. This is consistent with the philosophy of domain-oriented data-driven data mining.

## Rough Set Theory and Fuzzy Set Theory

Theories of rough set (Pawlak, 1982) and fuzzy set (Zadeh, 1965), as two important computing paradigm of granular computing, are both generalizations of classical set theory for modeling vagueness and uncertainty, which is a key issue in data mining. In this section, we will introduce rough set theory and fuzzy set theory briefly for the convenience of later discussion.

### Rough Set Theory

The theory of rough set is motivated by practical needs to interpret, characterize, represent, and process indiscernibility of individuals.

A decision information system is defined as $S =< U, A, V, f >$, where $U$ is a non-empty finite set of objects, called universe, $A$ is a non-empty finite set of attributes, $A = C \cup D$, where $C$ is the set of condition attributes and $D$ is the set of decision attributes. With every attribute $a \in A$, $V_a$ denotes the domain of attribute $a$. Each attribute has a determine function $f : U \times A \rightarrow V$.

Given a decision information system $S =< U, A, V, f >$, each subset of attribute $B \subseteq A$ determines an indiscernibility relation $IND(B) = \{(x, y) \mid (x, y) \in U \times U, \forall_{b \in B}(b(x) = b(y))\}$. Obviously, the indiscernibility relation $IND(B)$ is an equivalence relation on $U$ (reflexive, symmetric and transitive). The quotient set of equivalence classes induced by $IND(B)$, denoted by $U / IND(B)$, forms a partition of $U$, and each equivalence class of the quotient set is called an elementary set.

Let $S =< U, A, V, f >$ be a decision information system, for any subset $X \subseteq U$ and indiscernibility relation $IND (B)$, the $B$ lower and upper approximation of $X$ is defined as:

$$B_{-}(X) = \bigcup_{Y_i \in U / IND(B) \wedge Y_i \subseteq X} Y_i$$

$$B^{-}(X) = \bigcup_{Y_i \in U / IND(B) \wedge Y_i \cap X \neq \varnothing} Y_i.$$

If $B_{-}(X) = B^{-}(X)$, $X$ is definable with respect to $IND (B)$. Otherwise, $X$ is rough with respect to $IND (B)$. The lower approximation $B_{-}(X)$ is the union of elementary sets which are subsets of $X$, and the upper approximation $B^{-}(X)$ is the union of elementary sets which have a non-empty intersection with $X$. That is, $B_{-}(X)$ is the greatest definable set contained by $X$, while $B^{-}(X)$ is the least definable set containing $X$.

The lower approximation $B_{-}(X)$ is also called the positive region, the complement of the upper approximation $B^{-}(X)$ is called the negative region, and the difference of the upper approximation $B^{-}(X)$

*Figure 2. The positive region, negative region, and boundary region of a China map*

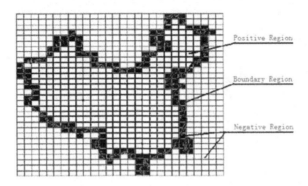

with the lower approximation $B\_(X)$ is called boundary region. The relationship among them is as Figure 2.

Rough set theory provides a systematic method for representing and processing vague concepts caused by indiscernibility in situations with incomplete information or a lack of knowledge. In the past years, many successful applications can be found in various fields, such as process control, economics, medical diagnosis, biochemistry, environmental science, biology, chemistry psychology, conflict analysis, emotion recognition, video retrieval, and so on.

## Fuzzy Set Theory

The notion of fuzzy set theory provides a convenient tool for representing vague concepts by allowing partial memberships.

In classical set theory, an object either belongs to a set or does not. That is:

$$A(x) = \begin{cases} 1 & x \in A \\ 0 & x \notin A \end{cases}, \text{ where } A(x) \text{ is a characteristic function of set } A.$$

An object can partially belong to a set in fuzzy set. Formally, consider a fuzzy set $A$, its domain $D$, and an object $x$. The membership function $\mu$ specifies the degree of membership of $x$ in $A$, such that $\mu_A(x){:}D \to [0, 1]$.

For example, given a real domain $\mathbb{R}$, let $A$ be a fuzzy set of numbers which are much greater than 0, the membership function with regard to $A$ is $\mu_A(x){:}\mathbb{R} \to [0, 1]$:

$$\mu_A(x) = \begin{cases} 0 & , x \leq 0 \\ \dfrac{1}{1+\dfrac{100}{x^2}} & , x > 0 \end{cases}.$$

*Figure 3. The membership function $\mu_A(x)$ of x in fuzzy set A*

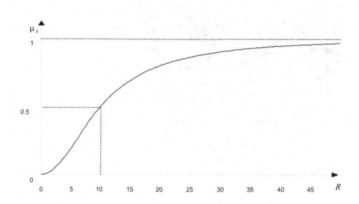

In Figure 3, it means $x$ does not belong to $A$ when $\mu_A(x) = 0$, whereas it means $x$ completely belongs to $A$ when $\mu_A(x) = 1$. Intermediate values represent varying degree of membership, for example, $\mu_A(10) = 0.5$.

The theory of fuzzy set provides an effective means for describing the behavior of systems which are too complex or ill-defined to be accurately analyzed using classical methods and tools. It has shown enormous promise in handling uncertainties to a reasonable extent, particularly in decision-making models under different kinds of risks, subjective judgment, vagueness, and ambiguity. Extensive applications of fuzzy set theory to various fields, e.g., expert systems, control systems, pattern recognition, and image processing, have already been well established.

From the introduction above, we could know that rough set and fuzzy set adopt different methods to address the boundary of an uncertain set. Rough set uses classical precise method, whereas fuzzy set uses imprecise method.

## 3. GRANULAR COMPUTING BASED DATA MINING

In granular computing, there are two important issues. One is the construction of granules, and the other is the computation with granules. Rough set uses equivalence relation to partition the universe into a granular space. However, it is difficult to define an equivalence relation in an incomplete information system. So, it is necessary to extend the classical rough set theory to non-equivalence relation. Different from an equivalence relation, a non-equivalence relation induces a covering of the universe. Therefore, studying the covering based granular computing is significant. In addition, developing high efficient algorithms and increasing the generalization ability of knowledge are another two important issues in data mining. In this section, we discuss these problems.

## Two Granular Models for Processing Incomplete Information Systems

Generally, the decision table to be processed is without any missing values or unknown values with each attribute, and many traditional data mining methods can only be applied to these cases, such as the classical rough set theory. However, due to inaccurate data measuring, inadequate comprehension or the limitation of acquiring data and so on, information systems with missing values or unknown values, called incomplete information systems, are actually unavoidable in knowledge acquisition (An, Shen, & Wang, 2003; Huang, Wang, & Wu, 2004; Liu, Hu, Jia, & Shi, 2004). In order to process incomplete information systems with rough set theory, two kinds of approaches were developed (Kryszkiewicz, 1999; Wang, 2001). One is filling the missing data, and then using the classical rough set theory to process it, but it may change the original information. The other is extending the classical rough set model to process incomplete information systems directly. Based on this idea, several extended rough set models are developed. Kryszkiewicz developed an extension based on tolerance relation (Kryszkiewicz, 1998, 1999), Slowinski developed an extension based on similarity relation (Slowinski & Vsnderpooten, 2000). Wang developed an extension based on limited tolerance relation (Wang, 2002). Wang find that both tolerance relation and similarity relation are two extremes for extensions, the condition of tolerance relation is too loose and that of similarity relation is too tight, and that of limited tolerance relation is moderate. In this section, according to the characteristics of incomplete information systems, two granular computing methods for incomplete information systems are introduced.

### Some Extended Models of Classical Rough Set Theory

For convenience of discussion, some typical extensions of rough set for incomplete information systems are introduced at first. We use * to denote unknown values or missing values.

Given an incomplete information system $S = < U, A, V, f >$. An attribute set $B$ is a subset of $A$, then a tolerance relation $T$ is defined as (Kryszkiewicz, 1998, 1999):

$$T = \{(x, y) \mid x \in U \wedge y \in U \wedge \forall_{c_j \in B} (c_j(x) = c_j(y) \vee c_j(x) = * \vee c_j(y) = *)\}$$

$T$ is reflexive and symmetric, but not always transitive. So, a tolerance relation $T$ is not an equivalence relation. The tolerance class is defined as:

$$I_B^T(x) = \{y \mid y \in U \wedge (x, y) \in T\}.$$

**Then**, the lower approximation $X_B^T$ and upper approximation $X_T^B$ of an object set $X$ with respect to an attribute set $B$ are defined as (Wang, 2001):

$$X_B^T = \{x \mid x \in U \wedge I_B^T(x) \subseteq X\},$$

$$X_T^B = \{x \mid x \in U \wedge I_B^T(x) \cap X \neq \varnothing\}.$$

Given an incomplete information system $S = <U, A, V, f>$. An attribute set $B$ is a subset of $A$, then a similarity relation $S$ is defined as(Slowinski & Vsnderpooten, 2000):

$$S = \{(x, y) \mid x \in U \wedge y \in U \wedge \forall_{c_j \in B}(c_j(x) = * \vee c_j(x) = c_j(y))\}$$

$S$ is reflexive and transitive, but not always symmetric. So, a similarity relation $S$ is not an equivalence relation. For an object $x \in U$, two sets for this extension of rough set theory are defined as:

$$R_B(x) = \{y \mid y \in U \wedge (y, x) \in S\},$$

$$R_B^{-1}(x) = \{y \mid y \in U \wedge (x, y) \in S\}.$$

**Then**, the lower approximation $X_B^S$ and upper approximation $X_S^B$ of an object set $X$ with respect to an attribute set $B$ are defined as(Wang, 2001):

$$X_B^S = \{x \mid x \in U \wedge R_B^{-1}(x) \subseteq X\},$$

$$X_S^B = \{x \mid x \in U \wedge R_B^{-1}(x) \cap X \neq \varnothing\}.$$

Given an incomplete information system $S = <U, A, V, f>$. An attribute set $B$ is a subset of $A$, then a limited tolerance relation $L$ is defined as (Wang, 2002):

$$L = \{(x, y) \mid x \in U \wedge y \in U \wedge (\forall_{b \in B}(b(x) = b(y) = *)$$
$$\vee((P_B(x) \cap P_B(y) \neq \varnothing) \wedge \forall_{b \in B}((b(x) \neq * \wedge b(y)$$

$$\neq *) \rightarrow (b(x) = b(y)))), \text{ where } P_B(x) = \{b \mid b \in B \wedge b(x) \neq *\}.$$

$L$ is reflexive and symmetric, but not always transitive. So, a limited tolerance relation $L$ is not an equivalence relation. The limited tolerance class $I_B^L(x)$ is defined as:

$$I_B^L(x) = \{y \mid y \in U \wedge (x, y) \in L\}.$$

**Then**, the lower approximation $X_B^L$ and upper approximation $X_L^B$ of an object set $X$ with respect to an attribute set $B$ are defined as(Wang, 2002):

$$X_B^L = \{x \mid x \in U \wedge I_B^L(x) \subseteq X\},$$

$$X_L^B = \{x \mid x \in U \wedge I_B^L(x) \cap X \neq \varnothing\}.$$

Given two sets $B \subseteq A$ and $X \subseteq U$. If $\forall_{x \in U}(P_B(x) \neq \varnothing)$, then $X_B^T \subseteq X_B^L \subseteq X_B^S$ and $X_S^B \subseteq X_L^B \subseteq X_T^B$ (Wang, 2002).

## Granular Computing Based on Tolerance Relation

For an object $x$ of an information system, let $a(x)$ be its value on attribute $a$, we can define the following rough logic formulas:

1. $(a,v)$ is an atomic formula. All atomic formulas are formula.
2. if $\phi$ and $\chi$ are both atomic formulas, then $\neg\phi$, $\phi \wedge \chi$, $\phi \vee \chi$, $\phi \rightarrow \chi$, $\phi \leftrightarrow \chi$ are also formulas.
3. Formulas resulted by using logic function $\neg, \wedge, \vee, \rightarrow, \leftrightarrow$ on formulas defined in (1) and (2) in finite steps are also formulas.

According to the above definition, in the extension of rough set theory based on tolerance relation, objects with same value or "*" on an attribute can constitute a set. Therefore, we can define granules with this set.

Let $f^{-1}(a,v)$ be a set of objects, $\forall_{x \in f^{-1}(a,v)}(a(x) = v \vee a(x) = *)$. Then, we can define a granule: $Gr^* = ((a,v), f^{-1}(a,v))$, where $(a,v)$ is called as the syntax of granular $Gr^*$ and $Gr^*$ an atomic granule. Suppose $\varphi$ be a logic combination of atomic formulas, $f^{-1}(\varphi)$ be an object set, and all the objects in $f^{-1}(\varphi)$ satisfy logic combination $\varphi$. Granule $Gr^* = (\varphi, f^{-1}(\varphi))$ is called a combination granular.

$gs(Gr^*)$ is a mapping function from granules to object sets,

$$\forall_{Gr^*}(Gr^* = (\varphi, f^{-1}(\varphi)) \Rightarrow gs(Gr^*) = f^{-1}(\varphi)) \text{ (Wang, Hu, Huang, \& Wu, 2005)}.$$

### Rules for Granular Computing

Suppose $Gr_1^* = (\varphi, f^{-1}(\varphi))$ and $Gr_2^* = (\psi, f^{-1}(\psi))$ be two granules, according to the five logic conjunctions in classic logic theory, the rules of granular computing can be defined as follows (Wang et al., 2005):

1. $\neg Gr_1^* = \neg(\varphi, f^{-1}(\varphi)) = (\neg\varphi, f^{-1}(\neg\varphi))$
2. $Gr_1^* \wedge Gr_2^* = (\varphi \wedge \psi, f^{-1}(\varphi \wedge \psi))$
3. $Gr_1^* \vee Gr_2^* = (\varphi \vee \psi, f^{-1}(\varphi \vee \psi))$

4.  $Gr_1^* \rightarrow Gr_2^* = (\varphi \rightarrow \psi, f^{-1}(\varphi) \subseteq f^{-1}(\psi))$

5.  $Gr_1^* \leftrightarrow Gr_2^* = (\varphi \leftrightarrow \psi, f^{-1}(\varphi) = f^{-1}(\psi))$

Here, the logic conjunction $\rightarrow$ is not an implication relation between granules, but an inclusion relation between granules.

In order to generate knowledge with granular computing theory, we should have enough granules from an incomplete information system. These granules should contain enough information about the original incomplete information system. That is, we need to decompose the original incomplete information system into granules.

Given an incomplete information system $S = <U, A, V, f>$, suppose $GrS$ be a set of granules. $\forall Gr^* \in GrS$, $Gr^* = (\varphi, f^{-1}(\varphi))$, where $\varphi = (a_1, v_1) \wedge (a_2, v_2) \wedge \ldots \wedge (a_m, v_m)$, $(m = |C|, v_i \neq *)$, and $\forall_{x \in U} \exists_{Gr^*} (x \in gs(Gr^*))$. We call this kind of granule sets as a granule space of the original information system $S$.

An algorithm for generating a granular space for an incomplete information system could be developed as follows. For an object $x(x \in U)$, we construct granule $Gr^* (x \in gs(Gr^*))$.

**Algorithm 1: Granular Space Generation for Incomplete Information Systems (Wang et al., 2005)**

**Input:** An incomplete information system $S$
**Output:** A granular space $GrS$ of $S$

- **Step1:** Let $GrS = \varnothing$, $m = |C|$, $n = |U|$, $i = 1$.
- **Step2:** For any object $x(x \in U)$, calculate its tolerance class $I_c^T(x)$.

- **Step3:** While ($i < n$)
  - Let $x$ be the $i$-th object in $U$.
  - If $\forall_{a_i \in C}(a_i(x) \neq *)$, then we construct a granule $Gr^* = (\varphi, f^{-1}(\varphi))$, where $\varphi = (a_1, v_1) \wedge (a_2, v_2) \wedge \ldots \wedge (a_m, v_m)$, $(m = |C|)$. $GrS = \cup \{Gr^*\}$, go to step 4.
  - If the value of $x$ are "*" on attribute $a_{i1}, a_{i2}, \ldots, a_{ik}$. Firstly, we find objects with non-null values on attribute $a_{i1}$ from the tolerance class $I_c^T(x)$. The values of these objects on attribute $a_{i1}$ construct a set $v_1$. For attributes $a_{i2}, \ldots, a_{ik}$, we can get similar sets $v_2, \ldots, v_k$ as $v_1$. The non-null values of $x$ and all combination of values from $v_1, v_2, \ldots, v_k$ are used to construct granules $Gr_1^*, Gr_2^*, \ldots, Gr_l^*$ $(l = \prod_{i=1}^{k} w_i, |v_1| = w_1, |v_2| = w_2, \ldots, |v_k| = w_k)$ $GrS = GrS \cup \{Gr_1^*\}$, $GrS = GrS \cup \{Gr_2^*\}, \ldots, GrS = GrS \cup \{Gr_l^*\}$

- ∘     If $v_i = \varnothing$, we let $v_i = \{p\}$ $(p \neq *)$, where $p$ is any value in attribute $v_i$.

- ∘     $i = i+1$.

Algorithm 1 could be illustrated with the following example.

## Example 1

An incomplete information table is shown in Table 1. Its object set is $U = \{x_1, x_2, ..., x_{12}\}$, the condition attribute set is $C = \{a_1, a_2, a_3, a_4\}$, and $D = \{d\}$ is the decision attribute.

For simplification, we only construct granules with object $x_1$ and $x_4$. All the attribute values of $x_1$ are not "*", so we can construct a granular $Gr^* = (\varphi, f^{-1}(\varphi))$, where

$$\varphi = (a_1, 3) \wedge (a_2, 2) \wedge (a_3, 1) \wedge (a_4, 0).$$

The values of $x_4$ are "*" on attribute $a_1$ and $a_3$, and $v_1 = \{1, 3\}$, $v_3 = \{1\}$. So, we can construct two granules from $x_4$, and their syntax are

$$\varphi = (a_1, 1) \wedge (a_2, 2) \wedge (a_3, 1) \wedge (a_4, 1) \text{ and } \psi = (a_1, 3) \wedge (a_2, 2) \wedge (a_3, 1) \wedge (a_4, 1).$$

## Granular Computing Based on Fuzzy-Clustering

Given an incomplete information system $S = \langle U, A, V, f \rangle$. Assuming $x$ and $y$ are two objects of $U$, we define a set $\delta(x, y)$ and $\Delta(x, y)$ as follows (Zhang, Wang, Hu, & Liu, 2006):

$$\delta(x, y) = \{a \mid a \in C \wedge a(x) \neq * \wedge a(y) \neq * \wedge a(x) = a(y)\}$$

$$\Delta(x, y) = \{a \mid a \in C \wedge a(x) \neq * \wedge a(y) \neq * \wedge a(x) \neq a(y)\}$$

Based on $\delta(x, y)$ and $\Delta(x, y)$, we define the similarity between $x_i$ and $x_j$, which are objects of $U$, as follows.

*Table 1. Incomplete information table*

| A | $x_1$ | $x_2$ | $x_3$ | $x_4$ | $x_5$ | $x_6$ | $x_7$ | $x_8$ | $x_9$ | $x_{10}$ | $x_{11}$ | $x_{12}$ |
|---|---|---|---|---|---|---|---|---|---|---|---|---|
| $a_1$ | 3 | 2 | 2 | * | * | 2 | 3 | * | 3 | 1 | * | 3 |
| $a_2$ | 2 | 3 | 3 | 2 | 2 | 3 | * | 0 | 2 | * | 2 | 2 |
| $a_3$ | 1 | 2 | 2 | * | * | 2 | * | 0 | 1 | * | * | 1 |
| $a_4$ | 0 | 0 | 0 | 1 | 1 | 1 | 3 | * | 3 | * | * | * |
| d | φ | φ | ψ | φ | ψ | ψ | φ | ψ | ψ | φ | ψ | φ |

$$s(x_i, x_j) = \begin{cases} 0 & \Delta(x_i, x_j) \neq \varnothing \\ 1 & i = j \\ |\delta(x_i, x_j)| / |A| & others \end{cases}$$

According to the formula $s(x_i, x_j)$, from the Example 1, we have $s(x_1, x_1) = 1$, $s(x_1, x_2) = 0$, ..., $s(x_1, x_{12}) = 3/4$, $s(x_2, x_1) = 0$, $s(x_2, x_2) = 1$, $s(x_2, x_3) = 1$, ..., $s(x_2, x_{12}) = 0$, ..., $s(x_{12}, x_1) = 3/4$, $s(x_{12}, x_2) = 0$, ..., $s(x_{12}, x_{11}) = 1/4$ and $s(x_{12}, x_{12}) = 1$. Then we get a fuzzy relation matrix $M = (r_{ij})_{m \times n}$, where $r_{ij} = s(x_i, x_j)$. From the definition of similarity, we can find that the matrix $M$ is reflexive and symmetric. We can have the transitive-closure matrix $\hat{M}$ of $M$. We use $\hat{M}_\lambda$ denoting $\lambda$-cut matrix of $\hat{M}$. When $\lambda = 0.25$, we have $\hat{M}_{0.25}$.

With fuzzy clustering we can divide the object set $U$ according to different $\lambda - cut$ sets. when $\lambda = 0.25$, we have a partition of $U$: $\{x_1, x_4, x_5, x_7, x_9, x_{11}, x_{12}\}, \{x_2, x_3\}, \{x_6\}, \{x_8\}, \{x_{10}\}$ For the convenience of description, this partition is denoted as $U / ind(C)_{0.25}$. In addition, we have a partition

$U / ind(D) = \{\{x_1, x_2, x_4, x_7, x_{10}, x_{12}\}, \{x_3, x_5, x_6, x_8, x_9, x_{11}\}\}$ induced by the decision attribute $D$.

So we have the positive region $POS_C(D)_{0.25} = \{x_6, x_8, x_{10}\}$ according to classical rough set theory, where $\varphi_C^J(\lambda = 0.25) = \{x_{10}\}$ $\varphi_J^C(\lambda = 0.25) = \{x_1, x_2, x_3, x_4, x_5, x_7, x_9, x_{10}, x_{12}\}$ $\psi_C^J(\lambda = 0.25) = \{x_6, x_8\}$ $\psi_J^C(\lambda = 0.25) = \{x_1, x_2, x_3, x_4, x_5, x_6, x_7, x_8, x_9, x_{11}, x_{12}\}$

$$M = \begin{bmatrix} 1 & 0 & 0 & 0 & 0 & 0 & 0 & 0 & 0 & 0 & \frac{1}{4} & \frac{3}{4} \\ 0 & 1 & 1 & 0 & 0 & 0 & 0 & 0 & 0 & 0 & 0 & 0 \\ 0 & 1 & 1 & 0 & 0 & 0 & 0 & 0 & 0 & 0 & 0 & 0 \\ 0 & 0 & 0 & 1 & \frac{1}{2} & 0 & 0 & 0 & 0 & 0 & \frac{1}{4} & \frac{1}{4} \\ 0 & 0 & 0 & \frac{1}{2} & 1 & 0 & 0 & 0 & 0 & 0 & \frac{1}{4} & \frac{1}{4} \\ 0 & 0 & 0 & 0 & 0 & 1 & 0 & 0 & 0 & 0 & 0 & 0 \\ 0 & 0 & 0 & 0 & 0 & 0 & 1 & 0 & \frac{1}{2} & 0 & 0 & \frac{1}{4} \\ 0 & 0 & 0 & 0 & 0 & 0 & 0 & 1 & 0 & 0 & 0 & 0 \\ 0 & 0 & 0 & 0 & 0 & 0 & \frac{1}{2} & 0 & 1 & 0 & \frac{1}{4} & \frac{3}{4} \\ 0 & 0 & 0 & 0 & 0 & 0 & 0 & 0 & 0 & 1 & 0 & 0 \\ \frac{1}{4} & 0 & 0 & \frac{1}{4} & \frac{1}{4} & 0 & 0 & 0 & \frac{1}{4} & 0 & 1 & \frac{1}{4} \\ \frac{3}{4} & 0 & 0 & \frac{1}{4} & \frac{1}{4} & 0 & \frac{1}{4} & 0 & \frac{3}{4} & 0 & \frac{1}{4} & 1 \end{bmatrix}$$

$$\hat{M} = \begin{bmatrix} 1 & 0 & 0 & \frac{1}{4} & \frac{1}{4} & 0 & \frac{1}{2} & 0 & \frac{3}{4} & 0 & \frac{1}{4} & \frac{3}{4} \\ 0 & 1 & 1 & 0 & 0 & 0 & 0 & 0 & 0 & 0 & 0 & 0 \\ 0 & 1 & 1 & 0 & 0 & 0 & 0 & 0 & 0 & 0 & 0 & 0 \\ \frac{1}{4} & 0 & 0 & 1 & \frac{1}{2} & 0 & \frac{1}{4} & 0 & \frac{1}{4} & 0 & \frac{1}{4} & \frac{1}{4} \\ \frac{1}{4} & 0 & 0 & \frac{1}{2} & 1 & 0 & \frac{1}{4} & 0 & \frac{1}{4} & 0 & \frac{1}{4} & \frac{1}{4} \\ 0 & 0 & 0 & 0 & 0 & 1 & 0 & 0 & 0 & 0 & 0 & 0 \\ \frac{1}{2} & 0 & 0 & \frac{1}{4} & \frac{1}{4} & 0 & 1 & 0 & \frac{1}{2} & 0 & \frac{1}{4} & \frac{1}{2} \\ 0 & 0 & 0 & 0 & 0 & 0 & 0 & 1 & 0 & 0 & 0 & 0 \\ \frac{3}{4} & 0 & 0 & \frac{1}{4} & \frac{1}{4} & 0 & \frac{1}{2} & 0 & 1 & 0 & \frac{1}{4} & \frac{3}{4} \\ 0 & 0 & 0 & 0 & 0 & 0 & 0 & 0 & 0 & 1 & 0 & 0 \\ \frac{1}{4} & 0 & 0 & \frac{1}{4} & \frac{1}{4} & 0 & \frac{1}{4} & 0 & \frac{1}{4} & 0 & 1 & \frac{1}{4} \\ \frac{3}{4} & 0 & 0 & \frac{1}{4} & \frac{1}{4} & 0 & \frac{1}{2} & 0 & \frac{3}{4} & 0 & \frac{1}{4} & 1 \end{bmatrix}$$

$$
\hat{M}_{0.25} =
\begin{bmatrix}
1 & 0 & 0 & 1 & 1 & 0 & 1 & 0 & 1 & 0 & 1 & 1 \\
0 & 1 & 1 & 0 & 0 & 0 & 0 & 0 & 0 & 0 & 0 & 0 \\
0 & 1 & 1 & 0 & 0 & 0 & 0 & 0 & 0 & 0 & 0 & 0 \\
1 & 0 & 0 & 1 & 1 & 0 & 1 & 0 & 1 & 0 & 1 & 1 \\
1 & 0 & 0 & 1 & 1 & 0 & 1 & 0 & 1 & 0 & 1 & 1 \\
0 & 0 & 0 & 0 & 0 & 1 & 0 & 0 & 0 & 0 & 0 & 0 \\
1 & 0 & 0 & 1 & 1 & 0 & 1 & 0 & 1 & 0 & 1 & 1 \\
0 & 0 & 0 & 0 & 0 & 0 & 0 & 1 & 0 & 0 & 0 & 0 \\
1 & 0 & 0 & 1 & 1 & 0 & 1 & 0 & 1 & 0 & 1 & 1 \\
0 & 0 & 0 & 0 & 0 & 0 & 0 & 0 & 0 & 1 & 0 & 0 \\
1 & 0 & 0 & 1 & 1 & 0 & 1 & 0 & 1 & 0 & 1 & 1 \\
1 & 0 & 0 & 1 & 1 & 0 & 1 & 0 & 1 & 0 & 1 & 1
\end{bmatrix}
$$

Using the same method, when $\lambda = 0.5$, we have the positive region $POS_C(D)_{0.5} = \{x_6,\ x_8, x_{10}, x_{11}\}$, where

$$\varphi_C^J(\lambda = 0.5) = \{x_{10}\}$$

$$\varphi_J^C(\lambda = 0.5) = \{x_1, x_2, x_3, x_4, x_5, x_7, x_9, x_{10}, x_{12}\}$$

$$\psi_C^J(\lambda = 0.5) = \{x_6, x_8, x_{11}\}$$

$$\psi_J^C(\lambda = 0.5) = \{x_1, x_2, x_3, x_4, x_5, x_6, x_7, x_8, x_9, x_{11}, x_{12}\}$$

When $\lambda = 0.75$, we have the positive region $POS_C(D)_{0.75} = \{x_6, x_7, x_8, x_{10}, x_{11}\}$, where

$$\varphi_C^J(\lambda = 0.75) = \{x_7, x_{10}\}$$

$$\varphi_J^C(\lambda = 0.75) = \{x_1, x_2, x_3, x_4, x_5, x_7, x_9, x_{10}, x_{12}\}$$

$$\psi_C^J(\lambda = 0.75) = \{x_6, x_8, x_{11}\}$$

$$\psi_J^C(\lambda = 0.75) = \{x_1, x_2, x_3, x_4, x_5, x_6, x_8, x_9, x_{11}, x_{12}\}$$

Obviously,

$$POS_C(D)_{0.75} \supseteq POS_C(D)_{0.5} \supseteq POS_C(D)_{0.25}$$

$$\varphi_J^C(\lambda = 0.75) \subseteq \varphi_J^C(\lambda = 0.5) \subseteq \varphi_J^C(\lambda = 0.25)$$

and

$$\psi_J^C(\lambda = 0.75) \subseteq \psi_J^C(\lambda = 0.5) \subseteq \psi_J^C(\lambda = 0.25)$$

It is not difficult to draw a conclusion that the partition $U \,/\, IND(C)_\lambda$ becomes more and more finer with the increasing of $\lambda$. That is, if $1 \ge \lambda_1 \ge \lambda_2 > 0$, then $POS_C(D)_{\lambda_1} \supseteq POS_C(D)_{\lambda_2}$

The main idea of this method is constructing equivalent relation by fuzzy-clustering, and then constructing the corresponding upper approximation and lower approximation with the classical rough set theory. From the introduction above, we can find that this method combines the advantages of fuzzy set and rough set, and it is more variable by selecting different $\lambda$ than other methods processing incomplete information systems in real world problems.

In this section, two granular computing methods for processing incomplete information system are introduced. One is based on tolerance relation for processing incomplete information system, and the other is based on fuzzy-clustering transforming nonequivalence relation into equivalence relation.

## Uncertainty in Covering Based Granular Computing

Granulation of a universe involves grouping of similar elements into granules to form coarse-grained views of the universe. Approximation of concept deals with the descriptions of concepts using granules. Rough set theory provides a method to approximate an unknown concept by a given knowledge base. The classical rough set theory is based on a partition of the universe. However, the knowledge base is often a covering of the universe. So, it is necessary to study the covering based granular computing, and its relationship with the partition based granular computing. In this section, we will mainly discuss the uncertainty measure in covering based rough set and its relationship with the uncertainty measure of classical rough set, or call as Pawlak's rough set.

### Uncertainty Measure of Pawlak's Rough Set

Let $U$ denote a finite and non-empty set called the universe, and let $R \subseteq U \times U$ denote an equivalence relation on $U$. The pair $(U, R)$ is called an approximation space. If two elements $x$, $y$ in $U$ belong to the same equivalence class, we say that they are indistinguishable. The equivalence relation $R$ partitions the set $U$ into disjoint subsets. This partition of the universe is called the quotient set induced by $R$ and is denoted by $U \,/\, R$. Each equivalence class may be viewed as a granule consisting of indistinguishable elements. It is also referred to as an equivalence granule. The granulation structure induced by an equivalence relation is a partition of the universe.

Let $(U, R)$ be an approximation space, $X$ be an arbitrary concept, i.e., a subset of $U$. Then the accuracy of $X$ in $(U, R)$ is defined as:

$$\alpha(X) = \frac{|R_{-}(X)|}{|R^{-}(X)|}.$$

Where $|.|$ denotes the cardinality of a set. For the empty set $\varnothing$, we define $\alpha(\varnothing) = 1$. The accuracy has the following properties:

1.   $0 \leq \alpha(X) \leq 1$;

2.   $\alpha(X) = 0$, iff the lower approximation of $X$ is empty;

3.   $\alpha(X) = 1$, iff $X$ is exact in $(U, R)$.

The roughness of knowledge is defined based on indiscernibility relation and inclusion degree, but its intension is not clear. For this reason, information entropy was applied into rough set theory to measure the roughness of knowledge by Miao (Miao & Wang, 1998).

Let $(U, R)$ be an approximation space. A measure of uncertainty in rough set theory is defined by(Miao & Wang, 1998):

$$H(R) = -\sum_{Y_i \in U/R} \frac{|Y_i|}{|U|} \log_2 \frac{|Y_i|}{|U|}.$$

Let $R$ and $S$ be two equivalence relations on $U$. If $\forall_{X_i \in U/R}(\exists_{Y_j \in U/S}(X_i \subseteq Y_j))$, then we say $R$ is coarser than $S$, denoted by $R \preceq S$. Especially, if $R \preceq S$, and $R \neq S$, then we say $R$ is strictly coarser than $S$, denoted by $R \prec S$.

Let $U$ be a universe, $R$ and $S$ be two equivalence relations on $U$. If $R \preceq S$, then $H(R) \geq H(S)$. Especially, if $R \prec S$, then $H(R) > H(S)$ (Miao & Wang, 1998).

**Example 2**
Let $U = \{x_1, x_2, x_3\}$, $R$ and $S$ be two equivalence relations on $U$, $U/R = \{\{x_1\}, \{x_2\}, \{x_3\}\}$ and $U/S = \{\{x_1, x_2\}, \{x_3\}\}$ be the quotient sets induced by $R$ and $S$ respectively. According the introduction above, one can find that $R$ is strictly coarser than $S$. In addition, $H(R) = \log_2 3$ and $H(S) = \log_2 3 - 2/3$, namely $H(R) > H(S)$. This is consistent with the above conclusion.

## Uncertainty Measure of Covering Based Rough Set

From the above introduction, we can see that Pawlak's rough set theory is based on an equivalence relation, which is too restrictive for many real problems, such as knowledge discovering from incomplete information system. In order to apply rough set in these fields, it is necessary to extend the classical rough set model. Therefore, some extended rough set models were proposed in recent years. Covering based rough sets is an important one of them (Bonikowski, Bryniarski, & Wybraniec, 1998; Mordeson, 2001; Zhu & Wang, 2003).

Let $U$ be a non-empty set, $C$ be a covering of $U$. We call the ordered pair $(U, C)$ a covering approximation space.

Let $(U, C)$ be a covering approximation space, $x$ an object of $U$, then the set family $Md(x) = \{K \in C \mid x \in K \wedge \forall S \in C(x \in S \wedge S \subseteq K \Rightarrow K = S)\}$ is called the minimal description of $x$ (Bonikowski et al., 1998).

The purpose of the minimal description concept is to describe an object using the essential characteristics related to this object, not all the characteristics for this object.

Let $(U, C)$ be a covering approximation space, for a set $X \subseteq U$, then $C_*(X)$ is called the covering lower approximation of the set $X$, and $C^*(X)$ is called the covering upper approximation of the set $X$. Their definitions are as follows (Bonikowski et al., 1998):

$$C_*(X) = \cup\{K \in C \mid K \subseteq X\}, \ C^*(X) = C_*(X) \cup \{K \in Md(x) \mid x \in X - C_*(X)\}$$

If $C_*(X) = C^*(X)$, then $X$ is called relatively exact to $C$, or definable, otherwise $X$ is called relatively inexact to $C$, or indefinable.

Let $C_1$ and $C_2$ be two coverings of the universe $U = \{x_1, x_2, ..., x_n\}$ and $r(C_1) = \{c_{11}, c_{12}, ..., c_{1p}\}$, $r(C_2) = \{c_{21}, c_{22}, ..., c_{2q}\}$ are the reductions of the covering $C_1$ and $C_2$ respectively. If for every $x_i \in U$, $x_i \in C_{1l}(1 \leq l \leq p)$, and $x_i \in C_{2l'}(1 \leq l' \leq q)$, $C_{1l} \subseteq C_{2l'}$ holds, then $r(C_1)$ is finer than $r(C_2)$, denoted by $r(C_1) \subseteq r(C_2)$. Especially, if $r(C_1) \subseteq r(C_2)$, and $r(C_1) \neq r(C_2)$ then $r(C_1)$ is called strictly finer than $r(C_2)$, denoted by $r(C_1) \subset r(C_2)$ (Huang, He, & Zhou, 2004).

**Example 3**

Let $U = \{x_1, x_2, x_3, x_4\}$ be a universe, $C = \{K_1, K_2, K_3\}$ be a covering of the universe, where $K_1 = \{x_1\}$, $K_2 = \{x_1, x_2, x_3\}$ and $K_3 = \{x_3, x_4\}$. In the covering approximation space, $x_1$ belongs to $K_1$ and $K_2$. Since $K_1 \subseteq K_2$, $Md(x_1) = \{K_1\}$. In the same way, we can get $Md(x_2) = \{K_2\}$, $Md(x_3) = \{K_2, K_3\}$, and $Md(x_4) = \{K_3\}$. For a subset $X = \{x_1, x_4\}$ of the universe, $C_*(X) = \{x_1\}$, and $C^*(X) = \{x_1, x_3, x_4\}$.

## Relationship of Covering Approximation Space and Its Transformed Pawlak's Approximation Space

Let $C$ be a covering of $U$. For any $x, y \in U$, $\bigcap\limits_{x \in A \wedge A \in C} A = \bigcap\limits_{y \in B \wedge B \in C} B$, if and only if $(x, y) \in \theta$, where $\theta$ is a binary relation on $U$, called equal domain relation on $U$ induced by $C$, or equal domain relation for short (Zhou, Zhang, & Chen, 2004).

Let $C$ be a covering of $U$. The equal domain relation $\theta$ on $U$ induced by $C$ is an equivalence relation. As we know, an equivalence relation on a universe can induce a partition. Since an equal domain relation is an equivalence relation, we can use it to convert a covering into a partition.

Let $C$ be a covering of $U$, $\theta$ be an equal domain relation on $U$ induced by $C$. For any set $X \subseteq U$, $\underline{\theta}(X)$ is called the general lower approximation, and $\overline{\theta}(X)$ is called the general upper approximation (Zhou et al., 2004). They are defined as follows:

$$\underline{\theta}(X) = \cup \{Y_i \in U / \theta \mid Y_i \subseteq X\},$$

$$\overline{\theta}(X) = \cup \{Y_i \in U / \theta \mid Y_i \cap X \neq \varnothing\}.$$

Let $C$ be a covering of $U$, $\theta$ be an equal domain relation on $U$ induced by $C$, $U / \theta = \{Y_1, Y_2, ..., Y_n\}$ be the partition induced by $\theta$, then the general rough entropy of $C$ can be defined as follows (Hu, Wang, & Zhang, 2006):

$$GE(C) = -\sum_{k=1}^{n} \frac{|Y_k|}{|U|} \log_2 \frac{|Y_k|}{|U|}.$$

Let $C_1$, $C_2$ be two coverings of $U$, $\theta_1$ and $\theta_2$ be the equal domain relations on $U$ induced by $C_1$ and $C_2$ respectively. If $r(C_1) \subseteq r(C_2)$, then $\theta_1 \preceq \theta_2$ (Hu et al., 2006).

**Example 4.**
Let $U = \{x_1, x_2, x_3, x_4\}$ be a universe, $C_1$ and $C_2$ be two coverings of $U$, where

$$C_1 = \{\{x_1, x_2,\}, \{x_3, x_4\}\}, \ C_2 = \{\{x_1, x_2, x_3, x_4\}, \{x_2\}, \{x_3\}, \{x_4\}, \{x_2, x_4\}, \{x_3, x_4\}\}$$

$\theta_1$ and $\theta_2$ be the equal domain relations on $U$ induced by $C_1$ and $C_2$ respectively. Then $U / \theta_1 = C_1$, $U / \theta_2 = \{\{x_1\}, \{x_2\}, \{x_3\}, \{x_4\}\}$. Thus, $\theta_2 \prec \theta_1$ holds, while $r(C_2) \not\subseteq r(C_1)$.

From the above introduction, we can conclude that if there is a partial order relation between reductions of two coverings, then there is the same partial order relation between the partitions induced by the equal domain relations of these two coverings. However, the reverse proposition does not hold according to Example 4.

Let $C_1$, $C_2$ be two coverings of $U$, and $\theta_{r(C_1)}$, $\theta_{r(C_2)}$ be the equal domain relation on $U$ induced by $C_1$ and $C_2$ respectively. If $r(C_1) \subseteq r(C_2)$, then $GE(C_1) \geq GE(C_2)$ (Hu et al., 2006).

Information entropy was applied into both classical rough set and extended rough set to measure the uncertainty separately, but their relationship is not clear. Based on equal domain relation, a covering approximation space is converted into a partition approximation space, and uncertainty measures of covering based rough set are introduced in this section.

## Attribute Reduction Based on Granular Computing

Attribute reduction is a very important issue in data mining and machine learning. It can reduce redundant attributes, simplify the structure of an information system, speed up the following process of rule induction, reduce the cost of instance classification, and even improve the performance of the generated rule systems. A lot of attribute reduction algorithms based on rough set theory have been developed in the last decades, which can be classified into two categories: (1)attribute reduction from the view of algebra(Chang, Wang, & Wu, 1999; Hu & Cercone, 1995; Hu & Cercone, 1996; Jelonek, Krawiec, & Slowinski, 1995) ; (2)attribute reduction from the view of information(Miao & Hu, 1999; Wang, Yu, & Yang, 2002; Wang, Yu, Yang, & Wu, 2001). No matter which method we choose, the challenging issue of these methods is multiple computing for equivalent classes. The objective of this section is to design an encoding method for granules based on bitmap, and develop an efficient method for attribute reduction.

### Encoding Granules with Bitmap Technique

The construction of granular computing and computation with granules are the two basic issues of GrC. The former issue deals with the formation, representation, and interpretation of granules. The later issue deals with the utilization of granules in problem solving (Yao, 2000). The bitmap technique was proposed in the 1960's (Bertino et al., 1997) and has been used by a variety of products since then. Recently, many attempts have been paid to applying bitmap techniques in knowledge discovery algorithms (Lin, 2000; Louie & Lin, 2000), for bitmaps improve the performance and reduce the storage requirement. In this section, we will introduce a method for encoding granules using bitmap.

An information table could be encoded using bitmap, called encoding information table (Hu, Wang, Zhang, & Liu, 2006).

Table 2 is an example of information table.

The encoding rule is as follows:

*Table 2. An information table*

| Object | Height | Hair | Eyes | class |
|--------|--------|-------|-------|-------|
| $O_1$ | short | blond | blue | + |
| $O_2$ | short | blond | brown | - |
| $O_3$ | tall | red | blue | + |
| $O_4$ | tall | dark | blue | - |
| $O_5$ | tall | dark | blue | - |
| $O_6$ | tall | blond | blue | + |
| $O_7$ | tall | dark | brown | - |
| $O_8$ | short | blond | brown | - |

*Table 3. Encoded information table*

| Object | Height | Hair | Eyes | class |
|--------|--------|------|------|-------|
| $O_1$ | 10 | 100 | 10 | 10 |
| $O_2$ | 10 | 100 | 01 | 01 |
| $O_3$ | 01 | 010 | 10 | 10 |
| $O_4$ | 01 | 001 | 10 | 01 |
| $O_5$ | 01 | 001 | 10 | 01 |
| $O_6$ | 01 | 100 | 10 | 10 |
| $O_7$ | 01 | 001 | 01 | 01 |
| $O_8$ | 10 | 100 | 01 | 01 |

1. For an attribute $a$, the code length of $a$ is equal to the cardinality of $V_a$;

2. Every bit of the code denotes a value in $V_a$

3. For every attribute value, its code can be represented by a $|V_a|$-length bitmap, in which the corresponding bit is set to be 1, other bits 0.

For example, the cardinality of *Height* is 2, so the length of its code is two. Let the first bit denote *short* and the second bit *tall*. The attribute value *tall* will be encoded as 01, and *short* as 10. According to this rule, the information table shown in Table 2 could be encoded like Table 3.

Each subset $A$ of condition attributes determines an equivalent relation on $U$, in which two objects are equivalent if and only if they have exact the same values under $A$. An equivalence relation divides a universal set into a family of pair-wise disjoint subsets, called the partition of the universe. Here we use a matrix to represent a partition induced by an attribute. For an attribute $a$ in an information system $S$, the partition matrix can be defined as $P(a) = \{P_a(i,j)\}_{|U|\times|U|}$, where

$$P_a(i,j) = \begin{cases} 1, a(i) = a(j) \\ 0, else \end{cases}$$

To generate the partition matrix on an attribute, the traditional way, according to above definition, is to compare the attribute values and $P_a(i,j)$ is set to be 1 if the object $i$ and $j$ have the same value on attribute $a$, otherwise $P_a(i,j)$ is set to be 0. Here we could have another way using bitmap. In terms of the definition of the encoded information table, if two objects have the same value on an attribute, then they have the same code value on this attribute. To judge whether two objects have the same code value, the logic operation *AND* can be applied, i.e., $P_a(i,j)$ is set to be 1 for the result of non-zero, otherwise is set to be 0. Because the partition is symmetrical, it can be simplified to reduce the storage. For example, Table 4 is the partition matrix on *Height*, and Table 5 is the partition matrix on *Eyes*.

Having the partition matrix on each attribute, the partition matrix on a subset of condition attributes can be further computed. For a subset $A$ of condition attributes, the partition matrix $P(A) = \{P_A(i,j)\}_{|U|\times|U|}$, can be computed using the following formula:

*Table 4. Partition matrix on Height*

| P | $O_1$ | $O_2$ | $O_3$ | $O_4$ | $O_5$ | $O_6$ | $O_7$ | $O_8$ |
|---|---|---|---|---|---|---|---|---|
| $O_1$ | 1 | | | | | | | |
| $O_2$ | 1 | 1 | | | | | | |
| $O_3$ | 0 | 0 | 1 | | | | | |
| $O_4$ | 0 | 0 | 1 | 1 | | | | |
| $O_5$ | 0 | 0 | 1 | 1 | 1 | | | |
| $O_6$ | 0 | 0 | 1 | 1 | 1 | 1 | | |
| $O_7$ | 0 | 0 | 1 | 1 | 1 | 1 | 1 | |
| $O_8$ | 1 | 1 | 0 | 0 | 0 | 0 | 0 | 1 |

*Table 5. Partition matrix on Eyes*

| P | $O_1$ | $O_2$ | $O_3$ | $O_4$ | $O_5$ | $O_6$ | $O_7$ | $O_8$ |
|---|---|---|---|---|---|---|---|---|
| $O_1$ | 1 | | | | | | | |
| $O_2$ | 0 | 1 | | | | | | |
| $O_3$ | 1 | 0 | 1 | | | | | |
| $O_4$ | 1 | 0 | 1 | 1 | | | | |
| $O_5$ | 1 | 0 | 1 | 1 | 1 | | | |
| $O_6$ | 1 | 0 | 1 | 1 | 1 | 1 | | |
| $O_7$ | 0 | 1 | 0 | 0 | 0 | 0 | 1 | |
| $O_8$ | 0 | 1 | 0 | 0 | 0 | 0 | 1 | 1 |

$$P_A(i, j) = AND \ P_{a_i}(i, j), \ a_i \in A.$$

For instance, we can get the partition on {*Height, Eyes*} based on the above two partition matrixes. It is shown in Table 6.

For convenience, we complement the partition matrix by symmetry. A partition matrix represents the equivalence relation holding between all the objects. In each line or column of a partition matrix, the subset consists of all objects which are equivalent to the object denoted by the line. In other words, every line or column represents an equivalence class. Using partition matrix, we can easily get all equivalent classes. For example,

$$U \ / \ \{Height, Eyes\} = \{\{O_1\}, \{O_2, O_8\}, \{O_3, O_4, O_5, O_6\}, \{O_7\}\}$$

## Attribute Reduction Based on Granular Computing

Attribute reductions based on algebra and information views were discussed in (Wang, Zhao, An, & Wu, 2004). Although their definitions are different, both of them need to compute equivalent classes, so we can use the methods developed in the last section. Moreover, the set operation can be replaced by logic operation, which could improve the performance.

Let $S$ be an information system. Using partition matrix we can get the codes of equivalent classes on condition attributes and decision attributes. Suppose they are $\{C_1, C_2, ..., C_i\}$ and $\{D_1, D_2, ..., D_j\}$, we can develop the following algorithm to compute the positive region of $C$ with respect to $D$.

**Algorithm 2: Computing Positive Region of C with respect to D**

**Input:** $IND(C)= \{C_1, C_2, ..., C_i\}$ and $IND(D)= \{D_1, D_2, ..., D_j\}$
**Output:** The positive region of $C$ with respect to $D$, $POS_C(D)$

- **Step 1**: Let $POS_C(D) = G_\varnothing$.

- **Step 2**: If $IND(C) \neq \varnothing$, then select an element $C_m$ from $IND(C)$, let $IND(C)=IND(C)-\{C_m\}$, $T = IND(D)$. Otherwise go to Step 5.

*Table 6. Partition matrix on {Height, Eyes}*

| P | $O_1$ | $O_2$ | $O_3$ | $O_4$ | $O_5$ | $O_6$ | $O_7$ | $O_8$ |
|---|---|---|---|---|---|---|---|---|
| $O_1$ | 1 | 0 | 0 | 0 | 0 | 0 | 0 | 0 |
| $O_2$ | 0 | 1 | 0 | 0 | 0 | 0 | 0 | 1 |
| $O_3$ | 0 | 0 | 1 | 1 | 1 | 1 | 0 | 0 |
| $O_4$ | 0 | 0 | 1 | 1 | 1 | 1 | 0 | 0 |
| $O_5$ | 0 | 0 | 1 | 1 | 1 | 1 | 0 | 0 |
| $O_6$ | 0 | 0 | 1 | 1 | 1 | 1 | 0 | 0 |
| $O_7$ | 0 | 0 | 0 | 0 | 0 | 0 | 1 | 0 |
| $O_8$ | 0 | 1 | 0 | 0 | 0 | 0 | 0 | 1 |

- **Step 3**: If $T \neq \varnothing$, then select an element $D_n$ from $IND(D)$, let $T = T - \{D_n\}$, $t = C_m \, AND$ $D_n$.
- **Step 4**: If $t = 0$, then go to Step 3. Otherwise if $t \, XOR \, C_m = 0$, then let $POS_C(D) = POS_C(D)$ $OR \, C_m$. Go to Step 2.
- **Step 5**: End.

According to the definition of attribute reduction in the algebra view, here we can develop a new attribute reduction algorithm.

**Algorithm 3: Attribute Reduction Based on Granular Computing (ARGrC)**

**Input**: An decision information system *S*
**Output**: A reduction of condition attribute *C*, *RED(C)*
- **Step 1**: Let *RED(C)*=$\varnothing$, *A=C*, compute the significance of each attribute $a \in A$, and sort the set of attributes based on significance.
- **Step 2**: Compute $POS_C(D)$ with algorithm 2.
- **Step 3**: Compute $POS_{RED(C)}(D)$ with algorithm 2.
- **Step 4**: If $(POS_{RED(C)}(D) \, XOR \, POS_C(D)) = 0$, then let *A = RED(C)*, go to Step 6.
- **Step 5**: Select an attribute *a* from *A* with the highest significant value, *RED(C)= RED(C)*$\cup\{a\}$, *A=A-{a}*, go to step 3.
- **Step 6**: If $A = \varnothing$, then go to Step 8. Otherwise, select an attribute *a* from *A*, *A=A-{a}*.
- **Step 7**: Compute $POS_{RED(C)-\{a\}}(D)$ with algorithm 2, if $POS_C(D) \, XOR \, POS_{RED(C)-\{a\}}(D)$=0, then let *RED(C)= RED(C)-{a}*. go to Step 6.
- **Step 8**: End.

The time complexity of ARBGrC is $O(mn^2)$, where *n* is the number of objects and *m* is the number of attributes. In order to test the efficiency of ARBGrC algorithm, we compare it with other two algorithms. One is the algorithm introduced in (Wang, 2001), the other is the algorithm developed in (Liu, Sheng, Wu, Shi, & Hu, 2003). From the simulation results (Hu et al., 2006), Table 7 demonstrates that ARBGrC is more efficient in time than other algorithms.

## Rule Generation Based on Granular Computing

The aim of data mining is to discover knowledge from data. Generally speaking, the more concise the knowledge is, the more powerful the generalized ability of the knowledge is. So, we want the rule set to be as small as possible, and each rule to be as short as possible. For this aim, we will introduce two rule generation algorithms based on granular computing. One is developed in (An, Wang, Wu, & Gan, 2005), but it can only process consistent information system. In order to process inconsistent information system, another algorithm based on data driving is proposed by Gan(Gan, Wang, & Hu, 2006).

*Table 7. Simulation results*

| Data set | NI | NOA | Wang's algorithm | | Liu's algorithm | | ARBGrC | |
|---|---|---|---|---|---|---|---|---|
| | | | NAR | TC(s) | NAR | TC(s) | NAR | TC(s) |
| Zoo | 101 | 16 | 5 | 0.0745323 | 5 | 0.0236871 | 5 | 0.0199314 |
| Wine | 178 | 13 | 2 | 0.1882960 | 2 | 0.1238230 | 2 | 0.0251350 |
| Bupa | 345 | 6 | 3 | 0.3069120 | 3 | 0.1986720 | 3 | 0.0435812 |
| Letter-recognition | 5000 | 16 | 9 | 202.7750 | 10 | 138.4930 | 9 | 58.9536 |

*where NI is the number of instances, NOA is the number of original attributes, NAR is the number of attributes after reduction and TC is the time consuming.

## A Rule Generation Algorithm Based on Granular Computing

An information table consists of some instances. If it represents the whole granule space, it can be divided into some small spaces. Each small space would be taken as a basic granule. These basic granules are further composed or decomposed into new granules so that new granules could describe the whole problem space or solve the problem at different hierarchies. During the process of problem solving, how to compose or decompose basic granules into new rule granules, and adjust the solution and granule space to improve the algorithm's efficiency, are two key aspects of the algorithm.

Considering the above two aspects, the rule generation algorithm based on granular computing can be developed(An et al., 2005). At first, an information table is divided into some basic granules with respect to atomic formulae of the decision logic language. Secondly, these basic granules are further composed or decomposed into new granules with boolean calculation, and the granule space is reduced correspondingly. In order to improve the performance of rule granule generation, RGAGC adjusts the solution space with the "false preserving" property of quotient space theory. That is, if RGAGC cannot generate rule granules from the granule space, it should enlarge the current solution space, so that it can generate rule granules from the granule space, otherwise it generates rule granules from the current solution space directly. The above steps are repeated until rule granules contain all instances of an information table. Finally, rules are generated from these rule granules.

**Algorithm 4: A rule generation algorithm based on granular computing (RGAGC)(An et al., 2005)**

**Input:** A decision information system
**Output:** Rule set

- **Step 1:** Initialize rule granule set $RGS = \{\varnothing\}$, condition attribute set ($CS$) with reference to rule granule set is set to be $\varnothing$, where, $CS$ represents the solution space. Set $m=1$, where $m$ is a counter for the times of dividing the whole granule space.
- **Step 2:** Divide the information table into basic granules with reference to atomic formulae. These basic granules are classified into two granule spaces, condition attribute granule set ($CG$) and decision attribute granule set ($DG$). If a granule with reference to atomic formula is ($a \in C, v$), it belongs to $CG$, otherwise $DG$.

*Table 8. Simulation results*

| Data set | Average rule length | | Recognition rate(%) | |
|---|---|---|---|---|
| | RGAGC | ID3 | RGAGC | ID3 |
| Abalone Data | 1.77 | 1.41 | 33.7 | 6.0 |
| Car Evaluation Database | 3.40 | 4.56 | 66.0 | 63.2 |
| German Credit Data | 2.64 | 1.96 | 99.8 | 39.2 |
| Nursery Database | 4.12 | 6.01 | 91.98 | 72.7 |
| Protein Localization Sites | 1.00 | 1.00 | 7.0 | 0.0 |

- **Step 3:** For each granule $Cg_i \in CG$ and $Dg_k \in DG$, calculate the certainty support $AS\ (Cg_i \Rightarrow Dg_k)$.

- **Step 4:** If $(CS == \varnothing)$\{For i=1 to n /* $n = |CG|$ is the number of granules in $CG$ */\{If $AS(Cg_i \in CG \Rightarrow Dg_k \in DG) == 1$)\{ $RGS = RGS \cup \{Cg_i\}$, $CS = CS \cup \{a_j \notin CS\}$ where granule $Cg_i$ with reference to atomic formula is $(a_j \in C, v).$\}\}\} Else \{For i=1 to $n$ /* $n = |CG|$ is the number of granules in $CG$ */\{If $((a_{1...m} \in CS)$ \&\&$(AS(Cg_1 \otimes ... \otimes Cg_{mk} \Rightarrow Dg) == 1))$/* Where granule $Cg_i$ with reference to atomic formula is $(a_j \in C, v)$. If RGAGC can generate rule granules from the current granule space directly, it need not adjusts the current solution space, otherwise, it should enlarge the current solution space so that it can generate rule granules from the granule space. */ $\{RGS = RGS \cup \{Cg_1 \otimes ... \otimes Cg_m\}\}$.
Else if $((AS(Cg_1 \in CG \otimes ... \otimes Cg_m \in CG \Rightarrow Dg_k \in DG) == 1)$\&\&$(Cg_1 \otimes ... \otimes Cg_m = Cg_1' \otimes ... \otimes Cg_m'))$ /*Where $Cg'$ is a granule at the previous granule hierarchy. After Step 5, the granule $Cg'$ is converted to granule $Cg$. */ $RGS = RGS \cup \{Cg_1 \otimes ... \otimes Cg_m\}$ $CS = CS \cup \{a_j \notin CS\}, j = 1...m\}\}\}\}$

- **Step 5:** Modify condition attribute granule set $CG$ and decision attribute granule set $DG$. That is, instances in both $CG$ and $RGS$ are removed from $CG$, instances in both $DG$ and $RGS$ are removed from $DG$. Set $m=m+1$.
- **Step 6:** Repeat step 3, 4 and 5 until $RGS$ contains all instances of the information table.
- **Step 7:** Output rule granule set $RGS$ and exit.

RGAGC is a valid method to generate rules from the granule space. Comparing with many classic decision tree algorithms, RGAGC generates a single rule granule in each step instead of selecting a suitable attribute. It is a more general algorithm for rule generation, since it could generate rules from the granule space without considering the problem of selecting an attribute according to some measure. On the other hand, in order to improve the performance of rule granule generation, the "false preserving" property of quotient space theory is used as a strategy to control the process of rule granule generation, so that RGAGC could generate rule granules from the granule space quickly. Table 8 indicates that our conclusion is true.

## A Self-Learning Algorithm Based on Granular Computing

Comparing with many traditional decision tree algorithms, RGAGC doesn't need to solve the problem of attribute selection, it's an efficient way to acquire knowledge from decision tables. However, RGAGC cannot deal with uncertain information tables.

Skowron proposed a rough set framework for mining propositional default rules, which can generate rules under uncertain conditions (Mollestad & Skowron, 1996). Unfortunately, its performance relies on a given threshold. In order to achieve the maximum recognition rate of the rule set and keep the number of the rules at an acceptable level, the idea of self learning, which is proposed by Wang(Wang, 2001), is applied in the default rules generating algorithm(Gan et al., 2006). The algorithm extracts rules in the granules at the 1st hierarchy at first, then extracts rules in the granules at the 2nd hierarchy, and so on. When a rule is generated from a granule, all the objects in this granule will be considered as "covered" by this rule, which means, this newly generated rule can explain these objects. As rules with good adaptability are obtained first, and the algorithm stops immediately when the whole decision table is covered by the rule set.

**Algorithm 5: A self-learning algorithm based on granular computing (ALG) (Gan et al., 2006)**

**Input**: An decision information system
**Output**: Rule set

- **Step 1**: Set $RS = \varnothing$, $Gr_{RS} = \varnothing$, $DFS = \varnothing$, $h = 1$, where, $Gr_{RS}$ is the set of objects already been covered by rules in $RS$, $DFS$ is the set of atomic formulae given by decision attribute $D = \{d\}$, $h$ is the length of formulae used to decompose $S$.

- **Step 2**: Calculate the minimum local certainty $a_c$ of $S$. Calculate the atomic formulae $\varphi_j$ given by decision attribute $D = \{d\}$, let $DFS = DFS \cup \varphi_j$, where $j = 1, ..., |U / IND(D)|$.

- **Step 3**: Calculate the decomposition of $S$ at the $h$th hierarchy, $\Psi_S^h = \{\{m(\phi_1^h)\}, ..., \{m(\phi_i^h)\}, ..., \{m(\phi_n^h)\}\}$, where $\phi_i^h$ is a formula with the length of $h$, $i = 1, ..., n$, $n$ is the number of granules in $\Psi_S^h$.

  For each $\varphi_j \in DFS$:

  Calculate ($AS(\phi_i^h \Rightarrow \varphi_j)$).

  If ($AS(\phi_i^h \Rightarrow \varphi_j) \geq a_c$) and $m(\phi_i^h) - Gr_{RS} \neq \varnothing$, then:

  $RS = RS \cup \{\phi_i^h \Rightarrow \varphi_j \mid AS(\phi_i^h \Rightarrow \varphi_j)\}$ $Gr_{RS} = Gr_{RS} \cup \{m(\phi_i^h \Rightarrow \varphi_j)\}$,

  $AS(\phi_i^h \Rightarrow \varphi_j)$ is the reliability of this rule.

- **Step 4**: If $U - Gr_{RS} \neq \varnothing$, then $h = h + 1$, go to Step3, otherwise stop the algorithm.

Table 9 shows that ALG is valid in processing uncertain information system. Moreover, the rule set generated by ALG is smaller than Skowron's default rule generation algorithm (Gan et al., 2006).

In the algorithms introduced above, decision tables are divided into granules with the same granularity in each hierarchy. Based on these granules, rules are generated. To process uncertain information, the minimum local certainty is used as a threshold to control the process of rule generation. These algorithms tend to search for rules in larger granularity, and rules with good adaptability are obtained at first. Thus, the rule sets generated by these algorithms are small.

## 4. CONCLUSION

In this chapter, a new understanding of data mining, domain-oriented data-driven data mining (3DM), is introduced. Moreover, its relationship with granular computing is analyzed. From the view of granular computing, data mining could be considered as a process of transforming the knowledge from a finer granularity to a coarser granularity. Rough set and fuzzy set are two important computing paradigms of granular computing. For their ability in processing vague information, they were often used in data mining. Some applications of granular computing in data mining are introduced in the views of rough set and fuzzy set. Although several problems in data mining have been partial solved by fuzzy set theory and rough set theory, there are some problems needed to be further studied.

Fuzzy set theory and rough set theory are two important extension of classical set theory. How to combine these two theories to solve problems that cannot be solved by any one of them? A good example has been illustrated in this chapter. The classical rough set theory is based on an equivalence relation, which restricts its application field. Although some extended rough set models have been proposed to process an incomplete information system, any one of them is developed for a special case. Therefore, fuzzy set theory and rough set theory were combined to get a flexible way in processing an incomplete information system in this chapter, viz. any one of the former extended models is a special case when a special $\lambda$ is applied.

Uncertainty measure is a key problem for computing significant of attribute, attribute core, and attribute reduction in rough set theory. The uncertainty measure can be classified into uncertainty of knowledge, uncertainty of rough set, and uncertainty of decision. The uncertainty measures in Pawlak approximation space have been studied deeply, while the uncertainty measures in covering approximation space have not obtain adequate attention. In addition, what are the axioms of uncertainty measures? This is still an open problem.

Bitmap technology is a method computing with bit string. Because it is machine oriented, it can improve the computation efficiency evidently. In this chapter, we encoded granules with bit strings, and then developed a high efficient attribute reduction algorithm by translating set operation of granules

*Table 9. Simulation results*

| Data set | Threshold | Recognition rate | | Number of rules | |
|---|---|---|---|---|---|
| | | ALG | DRGA | ALG | DRGA |
| Agaricus-lepiota | 0.38 | 62.43% | 62.93% | 22 | 240 |
| Breast-cancer-wisconsin | 0.5 | 99.71% | 93.43% | 39 | 251 |
| Dermatology | 0.33 | 62.84% | 59.56% | 11 | 59 |
| Letter-recognition | 0.2 | 42.7% | 40.3% | 27 | 128 |

into logical operation of bit strings. That is to say, if a problem could be converted into a bit computable problem, then the efficiency of this problem can be improved by bitmap technology.

To enhance the generalization of rule sets, simply rules are preferred. From the perspective of granularity, we should try our best to generate rules from the coarsest knowledge space. In this chapter, two rule generation algorithms were introduced. The basic idea is to generate rules from the coarsest knowledge space at first, and then thinner knowledge spaces. Through experiment analysis, we can find that the rule sets generated by these two algorithms are simpler than other similar algorithms. However, these two algorithms are not high efficiency. That may be improved with bitmap technology.

## 5. ACKNOWLEDGMENT

Thanks for the support of National Natural Science Foundation of P. R. China (No.60573068, No.60773113), Natural Science Foundation of Chongqing (No. 2005BA2041, No.2008BA2017), and Science & Technology Research Program of the Municipal Education Committee of Chongqing (No. KJ060517). In addition, the authors would like to thank the anonymous referees for their valuable suggestions for improving this chapter.

## REFERENCES

An, J. J., Wang, G. Y., Wu, Y., & Gan, Q. (2005). A rule generation algorithm based on granular computing, *2005 IEEE International Conference on Granular Computing (IEEE GrC2005)* (pp. 102-107). Beijing, P. R. China.

An, Q. S., Shen, J. Y., & Wang, G. Y. (2003). A clustering method based on information granularity and rough sets. *Pattern Recognition and Artificial Intelligence, 16*(4), 412–417.

Bargiela, A., & Pedrycz, W. (2005). Granular mappings. *IEEE trans. on systems. Man and Cybernetics SMC-A, 35*(2), 288–301.

Bargiela, A., & Pedrycz, W. (2006). The roots of granular computing, In *Proceedings of 2006 IEEE International Conference on Granular Computing* (pp. 806-809).

Bargiela, A., Pedrycz, W., & Hirota, K. (2004). Granular prototyping in fuzzy clustering. *IEEE Transactions on Fuzzy Systems, 12*(5), 697–709. doi:10.1109/TFUZZ.2004.834808

Bargiela, A., Pedrycz, W., & Tanaka, M. (2004). An inclusion/exclusion fuzzy hyperbox classifier. *International Journal of Knowledge based Intelligent Engineering Systems, 8*(2), 91-98.

Bertino, E., Chin, O. B., Sacks-Davis, R., Tan, K., Zobel, J., & Shidlovsky, B. (1997). *Indexing techniques for advanced database systems*. Amsterdam: Kluwer Academic Publishers Group.

Bonikowski, Z., Bryniarski, E., & Wybraniec, U. (1998). Extensions and intentions in the rough set theory. *Information Science, 107*, 149–167. doi:10.1016/S0020-0255(97)10046-9

Cao, L. B., Schurmann, R., & Zhang, C. Q. (2005). Domain-driven in-depth pattern discovery: a practical methodology, In *Proceedings of Australian Data Mining Conference* (pp. 101-114).

Chang, L. Y., Wang, G. Y., & Wu, Y. (1999). An approach for attribute reduction and rule generation based on rough set theory. *Chinese Journal of Software*, *10*(11), 1207–1211.

Dorado, A., Pedrycz, W., & Izquierdo, E. (2005). User-driven fuzzy clustering: on the road to semantic classification, In *Proceedings of RSFDGrc 2005* (Vol. LNCS3641, pp. 421-430).

Frawley, W. J., Piatetsky-Shapiro, G., & Matheus, C. (1991). *Knowledge discovery in databases: an overview*. Cambridge, MA: MIT Press.

Gan, Q., Wang, G. Y., & Hu, J. (2006). A self-learning model based on granular computing. In *Proceedings of the 2006 IEEE International Conference on Granular Computing* (pp. 530-533). Atlanta, GA.

Hu, J., Wang, G. Y., & Zhang, Q. H. (2006). Uncertainty measure of covering generated rough set, *2006 IEEE/WIC/ACM International Conference on Web Intelligence and Intelligent Agent Technology (WI-IAT 2006 Workshops) (WI-IATW'06)* (pp. 498-504). Hongkong, China.

Hu, J., Wang, G. Y., Zhang, Q. H., & Liu, X. Q. (2006). *Attribute reduction based on granular computing*. Paper presented at the The Fifth International Conference on Rough Sets and Current Trends in Computing (RSCTC2006), Kobe, Japan.

Hu, X., & Cercone, H. (1996). Mining knowledge rules from databases: a rough set approach, *Proceedings of the Twelfth International Conference on Data Engineering* (pp. 96-105).

Hu, X. H., & Cercone, N. (1995). Learning in relational database: a rough set approach. *International Journal of Computational Intelligence*, *11*(2), 323–338.

Hu, X. H., Liu, Q., Skowron, A., Lin, T. Y., Yager, R. R., & Zhang, B. (2005). *Proceedings of 2005 IEEE International Conference on Granular Computing* (pp. 571-574). Beijing, China.

Huang, B., He, X., & Zhou, X. Z. (2004). Rough entropy based on generalized rough sets covering reduction. *Journal of software, 15*(2), 215-220.

Huang, H., Wang, G. Y., & Wu, Y. (2004). A direct approach for incomplete information systems. In. *Proceedings of SPIE In Data Mining and Knowledge Discovery: Theory, Tools, and Technology VI, 5433*, 114–121.

Jelonek, J., Krawiec, K., & Slowinski, R. (1995). Rough set reduction of attributes and their domains for neural networks. *International Journal of Computational Intelligence, 11*(2), 339–347.

Kryszkiewicz, M. (1998). Rough set approach to incomplete information systems. *Information Science, 112*, 39–49. doi:10.1016/S0020-0255(98)10019-1

Kryszkiewicz, M. (1999). Rules in incomplete information system. *Information Sciences, 113*(3-4), 271–292. doi:10.1016/S0020-0255(98)10065-8

Kuntz, P., Guillet, F., Lehn, R., & Briand, H. (2000). A user-driven process for mining association rules. In *Proceedings of the 4th European Conference on Principles of Data Mining and Knowledge Discovery* (Vol. 1910, pp. 483-489).

Lin, T. Y. (1997). *Granular computing*. Announcement of the BISC Special Interest Group on Granular Computing.

Lin, T. Y. (2000). Data mining and machine oriented modeling: a granular computing approach. *Journal of Applied Intelligence, 13*(2), 113–124. doi:10.1023/A:1008384328214

Liu, S. H., Hu, F., Jia, Z. Y., & Shi, Z. Z. (2004). A rough set-based hierarchical clustering algorithm. *Journal of Computer research and Development, 41*(4), 552-557.

Liu, S. H., Sheng, Q. J., Wu, B., Shi, Z. Z., & Hu, F. (2003). Research on efficient algorithms for rough set methods. *Chinese Journal of Computers, 26*(5), 524–529.

Louie, E., & Lin, T. Y. (2000). Finding association rules using fast bit computation: machine-oriented modeling, In *Proceedings of the 12th International Symposium on Methodologies for Intelligent Systems,* (pp. 486-494). Charlotte, NC.

Miao, D. Q., & Hu, G. R. (1999). A heuristic algorithm for reduction of knowledge. *Journal of Computer Research & Development, 36*(6), 681–684.

Miao, D. Q., & Wang, J. (1998). On the relationships between information entropy and roughness of knowledge in rough set theory. *Pattern Recognition and Artificial Intelligence, 11*(1), 34–40.

Mollestad, T., & Skowron, A. (1996). A rough set framework for data mining of propositional default rules. In *Proceedings of the 9th International Symposium on Methodologies for Intelligent Systems. ISMIS* (pp. 448-457).

Mordeson, J. N. (2001). Rough set theory applied to (fuzzy) ideal theory. *Fuzzy Sets and Systems, 121*(2), 315–324. doi:10.1016/S0165-0114(00)00023-3

Patrick, J., Palko, D., Munro, R., & Zappavigna, M. (2002). User driven example-based training for creating lexical knowledgebases, Australasian Natural Language Processing Workshop,Canberra, Australia (pp. 17-24). Canberra, Australia.

Pawlak, Z. (1982). Rough sets. *International Journal of Computer and Information Sciences, 11*, 341–356. doi:10.1007/BF01001956

Skowron, A. (2001). Toward intelligent systems: calculi of information granules. *Bulletin of International Rough Set Society, 5*(1-2), 9–30.

Skowron, A., & Stepaniuk, J. (2001). Information granules: towards foundations of granular computing. *International Journal of Intelligent Systems, 16*(1), 57–85. doi:10.1002/1098-111X(200101)16:1<57::AID-INT6>3.0.CO;2-Y

Slowinski, R., & Vsnderpooten, D. (2000). A generalized definition of rough approximations based on similarity. *IEEE Transactions on Knowledge and Data Engineering, 12*(2), 331–326. doi:10.1109/69.842271

Wang, G. Y. (2001). *Rough set theory and knowledge acquisition.* Xi'an, China: Xi'an Jiaotong University Press.

Wang, G. Y. (2002). Extension of rough set under incomplete information systems. *Journal of Computer Research and Development, 39*(10), 1238–1243.

Wang, G. Y. (2006). Domain-oriented data-driven data mining based on rough sets. *Journal of Nanchang Institute of Technology, 25*(2), 46.

Wang, G. Y. (2007). Domain-oriented data-driven data mining (3dm): simulation of human knowledge understanding, *WImBI 2006* (Vol. *LNCS, 4845*, 278–290.

Wang, G. Y., Hu, F., Huang, H., & Wu, Y. (2005). A granular computing model based on tolerance relation. *Journal of China Universities of Posts and Telecommunications, 12*(3), 86–90.

Wang, G. Y., Yu, H., & Yang, D. C. (2002). Decision table reduction based on conditional information entropy. *Chinese Journal of Computers, 25*(7), 759–766.

Wang, G. Y., Yu, H., Yang, D. C., & Wu, Z. F. (2001). Knowledge reduction based on rough set and information entropy. In *Proceedings of the 5th World Multiconference on Systemics, Cybernetics and Informatics* (pp. 555-560). Orlando, FL: IIIS.

Wang, G. Y., Zhao, J., An, J. J., & Wu, Y. (2004). Theoretical study on attribute reduction of rough set theory: comparison of algebra and information views. In *Proceedings of the 3rd International Conference on Cognitive Informatics(ICCI'04)* (pp. 148-155).

Yao, J. T., & Yao, Y. Y. (2002). A granular computing approach to machine learning. In *Proceedings of the 1st International Conference on Fuzzy Systems and Knowledge Discovery (FSKD'02)* (pp. 732-736). Singapore.

Yao, J. T., & Yao, Y. Y. (2002). Induction of classification rules by granular computing. In *Proceedings of the 3rd International Conference on Rough Sets and Current Trends in Computing* (Vol. 2475, pp. 331-338).

Yao, Y. Y. (2000). Granular computing: basic issues and possible solutions. In *Proceedings of the 5th Joint Conference on Information Sciences* (Vol. 1, pp. 186-189). Atlantic City, NJ.

Yao, Y. Y. (2005). Perspectives of granular computing. In *Proceedings of 2005 IEEE International Conference on Granular Computing* (Vol. 1, pp. 85-90).

Yao, Y. Y. (2007). The art of granular computing. In *Proceedings of International Conference on Rough Sets and Emerging Intelligent System Paradigms* (RSEISP'07), (LNAI 4585, pp. 101-112).

Zadeh, L. A. (1965). Fuzzy sets. *Information and Control, 8*(3), 338–353. doi:10.1016/S0019-9958(65)90241-X

Zadeh, L. A. (1997). Towards a theory of fuzzy information granulation and its centrality in human reasoning and fuzzy logic. *Fuzzy Sets and Systems, 90*(2), 111–127. doi:10.1016/S0165-0114(97)00077-8

Zadeh, L. A. (1998). Some reflections on soft computing, granular computing and their roles in the conception, design and utilization of information/ intelligent systems. *Soft Computing, 2,* 23–25. doi:10.1007/s005000050030

Zadeh, L. A. (1998). Some reflections on soft computing, granular computing and their roles in the conception,design and utilization of information/intelligent systems. *Soft Computing, 2*(1), 23–25. doi:10.1007/s005000050030

Zadeh, L. A. (2006). Generalized theory of uncertainty (GTU) - principal concepts and ideas. *Computational Statistics & Data Analysis, 51*(1), 15–46. doi:10.1016/j.csda.2006.04.029

Zhang, C. Q., & Cao, L. B. (2006). Domain-driven data mining: methodologies and applications. In *Proceedings of the 4th International Conference on Active Media Technology*.

Zhang, Q. H., Wang, G. Y., Hu, J., & Liu, X. Q. (2006). Incomplete information systems processing based on fuzzy-clustering. In *Proceedings of the 2006 IEEE/WIC/ACM International Conference on Web Intelligence and Intelligent Agent Technology* (WI-IAT 2006 Workshops), (pp. 486-489). Hong Kong, China.

Zhang, Y. Q., & Lin, T. Y. (Eds.). (2006). *Proceedings of 2006 ieee international conference on granular computing*. Atlanta, GA.

Zhao, Y., & Yao, Y. Y. (2005). Interactive user-driven classification using a granule network. In *Proceedings of the 5th International Conference of Cognitive Informatics* (ICCI`05), (pp. 250-259). Irvine, CA.

Zhou, J., Zhang, Q. L., & Chen, W. S. (2004). Generalization of covering rough set. [Natural Science]. *Journal of Northeastern University, 25*(10), 954–956.

Zhu, W., & Wang, F. Y. (2003). Reduction and axiomization of covering generalized rough sets. *Information Science, 152*, 217–230. doi:10.1016/S0020-0255(03)00056-2

# Chapter 8
# Near Sets in Assessing Conflict Dynamics within a Perceptual System Framework

**Sheela Ramanna**
*University of Winnipeg, Canada*

**James F. Peters**
*University of Manitoba, Canada*

## ABSTRACT

*The problem considered in this chapter is how to assess different perceptions of changing socio-technical conflicts. Our approach to the solution to this problem of assessing conflict dynamics is to consider negotiation views within the context of perceptual information systems. Briefly, perceptual information systems (succinctly, perceptual systems) are real-valued, total, deterministic information systems. This particular form of an information system is a variant of the deterministic information system model introduced by Zdzisław Pawlak during the early 1980s. This leads to a near set approach to evaluating perceptual granules derived from conflict situations considered in the context of perceptual systems. A perceptual granule is a set of perceptual objects originating from observations of objects in the physical world. Conflict situations typically result from different sets of viewpoints (perceptions) about issues under negotiation. Perceptual systems provide frameworks for representing and reasoning about different perceptions of socio-technical conflicts. Reasoning about conflict dynamics is made possible with nearness relations and tolerance perceptual near sets used to define a measure of nearness. Several approaches to the analysis of conflict situations are presented in this paper, namely, conflict graphs, approximation spaces and risk patterns. An illustrative example of a requirements scope negotiation for an automated lighting system is presented. The contribution of this chapter is a new way of representing and reasoning about conflicts in the context of requirements engineering with near set theory.*

DOI: 10.4018/978-1-60566-324-1.ch008

# 1. INTRODUCTION

*All knowledge takes its place within the horizons opened up by perception. –Merleau-Ponty, Phenomenology of Perception, 1945.*

Conflict analysis and conflict resolution play an important role in negotiation during contract-management situations in many organizations. Conflict situations also result due to different sets of viewpoints about issues under negotiation. In other words, perceptions about issues play an important role in conflict analysis. The main problem considered in this chapter is how to discover perceptual granules useful in conflict analysis. A *perceptual granule* is a set of perceptual objects originating from observations of objects in the physical world. In this article, there is a shift in the view of information systems, where information extracted from perception of physical objects is contrasted with information in attribute-value tables may or may not originate in the physical world. The other distinguishing feature of the proposed approach is a reliance on probe functions (total, real-valued functions) representing features of perceptual granules rather than the traditional rough set approach, where there is as reliance on partial functions representing attributes defined by information tables. Granulation can be viewed as a human way of achieving data compression and it plays a key role in implementing the divide-and-conquer strategy in human problem-solving. A comprehensive study of granular computing can be found in Bargiela and Pedrycz (2003)Zadeh (1997), Yao, J.T. (2008) and Yao, Y.Y. (2008), Skowron, A., Peters, J. F. (2008). In this chapter, our approach to the solution to the problem of discovery and reasoning about conflict situations comes from near set theory (see, *e.g.*, Peters (2007b, 2007c), Peters and Wasilewski 2009).

The notion of a perceptual system was introduced by Peters (2007a, 2007b), Peters (2008) and elaborated in Peters and Wasilewski (2009). The idea of a perceptual system has its origins in earlier work on granulation by Peters, Skowron, Synak and Ramanna (2003) and in the study of rough set-based ethology by Peters, Henry and Ramanna (2005). Such a system is a new perception-based interpretation of the traditional notion of a deterministic information system by Zdzisław Pawlak(1981a, 1981b) as a real-valued, total, deterministic information system. Deterministic information systems were introduced independently by Zdzisław Pawlak (1981a) and elaborated by Ewa Orłowska (1998). It was also Orłowska (1982) who originally suggested that an approximation space provides a formal basis for perception or observation. This view of approximation spaces captures the kernel of near set theory, where perception is viewed at the level of classes in partitions of perceptual granules rather than at the level of individual objects (see, e.g., Peters (2007a, 2007b, 2007c) Peters, Skowron and Stepaniuk, 2007).

The earliest work on representing social conflicts as information systems using the HLAS can be found in Skowron, Ramanna and Peters (2006). Conflict situations modelled as decision systems that incorporate degree of conflict degrees as decisions were introduced in Ramanna, Peters, and Skowron (2006b). In the same paper, a discussion of assessing conflict dynamics with approximation spaces can be found. Assessing conflict dynamics with risk patterns can be found in Ramanna, Peters, and Skowron (2006c, 2006a). In Ramanna, and Skowron (2007c), the conflict model was expanded to incorporate technical conflicts which resulted in a socio-technical framework to represent and reason about conflicts during systems requirements gathering. Assessing conflict dynamics in the context of the socio-technical framework was presented in Ramanna, Peters, and Skowron (2007b, 2007c). Conflict analysis in the framework of rough sets and granular computing and near sets was introduced in Ramanna(2008). In addition, adaptive learning as a means of conflict resolution was presented in Ramanna(2008) and Ramanna, Peters, and Skowron (2007a).

In this chapter, we introduce perceptual information systems as a mechanism for representing and reasoning about different perceptions of socio-technical conflicts. Briefly, *perceptual information systems* (succinctly, *perceptual systems*) Peters and Ramanna(2009) are real-valued, total, deterministic information systems. This leads to a near set approach to deriving perceptual granules from conflict situations considered in the context of perceptual systems. A *perceptual granule*Peters (2007a, 2007b, 2007c,) is a set of perceptual objects originating from observations in the physical world. Reasoning about conflict dynamics is made possible with nearness relations and tolerance perceptual near sets that will be used in defining a measure of nearness. Perceptual information systems encapsulate behaviours and make it possible to extract pattern information. It is also possible to represent two different perceptions of social conflicts at different points in time as perceptual information systems. However, in this chapter, we have only considered socio-technical conflicts. The contribution of this chapter is a new way of representing and reasoning about conflicts in the context of requirements engineering with near set theory.

This chapter is organized as follows. An overview of several approaches used by the authors is described in Section 2. This is done for the sake of completeness of the chapter. In Section 3, conflict situations as perceptual information systems are described in detail. A new quantitative measure based on nearness which provides another means of assessing conflict dynamics are illustrated in Section 4.

## 2. APPROACHES TO ASSESSING CONFLICT DYNAMICS: AN OVERVIEW

This section briefly introduces approaches to modeling conflict situations. The basic concepts of conflict theory that we use in this paper are due to Pawlak (1984, 1987, 1993 1998, and 2007b).

### 2.1. Conflict Model

Information systems provide a practical basis for representation and reasoning in rough set theory. In a rough set approach to conflict analysis, an information system is represented by a table containing rows labeled by *objects* (*agents*), columns by *attributes* (*issues*). The entries of an information table are *values of attributes* (*votes*) that describe each agent, that is, each entry corresponds to a row *x* and column *a* representing opinion of an agent *x* about issue *a*. Formally, an *information system* can be defined as a pair S = (U, A), where U is a nonempty, finite set called the *universe* (elements of U are called *objects*) and A is a nonempty, finite set of *attributes* (Pawlak and Skowron, 2007a).

Decision systems provide yet another practical and powerful framework for representing knowledge, particularly for discovering patterns in objects and in classification of objects into decision classes. In addition, decision systems also make it possible to represent and reason about objects at a higher level of granularity. This is necessary for modeling complex conflict situations. The extension of the basic model of conflict to a decision system with complex decisions was introduced in Ramanna, Peters and Skowron(2006b). We recall some basic assumptions that agents in the complex conflict model are represented by conflict situations CS = (Ag,V), where Ag is the set of lower level agents, V is the set of voting functions $\{v_1,....v_k\}$ and v: Ag -> {-1,0,1}. Hence, agents in the complex conflict model are related to groups of lower level agents linked by a voting function. The voting functions in the complex conflict models are defined on such conflict situations. In this, way we obtain an information system (U, A), where U is the set of situations. Observe that any situation CS= (Ag,V) can be represented by a matrix.

$$\left[ v\left(ag\right)\right]_{ag \in Ag} \tag{1}$$

where v(ag) is the result of voting by the agent ag∈Ag.

## 2.2. Conflict Graphs

With every conflict situation CS=(Ag,v), we can associate a *conflict graph* which provides *quantitative* assessment of conflict dynamics between agents. In Figure 1, solid lines denote conflicts, dotted lines denote agreements, and for simplicity, neutrality is not shown explicitly in the graph.

As one can see agents B, C, and D form a coalition with respect to an issue v. A conflict degree Con(CS) of the conflict situation CS=(Ag,v) is defined by Equation (2):

$$\mathrm{Con(CS)} = \frac{\sum_{\{(ag,ag') \, : \, \varphi_v(ag,ag') \, = \, -1\}} \left|\varphi_v\left(ag,ag'\right)\right|}{2\left|\dfrac{n}{2}\right| \times \left(n - \left|\dfrac{n}{2}\right|\right)} \tag{2}$$

where n = Card(Ag), $\varphi_v(ag,ag')$ is an auxilliary function defined on the voting function v with the following interpretation: i) $\varphi_v(ag,ag') = 1$ means that agents ag and ag' have the same opinion about an issue v ii) $\varphi_v(ag,ag') = 0$ means that at least one of the agents has no opinion on issue v iii) $\varphi_v(ag,ag') = -1$ means that both agents have a different opinion on issue v. It should be noted that Con(CS) is a measure of discernibility between agents from Ag relative to the voting function v. For a more general conflict situation CS=(Ag,V) for different issues, the conflict degree in CS (*tension* generated by V) can be defined by Equation (3):

$$\mathrm{Con(CS)} = \frac{\sum_{i=1}^{k} \mathrm{Con(CS}_i)}{k} \tag{3}$$

We can extend the information system (U, A) to the decision system (U, A, d) assuming, that d(s)=Con(CS$_v$) for any CS=(Ag,v) where s ∈ U. For the constructed decision system (U, A, d) one can measure discernibility between compound decision values which correspond to conflict situations in the constructed decision table.

## 2.3. Approximation Spaces

The decision system representation of the conflict model is rather powerful in that it offers deeper insight into conflict dynamics whereby one can observe changes to the level of conflict whenever different *issues* (dimensions) are selected. This is made possible when we combine the model with approximation spaces. Let DS=(U, A, d), where U denotes a non-empty set of requirements (objects), A represents a non-empty set of scope negotiation parameters(attributes), and d denotes an estimated degree of conflict. Let $D_i$ denote the i[th] decision, that is, $\{D_i = u \in U \, d(u) = i\}$, which is set of requirements with conflict level i. For any boolean combination of descriptors over DS the semantics of α in DS is denoted by $\|\alpha\|_{DS}$, that is, the set of all objects from U satisfying α (Pawlak, 1991).

*Figure 1. Sample conflict graph*

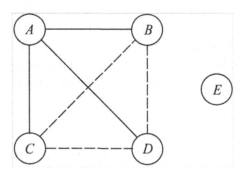

In what follows, assume that $i = L$ and $D_L$ denotes a decision class representing a low degree of conflict between stakeholders. Now, we can define a generalized approximation space GAS = $(U, N_B, v_B)$ where for any object $r \in U$, the neighborhood $N_B$ (r) is defined by Equation (4):

$$N_B(r) = \left\| \bigwedge_{a \in B} (a=a(r)) \right\|_{DS} \tag{4}$$

and the coverage function $v_B$ is defined by Equation (5):

$$\nu_B(X, Y) = \begin{cases} \dfrac{|X \cap Y|}{|Y|} & , if\ Y \neq \varnothing, \\ 1 & , \text{ otherwise,} \end{cases} \tag{5}$$

where $X, Y \subseteq U$. This form of specialization of a GAS is called a *lower approximation space* introduced by Peters and Henry (2006c). Assuming that the lower approximation $B_* D_i$ represents an acceptable (standard) level of conflict during negotiation, we are interested in the values given by Equation (6):

$$\nu_B\left(N_B(r), B_* D_L\right), \tag{6}$$

of the coverage function specialized in the context of a decision system DS for the neighborhoods $N_B(r)$ and the standard $B_* D_L$ for conflict negotiation. Computing the rough coverage value for issues extracted from a decision table representation, implicitly measures the extent to which an acceptable level of conflict for complex situations has been followed. Another conflict dynamic that can be observed is the effect on the level of conflict when the set of condition attributes B is changed.

## 2.4. Risk Patterns

Risk patterns offer a different yet complementary insight into conflict dynamics. Risk patterns are defined by specific reducts (and their approximations) of the conflict model. In this section, we assume that the distance between conflict degrees is defined by Equation (7):

$$\text{disc}_{\text{CS}^T}\left(v,v'\right) = \left|\text{Con}(\text{CS}_v)\text{-Con}(\text{CS}_{v'})\right| \tag{7}$$

Now, one can consider reducts of this decision table relative to a fixed distance $\delta$ between decision values. Let DT = (U,A, d) be a (consistent) decision table and let $\delta$ be a distance function between decisions from $V_d$. Any minimal set $B \subseteq A$ satisfying condition given by Equation (8)

$$\delta \, (d(x), d(y)) \geq \text{tr} \wedge (\text{non}(x \, \text{IND(A)} \, y) \Rightarrow \text{non}(x \quad \text{IND(B)} \, y)) \tag{8}$$

where IND(A), IND(B) are the indiscernibility relations relative to A, B respectively Pawlak (1991) and tr is a given threshold called a (d, tr)-reduct of DT.

One can use an approach presented in Skowron and Rauszer (1992) and define modified discernibility reducts making it possible to compute such reducts using a Boolean reasoning method. Any such reduct B defines a set of risk patterns. Such patterns are obtained by taking the values of attributes from B relative to any object x from DT, that is,

$$\underset{a \in B}{\wedge} \left(a = a(x)\right) \tag{9}$$

From the distance reduct definition, the deviation of the decision on the set of objects satisfying Formula (9) in DT, that is, on the set (10).

$$\left\|\underset{a \in B}{\wedge} \left(a = a(x)\right)\right\|_{DS} = \left\{y \in U : a(y) = A(x) \text{ for } a \in B\right\} \tag{10}$$

is at most tr.

One can analyze the dynamics of conflict degree changes by dropping conditions from defined risk patterns. Excluding certain conditions may cause small changes to the deviation of decisions, while excluding other conditions can lead to a substantial increase in the decision deviation. In other words, different sets of issues can lead to differing deviations in conflict degrees.

## 3. MODELLING CONFLICT SITUATIONS AS PERCEPTUAL INFORMATION SYSTEMS

*The better theory is the more precise description of the [object] it provides. –Ewa Orlowska, Studia Logica, 1990.*

The underlying philosophy in the conflict model is that, requirements for harmony in social interaction among project stakeholders and in the expression of technical specifications inevitably lead to conflicts that must be resolved during negotiation. It should also be observed that resolution of socio-technical conflicts can be aided by a fusion of the approximation spaces that takes advantage of the near set approach to perceptual synthesis (see Ramanna, 2008). It has been shown that it is possible to combine near sets and approximate adaptive learning (see Ramanna, Peters, Skowron, 2007a). In this chapter, we focus on measuring the degree of nearness of behaviours during negotiations. This entails a methodology for discovering perceptual granules (*i.e.*, sets of perceptual objects) that are, in some sense, close to each other. The proposed approach to comparing conflict behaviours and extracting pattern information takes advantage of recent studies of the nearness of objects and near sets. Behavior patterns are considered near each other if, and only if they have similar descriptions. The basic approach to comparing perceptual information systems is inspired by the early 1980s work by Zdzisław Pawlak on the classification of objects by means of attributes (see Pawlak, 1981a). Objects are classified by comparing descriptions of conflict behavior stored in information tables.

## 3.1. Perceptual Information Systems: Formal Definition

For representing different perceptions of conflict dynamics, we use the notion of a perceptual information system. In general, an *information system* is a triple $S = <Ob, At, \{Val_f\}_{f \in At}>$ where Ob is a set of objects, *At* is a set of functions representing either object features or object attributes, and each $Val_f$ is a value domain of a function $f \in At$, where $f: Ob \rightarrow P(Val_f)$ ($P(Val_f)$ is a power set of $Val_f$). If $f(x) \neq \varnothing$ for all $x \in Ob$ and $f \in At$, then *S* is *total*. If $card(f(x)) = 1$ for every $x \in Ob$ and $f \in At$, then *S* is *deterministic*. Otherwise *S* is *non-deterministic*. In the case where $f(x) = \{v\}$, $\{v\}$ is identified with v. An information system *S* is *real valued* iff $Val_f = R$ for every $f \in At$. Very often a more concise notation is used: $<Ob, At>$, especially when value domains are understood, as in the case of real valued information systems. An *object description* is defined by means of a tuple of function values $\varphi(x)$ associated with a perceptual object $x \in X$ (see Table 1).

The important thing to notice is the choice of functions $\varphi_i \in B$ used to describe an object of interest. Assume that $B \subseteq F$ is a given set of functions representing features of sample objects O. Let $X \subseteq O$ and let $\varphi_i \in B$, where $\varphi_i: O \rightarrow R$. In combination, the functions representing object features provide a basis for an *object description* $\varphi: O \rightarrow R^L$, a vector containing measurements (returned values) associated with each functional value $\varphi_i(x)$ for $x \in X$, where $|\varphi| = L$, that is the description length is L. In general, an object description has the form shown in Equation (11).

$$\varphi(x) = (\varphi_1(x), ..., \varphi_i(x), ..., \varphi_L(x)), \tag{11}$$

In Figure 2, the general form of a description in Equation (11) is instantiated by using particular probe functions $\varphi_1, ..., \varphi_i, ..., \varphi_L \in F$ where $\varphi_i: O \rightarrow R$ in an object description $\varphi: O \rightarrow R^L$ for a particular perceptual object such as $x_r$. In effect, the object description $\phi(x_r)$ in Equation (11) is a vector of probe function values. The descriptions represented in a table (see Figure 2) each have length $L = c$, where $c$ is the number of columns (not including column X).

## 3.2. Relations, Partitions, and Classes

Information granulation starts with the B-partition $\sim_B$ of a set of sample objects X gathered during conflict analysis. Each partition consists of equivalence classes called elementary sets that constitute fine-grained information granulation, where each elementary set contains objects with matching descriptions. The elementary sets in a partition are used to construct complex information granules of a decision class that reflects a perception of the sample objects relative a concept (such as conflict degree) impor-

*Table 1. Description of symbols*

| Symbol | Interpretation |
|---|---|
| R | Set of real numbers, |
| O | Set of perceptual objects, |
| X | $X \subseteq O$, a perceptual granule, |
| x | $x \in X$, sample object in perceptual granule X, |
| F | Set of functions representing object features, |
| B | $B \subseteq F$, set of sample functions representing object features(attributes), |
| $\varphi$ | $\varphi: O \rightarrow R^L$, probe function, |
| L | Description length, |
| $\varphi(x)$ | $\varphi(x) = (\varphi_1(x),..., \varphi_i(x),... \varphi_L(x))$ description, |
| $\varepsilon$ | $\varepsilon \in [0,1]$ |
| $\sim_B$ | indiscernibility relation, |
| $\cong_B$ | weak indiscernibility relation, |
| $\cong_{B,\varepsilon}$ | weak tolerance nearness relation, |
| $x/\sim_B$ | $x/\sim_B = \{ y \in X \mid y \sim_B x \}$, elementary set (class), |
| $O/\sim_B$ | $O/\sim_F = \{ x/\sim_B \mid x \in O \}$, quotient set, |
| $\bowtie_F$ | nearness relation, |
| $\underline{\bowtie}_F$ | weak nearness relation, |
| $\underline{\underline{\bowtie}}_F$ | weak tolerance nearness relation, |
| <X,F> | $\varphi_B(x) = (\varphi(x_1),...,\varphi_L(x|_{X_i}))$ perceptual information system |

*Figure 2. Representation of a perceptual system*

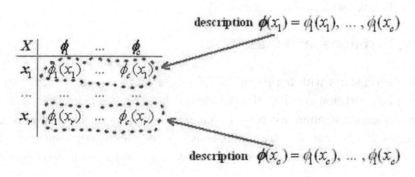

tant in conflict analysis and resolution. To establish a nearness relation, we first consider the traditional indiscernibility relation. Let $B \subseteq F$ denote a set of functions representing perceptual object features. The indiscernibility relation $\sim_B$ introduced by Zdzislaw Pawlak (1981a) is distinguished from weak indiscernibility $\simeq_B$ introduced introduced by Ewa Orlowska (1998). In keeping with the original indiscernibility relation symbol $\sim_F$ Zdzislaw Pawlak (1981a), the symbol $\bowtie$ is used to denote weak indiscernibility relation instead of the notation *weakind* (Ewa Orlowska, 1998). For the sake of completeness, we recall the following definitions:

## Definition 1. Indiscernibility Relation (Pawlak, 1981a)

Let $<O, F>$ be a perceptual system. For every $B \subseteq F$ the indiscernibility relation $\sim_B$ is defined as follows: $\sim_B = \{(x, y) \in O \times O \mid \forall \varphi_{ii} \in B. \varphi_i(x) = \varphi_i(y)\}$. If $B = \{\varphi\}$ for some $\varphi \in F$, instead of $\sim\{\varphi\}$ we write $\sim\varphi$.

## Definition 2. Weak Indiscernibility Relation (Ewa Orlowska, 1998)

Let $<O, F>$ be a perceptual system. For every $B \subseteq F$ the weak indiscernibility relation $\simeq_B$ is defined as follows: $\simeq_B = \{(x, y) \in O \times O \mid \exists \varphi_i \in B. \varphi_i(x) = \varphi_i(y)\}$. If $B = \{\varphi\}$ for some $\varphi \in F$, instead of $\simeq\{\phi\}$ we write $\simeq \phi$.

## Definition 3. Weak Tolerance Relation

Let $<O, F>$ be a perceptual system and let $\varepsilon \in R$. For every $B \subseteq F$ the weak tolerance relation $\simeq_{B,\varepsilon}$ is defined as follows:

$$\simeq_{B,\varepsilon} = \{(x, y) \in O \times O \mid \exists \varphi_i \in B. |\varphi_i(x) - \varphi_i(y)| \leq \varepsilon \}.$$

A more complete presentation on the formal definitions of the above three relations can be found in (Peters, 2008). Let O1 and O2 denote collections of perceptual objects.

## Definition 4

Let $P1 = <O1, F>$ denote perceptual system P1. Similarly, let $P2 = <O2, F>$ denote a second, distinct perceptual system. Also, let $\varepsilon \in R$. P1 has a weak tolerance relation to P2 if, and only if $O1 \simeq_{F,\varepsilon} O2$.

**Observation 1**

Let $Sys1 = <O1, F>$ denote perceptual system Sys1. Similarly, let $Sys2 = <O2, F>$ denote a second, distinct perceptual system with the same set of features F (issues). Let $B \subseteq F$ and choose $\varepsilon$. Then

$$Sys1 \simeq_{B,\varepsilon} Sys1 \Leftrightarrow O1 \simeq_{B,\varepsilon} O2 \qquad (12)$$

In the case of conflicts, these two systems represent two different perceptions of requirements at different points in time. They could also represent perceptions of social and technical conflicts (objective and subjective viewpoints). We now present nearness relations and tolerance perceptual near sets that will be used in defining a measure of nearness of perceptual objects.

## 3.3. Nearness Relations and Tolerance Perceptual Near Sets

*Thus the near-thing, as "the same", appears now from this "side", now from that; and the "visual perspectives" change.... –Edmund Husserl, Cartesian Meditations, 1929.*

Three basic nearness relations are briefly presented and illustrated in this section.

### Definition 5. Nearness Relation (Peters and Wasilewski, 2009)

Let $<O, F>$ be a perceptual system and let X, Y $\subseteq$ O. A set X is perceptually near to the set Y within the perceptual system ($X \bowtie_F Y$), if and only if there are F1, F2 $\subseteq$ F and f $\in$ F and there are A $\in$ O/$\sim_{F1}$, B$\in$ O/$\sim_{F2}$, C$\in$ O/$\sim_f$ such that A $\subseteq$ X, B $\subseteq$ Y and A,B $\subseteq$ C. If a perceptual system is understood, then we say briefly that a set X is near to a set Y.

### Definition 6. Weak Nearness Relation (Peters and Wasilewski, 2009)

Let $<O, F>$ be a perceptual system and let X, Y $\subseteq$ O. The set X is weakly near to the set Y *within* the perceptual system $<O, F>$ ($X \underline{\bowtie}_F Y$) iff there are x $\in$ X and y $\in$ Y and there is $B \subseteq F$ such that x $\sim_B$ y. If a perceptual system is understood, then we say shortly that a set X *is weakly near to* set Y.

### Definition 7. Weak Tolerance Nearness Relation (Peters, 2009)

Let $<O, F>$ be a perceptual system and let X, Y $\subseteq$ O, $\varepsilon \in [0, 1]$. The set X is perceptually near to the set *Y within* the perceptual system _$<O, F>$ ($X \underline{\underline{\bowtie}}_F Y$) iff there exists x $\in$ X and y $\in$ Y and there is $\varphi \in$ F, $\varepsilon \in$ R such that x $\simeq_{B,\varepsilon}$ y. If a perceptual system is understood, then we say that a set X is *perceptually near* to a set Y in a weak tolerance sense of *nearness*.

### Definition 8. Tolerance Perceptual Near Sets (Peters, 2009)

Let $<O, F>$ be a perceptual system and let $X \subseteq O$. A set X is a tolerance perceptual near set near iff there is $Y \subseteq O$ such that $X \underline{\underline{\bowtie}}_F Y$.

Obviously, the greater the number of perceptual objects in near sets that have matching descriptions, the greater the degree of nearness of the sets. This observation leads to the various measures of nearness of sets using the nearness relations. In this chapter, we introduce a nearness measure based on the weak tolerance nearness relation in Def. 7.

## Definition 9. Tolerance Nearness Measure

Let <O, F> be a perceptual system and let X, Y $\subseteq$ O, X $\neq$ Y. Let B $\subseteq$ F, $\varphi$ $\in$ B, $\varepsilon$ $\in$ [0, 1]. A measure of nearness of sets X and Y is computed using

$$\mu_{\phi,\varepsilon}(X,Y) = \frac{\left|\left\{(x, y) \in X \times Y \mid x \simeq_{\phi,\varepsilon} y\right\}\right|}{\left(\begin{array}{c}\left|X \cup Y\right| \\ 2\end{array}\right)} \qquad (13)$$

that is, for each (x, y) $\in$ X $\times$ Y, it is the case that $|\varphi(x) - \varphi(y)| \leq \varepsilon$.

## 4. ASSESSING CONFLICT DYNAMICS WITH NEAR SETS: ILLUSTRATION

A typical system requirements engineering process leads to conflicts between project stakeholders. A stakeholder is one who has a share or an interest in the requirements for a systems engineering project. Cost effective engineering of complex software systems involves a collaborative process of requirements identification through negotiation. This is one of the key ideas of the Win-Win[1] approach (see Boehm 2001) used in requirements engineering. This approach also includes a decision model where a minimal set of conceptual elements, such as win conditions, issues, options and agreements, serves as an agreed upon ontology for collaboration and negotiation defined by the Win-Win process. System requirements (goals) are viewed as conditions. If all members agree on a requirement (i.e., no conflicts), then that requirement becomes an agreement. Otherwise, the requirement becomes an issue for further negotiation. Each issue could have an option (i.e., an alternate requirement) suggested by the team. A complete example of the problem of achieving agreement on high-level system requirements for a home lighting automation system (HLAS) be found in Skowron, Ramanna and Peters (2006). To assess conflict dynamics, we consider the following objects and features (negotiation parameters):

- **Objects:**
  - s(t)1.1 - ability to control up to a maximum of 20 custom lighting scenes throughout the residence,
  - s(t)1.2 - each scene provides a preset level of illumination (max. of 3) for each lighting bank,
  - s(t)1.3 - maximum range of a scene is 20 meters, r1.4 - activated using Control Switch,
  - s(t)1.4 - activated using Control Switch,
  - s(t)1.5 - activated using Central Control Unit,
  - s(t)1.6 - Ability to control an additional 2 lighting scenes in the yard.
- **Features:**
  - *Level of effort(e)* which is a rough estimate of development effort
  - *Importance(I)* which determines whether a requirement is essential to the project

- ○ *Stability(S)* of a requirement which indicates its volatility
- ○ *Risk(R)* which indicates whether the requirement is technically achievable
- ○ *Testability(T)* indicating whether a requirement is testable
- ○ *cd* indicating degree of social conflict in Table 2 computed using Equation (2) (see section 2.2) indicating degree of technical conflict in Table 3 (Egyed and Grünbacher, P., Kepler, 2001 and 2004).

Table 2 and Table 3 show sample values for features (negotiation parameters) of high-level functionality of Custom Lighting Scene that stakeholders are planning to include in the software. The values for the parameters differ from our earlier work in that *all of the features* real-valued in keeping with the definition of $\varphi: O \rightarrow R^L$. Also, the values reflect a level of granularity that is fine rather than coarse. Qualitative values for each of the parameters were used in our previous work (e.g, high, medium or low). The qualitative features values make it possible to assess conflict dynamics using the traditional indiscernibility relation (see definition 1]). The introduction of the real-valued features facilitates reasoning using tolerance relation (see definition 3). Another distinguishing element in this work, is the introduction of two perceptual information systems, one for each type of conflict. We are interested in measuring the nearness of perceptions (or how far) of the two different types of conflict. Using definition 4, P1 = <X1, F> and P2 = <Y1, F>. Note that s1.1.. s1.6 and t1.1.. t1.6 are the same set of requirements (objects). They have been given different identifiers for the sake of illustration. In Tables 2 and 3, cd denotes *conflict degree*. Values for cd in Table 2 have been computed using Equation 2.

## Example 1. Comparing Perceptual ISs Representing Conflict

Let P1 = <X1, F> denote perceptual system X1 = {s1.1,..., s1.6}, F = {E, I, S, R, T}, where the values of probe functions from F are given in Table 2. Similarly, let P1 = <Y1, F> denote perceptual system Y1 = {t1.1,..., t1.6}, F = {E, I, S, R, T} where the values of the probe functions from F are given in Table 3. Now choose samples X and Y that are also weak tolerance near sets from Tables 2 and 3. The basic idea here is to look for sets of objects containing at least one pair of objects that satisfy the weak tolerance relation.

**Tolerance Perceptual Near Sets**

*Table 2. Perceptual IS: social conflict*

| X1 | E | I | S | R | T | cd |
|------|------|------|------|-----|---|------|
| s1.1 | 0.4 | 0.9 | 0.1 | 0.2 | 1 | 0.22 |
| s1.2 | 0.5 | 0.9 | 0.1 | 0.2 | 1 | 0.44 |
| s1.3 | 0.8 | 0.4 | 0.2 | 0.5 | 1 | 0.2 |
| s1.4 | 0.2 | 0.95 | 0.99 | 0.1 | 1 | 0 |
| s1.5 | 0.35 | 0.75 | 0.4 | 0.8 | 1 | 0.67 |
| s1.6 | 0.6 | 0.1 | 0.7 | 0.8 | 0 | 0.89 |

*Table 3. Perceptual IS: technical conflict*

| Y1 | E | I | S | R | T | cd |
|------|------|------|-----|------|---|------|
| t1.1 | 0.45 | 0.9 | 0.1 | 0.15 | 1 | 0.7 |
| t1.2 | 0.57 | 0.98 | 0.3 | 0.2 | 1 | 0.2 |
| t1.3 | 0.89 | 0.6 | 0.2 | 0.5 | 1 | 0 |
| t1.4 | 0.1 | 0.85 | 0.9 | 0.16 | 1 | 0.9 |
| t1.5 | 0.6 | 0.88 | 0.5 | 0.8 | 1 | 0.88 |
| t1.6 | 0.7 | 0.3 | 0.6 | 0.7 | 0 | 0.25 |

- Let $\varepsilon = 0.3$, B = {cd},
- X1 = {{s1.1, s1.3 s1.4}, {s1.5, 1.6}},
- Y1 = {{t1.2, t1.3, t1.6}, {t1.1, t1.4, t1.5}},
- $X1 \underline{\bowtie}_{cd} Y1$,

- since we can find x $\in$ X1, y $\in$ Y1, where $x \simeq_{cd,0.3} y$, since

- $|cd(s1.1) - cd(t1.2)| = |0 - 0| = 0 \leq 0.3$

Notice that s1.1and t1.2 denote tolerance classes and not individual objects.

**Tolerance Nearness Measure**

Consider the near sets from Example 1 where $\varepsilon = 0.3$, $|X1 \cup Y1| = 12$, where

$$\binom{12}{2} = \frac{12!}{2!10!} = \frac{12 \times 11}{2} = 66 ,$$

and let $cd \in F$. From example 1, X1 = {{s1.1, s1.3 s1.4}, {s1.5, 1.6}}, Y1 = {{t1.2, t1.3, t1.6}, {t1.1, t1.4, t1.5}}. The degree of nearness of X1 and Y1 is

$$\mu_{cd,\varepsilon}(X1,Y1) = \frac{\left|\left\{(s1.1,t1.2),(s1.5,t1.1)\right\}\right|}{\binom{12}{2}}$$

$$= 2 / 66$$
$$= 0.03$$

## Example 2. Comparing Perceptual ISs Representing Conflict

In this example, the setup in Example 1 is changed due to the selection of a new tolerance class threshold.

**Tolerance Perceptual Near Sets**

- Let $\varepsilon = 0.2$, B = {cd},
- X1 = {{s1.1, s1.3}, {s1.3 s1.4}, {s1.2} {s1.5} {s1.6}},
- Y1 = {{t1.2, t1.3}, {t1.1, t1.4, t1.5}, { t1.6}},
    $X1 \underline{\bowtie}_{cd} Y1$,

    since we can find x $\in$ X1, y $\in$ Y1, where $x \simeq_{cd,0.2} y$, since

- $|cd(s1.1) - cd(t1.2)| = |0 - 0| = 0 \leq 0.2$

Observe also that s1.1and t1.2 denote tolerance classes and not individual objects.

**Tolerance Nearness Measure**

Consider the tolerance perceptual near sets from Example 2 where $\varepsilon = 0.2$, $|X1 \cup Y1| = 12$, where

$$\binom{12}{2} = \frac{12!}{2!10!} = \frac{12 \times 11}{2} = 66 \text{, and let}$$

$cd \in F$. From example 1, $X1 = \{\{s1.1, s1.3\}, \{s1.3 \; s1.4\}, \{s1.2\} \; \{s1.5\} \; \{s1.6\}\}$, $Y1 = \{\{t1.2, t1.3\}, \{t1.1, t1.4, t1.5\}, \{t1.6\}\}$, The degree of nearness

$$\mu_{cd,\varepsilon}(X1,Y1) = \frac{\left| \left\{ (s1.1,t1.2),(s1.1,t1.6),(s1.4,t1.2),(s1.4,t1.6),(s1.6,t1.1) \right\} \right|}{\binom{12}{2}}$$

$$= 5 \,/\, 66$$
$$= 0.07$$

Example 1 and Example 2 illustrate that the choice of threshold $\varepsilon$ determines the "nearness" of the two perceptual systems for one negotiation feature (cd). One can see that as more negotiation features are considered, the nearness value changes. These changes reflect the dynamics of similar technical and social conflicts.

## 5. CONCLUSION

In this chapter, we have introduced a new framework to represent socio-technical conflicts during negotiation. This framework is in the form of a collection of perceptual information systems. The underlying assumption is that conflict situations result due to different sets of viewpoints (perceptions) about issues under negotiation. Reasoning about conflict dynamics is made possible with nearness relations and tolerance perceptual near sets used in defining measures of nearness. In the interest of completeness, we have presented a complete survey of rough set based conflict models and methodologies for conflict dynamics in the context of requirements engineering. The contribution of this chapter is a new way of representing and reasoning about conflicts in the context of requirements engineering using near set theory.

## ACKNOWLEDGMENT

The research of James F. Peters and Sheela Ramanna is supported by NSERC Canada grant 185986 and 194376. The authors gratefully acknowledge Andrzej Skowron for his insights and earlier co-authored work in conflict theory.

# REFERENCES

Bargiela, A., & Pedrycz, W. (2003). *Granular Computing*. Boston: Kluwer.

Boehm, B., Grünbacher, P., & Kepler, J. (2001, May/June). Developing groupware for requirements negotiation: Lessons learned. *IEEE Software*, 46–55. doi:10.1109/52.922725

Egyed, A., & Grünbacher, P. (2004, November/December). Identifying requirements conflicts and cooperation: how quality attributes and automated traceability can help. *IEEE Software*, 50–58. doi:10.1109/MS.2004.40

Foundations of Logic and Linguistics. (n.d.). *Problems and Solutions*. London: Plenum.

Orłowska, E. (1998). Incomplete Information: Rough Set Analysis. Studies in Fuzziness and Soft Computing, 13, 1-22. Berlin Heidelberg, Germany: Springer Verlag.

Orłowska, E. (1982). *Semantics of Vague Concepts, Applications of Rough Sets*. Polish Academy of Sciences Institute for Computer Science, (Report 469).

Pawlak, Z. (1981a). *Classification of Objects by Means of Attributes. (Report 429)*. Institute for Computer Science, Polish Academy of Sciences.

Pawlak, Z. (1981b). *Rough Sets. (Report 431)*. Institute for Computer Science, Polish Academy of Sciences.

Pawlak, Z. (1982). Rough sets. *International J. Comp. Inform. Science*, *11*, 341–356. doi:10.1007/BF01001956

Pawlak, Z. (1984). On Conflicts. *International Journal of Man-Machine Studies*, *21*, 127–134. doi:10.1016/S0020-7373(84)80062-0

Pawlak, Z. (1987). *On Conflicts*. Warsaw, Poland: Polish Scientific Publishers. (in Polish)

Pawlak, Z. (1991). *Rough Sets - Theoretical Aspects of Reasoning about Data*. Amsterdam: Kluwer Academic Publishers.

Pawlak, Z. (1993). Anatomy of conflict. *Bulletin of the European Association for Theoretical Computer Science*, *50*, 234–247.

Pawlak, Z. (1998). An inquiry into anatomy of conflicts. *Journal of Information Science*, *109*, 65–78. doi:10.1016/S0020-0255(97)10072-X

Pawlak, Z., & Skowron, A. (2007a). Rudiments of rough sets. *Information Sciences*, *177*, 3–27. doi:10.1016/j.ins.2006.06.003

Pawlak, Z., & Skowron, A. (2007b). Rough sets: Some extensions. *Information Sciences*, *177*, 28–40. doi:10.1016/j.ins.2006.06.006

Peters, J. F. (2007a). Classification of objects by means of features, In *Proceedings of the IEEE Symposium Series on Foundations of Computational Intelligence* (IEEE SCCI 2007). Honolulu, HI.

Peters, J. F. (2007b). Near sets. Special theory about nearness of objects. *Fundamenta Informaticae*, *75*(1-4), 407–433.

Peters, J. F. (2007c). Near sets. General theory about nearness of objects. *Applied Mathematical Sciences, 1*(53), 2609–2029.

Peters, J. F. (2008). Classification of perceptual objects by means of features. *Int. J. of Info. Technology & Intelligent Computing, 3*(2), 1–35.

Peters, J. F. (2008a). Approximation and perception in ethology-based reinforcement learning. In Pedrycz, W., Skowron, A., & Kreinovich, V. (Eds.), *Handbook on Granular Computing*. New York: Wiley. doi:10.1002/9780470724163.ch30

Peters, J. F. (2009). Tolerance near sets and image correspondence. Int. *J. of Bio-Inspired Computation, 1*(4), 239–245. doi:10.1504/IJBIC.2009.024722

Peters, J. F., & Henry, C. (2006c). Reinforcement Learning with Approximation Spaces. *Fundamenta Informaticae, 71*, 323–349.

Peters, J. F., Henry, C., & Ramanna, S. (2005). Rough ethograms: Study of intelligent system behaviour. In Kłopotek, M. A., Wierzcho'n, S., & Trojanowski, K. (Eds.), *New Trends in Intelligent Information Processing and Web Mining (IIS05)* (pp. 117–126). Gdansk, Poland. doi:10.1007/3-540-32392-9_13

Peters, J. F., & Ramanna, S. (2007). Feature Selection: Near Set Approach. In*Proceedings of MCDM'07*, (LNCS 4484), Springer- Verlag, Berlin 57-71.

Peters, J. F., & Ramanna, S. (2009). Affinities between perceptual information granules: Foundations and perspectives. In Bargiela, A., & Pedrycz, W. (Eds.), *Human-Centric Information Processing Through Granular Modelling. Studies in Computational Intelligence* (pp. 49–66). Berlin, Germany: Springer. doi:10.1007/978-3-540-92916-1_3

Peters, J. F., & Skowron, A. (2006a). Zdzislaw Pawlak: Life and Work. *Transactions on Rough Sets, 5*, 1–24. doi:10.1007/11847465_1

Peters, J. F., & Skowron, A. (2007). Zdzisław Pawlak life and work (1906-2006). *Information Sciences, 177*, 1–2. doi:10.1016/j.ins.2006.06.004

Peters, J. F., Skowron, A., & Stepaniuk, J. (2006b). Nearness in approximation spaces. In G. Lindemann, H. Schlilngloff et al. (Eds.), Proceedings of Concurrency, Specification & Programming (CS & P'2006), (pp. 434-445). Informatik-Berichte Nr. 206, Humboldt-Universität zu Berlin.

Peters, J. F., Skowron, A., & Stepaniuk, J. (2007). Nearness of objects: Extension of approximation space model. *Fundamenta Informaticae, 79*, 1–16.

Peters, J. F., Skowron, A., Synak, P., & Ramanna, S. (2003). Rough sets and information granulation. In Bilgic, T., Baets, D., Kaynak, O. (Eds.), *Tenth Int. Fuzzy Systems Assoc. World Congress IFSA*, Instanbul, Turkey (Lecture Notes in Artificial Intelligence 2715, pp. 370-377). Berlin Heidelberg, Germany: Springer Verlag.

Peters, J. F., & Wasilewski, P. (2009). *Foundations of near set theory*. Information Sciences. *International Journal, 179*(18), 3091–3109.

Ramanna, S. (2008). *Conflict analysis in the framework of rough sets and granular computing, Handbook of Granular Computing*. New York: Wiley.

Ramanna, S., Peters, J. F., & Skowron, A. (2006, September 27-29) Analysis of Conflict Dynamics by Risk Patterns. In *Proceedings of the Workshop on Concurrency, Specification and Programming* (CS&P 2006), Berlin, Germany.

Ramanna, S., Peters, J. F., & Skowron, A. (2006a). Approaches to Conflict Dynamics based on Rough Sets, *Fundamenta Informaticae,* (75), 1-16.

Ramanna, S., Peters, J. F., & Skowron, A. (2006b) Generalized conflict and resolution model with approximation spaces. In Iniuguchi, M., Greco, S., Nguyen, H.S. (Eds.), *Proceedings of RSCTC'06*, (LNAI, 4259, pp. 274-283). Berlin Heidelberg, Germnay: Springer-Verlag.

Ramanna, S., Peters, J. F., & Skowron, A. (2007a). Approximate Adaptive Learning During Conflict Resolution. *Journal of Information Technology and Intelligent Computing, 2.*

Ramanna, S., Peters, J. F., & Skowron, A. (2007b). Approximation Space-based Socio-Technical Conflict Model. In *Proceedings of RSKT'07*, (LNCS 4481, pp. 476-483). Berlin Heidelberg, Germany: Springer Verlag.

Ramanna, S., & Skowron, A. (2007c). Requirements Interaction and Conflicts: A Rough Set Approach. In *Proceedings of the IEEE Symposium Series on Foundations of Computational Intelligence* (IEEE SCCI 2007). Honolulu, HI.

Skowron, A., & Peters, J. F. (2008). Rough-granular computing. In Pedrycz, W., Skowron, A., Kreinovich, V. (Eds.), *Handbook on Granular Computing*, 285-328. New York. Wiley.

Skowron, A., Ramanna, S., & Peters, J. F. (2006). Conflict Analysis and Information Systems: A Rough Set Approach. In *Proceedings of RSKT'06*, (LNCS 4062, pp. 233-241). Berlin, Heidelberg, Germany: Springer Verlag.

Skowron, A., & Rauszer, C. (1992). The DiscernibilityMatrices and Functions in Information Systems. In Słowinski, R. (Ed.), *Intelligent Decision Support - Handbook of Applications and Advances of the Rough Sets Theory, System Theory, Knowledge Engineering and Problem Solving 11* (pp. 331–362). Dordrecht, The Netherlands: Kluwer.

Yao, J. T. (2008). Recent Developments in Granular Computing. In *Proceedings of the 2008 IEEE International Conference on Granular Computing*, (pp. 74-79).

Yao, Y. Y. (2008). Granular Computing: Past, Present and Future. In *Proceedings of the 2008 IEEE International Conference on Granular Computing*, (pp. 80-85).

Zadeh, L. A. (1997). Toward a theory of fuzzy information granulation and its certainty in human reasoning and fuzzy logic. *Fuzzy Sets and Systems*, *90*, 111–127. doi:10.1016/S0165-0114(97)00077-8

## ENDNOTE

[1]    The WINWIN Homepage: http://sunset.usc.edu/research/WINWIN

# Chapter 9
# Rule Extraction and Rule Evaluation Based on Granular Computing

**Jiye Liang**
*Shanxi University, P.R. China*

**Yuhua Qian**
*Shanxi University, P.R. China*

**Deyu Li**
*Shanxi University, P.R. China*

## ABSTRACT

*In rough set theory, rule extraction and rule evaluation are two important issues. In this chapter, the concepts of positive approximation and converse approximation are first introduced, which can be seen as dynamic approximations of target concepts based on a granulation order. Then, two algorithms for rule extraction called MABPA and REBCA are designed and applied to hierarchically generate decision rules from a decision table. Furthermore, to evaluate the whole performance of a decision rule set, three kinds of measures are proposed for evaluating the certainty, consistency and support of a decision-rule set extracted from a decision table, respectively. The experimental analyses on several decision tables show that these three new measures are adequate for evaluating the decision performance of a decision-rule set extracted from a decision table in rough set theory. The measures may be helpful for determining which rule extraction technique should be chosen in a practical decision problem.*

## 1. INTRODUCTION

*Granular computing* (GrC) is a new active area of current research in *artificial intelligence*, and is a new concept and computing formula for information processing. It has been widely applied to many branches of artificial intelligence such as problem solving, knowledge discovery, image processing, semantic web services [18, 29-31, 37].

DOI: 10.4018/978-1-60566-324-1.ch009

As follows, for our further development, we briefly review research on GrC. In 1979, the problem of fuzzy information granules was introduced by Zadeh. Then, in [47, 48] he introduced a concept of granular computing, as a term with many meanings, covering all the research of theory, methods, techniques and tools related to granulation. He identified three basic concepts that underlie the process of human cognition, namely, granulation, organization, and causation. "Granulation involves decomposition of whole into parts, organization involves integration of parts into whole, and causation involves association of causes and effects". Some authors [37, 45] examined granular computing in connection with the theory of rough sets. Yao [45, 46] suggested the use of hierarchical granulations for the study of stratified rough set approximations and studied granular computing through using neighborhood systems. The theory of quotient space had been extended into the theory of fuzzy quotient space based on fuzzy equivalence relation [50]. Liang and Shi [14, 15] established the relationship among knowledge granulation, information entropy, granularity measure and rough entropy in information systems. Liang and Qian [17] developed an axiomatic approach to knowledge granulation in information systems. Granular computing mainly has three important models: (1) computing with words, (2) *rough set theory*, and (3) quotient space theory. As applications of granular computing, in this chapter, we focus on *rule extraction* and *rule evaluation* based on granular computing.

In the view of granular computing, a target concept described by a set is always characterized via the so-called upper and lower approximations under static granulation in rough set theory, and a static boundary region of the concept is induced by the upper and lower approximations [22-25]. However, through this mechanism, we cannot improve the approximation measure of a rough set and more clearly analyze the approximation structure of a rough set [34, 38]. Based on these conclusions, one objective of this chapter is to establish two kinds of structures of the approximation of a target concept by introducing a notion of a granulation order, called positive approximation and converse approximation, and to apply them to rule extracting from decision tables.

Generally speaking, a set of decision rules can be generated from a decision table by adopting any kind of rule extracting methods. In recent years, how to evaluate the decision performance of a decision rule has become a very important issue in rough set theory. In [3], based on information entropy, Duntsch suggested some uncertainty measures of a decision rule and proposed three criteria for model selection. For a decision rule set consisting of every decision rule induced from a decision table, three parameters are traditionally associated: the strength, the certainty factor and the coverage factor of the rule [32, 33]. In many practical decision problems, we always adopt several rule-extracting methods for the same decision table. In this case, it is very important to check whether or not each of the rule-extracting approaches adopted is suitable for the given decision table. In other words, it is desirable to evaluate the decision performance of the decision-rule set extracted by each of the rule-extracting approaches. This strategy can help a decision maker to determine which of rule-extracting methods is preferred for a given decision table. However, all of the above measures for this purpose are only defined for a single decision rule and are not suitable for evaluating the *decision performance* of a decision-rule set. There are two more kinds of measures in the literature [26-28], which are approximation accuracy for decision classification and consistency degree for a decision table. Although these two measures, in some sense, could be regarded as measures for evaluating the decision performance of all decision rules generated from a complete decision table, they have some limitations. For instance, the certainty and consistency of a rule set could not be well characterized by the approximation accuracy and consistency degree when their values reaches zero. As we know, when the approximation accuracy or consistency degree is equal to zero, it is only implied that there is no decision rule with the certainty of one in the complete decision table. This shows that the approximation accuracy and consistency degree of a complete decision table cannot give elaborate depictions of the certainty and consistency for a rule set. To overcome the shortcomings of the existing measures, another objective of this chapter is to find some measures for evaluating the decision performance of a set of decision rules and analyze how each of these measures depends on the condition granulation and decision granulation of a decision table.

The rest of this chapter is organized as follows. Some preliminary concepts such as information systems, rough set approximation and decision tables are briefly reviewed in Section 2. In Section 3, *positive approximation* and *converse approximation* of a target concept based on *dynamic granulation* are presented, respectively, and two new approaches to extracting decision rules are obtained through using these two approximations. In Section 4, through classifying decision tables in rough set theory into three types according to their consistencies, we introduce three new measures for evaluating the decision performance of a decision-rule set extracted from a decision table and analyze how each of these three measures depends on the condition granulation and decision granulation of each of the three types of decision tables. Section 5 concludes this chapter with some remarks and discussions.

## 2. PRELIMINARIES

In this section, we review some basic concepts such as information systems, decision tables and rough set approximation.

An *information system* (sometimes called a data table, an attribute-value system, a knowledge representation system, etc.), as a basic concept in rough set theory, provides a convenient framework for the representation of objects in terms of their attribute values [7-10]. An information system $S$ is a pair $(U, A)$, where $U$ is a non-empty and finite set of objects and is called the universe and $A$ is a non-empty and finite set of attributes. For each $a \in A$, a mapping $a : U \rightarrow V_a$ is determined by a given decision table, where $V_a$ is the domain of $a$ [11].

Each non-empty subset $B \subseteq A$ determines an indiscernibility relation in the following way:

$$R_B = \{(x, y) \in U \times U \mid a(x) = a(y), \forall a \in B\}.$$

The relation $R_B$ partitions $U$ into some equivalence classes given by

$$U / R_B = \{[x]_B \mid x \in U\}, \text{ just } U / B,$$

where $[x]_B$ denotes the equivalence class determined by $x$ with respect to $B$, i.e.,

$$[x]_B = \{y \in U \mid (x, y) \in R_B\}.$$

Let $P, Q \in 2^A$ be two attribute subsets, where $2^A$ is a power set of $A$. By $IND(P)$ and $IND(Q)$ we denote the indiscernible relations induced by $P$ and $Q$, respectively. A partial relation $\preceq$ on $2^A$ is defined in [12, 16] as follows: $P \preceq Q (Q \succeq P)$ if and only if, for every $P_i \in U / IND(P)$, there exists $Q_j \in U / IND(Q)$ such that $P_i \subseteq Q_j$, where

$$U / IND(P) = \{P_1, P_2, \cdots, P_m\} \text{ and } U / IND(Q) = \{Q_1, Q_2, \cdots, Q_n\}$$

are partitions induced by $IND(P)$ and $IND(Q)$, respectively.

A decision table is an information system $S = (U, C \cup D)$ with $C \cap D = \varnothing$, where an element of $C$ is called a condition attribute, $C$ is called a condition attribute set, an element of $D$ is called a decision attribute, and $D$ is called a decision attribute set. If $U / C \preceq U / D$, then $S = (U, C \cup D)$ is said to be consistent, otherwise it is said to be inconsistent [19, 44, 35]. One can extract certain decision rules from a consistent decision table and uncertain decision rules from an inconsistent decision table [40].

Given an equivalence relation $R$ on $U$ and a subset $X \subseteq U$, one can define a lower approximation of $X$ and an upper approximation of $X$ by the following

$$\underline{R}X = \bigcup \{x \in U \mid [x]_R \subseteq X\},$$

$$\overline{R}X = \bigcup \{x \in U \mid [x]_R \cap X \neq \varnothing\}.$$

The $R$-positive region of $X$ is $POS_R(X) = \underline{R}X$, the $R$-negative region of $X$ is $NEG_R(X) = U - \overline{R}X$ and the boundary or $R$-borderline region of $X$ is $BN_R(X) = \overline{R}X - \underline{R}X$

## 3. RULE-EXTRACTING APPROACH UNDER DYNAMIC GRANULATION

### 3.1. Positive Approximation and Rule Extraction

In an information system, a partition induced by an equivalence relation provides a granulation world for describing a target concept. Thus, a sequence of granulation worlds from coarse to fine can be determined by a sequence of attribute sets with granulations from coarse to fine in the power set of $A$. The positive approximation gives the definition of the upper and lower approximations of a target concept under a given granulation order [13, 38]. It can be used to extract from a given decision table decision rules with granulations from coarse to fine. The definition of the positive approximation is as follows.

### Definition 3.1

Let $S = (U, A)$ be an information system, $X \subseteq U$ and $P = \{R_1, R_2, \cdots, R_n\}$ a family of attribute sets with $R_1 \succeq R_2 \succeq \cdots \succeq R_n (R_i \in 2^A)$. Let $P_i = \{R_1, R_2, \cdots R_i\}$, we define $P_i$-upper approximation $\overline{P_i}(X)$ and $P_i$-lower approximation $\underline{P_i}(X)$ of $P_i$-positive approximation of $X$ as

$$\overline{P_i}(X) = \overline{R_i}(X),$$

$$\underline{P_i}(X) = \bigcup_{k=1}^{i} \underline{R_k}(X_k),$$

where $X_1 = X$ and $X_k = X - \bigcup_{j=1}^{k-1} \underline{R_j} X_j$ for $k = 2, 3, \cdots, n$, $i = 1, 2, \cdots, n$.

## Theorem 3.1

Let $S = (U, A)$ be an information system, $X \subseteq U$ and $P = \{R_1, R_2, \cdots, R_n\}$ a family of attribute sets with $R_1 \succeq R_2 \succeq \cdots \succeq R_n (R_i \in 2^A)$. Let $P_i = \{R_1, R_2, \cdots, R_i\}$, then $\forall P_i (i = 1, 2, \cdots, n)$, we have

$$\underline{P_i}(X) \subseteq X \subseteq \overline{P_i}(X),$$

$$\underline{P_1}(X) \subseteq \underline{P_2}(X) \subseteq \cdots \subseteq \underline{P_n}(X).$$

Theorem 3.1 states that the lower approximation of the positive approximation of a target concept enlarges as a granulation order becomes longer through adding an equivalence relation, which will help to exactly describe the target concept.

## Theorem 3.2

Let $S = (U, A)$ be an information system, $X \subseteq U$ and $P = \{R_1, R_2, \cdots, R_n\}$ a family of attribute sets with $R_1 \succeq R_2 \succeq \cdots \succeq R_n (R_i \in 2^A)$. Let $P_i = \{R_1, R_2, \cdots, R_i\}$, then $\forall P_i (i = 1, 2, \cdots, n)$, we have

$$\alpha_{P_1}(X) \leq \alpha_{P_2}(X) \leq \cdots \leq \alpha_{P_n}(X),$$

where $\alpha_{P_i}(X) = \dfrac{|\underline{P_i}(X)|}{|\overline{P_i}(X)|}$ is the approximation measure of $X$ with respect to $P$.

The approximation measure was introduced to the positive approximation in order to describe the uncertainty of a target concept under a granulation order [13]. From this theorem, one can see that the approximation measure of a target concept enlarges as a granulation order becomes longer through adding an equivalence relation.

We apply rough set method for decision rule mining from decision tables. It is not always possible to extract laws from experimental data by computing first all reducts of a decision table and next decision rules on the basis of these reducts [1, 2, 6, 39, 41-43, 49, 51-53].

In the following, we propose an algorithm for decision-rule mining in consistent decision tables by using the positive approximation. The application will be helping for understanding the idea of positive approximation.

Let $S = (U, C \cup D)$ be a consistent decision table, where $C$ and $D$ are condition and decision attribute sets respectively, and $C \cap D = \varnothing$. The positive region of $D$ with respect to $C$ is defined as follows

$$pos_C(D) = \bigcup_{X \in U/D} \underline{C}X.$$

In a decision table $S = (U, C \cup D)$, the significance of $c \in C$ with respect to $D$ is defined as follows [49]:

$$sig^D_{C-\{c\}}(c) = \gamma_C(D) - \gamma_{C-\{c\}}(D),$$

where $\gamma_C(D) = \dfrac{|pos_C(D)|}{|U|}$.

In a decision table $S = (U, C \cup D)$, the significance of $c \in C - C'$ ($C' \subseteq C$) with respect to $D$ is defined as follows

$$sig^D_{C'}(c) = \gamma_{C' \cup \{c\}}(D) - \gamma_{C'}(D),$$

where $\gamma_{C'}(D) = \dfrac{|pos_{C'}(D)|}{|U|}$.

**Algorithm 3.1**

```
MABPA (mining rules in a consistent decision table)

Input: consistent decision table S = (U, C ∪ D)

Output: decision rules Rule .

For ∀c ∈ C, compute the significance and relative core
```

$$core_D(C) = \{c \in C \mid sig^D_{C-\{c\}}(c) > 0\};$$

If $core_D(C) \neq \varnothing$, let $P_1 = core_D(C)$; else, for $\forall c \in C$, compute the dependence $\gamma_C(D)$ of $D$ to $c$, let $\gamma_{c_1}(D) = \max\{\gamma_C(D) \mid c \in C\}$ and $P_1 = \{c_1\}$

Compute $U / D = \{Y_1, Y_2, \cdots, Y_d\}$;

Let $P = \{P_1\}$, $i = 1$, $U^* = U$, $\Gamma = \phi$, $Rule = \phi$;

Compute $U^* \neq IND(P_i) = \{X_{i1}, X_{i2}, \cdots, X_{is_i}\}$

Let $\Gamma' = \{X_k \in U^* / IND(P_i) \mid X_k \subseteq Y_j (Y_j \in U / D, j = \{1, 2, \cdots, d\})\}$ Let $Rule' =$, for $\forall X_k \in \Gamma'$, put $des_{P_i}(X_k) \rightarrow des_D(Y_j)(Y_j \in U / D, Y_j \supseteq X_k)$ into $Rule'$. Let $Rule = Rule \cup Rule'$, $\Gamma = \Gamma \cup \Gamma'$

If $\bigcup_{x \in \Gamma} x = U$, go to (8); else, $U^* = U^* - \bigcup_{x \in \Gamma} x$, for $\forall c \in C - P_i$. compute $sig_{P_i}^D(c)$, let $sig_{P_i}^D(c_2) = \max\{sig_{P_i}^D(c), c \in C - P_i\}$, $P_{i+1} = P_i \cup \{c_2\}$, let $P = P \cup \{P_{i+1}\}$, $i = i + 1$ go to (5);

Output $Rule$.

Obviously, generation of decision rules is not based on a reduct of a decision table, but $P$ (a granulation order) and $U^*$ in the MABPA. By using MABPA algorithm, the time complexity of extract rules is polynomial. At the first step, we need to compute $core_D(C)$, i.e., compute $sig_{C-\{c\}}^D(c)$ for all $c \in C$. The time complexity for computing $core_D(C)$ is $O(|C||U|^2)$. At step 3, the time complexity for computing $U / D$ is $O(|U|^2)$. At step 5, the time complexity for computing $U^* / IND(P_i)$ is $O(|U|^2)$. At step 7, the time complexity for computing all $sig_{P_i}^D(c)$ is $O(|C - P_i||C||U|^2)$; the time complexity to choose maximum for significance of attribute is $|C - P_i|$. From step 5 to step 7, $|C| - 1$ is the maximum value for the circle times. Therefore, the time complexity is

$$\sum_{i=1}^{|C|-1} O(|U|^2) + O(|C - P_i||C||U|^2) + O(|C - P_i|) = O(|C|^3|U|^2)$$

Other steps will not be considered because that their time complexity are all const. Thus the time complexity of the algorithm MABPA is as follows

$$O(|C||U|^2) + O(|U|^2) + O(|U|^2) + O(|C|^3|U|^2) = O(|C|^3|U|^2)$$

## 3.2. Converse Approximation and Rule Extraction

In some practical issues, we need to mining decision rules on the basis of keeping the approximation measure of a target concept. Obviously, the positive approximation appears not to be suited for rule extracting from decision tables on the basis of keeping the approximation measure of every decision class in decision partition on the universe. Therefore, in this section, we introduce a new set-approximation approach called a converse approximation and investigate some of its important properties.

Let $S = (U, A)$ be an information system and $R \in 2^A$. A partition induced by the equivalence relation $IND(R)$, provides a granulation world for describing a target concept $X$. So a sequence of attribute sets $R_i \in 2^A$ $(i = 1, 2, \cdots, n)$ with $R_1 \preceq R_2 \preceq \cdots \preceq R_n$ can determine a sequence of granulation worlds from fine to coarse. A converse approximation can give the definition of the upper and lover approximations of a target concept under a granulation order. In the following, we introduce the definition of the converse approximation of a target set under dynamic granulation.

### Definition 3.2

Let $S = (U, A)$ be an information system, $X \subseteq U$ and $P = \{R_1, R_2, \cdots, R_n\}$ a family of attribute sets with $R_1 \preceq R_2 \preceq \cdots \preceq R_n (R_i \in 2^A)$. Let $P_i = \{R_1, R_2, ..., R_i\}$, we define $P_i$-upper approximation $\overline{P_i}(X)$ and $P_i$-lower approximation $\underline{P_i}(X)$ of $P_i$-converse approximation of $X$ as

$$\overline{P_i}(X) = \overline{R_1}(X)$$

$$\underline{P_i}(X) = \underline{R_i}X_i \cup (\bigcup_{k=1}^{i-1}(\underline{R_k}X_k - \underline{R_{k+1}}X_k))$$

where $X_1 = X$ and $X_{k+1} = \underline{R_k}X_k$ for $k = 1, 2, \cdots, n$, $i = 1, 2, \cdots, n$.

Definition 3.2 shows that a target concept can be approached by the change in the lower approximation $\underline{P_i}(X)$ and the upper approximation $\overline{P_i}(X)$. In particular, we call $\overline{P_n}(X) = \overline{R_1}(X)$ and $\underline{P_n}(X) = \underline{R_n}X \cup (\bigcup_{k=1}^{n-1}\underline{R_k}X_k - \underline{R_{k+1}}X_k)$ $P$-upper approximation and $P$-lower approximation of $P$-converse approximation of $X$, respectively.

### Theorem 3.3

Let $S = (U, A)$ be an information system, $X \subseteq U$ and $P = \{R_1, R_2, \cdots, R_n\}$ a family of attribute sets with $R_1 \preceq R_2 \preceq \cdots \preceq R_n (R_i \in 2^A)$. Let $P_i = \{R_1, R_2, \cdots, R_i\}$, then $\forall P_i(i = 1, 2, \cdots, n)$, we have that

$$\underline{P_i}(X) \subseteq X \subseteq \overline{P_i}(X),$$

$$\underline{P_1}(X) = \underline{P_2}(X) = \cdots = \underline{P_n}(X).$$

**Proof**

It follows from Definition 3.2 that $\underline{R_i}X_i \subseteq X_i$ and $X_{i+1} \subseteq X_i$ hold for $\underline{R_i}X_i$. Therefore, one can obtain that

$$\underline{P_i}(X) = \underline{R_i}X \cup \left(\bigcup_{k=1}^{i-1}\underline{R_k}X_k - \underline{R_{k+1}}X_k\right)$$
$$= \underline{R_i}X \cup \underline{R_1}X_1 = \underline{R_1}X_1 = \underline{R_1}X$$

i.e., $\underline{P_1}(X) = \underline{P_2}(X)\cdots = \underline{P_n}(X) = \underline{R_1}(X)$.

Moreover, it is clear from Definition 3.2 that

$$\underline{P_i}(X) = \underline{R_1}X \subseteq X \subseteq \overline{P_1}(X) = \overline{P_i}(X).$$

Thus $\underline{P_i}(X) \subseteq X \subseteq \overline{P_i}(X)$. This completes the proof.

Theorem 3.3 states that the lower approximation and the upper approximation of $P$-converse approximation of a target concept do not change as a granulation order becomes longer through adding equivalence relations, which gives a new method of describing a target concept. In particular, the number of equivalence classes in $\underline{P_i}(X)$ decreases as the granulation order become longer. In other words,

some new equivalence classes under different granulations are induced by combining some known equivalence classes in the lower approximation of the target concept.

In order to illustrate the essence that the converse approximation is concentrate on the changes in the construction of the target concept $X$ (equivalence classes in lower approximation of $X$ with respect to $P$), we can redefine $P$-converse approximation of $X$ by using some equivalence classes on $U$. Therefore, the structure of $P$-upper approximation $\overline{P}(X)$ and $P$-lower approximation $\underline{P}(X)$ of $P$-converse approximation of $X$ are represented as follows:

$$[\overline{P}(X)] = \{\cup[x]_{R_1} \,|\, [x]_{R_1} \cap X \neq \varnothing\},$$

$$[\underline{P}(X)] = \left\{[x]_{R_1} \,|\, [x]_{R_1} \subseteq \underline{R_i}X_i \cup \left(\bigcup_{k=1}^{i-1}\underline{R_k}X_k - \underline{R_{k+1}}X_k\right), \ i = 1, 2, \cdots, n\right\}$$

where $X_1 = X$, $X_{k+1} = \underline{R_k} X_k$ for $i = 1, 2, \cdots, n$ and $[x]_{R_i}$ represents the equivalence class obtaining $x$ in the partition $U \, / \, R_i$. It follows from the structure of $[\underline{P}(X)]$ that

$$\underline{R_k} X_k - \underline{R_{k+1}} X_k = \{[x]_{R_k} \mid [x]_{R_k} \subseteq \underline{R_k} X_k \cap bn_{R_{k+1}}(X_k), x \in U\}$$

where $bn_{R_{k+1}} X_k = \overline{R_{k+1}} X_k - \underline{R_{k+1}} X_k$. That is to say, these objects in $\underline{R_k} X_k - \underline{R_{k+1}} X_k$ will result in a new boundary region if they are described by $R_{k+1}$. We only research new lower approximation induced by dynamic granulation order every time for describing the target concept.

## Example 3.2

Let $U = \{e_1, e_2, e_3, e_4, e_5, e_6, e_7, e_8\}$, $X = \{e_1, e_2, e_3, e_4, e_7, e_8\}$,

and $U \, / \, R_1 = \{\{e_1\}, \{e_2\}, \{e_3, e_4\}, \{e_5, e_6\}, \{e_7, e_8\}\}$, $U \, / \, R_2 = \{\{e_1\}, \{e_2\}, \{e_5, e_6\}, \{e_3, e_4, e_7, e_8\}\}$

be two partitions on $U$.

Obviously, $R_1 \underline{\prec} R_2$ holds. Thus, one can construct two granulation orders (a family of equivalence relations) $P_1 = \{R_1\}$ and $P_2 = \{R_1, R_2\}$.

By computing the converse approximation of $X$ with respect to $P$, one can easily obtain that

$$[\overline{P_1}(X)] = \{\{e_1\}, \{e_2\}, \{e_3, e_4\}, \{e_7, e_8\}\},$$

$$[\underline{P_1}(X)] = \{\{e_1\}, \{e_2\}, \{e_3, e_4\}, \{e_7, e_8\}\},$$

$$[\overline{P_2}(X)] = \{\{e_1\}, \{e_2\}, \{e_3, e_4\}, \{e_7, e_8\}\}$$

and

$$[\underline{P_2}(X)] = \{\{e_1\}, \{e_2\}, \{e_3, e_4, e_7, e_8\}\},$$

where $\{e_1\}, \{e_2\}$ can be induced by both equivalence relation $R_1$ and equivalence relation $R_2$, $\{e_3, e_4, e_7, e_8\}$ is only obtained by equivalence relation $R_2$. That is to say, the target concept $X$ is described by using granulation $P_1 = \{R_1\}$ and $P_2 = \{R_1, R_2\}$.

In order to discuss the properties of the converse approximation based on dynamic granulation, we need to introduce the definition of $\underline{\prec}$. Assume that $A, B$ be two families of classical sets, where

$A = \{A_1, A_2, \cdots, A_m\}$, $B = \{B_1, B_2, \cdots, B_n\}$. We say $A \preceq B$, if and only if, for any $A_i \in A$, there exists $B_j \in B$ such that $A_i \subseteq B_j$ $(i \leq m, j \leq n)$. From this denotation, we can obtain the following theorem.

## Theorem 3.4

Let $S = (U, A)$ be an information system, $X \subseteq U$ and $P = \{R_1, R_2, \cdots, R_n\}$ a family of attribute sets with $R_1 \preceq R_2 \preceq \cdots \preceq R_n (R_i \in 2^A)$. Let $P_i = \{R_1, R_2, \cdots, R_i\}$, then $\forall P_i (i = 1, 2, \cdots, n)$, we have that

$$[\underline{P_1}(X)] \preceq [\underline{P_2}(X)] \preceq \cdots \preceq [\underline{P_n}(X)].$$

**Proof**
It follows from Definition 3.2 and Theorem 3.3 that

$$\underline{P_1}(X) = \underline{P_2}(X) \cdots = \underline{P_n}(X) = \underline{R_1}(X).$$

Suppose $1 \leq i < j \leq n$, then $R_i \preceq R_j$. Therefore, one can get that

$$
\begin{aligned}
[\underline{P_i}(X)] &= \underline{R_i}X_i \cup \left( \bigcup_{k=1}^{i-1} (\underline{R_k}X_k - \underline{R_{k+1}}X_k) \right) \\
&\preceq \left( \bigcup_{k=1}^{i-1} (\underline{R_k}X_k - \underline{R_{k+1}}X_k) \right) \cup \left( \bigcup_{k=i}^{j-1} (\underline{R_k}X_k - \underline{R_{k+1}}X_k) \right) \cup \underline{R_j}X_j \\
&= \underline{R_j}X_j \cup \left( \bigcup_{k=i}^{j-1} (\underline{R_k}X_k - \underline{R_{k+1}}X_k) \right) \\
&= [\underline{P_j}(X)].
\end{aligned}
$$

Therefore $[\underline{P_1}(X)] \preceq [\underline{P_2}(X)] \preceq \cdots \preceq [\underline{P_n}(X)]$. This completes the proof.

Theorem 3.4 states that the number of classes in the lower approximation of $P$-converse approximation of a target concept decreases as the granulation order become longer through adding equivalence relations, and some new equivalence classes are induced by combing known equivalence classes in the lower approximation of the target concept. This mechanism can reduce the number of equivalence classes for describing a target concept on the basis of keeping the approximation measure $\alpha_P(X) = \dfrac{|\underline{P}(X)|}{|\overline{P}(X)|}$

which can simply the construction of the approximation of a target concept. In fact, through the converse approximation, we can more clearly understand the rough approximation of a target concept.

Let $S = (U, A)$ be an information system, $R \in 2^A$ a subset of attributes on $A$ and $\Gamma = \{X_1, X_2, \cdots, X_m\}$ a partition on $U$. Lower approximation and upper approximation of $\Gamma$ with respect to $R$ are defined by

$$\underline{R}\Gamma = \{\underline{R}X_1, \underline{R}X_2, \cdots, \underline{R}X_m\},$$

$$\overline{R}\Gamma = \{\overline{R}X_1, \overline{R}X_2, \cdots, \overline{R}X_m\}.$$

In the view of describing the target concept by using equivalence classes, we need to define a new measure to discuss the converge situation about equivalence classes in a lower approximation, which will be helpful in understanding the construction of the target concept in rough set theory. For this objective, we introduce the following notion called a converge degree.

## Definition 3.3

Let $S = (U, A)$ be an information system, $R \in 2^A$ a subset of attributes on $A$ and $\Gamma = \{X_1, X_2, \cdots, X_m\}$ a partition on $U$. Converge degree of $\Gamma$ with respect to $R$ as

$$c(R, \Gamma) = \sum_{i=1}^{m} \frac{|X_i|}{|U|} \sum_{j=1}^{s_i} p^2(X_i^j),$$

where $s_i$ is the number of equivalence classes in $\underline{R}X_i$, $p(X_i^j) = \dfrac{|X_i^j|}{|X_i|}$ and $X_i^j (1 \leq j \leq s_i)$ is an equivalence class in $\underline{R}X_i$.

Obviously, $0 \leq c(R, \Gamma) \leq 1$. In particular,

If $\Gamma = \{X\}$, then

$$c(R, \Gamma) = \sum_{i=1}^{m} \frac{|X_i|}{|U|} \sum_{j=1}^{s_i} p^2(X_i^j),$$

i.e., the converge degree of $\Gamma$ with respect to $R$ degenerates into the converge degree of $X$ with respect to $R$, denoted by $c(R, X)$;

If $U / R = \omega = \{\{x\} \mid x \in U\}$, then $c(R, \Gamma) = \sum_{i=1}^{m} \dfrac{|X_i|}{|U|} \times \dfrac{|X_i|}{|X_i|^2} = \dfrac{m}{|U|}$;

If $U / R = \delta = \{U\}$, then $c(R, \Gamma)$ achieves its minimum value $c(R, \Gamma) = \sum_{i=1}^{m} \dfrac{|X_i|}{|U|} \times 0 = 0$;

If $U / R = \Gamma$, then $c(R, \Gamma)$ achieves its maximum value $c(R, \Gamma) = \sum_{i=1}^{m} \dfrac{|X_i|}{|U|} \times 1 = 1$.

Let $S = (U, A)$ be an information system, $X \subseteq U$ and $P = \{R_1, R_2, \cdots, R_n\}$ a family of attribute sets with $R_1 \preceq R_2 \preceq \cdots \preceq R_n (R_i \in 2^A)$ and $\Gamma = \{X_1, X_2, \cdots, X_m\}$ be a partition on $U$. Lower approximation and upper approximation of $\Gamma$ with respect to $P$ are defined by

$$\underline{P}\Gamma = \{\underline{P}X_1, \underline{P}X_2, \cdots, \underline{P}X_m\},$$

$$\overline{P}\Gamma = \{\overline{P}X_1, \overline{P}X_2, \cdots, \overline{P}X_m\}.$$

Similar to Definition 3.3, one can define a converge degree of $\Gamma$ with respect to $P$ by

$$c(P,\Gamma) = \sum_{i=1}^{m} \frac{|X_i|}{|U|} \sum_{j=1}^{s_i} p^2(X_i^j),$$

where $s_i$ is the number of equivalence classes in $[\underline{P}X_i]$, $p(X_i^j) = \dfrac{|X_i^j|}{|X_i|}$ and $X_i^j (1 \le j \le s_i)$ is an equivalence class in $[\underline{P}X_i]$. It is clear that $0 \le c(P,\Gamma) \le 1$. In particular, $c(P,\Gamma)$ degenerated into $c(P,X)$ if $\Gamma = X$, i.e.,

$$c(P,\Gamma) = \sum_{j=1}^{s} \frac{|X_i|^2}{|X|^2},$$

where $s$ is the number of equivalence classes in $[\underline{P}(X)]$, which represents the converge degree of $X$ with respect to $P$.

In the following, we investigate two important properties of the converge degree.

## Theorem 3.5

Let $S = (U, A)$ be an information system, $X \subseteq U$ and $P = \{R_1, R_2, \cdots, R_n\}$ a family of attribute sets with $R_1 \preceq R_2 \preceq \cdots \preceq R_n (R_i \in 2^A)$. Let $P_i = \{R_1, R_2, \cdots, R_i\}$, then $\forall P_i (i = 1, 2, \cdots, n)$, we have

$$c(P_1, X) \le c(P_2, X) \le \cdots \le c(P_n, X).$$

**Proof**
From Theorem 3.4, it is clear that

$$[\underline{P_1}(X)] \preceq [\underline{P_2}(X)] \preceq \cdots \preceq [\underline{P_n}(X)].$$

Suppose $1 \le i < j \le n$, $[\underline{P_i}(X)] = \{A_1, A_2, \cdots, A_m\}$ and $[\underline{P_j}(X)] = \{B_1, B_2, \cdots, B_n\}$, then $[\underline{P_i}(X)] \preceq [\underline{P_j}(X)]$ and $m > n$. That is to say, there may exist a partition $\{C_1, C_2, \cdots, C_n\}$ of $\{1, 2, \cdots, m\}$ such that

$B_r = \bigcup_{l \in C_t} A_l$, $t = 1, 2, \cdots, n$. Therefore, one can obtain that

$$
\begin{aligned}
c(P_j, X) &= \frac{1}{|X|^2} \sum_{t=1}^{s_j} |B_t|^2 \\
&= \frac{1}{|X|^2} \sum_{t=1}^{s_j} \left| \bigcup_{l \in C_t} A_l \right|^2 = \frac{1}{|X|^2} \sum_{t=1}^{s_j} \left( \sum_{l \in C_t} |A_l| \right)^2 \\
&\geq \frac{1}{|X|^2} \sum_{t=1}^{s_j} \sum_{l \in C_t} |A_l|^2 = \frac{1}{|X|^2} \sum_{l=1}^{s_i} |A_l|^2 \\
&= c(P_i, X).
\end{aligned}
$$

Thus $c(P_1, X) \leq c(P_2, X) \leq \cdots \leq c(P_n, X)$. This completes the proof.

## Theorem 3.6

Let $S = (U, A)$ be an information system, $\Gamma = \{X_1, X_2, \cdots, X_m\}$ a partition on $U$ and $P = \{R_1, R_2, \cdots, R_n\}$ a family of attribute sets with $R_1 \preceq R_2 \preceq \cdots \preceq R_n$ ($R_i \in 2^A$). Let $P_i = \{R_1, R_2, \cdots, R_i\}$, then $\forall P_i (i = 1, 2, \cdots, n)$ we have

$$
c(P_1, \Gamma) \leq c(P_2, \Gamma) \leq \cdots \leq c(P_n, \Gamma).
$$

**Proof**

It follows that from Theorem 3.5 that $c(P_1, X_i) \leq c(P_2, X_i) \leq \cdots \leq c(P_n, X_i)$ for any $X_i (i \leq m)$. Suppose that $1 \leq k \leq t \leq n$, then $c(P_k, X_i) \leq c(P_t, X_i)$. Therefore, one can obtain that

$$
\begin{aligned}
c(P_j, \Gamma) &= \sum_{i=1}^{m} \frac{|X_i|}{|U|} \sum_{j=1}^{s_i} p^2(X_i^j) = \sum_{i=1}^{m} \frac{|X_i|}{|U|} \times c(P_k, X_i) \\
&\geq \sum_{i=1}^{m} \frac{|X_i|}{|U|} \times c(P_t, X_i) \\
&= c(P_t, \Gamma).
\end{aligned}
$$

Thus $c(P_1, \Gamma) \leq c(P_2, \Gamma) \leq \cdots \leq c(P_n, \Gamma)$. This completes the proof.

Theorems 3.5 and 3.6 show that the converge degree of $X_i \in \Gamma$ with respect to $P_i$ increases and the number of equivalence classes for describing the target concept $X_i$ decreases as a granulation order becomes longer through adding equivalence relations. Since the converse approximation can clearly describe and simply the structures of the lower and upper approximation of a target concept on the basis of keeping the approximation measure, it may have some potential applications in rough set theory, such as description of multi-targets concepts, approximation classification and rule extraction from decision tables.

In the following, as an application of the converse approximation, we apply this approach for decision-rule extracting from two types of decision tables (consistent decision tables and inconsistent decision tables). A rule-extracting algorithm based on the converse approximation called REBCA is designed to extract decision rules from a decision table, its time complexity is analyzed and two illustrative examples are also employed to show the mechanism of algorithm REBCA.

In general, we design different rule-extracting algorithms according to these two kinds of decision tables (consistent and inconsistent). In the view of the converse approximation based on dynamic granulation, the decision classification induced by decision attributes can be regarded as the target classification(some target concepts) and the condition attribute sets can be used to construct a granulation order.

Let $S = (U, C \cup D)$ be a decision table, the significance of $c \in C - C'(C' \subseteq C)$ with respect to $D$ is defined by

$$sig_{C'}^{D}(c) = \gamma_{C' \cup \{c\}}(D) - \gamma_{C'}(D),$$

where $\gamma_{C'}(D) = \dfrac{1}{|U|} \, | \, pos_{C'}(D) \, | = \dfrac{1}{|U|} \, | \bigcup_{X \in U/IND(D)} \underline{C'}X \, |$

Generally, we can obtain some more useful decision rules by combining rules through deleting some condition attributes in decision tables. Based on the target classes, the converse approximation gives a mechanism that can be used to combine decision rules on the basis of keeping the confidence of each decision rule. One can know how the mechanism works from the following algorithm.

**Algorithm 3.2**

```
REBCA (for extracting decision rules from a decision table)

Input: decision table S = (U, C ∪ D);

Output: decision rules Rule.
```

(1)    Computing decision classes $U/IND(D) = \{X_1, X_2, \cdots, X_m\}$

(2)    From $j = 1$ to $m$ Do

Let $C_1 \leftarrow C$, $P(1) \leftarrow \{\{C_1\}\}$.

i.    From $k = 1$ to $|C| - 1$ Do

For any $c \in C_k$, compute the significance $sig_{C_k}^{D}(c)$.

Let $C_{k+1} \leftarrow C_k - c_0$, where $c_0 : sig_{C_k}^{D}(c_0) = \min\{sig_{C_k}^{D}(c), c \in C_k\}$.

Let $P(k+1) \leftarrow P(k) \cup \{\{C_{k+1}\}\}$; $//\, P(k+1)$ is the granulation order induced by $C_k$ and $C_{k+1}$

ii.  Compute $[\underline{P(|C|)}(X_j)]$;

iii. Put every decision rule $des([x]) \rightarrow des(X_j)$ into the rule base $rule(j)$, where $[x] \in [\underline{P(|C|)}(X_j)]$.

(3)  Output $Rule = \bigcup_{j=1}^{m} rule(j)$

Obviously, the generation of decision rules is not based on a reduct of a decision table but $X_j \in U / IND(D)$ and a granulation order $P(j)$ induced by $X_j$ and $C$ in the algorithm REBCA. Furthermore, the number of decision rules can be largely reduced on the basis of keeping that all decision rules are all certain rules in a decision table.

By using REBCA algorithm, the time complexity to extract decision rules from a decision table is polynomial.

At step (1), the time complexity for computing a decision partition is $O(|U|^2)$.

At step (2), we need to compute the complexity of each of three steps respectively.

For (i.), since $|C| - 1$ is the maximum value for the circle times, the time complexity for constructing $P(j)$ is

$$O((|C|-1)|U|^2 + (|C|-2)|U|^2$$
$$+\cdots + |U|^2) = O(\frac{|C|(|C|-1)}{2}|U|^2)$$

For (ii.), the time complexity for computing $[\underline{P(|C|)}(X_j)]$ is $O(|C||U|^2)$;

For (iii.), the time complexity for putting each decision rule into rule base is $O(|X_j|)$;

Therefore, the time complexity for step (2) is

$$\sum_{j=1}^{m}\left[O\left(\frac{|C|(|C|-1)}{2}|U|^2\right)+O\left(|C||U|^2\right)+O(|X_j|)\right]$$
$$= O\left[\frac{m(|C|^2+|C|)}{2}|U|^2 + \sum_{j=1}^{m}|X_j|\right]$$
$$= O\left[\frac{m(|C|^2+|C|)}{2}|U|^2 + |U|\right]$$

At step (3), the time complexity is $O(|U|)$.

Thus, the time complexity of algorithm REBCA is

$$O(|U|^2) + O\left(\frac{m(|C|^2 + |C|)}{2} |U|^2 + |U|\right) + O(|U|)$$

$$= O\left(\frac{m}{2} |C|^2 |U|^2\right).$$

In fact, the time complexity of this algorithm can be reduced as $O\left(\frac{m}{2} |C|^2 |U| \log_2 |U|\right)$ if we

compute a classification by adopting ranking technique.

**Remark**

Algorithm REBCA is different from existing algorithms based on attribute reduct for extracting decision rules from decision tables. The time complexity of a rule-extracting algorithm based on attribute reduct is $O(|C|^3 |U|^2)$. Obviously, the time complexity of algorithm REBCA is much smaller than those of the existing algorithms based on attribute reduct. In particular, its size partially depend on the number of decision classes $m$. In many practical applications, $m$ is always smaller than the number of condition attributes $|C|$. Therefore, the time complexity of algorithm REBCA is largely reduced relative to those of the existing algorithms based on attribute reduct for extracting decision rules from decision tables.

In order to discuss applications of this algorithm, two types of decision tables will be examined, which are consistent decision tables and inconsistent decision tables. As follows, we show how algorithm REBCA to extract decision rules from decision tables by two illustrative examples. Firstly, we focus on a consistent decision table.

## Example 3.3

A consistent decision table $S_1 = (U, C \cup D)$ is given by Table 1, where $C = \{a, b, c, d\}$ is condition attribute set and $D = \{f\}$ is decision attribute set. By using algorithm REBCA, we can extract decision rules from table 1.

By computing, it follows that

$$U/D = \{\{1, 2, 3, 4, 5, 11\}, \{6, 7, 8, 9, 10, 12\}\}.$$

Let $X_1 = \{1, 2, 3, 4, 5, 11\}$ and $X_2 = \{6, 7, 8, 9, 10, 12\}$. From REBCA, we have that

$$P = \{\{a, b, c, d, e\}, \{a, b, c, e\}, \{a, c, e\}, \{a, e\}, \{e\}\}.$$

From the definition of converse approximation, one can obtain that

$$[\underline{P}(X_1)] = \{\{3, 11\}, \{1, 2, 4, 5\}\}, [\underline{P}(X_2)] = \{\{7, 12\}, \{9\}, \{6, 8, 10\}\}$$

Therefore, several decision rules can be extracted as follows:

$des(\{1,2,4,5\}) \rightarrow des(X_1)$, i.e., $(e = 2) \rightarrow (f = 1)$;

$des(\{3,11\}) \rightarrow des(X_1)$, i.e., $(a = 1, e = 2) \rightarrow (f = 1)$;

$des(\{6,8,10\}) \rightarrow des(X_2)$, i.e., $(e = 0) \rightarrow (f = 0)$;

$des(\{9\}) \rightarrow des(X_2)$, i.e., $(a = 2, e = 1) \rightarrow (f = 0)$;

$des(\{7,12\}) \rightarrow des(X_2)$, i.e., $(a = 3, e = 1) \rightarrow (f = 0)$.

For intuition, these five decision rules extracted by REBCA from the decision table $S_1$ are listed in Table 2.

This example shows the mechanism of the decision-rule extracting algorithm based on the converse approximation in a consistent decision table. In fact, attribute set $\{a, e\}$ is a relative reduct of condition attribute set $C$ in decision table $S_1$ (the notion of relative reduct is from the literature [49]) and these decision rules in Table 2 are also the same as the rule sets extracted from the algorithm based on attribute reduct. However, the time complexity of rule extracting algorithm based on the converse approximation is much smaller than the time complexity of the algorithm based on attribute reduct.

Then, we investigate how to extract decision rules from an inconsistent decision table through using algorithm REBCA. The following example will be helpful in understanding its mechanism.

*Table 1. A consistent decision table*

| U | Attributes | | | | | |
|---|---|---|---|---|---|---|
|   | a | B | c | d | e | f |
| 1 | 3 | 2 | 3 | 0 | 2 | 1 |
| 2 | 2 | 2 | 3 | 0 | 2 | 1 |
| 3 | 1 | 0 | 2 | 0 | 1 | 1 |
| 4 | 3 | 1 | 3 | 0 | 2 | 1 |
| 5 | 2 | 0 | 3 | 0 | 2 | 1 |
| 6 | 0 | 0 | 1 | 0 | 0 | 0 |
| 7 | 3 | 2 | 0 | 1 | 1 | 0 |
| 8 | 1 | 0 | 1 | 0 | 0 | 0 |
| 9 | 2 | 0 | 2 | 1 | 1 | 0 |
| 10 | 1 | 1 | 3 | 1 | 0 | 0 |
| 11 | 1 | 0 | 2 | 0 | 1 | 1 |
| 12 | 3 | 2 | 0 | 1 | 1 | 0 |

*Table 2. Decision rules extracted from the decision table $S_1$*

| Rule | Attributes | | |
|---|---|---|---|
|   | a | e | f |
| r1 |   | 2 | 1 |
| r2 | 1 | 1 | 1 |
| r3 |   | 0 | 0 |
| r4 | 3 | 1 | 0 |
| r5 | 2 | 1 | 0 |

## Example 3.4

An inconsistent decision table $S_2 = (U, C \cup D)$ is given by Table 3, where $C = \{a_1, a_2, a_3, a_4\}$ is condition attribute set and $D = \{d\}$ is decision attribute set. By using the algorithm REBCA, we can extract decision rules from Table 3.

By computing, it follows that

$$U / D = \{\{1, 5, 6\}, \{2, 3, 4\}\}.$$

Let $X_1 = \{1, 5, 6\}$ and $X_2 = \{2, 3, 4\}$. From REBCA, we have that

$$P = \{\{a_1, a_2, a_3, a_4\}, \{a_2, a_3, a_4\}, \{a_2, a_3\}, \{a_3\}\}$$

From the definition of converse approximation, one can obtain that

$$[\underline{P}X_1] = \{\{1\}\}, \ [\underline{P}X_2] = \{\{2, 4\}\}.$$

Therefore, two certain decision rules can be extracted as follows:

$des(\{1\}) \to des(X_1)$, i.e., $(a_2 = 0, a_3 = 0) \to (d = 1)$;

$des(\{2, 4\}) \to des(X_2)$, i.e., $(a_2 = 1, a_3 = 1) \to (d = 2)$.

And two uncertain decision rules are also acquired from the construction of $[\overline{P}(X_1)] - [\underline{P}(X_1)]$ and $[\overline{P}(X_2)] - [\underline{P}(X_2)]$ as follows:

$des(\{3, 5, 6\}) \to des(X_1)$, i.e., $(a_2 = 1, a_3 = 0) \to (d = 2)$ with $\mu = \dfrac{1}{3}$;

$des(\{3, 5, 6\}) \to des(X_2)$. i.e., $(a_2 = 1, a_3 = 0) \to (d = 1)$ with $\mu = \dfrac{2}{3}$;

where $\mu$ denotes the uncertain measure of a decision rule [49]. For intuition, these four decision rules extracted by REBCA from the decision table $S_2$ are listed in Table 4.

This example shows the mechanism of the decision-rule extracting algorithm based on the converse approximation in inconsistent decision tables. In fact, attribute set $a_2, a_3$ is a relative reduct of condition attribute set $C$ in this decision table(the notion of relative reduct is from the literature [49]), and these decision rules are also the same as rules sets obtained from the algorithm based on attribute reduct.

*Table 3. An inconsistent decision table*

| $U$ | Attributes | | | | |
|---|---|---|---|---|---|
| | $a_1$ | $a_2$ | $a_3$ | $a_4$ | $d$ |
| 1 | 1 | 0 | 0 | 0 | 1 |
| 2 | 0 | 1 | 1 | 1 | 2 |
| 3 | 0 | 1 | 0 | 0 | 2 |
| 4 | 0 | 1 | 2 | 0 | 2 |
| 5 | 0 | 1 | 0 | 0 | 1 |
| 6 | 0 | 1 | 0 | 0 | 1 |

*Table 4. Decision rules extracted from the decision table $S_2$*

| Rule | Attributes | | |
|---|---|---|---|
| | $a_2$ | $a_3$ | $d$ |
| $r_1$ | 0 | 0 | 1 |
| $r_2$ | 1 | 1 | 2 |
| $r_3$ | 1 | 0 | 2 |
| $r_4$ | 1 | 0 | 1 |

Therefore, we can extract decision rules from an inconsistent decision table through using REBCA algorithm with smaller time complexity.

Form the above analyses, it is easy to see that by using algorithm REBCA one can extract decision rules from both a consistent table and an inconsistent table. Unlike some rule-extracting approaches based on an attribute reduct, the time complexity of this algorithm is only $O(\frac{m}{2} \mid C \mid^2 \mid U \mid \log_2 \mid U \mid)$.

Hence, this approach may be used to effectively extract decision rules from practical data sets.

## 4. EVALUATING THE DECISION PERFORMANCE OF A DECISION TABLE

### 4.1. Decision Rule and Knowledge Granulation in Decision Tables

In the first part of this section, we briefly recall the notions of decision rules and certainty measure and support measure of a decision rule in rough set theory.

### Definition 4.1

Let $S = (U, C \cup D)$ be a decision table, $X_i \in U / C$, $Y_j \in U / D$ and $X_i \cap Y_j \neq \varnothing$. By $des(X_i)$ and $des(Y_j)$, we denote the descriptions of the equivalence classes $X_i$ and $Y_j$ in the decision table $S$. A decision rule is formally defined as

$$Z_{ij} : des(X_i) \rightarrow des(Y_j).$$

Certainty measure and support measure of a decision rule $Z_{ij}$ are defined as follows [23, 24]:

$$\mu(Z_{ij}) = \frac{\mid X_i \cap Y_j \mid}{\mid X_i \mid}, \ s(Z_{ij}) = \frac{\mid X_i \cap Y_j \mid}{\mid U \mid},$$

where $\mid \bullet \mid$ is the cardinality of a set. It is clear that the value of each of $\mu(Z_{ij})$ and $s(Z_{ij})$ of a decision

rule $Z_{ij}$ falls into the interval $\left[\frac{1}{\mid U \mid}, 1\right]$. In subsequent discussions, we denote the cardinality of the set

$X_i \cap Y_j$ by $\mid Z_{ij} \mid$, which is called the support number of the rule $Z_{ij}$.

In rough set theory, we can extract some decision rules from a given decision table [4, 5, 20, 21]. However, in some practical issues, it may happen that there does not exist any certain decision rule with the certainty of one in the decision-rule set extracted from a given decision table. In this situation, the lower approximation of the target decision is equal to an empty set in this decision table. To character-ize this type of decision tables, in the decision tables, conversely consistent decision tables and mixed decision tables.

As follows, we introduce several new concepts and notions, which will be applied in our further developments. For convenience, by $a(x)$ and $d(x)$ we denote the value of an object $x$ under a condition attribute $a \in C$ and a decision attribute $d \in D$, respectively.

## Definition 4.2

Let $S = (U, C \cup D)$ be a decision table, ,and $U / D = \{Y_1, Y_2, \cdots, Y_n\}$. A condition class $X_i \in U / C$ is said to be consistent if $d(x) = d(y), \forall x, y \in X_i$ and $\forall d \in D$ ; a decision class $Y_j \in U / D$ is said to be conversely consistent if $a(x) = a(y), \forall x, y \in Y_j$ and $\forall a \in C$.

It is easy to see that a decision table $S = (U, C \cup D)$ is consistent if every condition class $X_i \in U / C$ is consistent.

## Definition 4.3

Let $S = (U, C \cup D)$ be a decision table, ,and $U / D = \{Y_1, Y_2, \cdots, Y_n\}$. $S$ is said to be conversely con-sistent if every decision class $Y_j \in U / D$ is conversely consistent, i.e., $U / D \preceq U / C$. A decision table is called a mixed decision table if it is neither consistent nor conversely consistent.

In addition to the above concepts and notations, we say that $S = (U, C \cup D)$ is strictly consistent(or strictly and conversely consistent) if $U / C \prec U / D$ (or $U / D \prec U / C$).

A strictly and conversely consistent decision has some practical implications. A strictly and con-versely consistent decision table is inconsistent. In a strictly and conversely consistent decision table, there does not exist any condition class $X \in U / C$ and any decision class $Y \in U / D$ such that $X \subseteq Y$. In other words, one cannot extract any certain decision rule from a strictly and conversely consistent decision table. Furthermore, when a decision table is strictly and conversely consistent, two well-known classical evaluation measures, approximation accuracy and consistency degree, cannot be applied to measure its certainty and consistency. In the remaining part of this paper, one can see that the introduction of the conversely consistency will play an important role in revealing the limitations of the two classical measures and verifying the validity of the evaluation measures proposed in this paper.

In a mixed decision table, from Definition 4.3, one can see that there exist $X \in U / C$ and $Y \in U / D$ that $X$ is consistent and $Y$ is conversely consistent. We thus obtain the following results.

A decision table is strictly consistent iff there does not exist any $Y \in U / D$ such that $Y$ is conversely consistent, and

A decision table is strictly and conversely consistent iff there does not exist any $X \in U / C$ such that $X$ is consistent.

This implies that a mixed decision table can be transformed into a conversely consistent decision table (a consistent decision table) by deleting its strictly consistent part(by deleting its strictly and conversely consistent part). Hence, in a broad sense, a mixed decision table is a combination of a consistent decision table and a conversely consistent decision table. For this reason, we only focus on the properties of a consistent decision table and a conversely consistent decision table in this paper. For general decision tables, we investigate their characters by practical experimental analyses.

Granularity, a very an important concept in rough set theory, is often used to indicate a partition or a cover of the universe of an information system or a decision table [4,11,12,24-26,28,34]. The performance of a decision rule depends directly on the condition granularity and decision granularity of a decision table. In general, the changes of granulation of a decision table can be realized through two ways as follows: (1) refining/coarsening the domain of attributes and (2) adding/reducing attributes. The first approach is mainly used to deal with the case that the attribute values of some elements are imprecise in a decision table. For example, in Table1, the value of decision attribute Rheum of each element in the universe is either Yes or No. Hence, Rheum degree cannot be further analyzed, i.e., the decision values are imprecise. Obviously, decision rules extracting from this kind of decision tables are lack of practicability and pertinence. In the second approach, the certainty measure of a decision rule may be changed through adding or reducing some condition attributes or decision attributes in a decision table. For instance, in Table 1, the certainty measures of some decision rules can be increased by adding new condition attributes.

In general, knowledge granulation is employed to measure the discernibility ability of a knowledge in rough set theory. The smaller knowledge granulation of a knowledge is, the stronger its discernibility is. In [14, 15], Liang introduced a knowledge granulation $G(A)$ to measure the discernibility ability of a knowledge in an information system, which is given in the following definition.

## Definition 4.4

Let $S = (U, A)$ be an information system and $U / A = \{R_1, R_2, \cdots, R_m\}$. Knowledge granulation of $A$ is defined as

$$G(A) = \frac{1}{|U|^2} \sum_{i=1}^{m} |R_i|^2 .$$

Following this definition similarly, for a decision table $S = (U, C \cup D)$, we can call $G(C)$ and $G(D)$ and $G(C \cup D)$ condition granulation, decision granulation and granulation of $S$, respectively.

As a result of the above discussions, we come to the following two lemmas.

## Lemma 4.1

Let $S = (U, C \cup D)$ be a strictly consistent decision table, i.e., $U / C \prec U / D$. Then, there exists at least one decision class in $U / D$ such that it can be represented as the union of more than one condition classes in $U / C$.

**Proof**
Let $U / C = \{X_1, X_2, \cdots, X_m\}$ and $U / D = \{Y_1, Y_2, \cdots, Y_n\}$. By the consistency of $S$, a decision class $Y \in U / D$ is the union of some condition classes $X \in U / C$. Furthermore, sine $S$ is strictly consistent, there exist $X_0 \in U / C$ and $Y_0 \in U / D$ such that $X_0 \subseteq Y_0$. This indicates that $Y_0$ is equal to the union of more than one condition classes in $U / C$. This completes the proof.

## Lemma 4.2

Let $S = (U, C \cup D)$ be a strictly and conversely consistent decision table, i.e., $U / D \prec U / C$. Then, there exist at least one condition class in $U / C$ such that it can be represented as the union of more than one decision classes in $U / D$.

**Proof**
The proof is similar to that of Lemma 4.1.

By Lemma 4.1 and 4.2, one can easily obtain the following theorem.

## Theorem 4.1

Let $S = (U, C \cup D)$ be a decision table.

- If $S$ is strictly consistent, then $G(C) < G(D)$; and
- If $S$ is strictly and conversely consistent, then $G(C) > G(D)$.

It should be noted that the inverse propositions of Lemma 4.1 and 4.2 and Theorem 4.1 need not true.

## 4.2. Limitations of Classical Measures for Decision Tables

In this section, through several illustrative examples, we reveal the limitations of existing classical measures for evaluating the decision performance of a decision table.

In [23], several measures for evaluating a decision rule $Z_{ij} : des(X_i) \rightarrow des(Y_j)$ have been introduced, which are certainty measure

$$\mu(X_i, Y_j) = \frac{|X_i \cap Y_j|}{|X_i|} \text{ and } s(X_i, Y_j) = \frac{|X_i \cap Y_j|}{|U|}.$$

However, $\mu(X_i, Y_j)$ and $s(X_i, Y_j)$ are only defined for a single decision rule and are not suitable for measuring the decision performance of a decision-rule set.

In [23], approximation accuracy of a classification was introduced by Pawlak. Let $F = \{Y_1, Y_2, \cdots, Y_n\}$ be a classification of the universe $U$ and $C$ a condition attribute set. Then, $C$-lower and $C$-upper approximations of $F$ are given by $\underline{C}F = \{\underline{C}Y_1, \underline{C}Y_2, \cdots, \underline{C}Y_n\}$ and $\overline{C}F = \{\overline{C}Y_1, \overline{C}Y_2, \cdots, \overline{C}Y_n\}$, respectively, where

$$\underline{C}Y_i = \{x \in U \mid [x]_C \subseteq Y_i \in F\}, \ 1 \leq i \leq n, \text{ and } \overline{C}Y_i = \{x \in U \mid [x]_C \cap Y_i \neq \varnothing, Y_i \in F\}, \ 1 \leq i \leq n$$

The approximation accuracy of $F$ by $C$ is defined as

$$\alpha_C(F) = \frac{\sum_{Y_i \in U/D} |\underline{C}Y_i|}{\sum_{Y_i \in U/D} |\overline{C}Y_i|}.$$

The approximation accuracy expresses the percentage of possible correct decision when classifying objects by employing the attribute set $C$. In some situations, $\alpha_C(F)$ can be used to measure the certainty of a decision table. However, its limitations can be revealed by the following example.

## Example 4.1.

Let $S_1 = (U, C \cup D_1)$ and $S_1 = (U, C \cup D_2)$ be two decision tables with the same universe $U$. Support that

$$U / C = \{\{e_1, e_2\}, \{e_3, e_4, e_5\}, \{e_6, e_7\}\},$$

$$U / D_1 = \{\{e_1\}, \{e_2, e_3, e_4\}\{e_5, e_6\}, \{e_7\}\},$$

and

$$U \, / \, D_2 = \{\{e_1, e_3\}, \{e_2, e_4, e_6\}, \{e_5\}, \{e_7\}\}.$$

Then, six decision rules extracted from $S_1$ and their certainty measures and support measures corresponding to each individual rule are given by

$$r_1 : \quad des(\{e_1, e_2\}) \to des(\{e_1\}), \;\; \mu(r_1) = \frac{1}{2}, s(r_1) = \frac{1}{7};$$

$$r_2 : \quad des(\{e_1, e_2\}) \to des(\{e_2\}), \;\; \mu(r_2) = \frac{1}{2}, s(r_2) = \frac{1}{7};$$

$$r_3 : \quad des(\{e_3, e_4, e_5\}) \to des(\{e_3, e_4\}), \;\; \mu(r_3) = \frac{2}{3}, s(r_3) = \frac{2}{7};$$

$$r_4 : \quad des(\{e_3, e_4, e_5\}) \to des(\{e_5\}), \;\; \mu(r_4) = \frac{1}{3}, s(r_4) = \frac{1}{7};$$

$$r_5 : \quad des(\{e_6, e_7\}) \to des(\{e_6\}), \;\; \mu(r_5) = \frac{1}{2}, s(r_5) = \frac{1}{7};$$

$$r_6 : \quad des(\{e_6, e_7\}) \to des(\{e_7\}), \;\; \mu(r_6) = \frac{1}{2}, s(r_6) = \frac{1}{7};$$

Furthermore, seven decision rules extracted from $S_2$ and their certainty measures and support measures corresponding to each individual rule are given by

$$r_1' : \quad des(\{e_1, e_2\}) \to des(\{e_1\}), \;\; \mu(r_1') = \frac{1}{2}, s(r_1') = \frac{1}{7};$$

$$r_2' : \quad des(\{e_3, e_4, e_5\}) \to des(\{e_3\}), \;\; \mu(r_2') = \frac{1}{3}, s(r_2') = \frac{1}{7};$$

$$r_3' : \quad des(\{e_1, e_2\}) \to des(\{e_2\}), \;\; \mu(r_3') = \frac{1}{2}, s(r_3') = \frac{1}{7};$$

$$r_4' : \quad des(\{e_3, e_4, e_5\}) \to des(\{e_4\}), \;\; \mu(r_4') = \frac{1}{3}, s(r_4') = \frac{1}{7};$$

$$r_5' : \quad des(\{e_6, e_7\}) \to des(\{e_6\}), \;\; \mu(r_5') = \frac{1}{2}, s(r_5') = \frac{1}{7};$$

$$r_6' : \quad des(\{e_6, e_7\}) \to des(\{e_7\}), \;\; \mu(r_6') = \frac{1}{2}, s(r_6') = \frac{1}{7};$$

By formula the definition of approximation measure, we have that

$$\alpha_C(U / D_1) = \frac{\sum_{Y_i \in U/D} | \underline{CY}_i |}{\sum_{Y_i \in U/D} | \overline{CY}_i |} = \frac{0}{2+5+5+2} = 0,$$

$$\alpha_C(U / D_2) = \frac{\sum_{Y_i \in U/D} | \underline{CY}_i |}{\sum_{Y_i \in U/D} | \overline{CY}_i |} = \frac{0}{5+7+3+2} = 0.$$

That is to say $a_C(U / D_1) = a_C(U / D_2) = 0$.

Now, let us consider the average value of the certainty measure of each of the two rule sets extracted one from $S_1$ and the other from $S_2$. Taking the average of the certainty measure values corresponding to decision rules for each decision table, we have that

$$\frac{1}{6} \sum_{i=1}^{6} \mu(r_i) = \frac{1}{6}(\frac{1}{2} + \frac{1}{2} + \frac{2}{3} + \frac{1}{3} + \frac{1}{2} + \frac{1}{2}) = \frac{1}{2}$$

and

$$\frac{1}{7} \sum_{i=1}^{7} \mu(r_i') = \frac{1}{7}(\frac{1}{2} + \frac{1}{3} + \frac{1}{2} + \frac{1}{3} + \frac{1}{2} + \frac{1}{3} + \frac{1}{2}) = \frac{3}{7}$$

Obviously, $\frac{1}{2} = \frac{7}{14} > \frac{6}{14} = \frac{3}{7}$. It implies that the decision table $S_1$ has a higher certainty than $S_2$ on the average. However, this situation is not revealed by the approximation accuracy. Therefore, a more comprehensive and effective measure for evaluating the certainty of a decision table is needed.

The consistency degree of a decision table $S = (U, C \cup D)$, another classical measure proposed in [23], is defined as

$$c_C(D) = \frac{\sum_{i=1}^{n} | \underline{CY}_i |}{| U |}.$$

The consistency degree expresses the percentage of objects which can be correctly classified into decision classes of $U / D$ by a condition attribute set $C$. In some situations, $c_C(D)$ can be employed to measure the consistency of a decision table. Similar to Example 4.1, however, the consistency of a decision table also cannot be well characterized by the classical consistency degree because it only considers the lower approximation of a target decision. Therefore, a more comprehensive and effective measure for evaluating the consistency of a decision table is also needed.

From the definitions of the approximation accuracy and consistency degree, one can easily obtain the following property.

## Property 4.1

If $S = (U, C \cup D)$ is a strictly and conversely consistent decision table, then $\alpha_C(U / D) = 0$ and $c_C(D) = 0$.

Property 4.1 shows that the approximation accuracy and consistency degree cannot well characterize the certainty and consistency of a strictly and conversely consistent decision table.

**Remark**

From the above analyses, it is easy to see that the shortcomings of the two classical measures are mainly caused by the condition equivalence classes that cannot be induced in the lower approximation of the target decision in a given decision table. As we know, in an inconsistent decision table, there must exist some condition equivalence classes that cannot be included in the lower approximation of the target decision. In fact, for a strictly and conversely consistent decision table, the lower approximation of the target decision is an empty set. Hence, we can make a conclusion that the approximation accuracy and consistency degree cannot be employed to effectively characterize the decision performance of an inconsistent decision table. To overcome this shortcoming of the two classical measures, the effect of the condition equivalence classes that are not included in the lower approximation of the target decision should be taken into account in evaluating the decision performance of an inconsistent decision table [36].

## 4.3. Evaluation of the Decision Performance of a Rule Set

To overcome the shortcomings of the two classical measures, in this section, we introduce three new measures ($\alpha$, $\beta$ and $\gamma$) for evaluating the decision performance of a decision table and analyze how each of these three measures depends on the condition granulation and decision granulation of each of consistent decision tables and conversely consistent decision tables. For general decision tables, by employing three decision tables from real world, we illustrate the advantage of these three measure for evaluating the decision performance of a decision rule set extracted from a decision table.

## Definition 4.5

Let $S = (U, C \cup D)$ be a decision table, and

$$RULE = \{Z_{ij} : des(X_i) \rightarrow des(Y_j) \; X_i \in U / C, Y_j \in U / D\}.$$

Certainty measure of $S$ is defined as $\alpha(S) = \sum_{i=1}^{m} \sum_{j=1}^{n} s(Z_{ij}) \mu(Z_{ij}) = \sum_{i=1}^{m} \sum_{j=1}^{n} \dfrac{|X_i \cap Y_j|^2}{|U| \, |X_i|}$, where $s(Z_{ij})$

and $\mu(Z_{ij})$ are the certainty measure and support measure of the rule $Z_{ij}$, respectively.

## Theorem 4.2. (Extremum)

Let $S = (U, C \cup D)$ be a decision table, and

$$RULE = \{Z_{ij} : des(X_i) \to des(Y_j), X_i \in U / C, Y_j \in U / D\}.$$

For any $Z_{ij} \in RULE$, If $\mu(Z_{ij}) = 1$, then the measure $\alpha$ achieves its maximum value 1.

If $m = 1$ and $n = |U|$, then the measure $\alpha$ achieves its minimum value $\dfrac{1}{|U|}$.

**Proof**

From the definitions of $\mu(Z_{ij})$ and $s(Z_{ij})$, it follows that $\dfrac{1}{|U|} \le \mu(Z_{ij}) \le 1$ and

$$\sum_{i=1}^{m} \sum_{j=1}^{n} s(Z_{ij}) = \sum_{i=1}^{m} \sum_{j=1}^{n} \frac{|X_i \cap Y_j|}{|U|} = 1.$$

- If $\mu(Z_{ij}) = 1$ for any $Z_{ij} \in RULE$, then we have that

$$\alpha(S) = \sum_{i=1}^{m} \sum_{j=1}^{n} s(Z_{ij})\mu(Z_{ij}) = \sum_{i=1}^{m} \sum_{j=1}^{n} \frac{|X_i \cap Y_j|^2}{|U||X_i|} = \sum_{i=1}^{m} \sum_{j=1}^{n} \frac{|X_i \cap Y_j|}{|U|} \times 1 = 1.$$

- If $m = 1$ and $n = |U|$, then $\mu(Z_{ij}) = \dfrac{1}{|U|}$ for any $Z_{ij} \in RULE$. In this case, we have that

$$\alpha(S) = \sum_{i=1}^{m} \sum_{j=1}^{n} s(Z_{ij})\mu(Z_{ij}) = \sum_{i=1}^{m} \sum_{j=1}^{n} \frac{|X_i \cap Y_j|^2}{|U||X_i|} = \sum_{i=1}^{m} \sum_{j=1}^{n} \frac{|X_i \cap Y_j|}{|U|} \times \frac{1}{|U|} = \frac{1}{|U|}.$$

This completes the proof.

**Remark**

In fact, a decision table $S = (U, C \cup D)$ is consistent if and only if every decision rule from $S$ is certain, i.e., the certainty measure of each of these decision rules is equal to one. So, (1) of Theorem 4.2 shows that the measure $\alpha$ achieves its maximum value 1 when $S$ is consistent. When we want to distinguish any two objects of $U$ without any condition information, (2) of Theorem 4.2 shows that a achieves its minimum value $1/|U|$.

In the following example, how the measure $\alpha$ overcomes the limitation of the classical measure $\alpha_C(U / D)$ can be illustrated.

## Example 4.2

(Continued from Example 4.1). Computing the measure $\alpha$, we have that

$$
\begin{aligned}
\alpha(S_1) &= \sum_{i=1}^{m}\sum_{j=1}^{n} s(Z_{ij})\mu(Z_{ij}) \\
&= \frac{1}{7}\cdot\frac{1}{2} + \frac{1}{7}\cdot\frac{1}{2} + \frac{2}{7}\cdot\frac{2}{3} + \frac{1}{7}\cdot\frac{1}{3} + \frac{1}{7}\cdot\frac{1}{2} + \frac{1}{7}\cdot\frac{1}{2} \\
&= \frac{11}{21}
\end{aligned}
$$

$$
\begin{aligned}
\alpha(S_2) &= \sum_{i=1}^{m}\sum_{j=1}^{n} s(Z_{ij})\mu(Z_{ij}) \\
&= \frac{1}{7}\cdot\frac{1}{2} + \frac{1}{7}\cdot\frac{1}{2} + \frac{1}{7}\cdot\frac{1}{3} + \frac{1}{7}\cdot\frac{1}{3} + \frac{1}{7}\cdot\frac{1}{3} + \frac{1}{7}\cdot\frac{1}{2} + \frac{1}{7}\cdot\frac{1}{2} \\
&= \frac{9}{21}
\end{aligned}
$$

Therefore, $\alpha(S_1) > \alpha(S_2)$.

Example 4.2 indicates that unlike the approximation accuracy $\alpha_C(U / D)$, the measure $\alpha$ can be used to measure the certainty of a decision-rule set when $\alpha_C(U / D) = 0$, i.e., the lower approximation of each decision class is equal to an empty set.

**Remark**

From the definition of approximation measure, it follows that $\alpha_C(U / D) = 0$ if $\bigcup_{Y_i \in U/D} \underline{C}Y_i = \phi$. In fact, in a broad sense, $\underline{C}Y_i = \phi$ does not imply that the certainty of a rule concerning $Y_i$ is equal to 0. So the measure $\alpha$ is much better than the approximation accuracy for measuring the certainty of a decision-rule set when a decision table is strictly and conversely consistent.

In the following, we discuss the monotonicity of the measure $\alpha$ in a conversely consistent decision table.

## Theorem 4.3.

Let $S_1 = (U, C_1 \cup D_1)$ and $S_2 = (U, C_2 \cup D_2)$ be two conversely consistent decision tables. If $U / C_1 = U / C_2$ and $U / D_2 \prec U / D_1$, then $\alpha(S_1) > \alpha(S_2)$.

**Proof**

From $U / C_1 = U / C_2$ and the converse consistencies of $S_1$ and $S_2$, it follows that there exist $X_p \in U / C_1$ and $Y_q \in U / D_1$ such that $Y_q \subseteq X_p$ Since $U / D_2 \prec U / D_1$, there exist $Y_q^1, Y_q^2, \cdots, Y_q^s \in U / D_2 (s > 1)$

such that $Y_q = \bigcup_{k=1}^{s} Y_q^k$. In other words, the rule $Z_{pq}$ in $S_1$ can be decomposed into a family of rules $Z_{pq}^1, Z_{pq}^2, \cdots, Z_{pq}^s$ in $S_2$. It is clear that $|Z_{pq}| = \sum_{k=1}^{s} Z_{pq}^k$. Thus, $|Z_{pq}|^2 > \sum_{k=1}^{s} |Z_{pq}^k|^2$. Therefore, from the definition of $\alpha(S)$, it follows that $\alpha(S_1) > \alpha(S_2)$. This completes the proof.

Theorem 4.3 states that the certainty measure $\alpha$ of a conversely consistent decision table decreases with its decision classes becoming finer.

## Theorem 4.4

Let $S_1 = (U, C_1 \cup D_1)$ and $S_2 = (U, C_2 \cup D_2)$ be two conversely consistent decision tables. If $U / D_1 = U / D_2$ and $U / C_2 \prec U / C_1$, then $\alpha(S_1) < \alpha(S_2)$.

**Proof**
From $U / C_2 \prec U / C_1$, there exist $X_l \in U / C_1$ and an integer $s > 1$ such that $X_l = \bigcup_{k=1}^{s} X_l^k$, where $X_l^k \in U / C_2$. It is clear that $|X_l| = \sum_{k=1}^{s} |X_l^k|$. Therefore

$$\frac{1}{|X_l|} < \frac{1}{|X_l^1|} + \frac{1}{|X_l^2|} + \cdots + \frac{1}{|X_l^s|}.$$

Noticing that both $S_1$ and $S_2$ are conversely consistent, we have $|Z_{lq}| = |Z_{lq}^k|$ $(k = 1, 2, \cdots, s)$. Thus, we find Box 1.

This completes the proof.

Theorem 4.4 states that the certainty measure $\alpha$ of a conversely consistent decision table increases with its condition classes becoming finer.

For a general decision table, in the following, through experimental analyses, we illustrate the validity of the measure $\alpha$ for assessing the decision performance of a decision-rule set extracted from the decision table. In order to verify the advantage of the measure $\alpha$ over the approximation accuracy $\alpha_C(U / D)$, we have downloaded three public data sets with practical applications from UCI Repository of machine learning databases [54], which are described in Table 5. All condition attributes and decision attributes in the three data sets are discrete.

In Table 5, the data set Tie-tac-toe is the encoding of the complete set of possible board configurations at the end of tie-tac-toe games, which is used to obtain possible ways to create a "three-in-a-row"; the

*Table 5. Data sets description*

| Data sets | Samples | Condition features | Decision classes |
| --- | --- | --- | --- |
| Tic-tac-toe | 958 | 9 | 2 |
| Dermatology | 366 | 33 | 6 |
| Nersery | 12960 | 8 | 5 |

data set Dermatology is a decision table about diagnosing dermatitis according to some clinical features, which is used to extract general diagnosing rules; and Nursery data set is derived from a hierarchical decision model originally developed to rank applications for nursery schools.

Here, we compare the certainty measure a with the approximation accuracy $\alpha_C(D)$ on these three practical data sets. The comparisons of values of two measures with the numbers of features in these three data sets are shown in Tables 6-8.

It can be seen from Tables 6-8 that the value of the certainty measure $\alpha$ is not smaller than that of the approximation accuracy $\alpha_C(D)$ for the same number of selected features, and this value increases as the number of selected features becomes bigger in the same data set. The measure $\alpha$ and approximation accuracy will achieve the same value 1 if the decision table becomes consistent through adding the number of selected features. However, from Table 6, it is easy to see that the values of approximation accuracy equal to zero when the number of features equals 1 or 2. In this situation, the lower approximation of the target decision equals an empty set in the decision table. Hence, the approximation accuracy cannot be used to effectively characterize the certainty of the decision table when the value of approximation accuracy equals 0. But, for the same situation as that the numbers of features equal 1 and 2, the values of the certainty measure a equal 0.557 and 0.5661, respectively. It shows that unlike the ap-

*Table 6. $\alpha_C(D)$ and $\alpha$ with different numbers of features in the data set tie-tac-toe*

| Measure | features | | | | | | | | |
|---|---|---|---|---|---|---|---|---|---|
| | 1 | 2 | 3 | 4 | 5 | 6 | 7 | 8 | 9 |
| $\alpha_C(D)$ | 0.0000 | 0.0000 | 0.0668 | 0.0886 | 0.2647 | 0.6348 | 0.8933 | 1.0000 | 1.0000 |
| $\alpha$ | 0.5557 | 0.5661 | 0.6414 | 0.6650 | 0.7916 | 0.9000 | 0.9718 | 1.0000 | 1.0000 |

*Table 7. $\alpha_C(D)$ and $\alpha$ with different numbers of features in the data set Dernatology*

| Measure | features | | | | | | | | | | |
|---|---|---|---|---|---|---|---|---|---|---|---|
| | 3 | 6 | 9 | 12 | 15 | 18 | 21 | 24 | 27 | 30 | 33 |
| $\alpha_C(D)$ | 0.0000 | 0.0000 | 0.0668 | 0.0886 | 0.2647 | 0.6348 | 0.8933 | 1.0000 | 1.0000 | 1.0000 | 1.0000 |
| $\alpha$ | 0.5557 | 0.5661 | 0.6414 | 0.6650 | 0.7916 | 0.9000 | 0.9718 | 1.0000 | 1.0000 | 1.0000 | 1.0000 |

*Table 8. $\alpha_C(D)$ and $\alpha$ with different numbers of features in the data set Nursery*

| Measure | features | | | | | | | |
|---|---|---|---|---|---|---|---|---|
| | 1 | 2 | 3 | 4 | 5 | 6 | 7 | 8 |
| $\alpha_C(D)$ | 0.0000 | 0.0000 | 0.0000 | 0.0000 | 0.0000 | 0.0000 | 0.0000 | 1.0000 |
| $\alpha$ | 0.3425 | 0.4292 | 0.4323 | 0.4437 | 0.4609 | 0.4720 | 0.4929 | 1.0000 |

proximation accuracy, the certainty measure of the decision table with two features is higher than that of the decision table with only one feature. Hence, the measure $\alpha$ is much better than the approximation accuracy for an inconsistent decision table. We can make the same conclusion from Table 7 and 8. In other words, when $\alpha_C(D) = 0$ in Tables 6-8, the measure $\alpha$ is still valid for evaluating the certainty of the set of decision rules obtained by using these selected features. Hence, the measure $\alpha$ may be better than the approximation accuracy for evaluating the certainty of a decision table.

Based on the above analyses, we conclude that if $S$ is consistent, the measure $\alpha$ has the same evaluation ability as the accuracy measure $\alpha_C(D)$ and that if S is inconsistent, the measure $\alpha$ has much better evaluation ability than the accuracy measure $\alpha_C(D)$.

Now, we introduce a measure $\beta$ to evaluate the consistency of a set of decision rules extracted from a decision table.

## Definition 4.6

Let $S = (U, C \cup D)$ be a decision table, and

$$RULE = \{Z_{ij} : des(X_i) \rightarrow des(Y_j),\ X_i \in U \ / \ C, Y_j \in U \ / \ D\}.$$

Consistency measure $\beta$ of $S$ is defined as

$$\beta(S) = \sum_{i=1}^{m} \frac{|X_i|}{|U|}[1 - \frac{4}{|X_i|}\sum_{j=1}^{N_i}|X_i \cap Y_j| \mu(Z_{ij})(1 - \mu(Z_{ij}))]$$

where $N_i$ is the number of decision rules determined by the condition class $X_i$ and $\mu(Z_{ij})$ is the certainty measure of the rule $Z_{ij}$.

## Theorem 4.5 (Extremum)

Let $S = (U, C \cup D)$ be a decision table, and

$$RULE = \{Z_{ij} : des(X_i) \rightarrow des(Y_j)\ X_i \in U \ / \ C, Y_j \in U \ / \ D\}.$$

For every $Z_{ij} \in RULE$, if $\mu(Z_{ij}) = 1$, then the measure $\beta$ achieves its maximum value 1.

For every $Z_{ij} \in RULE$, if $\mu(Z_{ij}) = \frac{1}{2}$, then the measure $\beta$ achieves its minimum value 0.

**Proof**

From the definitions of $\mu(Z_{ij})$, it follows that $\frac{1}{|U|} \leq \mu(Z_{ij}) \leq 1$

If $\mu(Z_{ij}) = 1$ for all $Z_{ij} \in RULE$, then we have that

$$\beta(S) = \sum_{i=1}^{m} \frac{|X_i|}{|U|} [1 - \frac{4}{|X_i|} \sum_{j=1}^{N_i} |X_i \cap Y_j| \mu(Z_{ij})(1 - \mu(Z_{ij}))]$$

$$= \sum_{i=1}^{m} \frac{|X_i|}{|U|} [1 - \frac{4}{|X_i|} \sum_{j=1}^{N_i} |X_i \cap Y_j| \times 1 \times (1 - 1)]$$

$$= \sum_{i=1}^{m} \frac{|X_i|}{|U|} = 1$$

If $\mu(Z_{ij}) = \frac{1}{2}$ for all $Z_{ij} \in RULE$. In this case, we have that

$$\beta(S) = \sum_{i=1}^{m} \frac{|X_i|}{|U|} [1 - \frac{4}{|X_i|} \sum_{j=1}^{N_i} |X_i \cap Y_j| \mu(Z_{ij})(1 - \mu(Z_{ij}))]$$

$$= \sum_{i=1}^{m} \frac{|X_i|}{|U|} [1 - \frac{4}{|X_i|} \sum_{j=1}^{N_i} |X_i \cap Y_j| \times \frac{1}{4}]$$

$$= \sum_{i=1}^{m} \frac{|X_i|}{|U|} [1 - \frac{1}{|X_i|} \sum_{j=1}^{N_i} |X_i \cap Y_j| ]$$

$$= \sum_{i=1}^{m} \frac{|X_i|}{|U|} [1 - 1] = 0$$

This completes the proof.

It should be noted that the measure $\beta$ achieves its maximum one when $S = (U, C \cup D)$ is a consistent decision table.

**Remark**

Unlike the consistency degree $\alpha_C(U / D)$, the measure $\beta$ can be used to evaluate the consistency of a decision-rule set when $\alpha_C(U / D) = 0$ i.e., the lower approximation of each decision class is equal to an empty set. From the definition of consistency degree, it follows that $\alpha_C(U / D) = 0$ if $\bigcup_{Y_i \in U/D} \underline{C}Y_i = \phi$. In fact, as we know, $\underline{C}Y_i = \phi$ does not imply that the certainty of a rule concerning $Y_i$ is equal to 0. So the measure $\beta$ is much better than the classical consistency degree for measuring the consistency of a decision-rule set when decision tables are strictly and conversely consistent.

The monotonicity of the measure $\beta$ on conversely consistent decision tables can be found in the following Theorem 4.6 and 4.7.

## Theorem 4.6

Let $S_1 = (U, C_1 \cup D_1)$ and $S_2 = (U, C_2 \cup D_2)$ be two conversely consistent decision tables. If $U / C_1 = U / C_2$ and $U / D_2 \prec U / D_1$, then $\beta(S_1) < \beta(S_2)$ $\beta(S_1) > \beta(S_2)$ when $\forall \mu(Z_{ij}) \geq \dfrac{1}{2}$

**Proof**

Since $U / C_1 = U / C_2$ and the converse consistencies of $S_1$ and $S_2$, there exist $X_p \in U / C_1$ and $Y_q \in U / D_1$ such that $Y_q \subseteq X_p$. By $U / D_2 \prec U / D_1$, there derive that there exist $Y_q^1, Y_q^2, \cdots, Y_q^s \in U / D_2 (s > 1)$ such that $Y_q = \bigcup_{k=1}^s Y_q^k$. In other words, the rule $Z_{pq}$ in $S_1$ can be decomposed into a family of rules $Z_{pq}^1, Z_{pq}^2, \cdots, Z_{pq}^s$ in $S_2$. It is clear that $|Z_{pq}| = \sum_{k=1}^s Z_{pq}^k$.

Let $\delta_D(Z_{il}) = \dfrac{|X_i \cap [X_l]_D|}{|X_i|} (x_l \in X_i)$, where $[X_l]_D$ is the decision class of $X_l$ induced by $D$. So we know that if $x_l \in X_i \cap X_j$, then $\delta_D(Z_{il}) = \mu(Z_{ij})$ holds. Hence, it follows that

$$
\begin{aligned}
\beta(S) &= \sum_{i=1}^m \frac{|X_i|}{|U|}[1 - \frac{4}{|X_i|}\sum_{j=1}^{N_i} |X_i \cap Y_j| \mu(Z_{ij})(1 - \mu(Z_{ij}))] \\
&= \sum_{i=1}^m \frac{|X_i|}{|U|}[1 - \frac{4}{|X_i|}\sum_{l=1}^{|X_i|}\delta_D(Z_{il})(1 - \delta_D(Z_{il}))] \\
&= \sum_{i=1}^m \frac{|X_i|}{|U|}\frac{4}{|X_i|}\sum_{l=1}^{|X_i|}\left(\delta_D(Z_{il}) - \frac{1}{2}\right)^2 \\
&= \frac{4}{|U|}\sum_{i=1}^m \sum_{l=1}^{|X_i|}\left(\delta_D(Z_{il}) - \frac{1}{2}\right)
\end{aligned}
$$

Therefore, when $\forall \mu(Z_{ij}) \leq \dfrac{1}{2}$, we have that

$$
\begin{aligned}
\beta(S_1) &= \sum_{i=1}^m \frac{|X_i|}{|U|}[1 - \frac{4}{|X_i|}\sum_{j=1}^{N_i} |X_i \cap Y_j| \mu(Z_{ij})(1 - \mu(Z_{ij}))] \\
&= \frac{4}{|U|}\sum_{i=1}^m \sum_{l=1}^{|X_i|}\left(\delta_{D_1}(Z_{il}) - \frac{1}{2}\right)^2 \\
&= \frac{4}{|U|}\sum_{i=1,i\neq p}^m \sum_{l=1}^{|X_i|}\left(\delta_{D_1}(Z_{il}) - \frac{1}{2}\right)^2 + \frac{4}{|U|}\sum_{l=1}^{|X_p|}\left(\delta_{D_1}(Z_{pl}) - \frac{1}{2}\right)^2 \\
&< \frac{4}{|U|}\sum_{i=1,i\neq p}^m \sum_{l=1}^{|X_i|}\left(\delta_{D_2}(Z_{il}) - \frac{1}{2}\right)^2 + \frac{4}{|U|}\sum_{l=1}^{|X_p|}\left(\delta_{D_2}(Z_{pl}) - \frac{1}{2}\right)^2 \\
&= \beta(S_2)
\end{aligned}
$$

Similar to this idea, $\beta(S_1) > \beta(S_2)$ when $\forall \mu(Z_{ij}) \geq \frac{1}{2}$ can be proved. This completes the proof.

Theorem 4.6 states that the consistency measure $\beta$ of a conversely consistent decision table increases with its decision classes becoming finer when $\forall \mu(Z_{ij}) \leq \frac{1}{2}$, and decreases with its decision classes becoming finer when $\forall \mu(Z_{ij}) \geq \frac{1}{2}$.

## Theorem 4.7

Let $S_1 = (U, C_1 \cup D_1)$ and $S_2 = (U, C_2 \cup D_2)$ be two conversely consistent decision tables. If $U / D_1 = U / D_2$ and $U / C_2 \prec U / C_1$, then $\beta(S_1) > \beta(S_2)$ when $\forall \mu(Z_{ij}) \leq \frac{1}{2}$, and $\beta(S_1) < \beta(S_2)$ when $\forall \mu(Z_{ij}) \geq \frac{1}{2}$.

**Proof**

Let $\delta_C(Z_{il}) = \frac{|X_i \cap [x_l]_D|}{|X_i|} (x_l \in X_i, X_i \in U / C)$, where $[x_l]_D$ is the decision class of $x_l$ induced by $D$. So, we know that if $x_l \in X_i \cap Y_j$, then $\delta_C(Z_{il}) = \mu(Z_{ij})$ holds.

From $U / C_2 \prec U / C_1$, we know there exist $X_p \in U / C_1$ and an integer $s > 1$ such that $X_p = \bigcup_{k=1}^{s} X_p^k$, where $X_p^k \in U / C_2$. It is clear that $X_l = \sum_{k=1}^{s} |X_l^k|$, and $|X_p^k| < |X_p|$ for every $X_p^k \in U / C_2$. From the converse consistencies of $S_1$ and $S_2$, it follows that

$$\mu(Z_{pj}) = \frac{|X_p \cap Y_j|}{|X_p|} < \frac{|Y_j|}{|X_p|} < \frac{|Y_j|}{|X_p^k|} = \mu(Z_{pj}^k), k = \{1, 2, \cdots, s\}$$

That is $\delta_{C_1}(Z_{il}) < \delta_{C_2}(Z_{il})$.

Then, when $\forall \mu(Z_{ij}) \leq \frac{1}{2}$, we can get that

*Table 9. $c_C(D)$ and $\beta$ with different numbers of features in the data set tie-tac-toe*

| Measure | features | | | | | | | | |
|---------|----------|--------|--------|--------|--------|--------|--------|--------|--------|
| | 1 | 2 | 3 | 4 | 5 | 6 | 7 | 8 | 9 |
| $c_C(D)$ | 0.0000 | 0.0000 | 0.1253 | 0.1682 | 0.4186 | 0.7766 | 0.9436 | 1.0000 | 1.0000 |
| $\beta$ | 0.1114 | 0.1322 | 0.2827 | 0.3300 | 0.5832 | 0.8000 | 0.9436 | 1.0000 | 1.0000 |

$$\beta(S_1) = \sum_{i=1}^{m} \frac{|X_i|}{|U|} [1 - \frac{4}{|X_i|} \sum_{j=1}^{N_i} |X_i \cap Y_j| \mu(Z_{ij})(1 - \mu(Z_{ij}))]$$

$$= \frac{4}{|U|} \sum_{i=1}^{m} \sum_{l=1}^{|X_i|} \left( \delta_{C_1}(Z_{il}) - \frac{1}{2} \right)^2$$

$$= \frac{4}{|U|} \sum_{i=1, i \neq p}^{m} \sum_{l=1}^{|X_i|} \left( \delta_{C_1}(Z_{il}) - \frac{1}{2} \right)^2 + \frac{4}{|U|} \sum_{l=1}^{|X_p|} \left( \delta_{C_1}(Z_{pl}) - \frac{1}{2} \right)^2$$

$$> \frac{4}{|U|} \sum_{i=1, i \neq p}^{m} \sum_{l=1}^{|X_i|} \left( \delta_{C_2}(Z_{il}) - \frac{1}{2} \right)^2 + \frac{4}{|U|} \sum_{l=1}^{|X_p|} \left( \delta_{C_2}(Z_{pl}) - \frac{1}{2} \right)^2$$

$$= \frac{4}{|U|} \sum_{i=1, i \neq p}^{m} \sum_{l=1}^{|X_i|} \left( \delta_{C_2}(Z_{il}) - \frac{1}{2} \right)^2 + \frac{4}{|U|} \sum_{k=1}^{s} \sum_{l=1}^{|X_p^k|} \left( \delta_{C_2}(Z_{pl}) - \frac{1}{2} \right)^2$$

$$= \beta(S_2)$$

Similarly, we can prove that $\beta(S_1) < \beta(S_2)$ when $\forall \mu(Z_{ij}) \geq \frac{1}{2}$. This completes the proof.

Theorem 4.7 states that the consistency measure $\beta$ of a conversely consistent decision table decreases with its condition classes becoming finer when $\forall \mu(Z_{ij}) \leq \frac{1}{2}$, and increases with its condition classes becoming finer when $\forall \mu(Z_{ij}) \geq \frac{1}{2}$.

For general decision tables, to illustrate the differences between the consistency measure $\beta$ and the consistency degree $c_C(D)$, the three practical data sets in Table 2 will be used again. The comparisons of values of the two measures with the numbers of features in these three data sets are shown in Tables 9–11.

From Tables 9–11, it can be seen that the value of the consistency measure $\beta$ is not smaller than that of the consistency degree $c_C(D)$ for the same number of selected features, and this value increases as the number of selected features becomes bigger in the same data set. In particular, if the decision table becomes consistent through adding the number of selected features, the measure $\beta$ and the consistency degree will have the same value 1.

Whereas, from Table 9, it is easy to see that the values of the consistency degree equal 0 when the number of features equals 1 or 2. In this situation, the lower approximation of the target decision in the decision table equals an empty set. Hence, the consistency degree cannot be used to effectively characterize the consistency of the decision table when the value of the consistency degree equals 0. But, for the same situation as that the numbers of features equal 1 and 2, the values of the consistency measure $\beta$ equal 0.1114 and 0.1322, respectively. It shows that unlike the consistency degree, the consistency measure $\beta$ of the decision table with two features is higher than that of the decision table with only one feature. Therefore, the measure $\beta$ is much better than the consistency degree for an inconsistent decision table. Obviously, we can make the same conclusion from Table 10 and 11. In other words, the measure $\beta$ is still valid for evaluating the consistency of a set of decision rules obtained by using these selected features when the value of the consistency degree $c_C(D)$ is equal to 0. Given this advantage, we may conclude that the measure $\beta$ is much better than the classical consistency degree for evaluating the consistency of a decision table.

Based on the above analyses, we can draw conclusions that if $S$ is consistent, the measure $\beta$ has the same evaluation ability as the consistency degree $c_C(D)$ and that if $S$ is inconsistent, the measure $\beta$ has much better evaluation ability than the consistency degree $c_C(D)$. Finally, we consider how to define a better support measure for evaluating a decision-rule set.

Let $S = (U, C \cup D)$ be a decision table and

$$RULE = \{Z_{ij} : des(X_i) \rightarrow des(Y_j),\ X_i \in U / C, Y_j \in U / D\}.$$

Intuitively, the mean value of the support measures $s(Z_{ij})$ of all rules $Z_{ij}$ seems to be suitable for this task. However, the following example indicates our intuition unreliable.

## Example 4.3

Let $S_1 = (U, C_1 \cup D_1)$ and $S_2 = (U, C_2 \cup D_2)$ be two decision tables with the same universe $U$. Suppose that

*Table 10. $c_C(D)$ and $\beta$ with different numbers of features in the data set Dernatology*

| Measure | features | | | | | | | | | | |
|---|---|---|---|---|---|---|---|---|---|---|---|
| | 3 | 6 | 9 | 12 | 15 | 18 | 21 | 24 | 27 | 30 | 33 |
| $c_C(D)$ | 0.0055 | 0.4372 | 0.8060 | 0.9290 | 0.9809 | 1.0000 | 1.0000 | 1.0000 | 1.0000 | 1.0000 | 1.0000 |
| $\beta$ | 0.3101 | 0.5285 | 0.8471 | 0.9429 | 0.9818 | 1.0000 | 1.0000 | 1.0000 | 1.0000 | 1.0000 | 1.0000 |

*Table 11. $c_C(D)$ and $\beta$ with different numbers of features in the data set Nursery*

| Measure | features | | | | | | | |
|---|---|---|---|---|---|---|---|---|
| | 1 | 2 | 3 | 4 | 5 | 6 | 7 | 8 |
| $c_C(D)$ | 0.00000 | 0.00000 | 0.00000 | 0.00000 | 0.00000 | 0.00000 | 0.00000 | 1.00000 |
| $\beta$ | 0.13777 | 0.11119 | 0.11122 | 0.11126 | 0.11120 | 0.11111 | 0.11111 | 1.00000 |

$$U \, / \, C_1 = \{\{e_1, e_2\}, \{e_3, e_4\}, \{e_5, e_6, e_7, e_8, e_9\}\},$$

$$U \, / \, D_1 = \{\{e_1, e_2, e_3, e_4\}, \{e_5, e_6, e_7, e_8, e_9\}\},$$

$$U \, / \, C_2 = \{\{e_1, e_2, e_3, e_4, e_5, e_6\}, \{e_7, e_8, e_9\}\},$$

$$U \, / \, D_2 = \{\{e_1, e_2, e_3\}\{e_4, e_5, e_6\}, \{e_7, e_8, e_9\}\}.$$

By taking the average value, it follows that

$$\beta(S_1) = \frac{1}{|\,RULE\,|} \sum_{i=1}^{m} \sum_{j=1}^{n} s(Z_{ij}) = \frac{1}{3}\left(\frac{2}{9} + \frac{2}{9} + \frac{5}{9}\right) = \frac{1}{3}$$

$$\beta(S_2) = \frac{1}{|\,RULE\,|} \sum_{i=1}^{m} \sum_{j=1}^{n} s(Z_{ij}) = \frac{1}{3}\left(\frac{3}{9} + \frac{3}{9} + \frac{3}{9}\right) = \frac{1}{3}$$

Therefore, in this case, $\beta(S_1) = \beta(S_2)$.

In fact, the weight information of each decision rule has not been considered in this measure. Hence, it may not be able to effectively characterize the support measure of a complete decision table.

In this following, we defined a more effective support measure $\gamma$ for evaluating the support of a decision rule set.

## Definition 4.7

Let $S = (U, C \cup D)$ be a decision table, and

$$RULE = \{Z_{ij} : des(X_i) \rightarrow des(Y_j), \ X_i \in U \, / \, C, Y_j \in U \, / \, D\}.$$

Support measure $\gamma$ of $S$ is defined as $\gamma(S) = \sum_{i=1}^{m} \sum_{j=1}^{n} s^2(Z_{ij}) = \sum_{i=1}^{m} \sum_{j=1}^{n} \frac{|\,X_i \cap Y_j\,|^2}{|\,U\,|^2}$, where $s(Z_{ij})$ is

the support measure of the rule $Z_{ij}$.

## Theorem 4.8. (Extremum)

Let $S = (U, C \cup D)$ be a decision table, and

$$RULE = \{Z_{ij} : des(X_i) \rightarrow \quad des(Y_j), \ X_i \in U \, / \, C, Y_j \in U \, / \, D\}.$$

If $m = n = 1$, then the measure $\gamma$ achieves its maximum value 1, and

If $m = |U|$ or $n = |U|$, then the measure $\gamma$ achieves its minimum value $\dfrac{1}{|U|}$.

**Proof**

From the definitions of $s(Z_{ij})$, it follows that $\dfrac{1}{|U|} \leq s(Z_{ij}) \leq 1$ and

$$\sum_{i=1}^{m}\sum_{j=1}^{n} s(Z_{ij}) = \sum_{i=1}^{m}\sum_{j=1}^{n}\frac{|X_i \cap Y_j|}{|U|} = 1$$

If $m = n = 1$, then $s(Z_{ij}) = \dfrac{|X_i \cap Y_j|}{|U|} = \dfrac{|U|}{|U|} = 1$. Therefore, one can obtain that

$$\gamma(S) = \sum_{i=1}^{m}\sum_{j=1}^{n} s^2(Z_{ij}) = 1$$

If $m = |U|$ or $n = |U|$, then $s(Z_{ij}) = \dfrac{1}{|U|}$ for all $Z_{ij} \in RULE$. Hence,

$$\gamma(S) = \sum_{i=1}^{m}\sum_{j=1}^{n} s^2(Z_{ij}) = \sum_{i-1}^{m}\frac{1}{|U|^2} = \frac{1}{|U|}.$$

This completes the proof.

## Example 4.4 (Continued from Example 4.3)

From the definition of the measure $\gamma$, it follows that

$$\gamma(S_1) = \sum_{i=1}^{m}\sum_{j=1}^{n} s^2(Z_{ij}) = \left(\frac{2}{9}\right)^2 + \left(\frac{2}{9}\right)^2 + \left(\frac{5}{9}\right)^2 = \frac{34}{81}$$

and

$$\gamma(S_1) = \sum_{i=1}^{m}\sum_{j=1}^{n} s^2(Z_{ij}) = \left(\frac{3}{9}\right)^2 + \left(\frac{3}{9}\right)^2 + \left(\frac{3}{9}\right)^2 = \frac{27}{81}$$

Therefore, $\gamma(S_1) > \gamma(S_2)$.

Example 4.4 indicates that the measure $\gamma$ may be better than the measure $\beta$ used in Example 4.3 for evaluating a decision-rule set.

## Theorem 4.9

Let $S_1 = (U, C_1 \cup D_1)$ and $S_2 = (U, C_2 \cup D_2)$ be two decision tables. Then, $\gamma(S_1) < \gamma(S_2)$ if and only if $G(C_1 \cup D_1) < G(C_2 \cup D_2)$.

**Proof**

Suppose that

$$U / (C \cup D) = \{X_i \cap Y_j \mid X_i \cap Y_j \neq \varnothing, X_i \in U / C, Y_j \in U / D\}$$

and

$$RULE = \{Z_{ij} : X_i \rightarrow Y_j, X_i \in U / C, Y_j \in U / D\}$$

From Definition 4.4 and $s(Z_{ij}) = \dfrac{|X_i \cap Y_j|}{|U|}$ it follows that

$$G(C \cup D) = \frac{1}{|U|^2} \sum_{i=1}^{m} \sum_{j=1}^{n} |X_i \cap Y_j|^2$$

$$= \sum_{i=1}^{m} \sum_{j=1}^{n} \left( \frac{|X_i \cap Y_j|}{|U|} \right)^2 = \sum_{i=1}^{m} \sum_{j=1}^{n} s^2(Z_{ij}) = \gamma(S).$$

Therefore, $\gamma(S_1) < \gamma(S_2)$ if and only if $G(C_1 \cup D_1) < G(C_2 \cup D_2)$. This completes the proof.

Theorem 4.9 states that the support measure $\gamma$ of a decision table increases with the granulation of the decision table becoming bigger. As a direct result of Theorem 4.9, we obtain

## Corollary 4.1

Let $S_1 = (U, C_1 \cup D_1)$ and $S_2 = (U, C_2 \cup D_2)$ be two decision tables. If $U / (C_1 \cup D_1) \prec U / (C_2 \cup D_2)$, then $\gamma(S_1) < \gamma(S_2)$.

## Theorem 4.10

Let $S_1 = (U, C_1 \cup D_1)$ and $S_2 = (U, C_2 \cup D_2)$ be two conversely consistent decision tables. If $U / C_1 = U / C_2$ and $U / D_1 \prec U / D_2$, then $\gamma(S_1) < \gamma(S_2)$.

**Proof**

From $U / C_1 = U / C_2$ and the converse consistencies of $S_1$ and $S_2$, it follows that there exist $X_l \in U / C_1$ and $Y_{j_0} \in U / D_2$ such that $Y_{j_0} \subseteq X_l$. By $U / D_1 \prec U / D_2$, we derive that there exist

$Y_{j_0}^1, Y_{j_0}^2, \cdots, Y_{j_0}^s, \in U / D_1 (s > 1)$ such that $Y_{j_0} = \bigcup_{k=1}^{s} Y_{j_0}^k$ and $|Y_{j_0}| = \sum_{k=1}^{s} |Y_{j_0}^k|$. It is clear that $|Z_{lj_0}| = \sum_{k=1}^{s} |Z_{lj_0}^k|$. Hence,

$$
\begin{aligned}
\gamma(S_2) &= \sum_{i=1}^{m} \sum_{j=1}^{n} s^2(Z_{ij}) = \sum_{i=1}^{l-1} \sum_{j=1}^{n} s^2(Z_{ij}) + \sum_{j=1}^{n} s^2(Z_{lj}) + \sum_{i=l+1}^{m} \sum_{j=1}^{n} s^2(Z_{ij}) \\
&= \sum_{i=1}^{l-1} \sum_{j=1}^{n} s^2(Z_{ij}) + \sum_{j=1, j \neq j_0}^{n} s^2(Z_{lj}) + s^2(Z_{lj_0}) + \sum_{i=l+1}^{m} \sum_{j=1}^{n} s^2(Z_{ij}) \\
&= \sum_{i=1}^{l-1} \sum_{j=1}^{n} s^2(Z_{ij}) + \sum_{j=1, j \neq j_0}^{n} s^2(Z_{lj}) + \frac{|X_l \cap Y_{j_0}|^2}{|U|^2} + \sum_{i=l+1}^{m} \sum_{j=1}^{n} s^2(Z_{ij}) \\
&= \sum_{i=1}^{l-1} \sum_{j=1}^{n} s^2(Z_{ij}) + \sum_{j=1, j \neq j_0}^{n} s^2(Z_{lj}) + \frac{|X_l \cap \bigcup_{k=1}^{s} Y_{j_0}^k|^2}{|U|^2} + \sum_{i=l+1}^{m} \sum_{j=1}^{n} s^2(Z_{ij}) \\
&> \sum_{i=1}^{l-1} \sum_{j=1}^{n} s^2(Z_{ij}) + \sum_{j=1, j \neq j_0}^{n} s^2(Z_{lj}) + \frac{\sum_{k=1}^{s} |X_l \cap Y_{j_0}^k|^2}{|U|^2} + \sum_{i=l+1}^{m} \sum_{j=1}^{n} s^2(Z_{ij}) \\
&= \sum_{i=1}^{l-1} \sum_{j=1}^{n} s^2(Z_{ij}) + \sum_{j=1, j \neq j_0}^{n} s^2(Z_{lj}) + \sum_{k=1}^{s} s^2(Z_{lj_0}^k) + \sum_{i=l+1}^{m} \sum_{j=1}^{n} s^2(Z_{ij}) = \gamma(S_1)
\end{aligned}
$$

That is $\gamma(S_1) < \gamma(S_2)$. This completes the proof.

Theorem 4.10 states that the support measure $\gamma$ of a decision table decreases with its decision classes becoming finer.

## Theorem 4.11

Let $S_1 = (U, C_1 \cup D_1)$ and $S_2 = (U, C_2 \cup D_2)$ be two consistent decision tables. If $U / C_1 \prec U / C_2$ and $U / D_1 = U / D_2$, then $\gamma(S_1) < \gamma(S_2)$.

**Proof**
The proof is similar to that of Theorem 4.10.

Theorem 4.11 states that the support measure $\gamma$ of a decision table decreases as the condition classes becomes finer. As a result of Theorem 4.11, we obtain the following two corollaries.

## Corollary 4.2

Let $S_1 = (U, C_1 \cup D_1)$ and $S_2 = (U, C_2 \cup D_2)$ be two consistent decision tables. If $U / C_1 = U / C_2$, then $\gamma(S_1) = \gamma(S_2)$.

**Proof**

Suppose $U / (C \cup D) = \{X_i \cap Y_j \mid X_i \cap Y_j \neq \varnothing, X_i \in U / C, Y_j \in U / D\}$.

Since both $S_1$ and $S_2$ are consistent, we have that $U / C_1 \preceq U / D_1$ and $U / C_2 \preceq U / D_2$, i.e., $U / (C_1 \cup D_1) = U / C_1$ and $U / (C_2 \cup D_2) = U / C_2$.

It follows from $U / C_1 = U / C_2$ and $s(Z_{ij}) = \dfrac{\mid X_i \cap Y_j \mid}{\mid U \mid}$ that $\gamma(S_1) = \gamma(S_2)$. This completes the proof.

## Corollary 4.3

Let $S_1 = (U, C_1 \cup D_1)$ and $S_2 = (U, C_2 \cup D_2)$ be two conversely consistent decision tables. If $U / D_1 = U / D_2$, then $\gamma(S_1) = \gamma(S_2)$.

**Proof**

The proof is similar to that of Corollary 4.2.

Finally, we investigate the variation of the values of the support measure $\gamma$ with the numbers of features in the three practical data sets in Table 6. The values of the measure with the numbers of features in these three data sets are shown in Tables 12–14.

From these tables, one can see that the value of the support measure $\gamma$ decreases with the number of condition features becoming bigger in the same data set. Note that we may extract more decision rules

*Table 12. $\gamma$ with different numbers of features in the data set tie-tac-toe*

| Measure | features | | | | | | | | |
|---------|----------|---|---|---|---|---|---|---|---|
|         | 1 | 2 | 3 | 4 | 5 | 6 | 7 | 8 | 9 |
| $\gamma$ | 0.1998 | 0.0695 | 0.0304 | 0.0120 | 0.0060 | 0.0030 | 0.0016 | 0.0010 | 0.0010 |

*Table 13. $\gamma$ with different numbers of features in the data set Dernatology*

| Measure | features | | | | | | | | | | |
|---------|----------|---|---|----|----|----|----|----|----|----|----|
|         | 3 | 6 | 9 | 12 | 15 | 18 | 21 | 24 | 27 | 30 | 33 |
| $\gamma$ | 0.0593 | 0.0080 | 0.0052 | 0.0038 | 0.0032 | 0.0029 | 0.0028 | 0.0028 | 0.0028 | 0.0027 | 0.0027 |

*Table 14. $\gamma$ with different numbers of features in the data set Nursery*

| Measure | features | | | | | | | |
|---------|----------|---|---|---|---|---|---|---|
|         | 1 | 2 | 3 | 4 | 5 | 6 | 7 | 8 |
| $\gamma$ | 0.11418 | 0.02861 | 0.00721 | 0.00185 | 0.00064 | 0.00033 | 0.00011 | 0.00007 |

through adding the number of condition features in general. In fact, the bigger the number of decision rules is, the smaller the value of the support measure is in the same data set. Therefore, the measure $\gamma$ is able to effectively evaluate the support of all decision rules extracted from a given decision table.

From the above experimental results and analyses, the proposed measures $\alpha$, $\beta$ and $\gamma$ appear to be well suited for evaluating the decision performance of a decision table and a decision-rule set. These measures will be helpful for selecting a preferred rule-extracting method for a particular application.

## 5. CONCLUSION

The contribution of this chapter is twofold. On one side, a kind of dynamic approximation method of target concepts based on a granulation order is presented, which are the positive approximation and converse approximation. Two algorithms for rule extracting called MABPA and REBCA are designed and applied to hierarchically generate decision rules from a decision table. On the other side, to evaluate the whole performance of a decision rule set, three kinds of measures are proposed for evaluating the certainty, consistency and support of a decision-rule set extracted from a decision table, respectively. It has been analyzed how each of these three new measures depends on the condition granulation and decision granulation of each of the three types of decision tables. The experimental analyses on three practical decision tables show that these three new measures are adequate for evaluating the decision performance of a decision-rule set extracted from a decision table in rough set theory. These three kinds of measures may be helpful in determining which rule extraction technique should be chosen in a practical decision problem.

## ACKNOWLEDGMENT

This work was supported by the national natural science foundation of China (No. 60773133, No. 70471003, No. 60573074), the high technology research and development program of China (No. 2007AA01Z165), the foundation of doctoral program research of the ministry of education of China (No. 20050108004) and key project of science and technology research of the ministry of education of China.

## REFERENCES

[1] Bazan, J., Peters, J. F., Skowron, A., Nguyen, H. S., & Szczuka, M. (2003). Rough set approach to pattern extraction from classifiers. *Electronic Notes in Theoretical Computer Science, 82*(4), 1–10. doi:10.1016/S1571-0661(04)80702-3

[2] Beynon, M. (2001). Reducts within the variable precision rough sets model: a further investigation. *European Journal of Operational Research, 134*(3), 592–605. doi:10.1016/S0377-2217(00)00280-0

[3] Düntsch, I., & Gediaga, G. (1998). Uncertainty measures of rough set prediction. *Artificial Intelligence, 106*(1), 109–137. doi:10.1016/S0004-3702(98)00091-5

[4] Greco, S., Pawlak, Z., & Slowinski, R. (2004). Can Bayesian confirmation measures be useful for rough set decision rules. *Engineering Applications of Artificial Intelligence, 17*, 345–361. doi:10.1016/j.engappai.2004.04.008

[5] Huynh, V. N., & Nakamori, Y. (2005). A roughness measure for fuzzy sets. *Information Sciences, 173*, 255–275. doi:10.1016/j.ins.2004.07.017

[6] Komorowski, J., Pawlak, Z., Polkowski, L., & Skowron, A. (1999). Rough sets: a tutuorial. In Pal, S. K., & Skowron, A. (Eds.), *Rough fuzzy hybridization: a new trend in decision making* (pp. 3–98). Berlin, Germany: Springer.

[7] Kryszkiewicz, M. (2001). Comparative study of alternative type of knowledge reduction in inconsistent systems. *International Journal of Intelligent Systems, 16*, 105–120. doi:10.1002/1098-111X(200101)16:1<105::AID-INT8>3.0.CO;2-S

[8] Leung, Y., & Li, D. Y. (2003). Maximal consistent block technique for rule acquisition in incomplete information systems. *Information Sciences, 153*, 85–106. doi:10.1016/S0020-0255(03)00061-6

[9] Li, D. Y., & Ma, Y. C. (2000). Invariant characters of information systems under some homomorphisms. *Information Sciences, 129*, 211–220. doi:10.1016/S0020-0255(00)00017-7

[10] Li, D. Y., Zhang, B., & Leung, Y. (2004). On knowledge reduction in inconsistent decision information systems. *International Journal of Uncertainty. Fuzziness and Knowledge-Based Systems, 12*(5), 651–672. doi:10.1142/S0218488504003132

[11] Liang, J. Y., & Xu, Z. B. (2002). The algorithm on knowledge reduction in incomplete information systems. *International Journal of Uncertainty. Fuzziness and Knowledge-Based Systems, 24*(1), 95–103. doi:10.1142/S021848850200134X

[12] Liang, J. Y., & Li, D. Y. (2005). *Uncertainty and Knowledge Acquisition in Information Systems.* Beijing, China: Science Press.

[13] Liang, J. Y., Qian, Y. H., Chu, C. Y., Li, D. Y., & Wang, J. H. (2005). Rough set approximation based on dynamic granulation. *Lecture Notes in Artificial Intelligence, 3641*, 701–708.

[14] Liang, J. Y., Shi, Z. Z., & Li, D. Y. (2004). The information entropy, rough entropy and knowledge granulation in rough set theory. *International Journal of Uncertainty. Fuzziness and Knowledge-Based Systems, 12*(1), 37–46. doi:10.1142/S0218488504002631

[15] Liang, J. Y., Shi, Z. Z., Li, D. Y., & Wierman, W. J. (2006). The information entropy, rough entropy and knowledge granulation in incomplete information systems. *International Journal of General Systems, 35*(6), 641–654. doi:10.1080/03081070600687668

[16] Liang, J. Y., Chin, K. S., Dang, C. Y., & Richard, C. M. Yam. (2002). A new method for measuring uncertainty and fuzziness in rough set theory. *International Journal of General Systems, 31*(4), 331–342. doi:10.1080/0308107021000013635

[17] Liang, J. Y., & Qian, Y. H. (2008). Information granules and entropy theory in information systems. *Science in China-Series F.* doi:10.1007/s11432-008-0113-2

[18] Marczewski, E. (1958). A general scheme of independence in mathematics. *Bulletin de 1 Academie Polonaise des Sciences-Serie des Sciences Mathematiques Astronomiques et Physiques, 6,* 331-362.

[19] Mi, J. S., Wu, W. Z., & Zhang, W. X. (2003). Comparative studies of knowledge reductions in inconsistent systems. *Fuzzy Systems and Mathematics, 17*(3), 54–60.

[20] Nguyen, H. S., & Slezak, D. (1999). Approximate reducts and association rules correspondence and complexity results. *Lecture Notes in Artificial Intelligence, 1711,* 137–145.

[21] Pal, S. K., Pedrycz, W., Skowron, A., & Swiniarski, R. (2001). Presenting the special issue on rough-neruo computing. *Neurocomputing, 36,* 1–3. doi:10.1016/S0925-2312(00)00332-5

[22] Pawlak, Z. (1982). Rough sets. *International Journal of Computer and Information Science, 11,* 341–356. doi:10.1007/BF01001956

[23] Pawlak, Z. (1991). *Rough sets: theoretical aspects of reasoning about data.* Dordrecht, The Netherlands: Kluwer Academic.

[24] Pawlak, Z. (1998). Rough set theory and its applications in data analysis. *Cybernetics and Systems, 29,* 661–688. doi:10.1080/019697298125470

[25] Pawlak, Z. (2005). Some remarks on conflict analysis. *Information Sciences, 166,* 649–654.

[26] Pawlak, Z., & Skowron, Z. (2007). Rudiments of rough sets. *Information Sciences, 177,* 3–27. doi:10.1016/j.ins.2006.06.003

[27] Pawlak, Z., & Skowron, Z. (2007). Rough sets: some extensions. *Information Sciences, 177,* 28–40. doi:10.1016/j.ins.2006.06.006

[28] Pawlak, Z., & Skowron, Z. (2007). Rough sets and Boolean reasoning. *Information Sciences, 177,* 41–73. doi:10.1016/j.ins.2006.06.007

[29] Pedrycz, W., & Vukovick, G. (2000). Granular worlds: representation and communication problems. *International Journal of Intelligent Systems, 15,* 1015–1026. doi:10.1002/1098-111X(200011)15:11<1015::AID-INT3>3.0.CO;2-9

[30] Pedrycz, W. (2002). Relational and directional in the construction of information granules. *IEEE Transactions on Systems, Man, and Cybernetics. Part A, Systems and Humans, 32*(5), 605–614. doi:10.1109/TSMCA.2002.804790

[31] Qian, Y. H., & Liang, J. Y. (2006). Combination entropy and combination granulation in incomplete information system. *Lecture Notes in Artificial Intelligence, 4062,* 184–190.

[32] Qian, Y. H., Dang, C. Y., & Liang, J. Y. (2008). Consistency measure, inclusion degree and fuzzy measure in decision tables. *Fuzzy Sets and Systems, 159,* 2353–2377. doi:10.1016/j.fss.2007.12.016

[33] Qian, Y. H., Dang, C. Y., Liang, J. Y., Zhang, H. Y., & Ma, J. M. (2008). On the evaluation of the decision performance of an incomplete decision table. *Data & Knowledge Engineering, 65*(3), 373–400. doi:10.1016/j.datak.2007.12.002

[34] Qian, Y. H., Liang, J. Y., & Dang, C. Y. (2008). Converse approximation and rule extracting from decision tables in rough set theory. *Computers & Mathematics with Applications (Oxford, England)*, *55*(8), 1754–1765. doi:10.1016/j.camwa.2007.08.031

[35] Qian, Y. H., Liang, J. Y., Dang, C. Y., Wang, F., & Xu, W. (2007). Knowledge distance in information systems. *Journal of Systems Science and Systems Engineering*, *16*(4), 434–449. doi:10.1007/s11518-007-5059-1

[36] Qian, Y. H., Liang, J. Y., Li, D. Y., Zhang, H. Y., & Dang, C. Y. (2008). Measures for evaluating the decision performance of a decision table in rough set theory. *Information Sciences*, *178*, 181–202. doi:10.1016/j.ins.2007.08.010

[37] Qian, Y. H., & Liang, J. Y. (2008). Combination entropy and combination granulation in rough set theory. *International Journal of Uncertainty. Fuzziness and Knowledge-Based System*, *16*(2), 179–193. doi:10.1142/S0218488508005121

[38] Qian, Y. H., & Liang, J. Y. (2008). Positive approximation and rule extracting in incomplete information systems. *International Journal of Computer Science and Knowledge Engineering*, *2*(1), 51–63.

[39] Quafatou, M. (2000). -RST: a generalization of rough set theory. *Information Sciences*, *124*, 301–316. doi:10.1016/S0020-0255(99)00075-4

[40] Skowron, A. (1995). Extracting laws from decision tables: a rough set approach. *Computational Intelligence*, *11*, 371–388. doi:10.1111/j.1467-8640.1995.tb00039.x

[41] Skowron, A., & Rauszer, C. (1992). The discernibility matrices and functions in information systems. In Slowinski, R. (Ed.), *Intelligent decision support, handbook of applications and advances of the rough sets theory* (pp. 331–362). Dordrecht, The Netherlands: Kluwer Academic.

[42] Slezak, D. (1996). Approximate reducts in decision tables. In Bouchon-Meunier, B., Delgado, M., Verdegay, J. L., Vila, M. A., & Yager, R. (Eds.), *Proceeding of IPMU'96* (*Vol. 3*, pp. 1159–1164). Granada, Spain.

[43] Wu, W. Z., Zhang, M., Li, H. Z., & Mi, J. S. (2005). Knowledge reduction in random information systems via Dempster-Shafer theory of evidence. *Information Sciences*, *174*, 143–164. doi:10.1016/j.ins.2004.09.002

[44] Xu, Z. B., Liang, J. Y., Dang, C. Y., & Chin, K. S. (2002). Inclusion degree: a perspective on measures for rough set data analysis. *Information Sciences*, *141*, 229–238. doi:10.1016/S0020-0255(02)00174-3

[45] Yao, Y. Y. (2001). Information granulation and rough set approximation. *International Journal of Intelligent Systems*, *16*(1), 87–104. doi:10.1002/1098-111X(200101)16:1<87::AID-INT7>3.0.CO;2-S

[46] Yao, Y. Y. (2007). Neighborhood systems and approximate retrieval. *Information Sciences*, *174*, 143–164.

[47] Zadeh, L. A. (1997). Toward a theory of fuzzy information granulation and its centrality in human reasoning and fuzzy logic. *Fuzzy Sets and Systems*, *90*, 111–127. doi:10.1016/S0165-0114(97)00077-8

[48] Zadeh, L. A. (1998). Some reflections on soft computing, granular computing and their roles in the conception, design and utilization of information/intelligent systems. *Soft Computing*, *2*(1), 23–25. doi:10.1007/s005000050030

[50] Zhang, L., & Zhang, B. (2005). Fuzzy reasoning model and under quotient space structure. *Information Sciences*, *173*, 353–364. doi:10.1016/j.ins.2005.03.005

[51] Zhang, P., Germano, R., Arien, J., Qin, K. Y., & Xu, Y. (2006). Interpreting and extracting fuzzy decision rules from fuzzy information systems and their inference. *Information Sciences*, *176*, 1869–1897. doi:10.1016/j.ins.2005.04.003

[49] Zhang, W. X., Wu, W. Z., Liang, J. Y., & Li, D. Y. (2001). *Theory and method of rough sets*. Beijing, China: Science Press.

[52] Zhu, W., & Wang, F. Y. (2003). Reduction and axiomization of covering generalized rough sets. *Information Sciences*, *152*, 217–230. doi:10.1016/S0020-0255(03)00056-2

[53] Ziarko, W. (1993). Variable precision rough set model. *Journal of Computer and System Sciences*, *46*, 39–59. doi:10.1016/0022-0000(93)90048-2

[54] The UCI machine learning repository. http://mlearn.ics.uci.edu/MLRepositroy.html.

# Chapter 10
# Granular Models:
## Design Insights and Development Practices

**Witold Pedrycz**
*Polish Academy of Sciences, Poland*

**Athanasios Vasilakos**
*Polish Academy of Sciences, Poland*

## ABSTRACT

*In contrast to numeric models, granular models produce results coming in a form of some information granules. Owing to the granularity of information these constructs dwell upon, such models become highly transparent and interpretable as well as operationally effective. Given also the fact that information granules come with a clearly defined semantics, granular models are often referred to as linguistic models. The crux of the design of the linguistic models studied in this paper exhibits two important features. First, the model is constructed on a basis of information granules which are assembled in the form of a web of associations between the granules formed in the output and input spaces. Given the semantics of information granules, we envision that a blueprint of the granular model can be formed effortlessly and with a very limited computing overhead. Second, the interpretability of the model is retained as the entire construct dwells on the conceptual entities of a well-defined semantics. The granulation of available data is accomplished by a carefully designed mechanism of fuzzy clustering which takes into consideration specific problem-driven requirements expressed by the designer at the time of the conceptualization of the model. We elaborate on a so-called context – based (conditional) Fuzzy C-Means (cond-FCM, for brief) to demonstrate how the fuzzy clustering is engaged in the design process. The clusters formed in the input space become induced (implied) by the context fuzzy sets predefined in the output space. The context fuzzy sets are defined in advance by the designer of the model so this design facet provides an active way of forming the model and in this manner becomes instrumental in the determination of a perspective at which a certain phenomenon is to be captured and modeled. This stands in a sharp contrast with most modeling approaches where the development is somewhat passive by being predominantly based on the existing data. The linkages between the fuzzy clusters induced by the given context fuzzy set in the output space are combined by forming a blueprint of the overall granular*

DOI: 10.4018/978-1-60566-324-1.ch010

*model. The membership functions of the context fuzzy sets are used as granular weights (connections) of the output processing unit (linear neuron) which subsequently lead to the granular output of the model thus identifying a feasible region of possible output values for the given input. While the above design is quite generic addressing a way in which information granules are assembled in the form of the model, we discuss further refinements which include (a) optimization of the context fuzzy sets, (b) inclusion of bias in the linear neuron at the output layer.*

## 1. INTRODUCTION

Human centric systems and human centric computing are concerned with a functionality that makes systems highly responsive to the needs of human users. We fully acknowledge a fact that there could be a genuine diversity of requirements and preferences that might well vary from user to user. How could we build systems that are capable of accommodating such needs and offering in this way a high level of user-friendliness? There are numerous interesting scenarios one can envision in which human centricity plays a vital role. For instance, in system modeling, a user may wish to model the reality based on a unique modeling perspective. In this sense the data being available for modeling purposes are to be looked at and used in the construction of the model within a suitable context established by the user. In information retrieval and information organization (no matter whether we are concerned with audio, visual or hypermedia information), the same collection of objects could be structured and looked at from different standpoints depending upon the preferences of the individual user. In this case, an ultimate functionality of human-centric systems is to achieve an effective realization of relevance feedback provided by the user.

In this study, we are concerned with a category of fuzzy modeling that directly explores the underlying ideas of fuzzy clustering and leads to the concept of granular models. The essence of these models is to describe associations between information granules; viz. fuzzy sets formed both in the input and output spaces. The context within which such relationships are being formed is established by the system developer. Information granules are built using specialized, conditional (context-driven) fuzzy clustering. This emphasizes the human-centric character of such models: it is the designer who assumes an active role in the process of forming information granules and casting all modeling pursuits in a suitable, customized framework. Owing to the straightforward design process, granular models become particularly useful in *rapid* system prototyping. All of these features bring a significant component of novelty and uniqueness to the concept of granular modeling.

The study is arranged in a way it made self-contained to a significant extent. We start with some generic constructs such as information granules and elaborate on their origin (Section 2). The context-based clustering presented in Section 3 forms a viable vehicle to build information granules when considering their further usage in some input-output mapping. The proposed category of models is inherently granular and this facet of processing is captured by a generalized version of so-called granular neurons (Section 4) in which the connections are represented as fuzzy numbers rather than single numeric entities. By bringing the concept of conditional clustering along with the granular neuron as some aggregation mechanism we show that granular models are easily assembled into a web of connections between information granules and these architectural considerations are presented in Section 5. The consecutive part of the study is devoted to two further refinements of granular models where we introduce a bias term and elaborate on optimization of fuzzy sets of context. Incremental granular models are studied in Section 7.

## 2. THE CLUSTER-BASED REPRESENTATION OF THE INPUT–OUTPUT MAPPINGS

Clusters [2] and fuzzy clusters [1][3][4][6][10][19][20] establish a sound basis for constructing fuzzy models [17][18]. By forming fuzzy clusters in the input and output spaces (spaces of input and output variables), we span the fuzzy model over a collection of prototypes. More descriptively, these prototypes are regarded as a structural *skeleton* or a design *blueprint* of the resulting model. Once the prototypes have been formed, there are several ways of developing the detailed expressions governing the detailed relationships of the model. The one commonly encountered in the literature takes the prototypes formed in the output space, that is $z_1, z_2, ..., z_c \in \mathbf{R}$ and combines them linearly by using the membership grades of the corresponding degrees of membership of the fuzzy clusters in the input space. Consider some given input $\mathbf{x}$. Denote the corresponding grades of membership produced by the prototypes $\mathbf{v}_1, \mathbf{v}_2, ...,$ and $\mathbf{v}_c$ located in the input space by $u_1(\mathbf{x}), u_2(\mathbf{x}),..., u_c(\mathbf{x})$. The output of the model reads as follows

$$y = \sum_{i=1}^{c} z_i u_i(\mathbf{x}) \tag{1}$$

The value of $u_i(\mathbf{x})$ being the degree at which $\mathbf{x}$ is compatible with the i-th cluster in the input space, is computed in a similar way as encountered in the FCM algorithm, that is

$$u_i(\mathbf{x}) = \cfrac{1}{\sum_{j=1}^{c} \left( \cfrac{\|\mathbf{x} - \mathbf{v}_i\|}{\|\mathbf{x} - \mathbf{v}_j\|} \right)^{\frac{2}{m-1}}} \tag{2}$$

where "m" is a fuzzification factor (fuzzification coefficient). The reader familiar with radial basis function (RBF) neural networks [5][8][9] can easily recognize that a structure of (1) closely resembles the architecture of RBF neural networks. There are some striking differences. First, the receptive fields provided by (2) are automatically constructed without any need for their further adjustments (which is usually not the case in standard RBFs). Second, the form of the RBF is far more flexible than the commonly encountered RBFs such as, for example, Gaussian functions.

It is instructive to visualize the characteristics of the model, which realizes some nonlinear mapping between the input to output space. The character of resulting nonlinearity depends upon the distribution of the prototypes. It could be also impacted by the values of the fuzzification factor "m". Figure 1 illustrates some input-output characteristics for the fixed values of the prototypes and varying values of the fuzzification factor. The commonly chosen value of "m" equal to 2.0 is also included in these graphs. Undoubtedly, we see that this design parameter exhibits a significant impact on the character of nonlinearity being developed. The values of "m" close to 1 produce a stepwise (Boolean) character of the mapping; we observe significant jumps located at the points where we switch between the individual clusters in input space. In this manner the impact coming from each rule is very clearly delineated. The typical value of the fuzzification coefficient set up to 2.0 yields a gradual transition between the rules and this shows up through smooth nonlinearities of the input-output relationships of the model. The increase in the values of "m", as shown in Figure 1, yields quite *spiky* characteristics: we quickly reach

*Figure 1. Nonlinear input-output characteristics of the cluster-based model (1). Prototypes are fixed $(v_1 = -1, v_2 = 2.5 \, v_3 = 6.1; z_1 = 6, z_2 = -4, z_3 = 2)$ while the fuzzification coefficient (m) assumes several selected values ranging from 1.2 to 4.0*

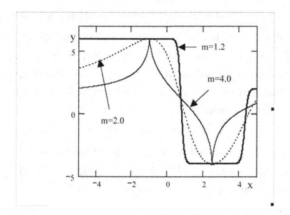

some modal values when moving close to the prototypes in the input space while in the remaining cases the characteristics switch between them in a relatively abrupt manner positioning close to the averages of the modes.

Figure 2 illustrates the characteristics of the model in case of different values of the prototypes. Again it becomes apparent that by moving the prototypes we are able to adjust the nonlinear mapping of the model to the existing experimental data.

It is helpful to contrast this fuzzy model with the RBF network equipped with Gaussian receptive fields, which is governed by the expression

$$y = \frac{\sum_{i=1}^{c} z_i G(x; v_i, \sigma)}{\sum_{i=1}^{c} G(x; v_i, \sigma)} \tag{3}$$

*Figure 2. Nonlinear input-output characteristics of the cluster-based model (1). The prototypes in the input space vary; the distribution of the prototypes in the output space are equal to $z_1 = 6, z_2 = -4, z_3 = 8; m = 2$*

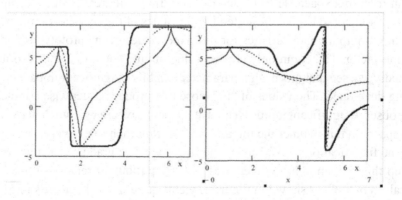

*Figure 3. Nonlinear input-output characteristics of RBF network; the changes in the spread values of the receptive fields show somewhat a similar effect to the one produced by the fuzzification factor. The remaining parameters of the model are fixed and equal to $z_1 = 6$, $z_2 = -4$, $z_3 = 8$; $v_1 = 1$; $v_2 = 5.2$, $v_3 = 5.1$*

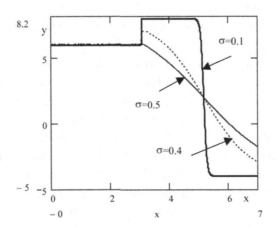

where $G(x;m,\sigma)$ denotes a certain Gaussian function (receptive field) characterized by its modal value (m) and spread ($\sigma$).Note that in (3) we usually require some normalization as the sum of these receptive fields may not always generate the value equal to 1. As shown in Figure 3, there is also no guarantee that for the prototypes the model coincides with the prototypes defined in the output space. This effect can be attributed to the smoothing effect of the Gaussian receptive fields. This stands in sharp contrast to the nonlinear nature of the relationship formed by the fuzzy partition.

## 3. CONTEXT-BASED CLUSTERING IN THE DEVELOPMENT OF GRANULAR MODELS

Clustering plays a crucial role in granular modeling. First, it helps convert numeric data into information granules. The produced information granules form a conceptual backbone or a *blueprint* of the model. While the model could be carefully refined further on, it is predominantly aimed at capturing the most essential, numerically dominant features of data by relying on their prudent summarization. The more clusters we intend to capture, the more detailed the resulting blueprint becomes. It is important to note that clustering helps manage dimensionality problem that is usually a critical issue in rule-based modeling. As being naturally based on Cartesian products of input variables rather than individual variables, they offer a substantial level of dimensionality reduction. Let us remind that in any rule-based system the number of input variables plays a pivotal role when it comes to the dimensionality of the resulting rule base. A complete rule base consists of $p^n$ where "p" is the number of information granules in each input variable and "n" denotes the total number of the input variables. Even in case of a fairly modest dimensionality of the problem, (say, n =10) and very few information granules defined for each variable (say, p = 4), we end up with a significant number of rules that is $4^{10} = 1,049 \times 10^6$. By keeping the same number of variables and using 8 granular terms (information granules) we observe a tremendous increase in the size of the rule base; here we end up with $2.825 \times 10^8$ different rules which amounts to substantial increase. There is no doubt that such rule bases are not practical. The effect of this combinatorial explosion becomes very apparent.

There are several ways of handling the dimensionality problem. An immediate one is to acknowledge that we do not need a complete rule base because there are various combinations of conditions that never occur in practice and are not supported by any experimental evidence. While this sounds very straightforward it is not that easy to gain sufficient confidence as to the nature of such unnecessary rules. The second more feasible approach would be to treat all variables at the same time by applying fuzzy clustering. The number of clusters is far smaller than the number of rules involving individual variables.

In what follows, we discuss various modes of incorporating clustering results into the blueprint of the fuzzy model. It becomes essential to understand the implications of the use of the clustering technique in forming information granules especially in the setting of the models. The most critical observation concerns a distinction between relational aspects of clustering and directional features of models. By their nature, unless properly endowed, clustering looks at multivariable data as relational constructs so the final product of cluster analysis results in a collection of clusters as concise descriptors of data where each variable is treated in the same manner irrespectively where it is positioned as a modeling entity. Typical clustering algorithms do not distinguish between input and output variables. This stands in contrast with what we observe in system modeling. The role of the variable is critical as most practical models are directional constructs, viz. they represent a certain mapping from independent to dependent variables. The distinction between these two categories of variables does require some modifications to the clustering algorithm to accommodate this requirement. To focus attention, let us consider a many input – many output (MIMO) model involving input and output variables $\mathbf{x}$ and $\mathbf{y}$, respectively, that is $\mathbf{y} = f(\mathbf{x})$. The experimental data come in the format of ordered tuples $\{(\mathbf{x}_k, \mathbf{target}_k)\}$, k=1, 2,,..N. If we are to ignore the directionality aspect, the immediate approach to clustering the data would be to concatenate the vectors in the input and output space so that $\mathbf{z}_k = [\mathbf{x}_k \mathbf{target}_k]$ and carry our clustering in such augmented feature space. By doing that we have concentrated on the relational aspects of data and the possible mapping component that is of interest has been completely ignored. To alleviate the problem, we may like to emphasize a role of the output variables by assigning to them higher values of weights. In essence, we emphasize that the clustering needs to pay more attention to the differences (and similarities) occurring in the output spaces (that is vectors $\mathbf{target}_1$, $\mathbf{target}_2$, ..., $\mathbf{target}_n$). This issue was raised in the past and resulted in a so-called directional fuzzy clustering, D-fuzzy clustering, for short [7]. An easy realization of the concept would be to admit that the distance function has to be computed differently depending upon the coordinates of $\mathbf{z}$ by using a certain positive weight factor $\gamma$. For instance, the Euclidean distance between $\mathbf{z}_k$ and $\mathbf{z}_l$ would read as $\|\mathbf{x}_k - \mathbf{x}_l\|^2 + \gamma \|\mathbf{target}_k - \mathbf{target}_l\|^2$ where $\gamma > 0$. The higher the value of $\gamma$, the more attention is being paid to the distance between the output variables. As usual, the dimensionality of the input space is far higher than the output one, the value of $\gamma$ needs to be properly selected to reach a suitable balance. Even though the approach might look sound, the choice of the weight factor becomes a matter of intensive experimentation.

Conditional fuzzy clustering [11][12] [14][15] is naturally geared towards dealing with direction-sensitive (direction-aware) clustering. The context variable(s) are those being the output variables and used in the modeling problem. Defining contexts over these variables become an independent task. Once the contexts have been formed, the ensuing clustering is induced (or directed) by the provided fuzzy set (relation) of context. Let us link this construct to rule-based modeling. In context-based clustering, the role of the conclusion is assumed by the context fuzzy set. The clusters formed in the input space form the conditions of the rule. Being more specific, the rule is of the form

*Figure 4. Examples of fuzzy sets of context reflecting a certain focus of the intended model: (a) low speed traffic, (b) high speed traffic*

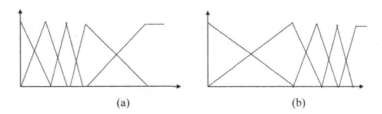

(a)                                        (b)

- if **x** is $A_1$ *or* $A_2$ *or* ... *or* $A_c$ then y is B

where B is a context fuzzy set and $A_1$, $A_2$, ..., $A_c$ are fuzzy sets (clusters) formed in the input space.

Given the context, we focus the pursuits of fuzzy clustering on the pertinent portion of data in the input space and reveal a conditional structure there. By changing the context we continue search by focusing on some other parts of the data. In essence, the result produced in this manner becomes a web of information granules developed conditionally upon the assumed collection of the contexts. Hence the directional aspects of the model we want to develop on the basis of the information granules become evident. The design of contexts is quite intuitive. First, these are fuzzy sets whose semantics is well defined. We may use terms such as *low*, *medium*, and *large* output. Second, we can choose fuzzy sets of context so that they reflect the nature of the problem and our perception of it. For instance, if for some reason we are interested in modeling a phenomenon of a slow traffic on a highway, we would define a number of fuzzy sets of context focused on low values of speed. To model highway traffic with focus on high speed we would be inclined to locate a number of fuzzy sets at the high end of the output space. The customization of the model by identifying its major focus is thus feasible through setting the clustering activities in a suitable context.

We can move on with some further refinements of context fuzzy sets and, if required, introduce a larger number of granular categories. Their relevance could be assessed with regard to the underlying experimental evidence. To assure full coverage of the output space, it is highly advisable that fuzzy sets of context form a fuzzy partition. Obviously, we can carry out clustering of data in the output space and arrive at some membership functions being generated in a fully automated fashion. This option is particularly attractive in the cases many output variables are treated together where the manual definition of the context fuzzy relations could be too tedious or even quite impractical.

In what follows, we briefly recall the essence of conditional (context-based) clustering and elaborate on the algorithmic facet of the optimization process. This clustering, which is a variant of the FCM, is realized for individual contexts, $W_1$, $W_2$,..., $W_p$. Let us consider a certain fixed context (fuzzy set) $W_j$ described by some membership function (the choice of its membership will be discussed later on). For the sake of convenience, we consider here a single output variable. A certain data point ($target_k$) located in the output space is then associated with the corresponding membership value of $W_j$, $w_{jk} = W_j(target_k)$. Let us introduce a family of the partition matrices induced by the j-th context and denote it by $U(W_j)$

$$U(W_j) = \left\{ u_{ik} \in [0,1] \Big| \sum_{i=1}^{c} u_{ik} = w_{jk} \ \forall k \ \text{and} \ 0 < \sum_{k=1}^{N} u_{ik} < N \ \forall i \right\} \tag{4}$$

where $w_{jk}$ denotes a membership value of the k-th data point to the j-th context (fuzzy set). The number of data is denoted by "N". The objective function guiding clustering is defined as the following weighted sum of distances

$$Q = \sum_{i=1}^{c} \sum_{k=1}^{N} u_{ik}^{m} ||\mathbf{x}_k - \mathbf{v}_i||^2 \tag{5}$$

The minimization of Q is realized with respect to the prototypes $\mathbf{v}_1, \mathbf{v}_2, \ldots, \mathbf{v}_c$ and the partition matrix $U \in U(W_j)$. The optimization is realized iteratively by updating the partition matrix and the prototypes in a consecutive manner [12]. More specifically, the partition matrix are computed as follows

$$u_{ik} = \frac{w_{jk}}{\sum_{j=1}^{c} \left( \frac{||\mathbf{x}_k - \mathbf{v}_i||}{||\mathbf{x}_k - \mathbf{v}_j||} \right)^{\frac{2}{m-1}}} \tag{6}$$

Let us emphasize here that the values of $u_{ik}$ pertain here to the partition matrix induced by the j-th context. The prototypes $\mathbf{v}_i$, i =1, 2,…, c are calculated in the well known form of the weighted average

$$\mathbf{v}_i = \frac{\sum_{k=1}^{N} u_{ik}^{m} \mathbf{x}_k}{\sum_{k=1}^{N} u_{ik}^{m}} \tag{7}$$

We iterate (6)-(7) until some predefined termination criterion has been satisfied.

The blueprint of the model, see Figure 5, has to be further formalized to explicitly capture the mapping between the information granules. This leads us to a detailed architecture of an inherently granular network whose outputs are information granules. The concept of a granular or granular neuron becomes an interesting construct worth exploring in this setting.

## 4. GRANULAR NEURON AS A GENERIC PROCESSING ELEMENT IN GRANULAR NETWORKS

As the name suggests, by the granular neuron we mean a neuron with granular connection. More precisely, we consider the transformation of many numeric inputs $u_1, u_2, \ldots, u_c$ (whose values are confined to the unit interval) of the form

*Figure 5. A blueprint of a granular model induced by some predefined fuzzy sets or relations of context defined in the input space (a); and a detailed view at the model in case of three contexts and two clusters per context (b)*

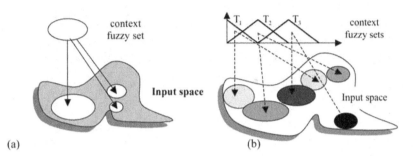

(a)                               (b)

$$Y = N(u_1, u_2, .., u_c, W_1, W_2, .., W_c) = \sum_{\oplus} (W_i \otimes u_i) \tag{8}$$

with $W_1, W_2, \ldots W_c$ denoting granular weights (connections), see Figure 6. The symbols of generalized (granular) addition and multiplication (that is $\oplus, \otimes$) are used here to emphasize a granular nature of the arguments being used in this aggregation. When dealing with interval-valued connections, $W_i = [w_{i-}, w_{i+}]$, the operations of their multiplication by some positive real input $u_i$ produce the results in the form of the following interval

$$W_i \otimes u_i = [w_{i-} u_i, w_{i+} u_i] \tag{9}$$

When adding such intervals being produced at the level of each input of the neuron, we obtain

$$Y = [\sum_{i=1}^{n} w_{i-} u_i, \sum_{i=1}^{n} w_{i+} u_i] \tag{10}$$

For the connections represented as fuzzy sets, the result of their multiplication by a positive scalar $u_i$ is realized through the use of the extension principle

$$(W_i \otimes u_i)(y) = \sup_{w:y=wu_i} [W_i(w)] = W_i(y/u_i) \tag{11}$$

Next, the extension principle is used to complete additions of fuzzy numbers being the partial results of this processing. Denote by $Z_i$ the fuzzy number $Z_i = W_i \otimes u_i$. We obtain

$$Y = Z_1 \oplus Z_2 \oplus \ldots \oplus Z_n \tag{12}$$

that is

$$Y(y) = \sup \{\min(Z_1(y_1), Z_2(y_2), \ldots, Z_n(y_n))\}$$

Figure 6. Computational model of a granular neuron; note a granular character of the connections and ensuing output Y

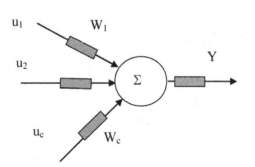

Figure 7. The overall architecture of the granular models

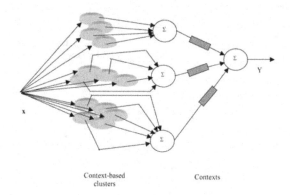

Context-based clusters

Contexts

Subject to

$$y = y_1 + y_2 + \ldots + y_n \tag{13}$$

Depending on a specific realization, these connections can be realized as intervals, fuzzy sets, shadowed sets, rough sets, etc. In spite of the evident diversity of the formalisms of granular computing under consideration, the output Y is also a granular construct as illustrated in Figure 6.

In case of fuzzy sets used to implement the connections, we end up with more complicated formulas for the resulting output. They simplify quite profoundly, though, if we confine ourselves to triangular fuzzy sets (fuzzy numbers) of the connections. Following the generic calculus of fuzzy numbers, we note that the multiplication of $W_i$ by a positive constant scales the fuzzy number yet retains the piecewise character of the membership function. Furthermore the summation operation does not affect the triangular shapes of the membership function so at the end the final result can be again described in the following format

The granular neuron exhibits several interesting properties that generalize the characteristics of (numeric) neurons. Adding a nonlinearity component (g) to the linear aggregation does not change the essence of computing; in case of monotonically increasing relationship (g(Y)), we end up with a transformation of the original output interval or fuzzy set (in this case we have to follow the calculations using the well known extension principle).

## 5. ARCHITECTURE OF GRANULAR MODELS BASED ON CONDITIONAL FUZZY CLUSTERING

The conditional fuzzy clustering has provided us with a backbone of the granular model [13], see also [16]. Following the principle of conditional clustering, we end up with a general topology of the model shown in Figure 7. It reflects a way in which the information granules are put together following the way the information granules have been formed.

The computations of the output fuzzy sets are completed in two successive steps: (a) aggregation of activation levels (membership grades) of all clusters associated with a given context, and (b) linear combination of the activation levels with the parameters of the context fuzzy sets. In case of triangular membership functions of the context fuzzy sets, the calculations follow the scheme described by (10).

The development of the granular model comprises two key phases, that is

1.  forming fuzzy sets of context, and
2.  running conditional clustering for the already available collection of contexts.

These two processing phases are tied together: once fuzzy sets of context have been provided, the clustering uses this information in the directed development of the structure in the input space.

The granular models come with several important features:

*   in essence, the granular model is nothing but a web of associations between information granules that have been constructed,
*   the model is inherently granular; even for a numeric input the model return some information granule, in particular some triangular fuzzy set (fuzzy number), and
*   third, the model is built following a design scheme of rapid prototyping. Once the information granules have been defined in the output space and constructed in the input space, no further design effort is required. Simply, we organize them in the topology as presented in Figure 7.

Noticeably, by changing the granularity of the contexts as well as their distribution across the output space, we can control the size of the fuzzy set of the output and adjust the specificity of the overall modeling process. The adjustments of the contexts could be helpful in further enhancements of granular models.

## 6. REFINEMENTS OF GRANULAR MODELS

The granular model can be augmented by several features with intension of improving its functionality and accuracy. The first modification is straightforward and concerns a bias component of the granular neuron. The second one focuses on an iterative scheme of optimization of the fuzzy sets of context.

### 6.1. Bias Term of Granular Neurons

So far the web of the connections between the contexts and their induced clusters was very much reflective of how the clustering has been realized. While the network can be assembled without any further computing effort, it becomes useful to look into its further refinement. In particular, we would look whether the model is not biased by a systematic error and if so, make some modifications to the topology of the granular model to alleviate this shortcoming. A numeric manifestation of the granular model can be viewed in the form of the modal value of the output fuzzy set of the granular model, see Figure 8. Denote it by $y_k$ considering that the fuzzy set itself is given as $Y(\mathbf{x}_k)$. If the mean of the error being computed as $target_k - y_k$ $k=1, 2, \ldots, N$ is nonzero, we are faced with a systematic error. Its elimination can be realized by involving a bias term as illustrated in Figure 8. This bias augments the summation node at the output layer of the network.

The bias is calculated in a straightforward manner

*Figure 8. Inclusion of the bias term in the granular model*

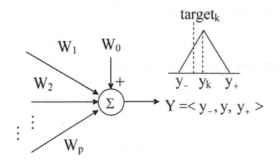

*Figure 9. An optimization scheme of the granular model*

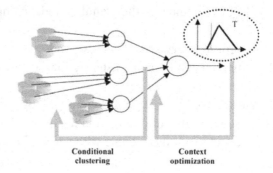

$$w_0 = -\frac{1}{N}\sum_{k=1}^{N}\left(\text{target}_k - y_k\right) \tag{14}$$

In terms of granular computing, the bias is just a numeric singleton which could be written down as a degenerated fuzzy number (singleton) of the form $W_0 = (w_0, w_0, w_0)$.

Subsequently, the resulting granular output Y reads in the form

1.  the lower bound $\sum_{t=1}^{p} z_t w_{t-} + w_0$

2.  modal value $\sum_{t=1}^{p} z_t w_t + w_0$

3.  the upper bound $\sum_{t=1}^{p} z_t w_{t+} + w_0$

## 6.2. Refinement of the Contexts

The conditional FCM has produced the prototypes or, equivalently, clusters in the input space. Using them we generate inputs to the granular neuron. The connections of the neuron are the fuzzy sets of context. In essence, the parameters of the network are downloaded from the phase of fuzzy clustering. This constitutes an essence of rapid prototyping.

There is however some room for improvement if one might involve in further optimization activities. The refinement may be necessary because of the fact that each conditional FCM is realized for some specific context and these developments tasks are independent. As a consequence of putting all pieces together, the prototypes may need some shifting. Furthermore the contexts themselves may require refinement and refocus. Note also that the result of the granular model is an information granule (interval, fuzzy set, fuzzy relation, etc.) and this has to be compared with a numeric datum $y_k$. Again, for illustrative purposes we have to confine ourselves to a single output granular model. Thus in the optimization we have to take this into account. As we are concerned with numeric and granular entities, there could be several ways of assessing the quality of the granular model and its further refinement, see Figure 9.

We put forward two optimization problems in which the minimization (and maximization, respectively) is carried out with respect to the parameters (modal values) of the fuzzy sets of context. The maximization of the average agreement of the granular output of the model with available numeric data is a straightforward one. Let us consider that Y is a granular output of the granular model produced for input $\mathbf{x}_k$, $Y(\mathbf{x}_k)$. As it is described by the membership function defined in the output space, we compute the membership degree at the value target$_k$, that is $Y(\mathbf{x}_k)$ (target$_k$)

$$\max_P \; \frac{1}{N} \sum_{k=1}^{N} Y(\mathbf{x}_k)(\text{target}_k) \tag{15}$$

As mentioned earlier, the maximization of (15) is completed with respect to the parameters of the context fuzzy sets where these parameters are collectively denoted by $\mathbf{P}$.

Alternatively we can consider a minimization of the average spread of the granular output of the network obtained for the corresponding inputs

$$\min_P \; \frac{1}{N} \sum_{k=1}^{N} (b_k - a_k) \tag{16}$$

where $a_k$ and $b_k$ are the lower and upper bounds of the triangular fuzzy number produced for $\mathbf{x}_k$. In both cases the optimization can be confined to the portion of the network requiring the refinement of the context fuzzy sets. Furthermore we can make the optimization more manageable by assuming that the successive contexts overlap at the level of ½. Given this condition, the optimization concentrates on the modal values of the triangular fuzzy sets of context. Once these values have been adjusted, the conditional FCM is repeated and the iteration loop of optimization is repeated.

## 7. INCREMENTAL GRANULAR MODELS

We can take another, less commonly adopted principle of granular modeling whose essence could be succinctly captured in the following manner

*Adopting a construct of a linear regression as a first-principle global model, refine it through a series of local fuzzy rules that capture remaining and more localized nonlinearities of the system*

More schematically, we could articulate the essence of the resulting fuzzy model by stressing the existence of the two essential modeling structures that are combined together using the following symbolic relationship

fuzzy model = linear regression & local granular models

By endorsing this principle, we emphasize the tendency that in system modeling we always proceed with the simplest possible model (Occam's principle), assess its performance and afterwards complete a series of necessary refinements. The local granular models handling the residual part of the model are conveniently captured through some rules.

Let us proceed with some illustrative examples, shown in Figure 10, that help underline and exemplify the above development principle. In the first case, Figure 10 (a), the data are predominantly governed by a linear relationship while there is only a certain cluster of points that are fairly dispersed within some region. In the second one, Figure 10 (b), the linearity is visible yet there are two localized clusters of data that contribute to the local nonlinear character of the relationship. In Figure 10 (c) there is a nonlinear function yet it exhibits quite dominant regions of linearity. This is quite noticeable when completing a linear approximation; the linear regression exhibits a pretty good match with a clear exception of the two very much compact regions. Within such regions, one could accommodate two rules that capture the experimental relationships present there. The nonlinearity and the character of data vary from case to case. In the first two examples, we note that the data are quite dispersed and the regions of departure from the otherwise linear relationship could be modeled in terms of some rules. In the third one, the data are very concentrated and with no scattering yet the nonlinear nature of the relationship is predominantly visible.

## 7.1. The Principle of Incremental Fuzzy Model and Its Design and Architecture

The fundamental scheme of the construction of the incremental granular model is covered as illustrated in Figure 11. There are two essential phases: the development of the linear regression being followed by the construction of the local granular rule-based constructs that attempt to eliminate errors (residuals) produced by the regression part of the model.

Before proceeding with the architectural details, it is instructive to start with some required notation. The experimental data under discussion are the pairs of the "n"-dimensional inputs and scalar inputs. They come in the following form $\{\mathbf{x}_k, \text{target}_k\}$ k=1,2,...,N, where $\mathbf{x}_k \in \mathbf{R}^n$ and $\text{target}_k \in \mathbf{R}$. The first principle linear regression model comes in the standard form of $z_k = L(\mathbf{x}, \mathbf{b}) = \mathbf{a}^T\mathbf{x}_k + a_0$ where the values of the coefficients of the regression plane, denoted here by $a_0$ and $\mathbf{a}$, namely $\mathbf{b} = [\mathbf{a}\ a_0]^T$, are determined through the standard least-square error method as encountered in any statistics textbooks. The enhancement of the model at which the granular part comes into the play is based on the transformed data $\{\mathbf{x}_k,$

*Figure 10. Examples of nonlinear relationships and their modeling through a combination of linear models of global character and a collection of local rule-based models*

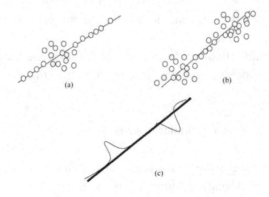

*Figure 11. A general flow of the development of the incremental granular models*

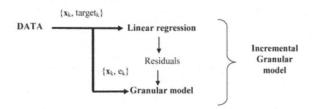

$e_k\}$, k=1, 2,…,N where the residual part manifests through the expression $e_k$ = target$_k$ – $z_k$ which denotes the error of the linear model. In the sequel, those data pairs are used to develop the incremental and granular rule-based part of the model. Given the character of the data, this rule-based augmentation of the model associates input data with the error produced by the linear regression model in the form of the rules *if input then error*. The rules and the information granules are constructed by means of the context –based clustering.

Let us recall the main design phases of the model, refer also to Figure 11 showing how the two functional modules operate.

Initial setup of the modeling environment. Decide upon the granularity of information to be used in the development of the model, viz. the number of contexts and the number of clusters formed for each context. Similarly, decide upon the parameters of the context-based clustering, especially the value of the fuzzification coefficient. The choice of the (weighted) Euclidean distance is a typical choice in the clustering activities.

1. Design of a linear regression in the input–output space, $z = L(\mathbf{x},\mathbf{b})$ with $\mathbf{b}$ denoting a vector of the regression hyperplane of the linear model, $\mathbf{b} =[\mathbf{a}\ a_0]^T$. On the basis of the original data set formed is a collection of input-error pairs, $(\mathbf{x}_k, e_k)$ where $e_k$ = target$_k$-$L(\mathbf{x}_k,\mathbf{a})$

2. Construction of the collection of contexts- fuzzy sets in the space of error of the regression model $E_1, E_2, …,E_p$. The distribution of these fuzzy sets is optimized through the use of fuzzy equalization while the fuzzy sets are characterized by triangular membership functions with a 0.5 overlap between neighboring fuzzy sets (recall that such arrangement of fuzzy sets leads to a zero decoding error, cf.[16]).

3. Context-based FCM completed in the input space and induced by the individual fuzzy sets of context. For "p" contexts and "c" clusters for each context, obtained are c×p clusters.

4. Summation of the activation levels of the clusters induced by the corresponding contexts and their overall aggregation through weighting by fuzzy sets (triangular fuzzy numbers) of the context leading to the triangular fuzzy number of output, $E = F(\mathbf{x}; E_1, E_2, …, E_p)$ where F denotes the overall transformation realized by the incremental granular model. Furthermore note that we eliminated eventual systematic shift of the results by adding a numeric bias term. These two functional modules are also illustrated in Figure 12.

5. The granular result of the incremental model is then combined with the output of the linear part; the result is a shifted triangular number Y, $Y = z \oplus E$.

*Figure 12. The overall flow of processing realized in the design of the incremental granular model. Note a flow of numeric and granular computing*

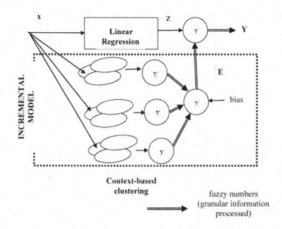

As an illustrative example, consider a one-dimensional spiky function, call it spiky(x), used in this experiment is a linear relationship augmented by two Gaussian functions described by their modal values m and spreads σ,

$$G(x) = \exp\left(\frac{-(x-c)^2}{2\sigma^2}\right) \tag{17}$$

This leads to the overall expression of the function to be in the form

$$\text{spiky}(x) = \begin{cases} \max(x, G(x)) & \text{if } 0 \le x \le 1 \\ \min(x, -G(x) + 2) & \text{if } 1 < x \le 2 \end{cases} \tag{18}$$

with c =0.5 and σ =0.1, refer to Figure 13. Each training and test data set consists of 100 pairs of input-output data.

As could have been anticipated, the linear regression is suitable for some quite large regions of the input variable but becomes quite insufficient in the regions where these two spikes are positioned. As a result of these evident departure from the linear dependency, the linear regression produces a high approximation error of $0.154 \pm 0.014$ and $0.160 \pm 0.008$ for the training and testing set, respectively. The augmented granular modification of the model was realized by experimenting with the two essential parameters controlling the granularity of the construct in the input and output space, that is "p" and "c". The corresponding results are summarized in Table 1 and 2. All of them are reported for the optimal values of the fuzzification coefficient as listed in Table 3, viz. its values for which the root mean squared error (RMSE) attained its minimum,

*Figure 13. Example spiky function used in the experiment*

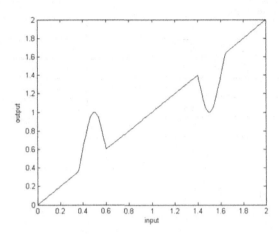

*Table 1. RMSE values (mean and standard deviation)-training data*

|  |  | No. of contexts (p) | | | |
|  |  | 3 | 4 | 5 | 6 |
|---|---|---|---|---|---|
| No. of clusters per context (c) | 2 | 0.148 ± 0.013 | 0.142 ± 0.018 | 0.136 ± 0.005 | 0.106 ± 0.006 |
|  | 3 | 0.141 ± 0.012 | 0.131 ± 0.008 | 0.106 ± 0.008 | 0.087 ± 0.006 |
|  | 4 | 0.143 ± 0.006 | 0.124 ± 0.007 | 0.095 ± 0.007 | 0.078 ± 0.005 |
|  | 5 | 0.131 ± 0.012 | 0.111 ± 0.007 | 0.077 ± 0.008 | 0.073 ± 0.006 |
|  | 6 | 0.126 ± 0.011 | 0.105 ± 0.005 | 0.072 ± 0.007 | 0.061 ± 0.007 |

*Table 2. RMSE values (mean and standard deviation)-testing data*

|  |  | No. of contexts (p) | | | |
|  |  | 3 | 4 | 5 | 6 |
|---|---|---|---|---|---|
| No. of clusters per context (c) | 2 | 0.142 ± 0.016 | 0.139 ± 0.028 | 0.139 ± 0.012 | 0.114 ± 0.007 |
|  | 3 | 0.131 ± 0.007 | 0.125 ± 0.017 | 0.115 ± 0.009 | 0.096 ± 0.009 |
|  | 4 | 0.129 ± 0.014 | 0.126 ± 0.014 | 0.101 ± 0.009 | 0.085 ± 0.012 |
|  | 5 | 0.123 ± 0.005 | 0.119 ± 0.016 | 0.097 ± 0.008 | 0.082 ± 0.010 |
|  | 6 | 0.119 ± 0.016 | 0.114 ± 0.015 | 0.082 ± 0.011 | 0.069 ± 0.007 |

*Table 3. Optimal values of the fuzzification coefficient for selected number of contexts and clusters*

| | | No. of contexts (p) | | | |
|---|---|---|---|---|---|
| | | 3 | 4 | 5 | 6 |
| No. of clusters per context (c) | 2 | 3.5 | 4.0 | 3.8 | 3.1 |
| | 3 | 3.2 | 3.9 | 3.5 | 3.1 |
| | 4 | 3.0 | 2.7 | 2.6 | 2.6 |
| | 5 | 3.1 | 2.8 | 2.2 | 2.4 |
| | 6 | 3.0 | 2.5 | 2.2 | 2.0 |

$$\text{RMSE} = \sqrt{\frac{1}{N} \sum_{k=1}^{N} (y_k - \text{target}_k)^2} \qquad (19)$$

where $y_k$ is the modal value of Y produced for input $\mathbf{x}_k$. The numeric range of this coefficient used in the experiments is between 1.5 and 4.0 with the incremental step of 0.1. The increase in the specificity of the granular constructs (either in the output space – via the number of contexts and the input space when increasing the number of the clusters) leads to the reduction of the RMSE values. The number of clusters for a fixed number of contexts exhibits a less significant effect on the reduction of the performance index in comparison to the case when increasing the number of the contexts. Figure 14 shows the variation of the RMSE values caused by the values of the fuzzification factor for these four cases. Here the optimal values of the parameters are such for which the testing error becomes minimal. As shown there, the values of the optimal fuzzification coefficient depend on the number of context and cluster but there is a quite apparent tendency: the increase in the values of "p" and "m" implies lower values of the fuzzification coefficient. This means that the preferred shape of the membership functions becomes more s*piky*.

As Figure 14 depicts, the increase in the number of the contexts and clusters leads to higher optimal values of the fuzzification factor. The optimal results along with the visualization of the prototypes when c =5 and p =5 are displayed in Figure 15 (this is one of the 10 runs). The plot shows the modal values as well as the lower and upper bound of the resulting fuzzy number produced by the incremental model. Here we have used the optimal value of the fuzzification factor (with the value being equal to 2.2).

## 8. CONCLUSION

The technology of granular modeling is rooted in the fundamental concept of information granules regarded as semantically meaningful conceptual entities that are crucial to the overall framework of user-centric modeling. The user is at position to cast modeling activities in a particular way that becomes a direct reflection of the main purpose of the given modeling problem. For instance, in data mining the user is ultimately interested in revealing relationships that could be of potential interest given the problem under consideration.

The algorithmic diversity of fuzzy clustering is particularly well suited to address the key objectives of granular modeling. Fuzzy clusters fully reflect the character of the data. The search for the structure is

*Figure 14. Performance index (RMSE) versus values of the fuzzification coefficient for some selected combinations of "p" and "m": (a) p = c = 6, (b) p = c = 5, (c) p = c = 4, (d) p = c = 3, solid line: training data, dotted line: testing data*

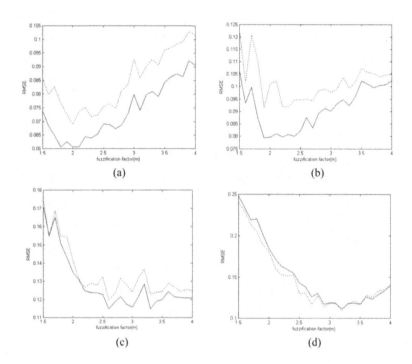

ultimately affected by some specific well-articulated modeling needs of the user. We have demonstrated that fuzzy sets of context can play an important role in shaping up modeling activities and help handle dimensionality issues decomposing the original problem into a series of sub-problems guided by specific contexts. By linking context fuzzy sets and the induced clusters we directly form the modeling blueprint of the model. It is relevant to note that granular models are expressed at a certain level of granularity. Instead of single numeric results that are typical for numeric models, the user is provided with a fuzzy set of result that can be communicated in some granular format, compatible with the vocabulary of granular terms being originally exploited in the design of the model, and presented visually in terms of the resulting membership functions.

The functionality and the underlying design methodology of the linguistic models presented here are in line with a variety of modeling tasks we encounter in practice. To make models relevant and user-centric, it becomes imperative to allow the designer to establish a certain perspective at the system through a suitable selection of information granules both in terms of their number as well as the distribution in the output space. It is also crucial that one builds a suitable, well-balanced position in which the available experimental evidence (conveyed by data) is fully utilized and the information granules forming the conceptual blueprint of the model are endowed with a well-defined semantics. The context fuzzy sets offer an important possibility to accentuate the regions of data on which the model should focus on and in this way making the model customized to the needs of the specific users (say, one might be interested in an accurate view at the relationships between inputs and output in case output is *low*). The granular nature of the models brings another very desirable feature that is their hierarchical extension.

*Figure 15. Modeling results for c = 5 and p =5 (m = 2.2); shown is also a distribution of the prototypes in the input space. Note that most of them are located around the spikes which is quite legitimate as they tend to capture the nonlinearities existing in these regions*

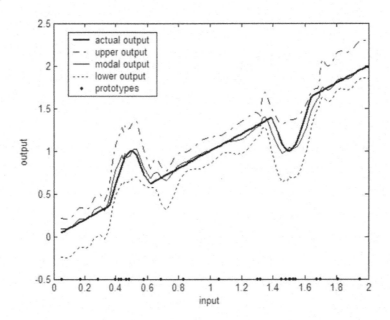

In the region of interest, one can define more specific, less abstract information granules and determine relationships between them. In this way, a structured and systematic expansion of the model is carried out.

# REFERENCES

Bezdek, J. C., & Pal, S. K. (1992). *Fuzzy Models for Pattern Recognition: Methods that Search for Structures in Data*. New York: IEEE Press.

Duda, R., & Hart, P. (1973). *Pattern Classification and Scene Analysis*. New York: Wiley.

Gath, I., & Geva, A. (1989). Unsupervised optimal fuzzy clustering. *IEEE Transactions on Pattern Analysis and Machine Intelligence*, *11*(7), 773–781. doi:10.1109/34.192473

Gath, I., Iskoz, A., Cutsem, B., & Van, M. (1997). Data induced metric and fuzzy clustering of non-convex patterns of arbitrary shape. *Pattern Recognition Letters*, *18*, 541–553. doi:10.1016/S0167-8655(97)00043-3

Gonzalez, J., Rojas, I., Pomares, H., Ortega, J., & Prieto, A. (2002). A new clustering technique for function approximation. *IEEE Transactions on Neural Networks*, *13*, 132–142. doi:10.1109/72.977289

Gustafson, D., & Kessel, W. (1992). Fuzzy clustering with a fuzzy covariance matrix. In Bezdek, J., & Pal, S. (Eds.), *Fuzzy models for Pattern Recognition: Methods that Search for Structures in Data*. New York: IEEE Press.

Hirota, K., & Pedrycz, W. (1995). D-fuzzy clustering. *Pattern Recognition Letters*, *16*, 193–200. doi:10.1016/0167-8655(94)00090-P

Karyannis, N. B., & Mi, G. W. (1997). Growing radial basis neural networks: merging supervised and unsupervised learning with network growth techniques. *IEEE Transactions on Neural Networks*, *8*, 1492–1506. doi:10.1109/72.641471

Kim, E., Park, M., Ji, S., & Park, M. (1997). A new approach to fuzzy modeling. *IEEE Transactions on Fuzzy Systems*, *5*, 328–337. doi:10.1109/91.618271

Lazzerini, B., & Marcelloni, F. Classification based on neural similarity. *Electronics Letters*, *38*(15), 810–812. doi:10.1049/el:20020549

Pedrycz, W. (1985). Algorithms of fuzzy clustering with partial supervision. *Pattern Recognition Letters*, *3*, 13–20. doi:10.1016/0167-8655(85)90037-6

Pedrycz, W. (1996). Conditional fuzzy C-Means. *Pattern Recognition Letters*, 17, 625-632.Pedrycz, W. (1998). Conditional fuzzy clustering in the design of radial basis function neural networks. *IEEE Transactions on Neural Networks*, *9*, 601–612. doi:10.1109/72.701174

Pedrycz, W., & Kwak, K. (2006). Granular models as a framework of user-centric system modeling. *IEEE Trans. on Systems, Mans, and Cybernetics – Part A,*, 727-745.

Pedrycz, W., & Vasilakos, A. (1999). Linguistic models and linguistic modeling. *IEEE Transactions on Systems, Man, and Cybernetics*, *29*, 745–757. doi:10.1109/3477.809029

Pedrycz, W., & Waletzky, J. (1997). Fuzzy clustering with partial supervision. *IEEE Transactions on Systems, Man, and Cybernetics*, *5*, 787–795.

Sugeno, M., & Yasukawa, T. (1993). A fuzzy-logic-based approach to qualitative modeling. *IEEE Transactions on Fuzzy Systems*, *1*, 7–31. doi:10.1109/TFUZZ.1993.390281

Takagi, T., & Sugeno, M. (1985). Fuzzy identification of systems and its applications to modeling and control. *IEEE Transactions on Systems, Man, and Cybernetics*, *15*, 116–132.

Zadeh, L. A. (1979). Fuzzy sets and information granularity. In Gupta, M., Ragade, R., & Yager, R. (Eds.), *Advances in Fuzzy Set Theory and Applications* (pp. 3–18). Amsterdam.

Zadeh, L. A. (1997). Toward a theory of fuzzy information granulation and its centrality in human reasoning and fuzzy logic. *Fuzzy Sets and Systems*, *90*, 111–127. doi:10.1016/S0165-0114(97)00077-8

# Chapter 11
# Semantic Analysis of Rough Logic

**Qing Liu**
*Nanchang University, China*

## ABSTRACT

*In this Chapter, we analyse the semantics of the rough logic. Related operations and related properties of semantics based on the rough logic are also discussed. Related reasoning of the semantis are also studied. Significant of studying semantics of the rough logic will hopefully offer a new idea for the applications to classical logic and other nonstandard logic, also hopefully offer a new theory and methodology for problem resolving in artificial intelligence.*

## 1. INTRODUCTION

Rough logic in this chapter is viewed as a nonstandard logic defined on a given information system $IS = (U, A)^{[1,2]}$. Atomic formulae of the logic are defined as $a = v$ or $a_v$. It is interpreted as $a(x) = v$ where $a$ is an attribute in $A$, $x$ is a individual variable on $U$, and $v$ is an attribute value. The compound formulae are consisted of the atomic formulae and usual logical connectives. The rough logic is abbreviated as $RL_{IS}^{[3-5]}$. Its truth value is the multi-valued.

Senmantic analysis of logic is a means of studying logic. Kripks tried to study modal logic through Semantic Analysis of Modal Logic[6], Luis try also to define semantics of Modal Logic as a subset of state space, to study the resolution of Modal Logic by semantics of modal logic[7]. Zadeh tried to change his research from Fuzzy Logic to its semantic, he defined the meaning of fuzzy propositional logical formula as a set of elements of satisfying this fuzzy propositional logical formula in 1979[8-10]. In this

DOI: 10.4018/978-1-60566-324-1.ch011

Chapter, we analyse related properties and approximate reasoning of the rough logical semantics. Pawlak proposed Rough Sets based on the semantics of indiscernibility relation, to define the upper and the lower approximations of a undefinable set[1,2], so Pawlak's rough set approach solved the problem of computing elements on boundary by Frege in 1914[10]. From the view of problem solving in artificial intelligence, Hobbs tried to define indiscernibility relation based on the semantics of predicates in logical formulae[11], he offer a new theoretical tool and methodology for problem solving in artificial intelligence.

In the Chapter, rough logic is described in Section 2. Truth values of the rough logical formulae are defined in Section 3. Sematic model of the rough logic is described in Section 4. Satisfiability of meaning based on rough logical formulae is also described in Section 5. The Related operations of semantics based the rough logic are presented in Section 6. Related properties of semantics based on the rough logic are given in Section 7. The normal forms of meaning of rough logical formulae are discussed in Section 8. Reasoning based on semantics of rough logical formula is discussed in Section 9. Applications of the semantics based on rough logic are presented in Section 10. Final Section is the perspective of studying the semantics of rough logic.

## 2. BASIC CONCEPT OF ROUGH LOGIC

### Definition 1

Well-formed formulae (wffs) of the Rough Logic (RL) are recursively defined as follows[8-20]:

(1)   All atoms of form $a_v$ are wffs in $RL_{IS}$, where $a \in A$, $v \in V_a$;

(2)   Let $F_1$, $F_2$ be wffs in $RL_{IS}$, then $\neg F_1$, $F_1 \vee F_2$, $F_1 \wedge F_2$, $F_1 \rightarrow F_2$ and $F_1 \leftrightarrow F_2$ are also wffs in

$RL_{IS}$;

(3)   The obtainable formulae what (1)-(2) are quoted finite times are wffs in $RL_{IS}$.

Noteworthiness, the predicates to occur in rough logical formulae are the attribute in a given information system. Therefore, $a_5 \rightarrow c_0$ in following Table 1 is a rough logical formula defined in a given Information System (IS), where predicate symbol $a$ and $c$ are the attribute in $A$ on $IS^{[8,13,20-25]}$.

## 3. TRUTH VALUES OF ROUGH LOGICAL FORMULAE

Meaning of the rough logical formula $F(\bullet)$ defined in a given information system $IS = (U, A)$ is a subset on $U$, denoted by

*Table 1. Information system* $IS = (U, A)$

| U | A | | | | |
|---|---|---|---|---|---|
| | | b | c | d | e |
| 1 | 5 | 4 | 0 | 1 | 1 |
| 2 | 3 | 4 | 0 | 2 | 1 |
| 3 | 3 | 4 | 0 | 2 | 2 |
| 4 | 0 | 2 | 0 | 1 | 2 |
| 5 | 3 | 2 | 1 | 2 | 2 |
| 6 | 5 | 2 | 1 | 1 | 0 |

$$m(F(\bullet)) = \{u \in U : u \models_{IS} F(\bullet)\}$$

where $\models_{IS}$ is a satisfiable symbol on $IS$. Truth values of the rough logical formulae are defined as follows.

## Definition 2

Let $F_1, F_2 \in RL_{IS}$ be rough logical formulae defined in a given information system $IS$. $I$ and $u$ are the interpretation and the assignment to the formula defined in $IS$ respectively. Thus the truth values are computed by following rules:

(1)   $T_{I_u}(F_1) = K(m(F_1)) / K(U) = \lambda$, $K(\bullet)$ denotes the base number of set $\bullet$. $m(\bullet)$ is a set from the propositional variable $\bullet$ or the formula $\bullet$ into a subset on $U$, $\lambda \in [0,1]$ is a real number, It means that is true to degree at lest $\lambda$ in interpretion I and assignment u.;

(2)   $T_{I_u}(\neg F_1) = T_{I_{u_\lambda}}(F_1)$;

(3)   $T_{I_u}(F_1 \vee F_2) = \max\{T_{I_u}(F_1), T_{I_u}(F_2)\}$;

(4)   $T_{I_u}(F_1 \wedge F_2) = \min\{T_{I_u}(F_1), T_{I_u}(F_2)\}$;

(5)   $T_{I_u}((\forall x)F_1(x)) = \min\{T_{I_u}(F_1(e_1)), ..., T_{I_u}(F_1(e_n))\}$.

In (5) $U$ is limited to be a finite universe of objects[34], $x$ is an individual variable on $U$. $e_i$ is a value of $x$ on $U$. It is an entity (concrete studying object) on $U$.

# 4. SEMANTIC MODEL OF ROUGH LOGIC

Semantics model of the rough logic is denoted by 6-tuple

$$M = (U, A, T_{I_u}, I, u, m)$$

- $U$ is a universe set of discourse objects on $IS = (U, A)$.

- $A$ is a set of attributes on $IS$.

- $T_{I_u}$ is a united assignment symbol to individual constant, individual variable, function and predicate to occur in the formula.

- $I$ is an interpretation symbol to individual constant, function and predicate to occur in the formula.

- $u$ is an assignment symbol to individual variable to occur in the formula.

- $m$ is a mapping from the formula defined on $IS$ to the subset on $U$.

Given a model $M$, formula $F(x) \in RL_{IS}$ is $\lambda$ − satisfiable to degree at least $\lambda$ in the model $M$, denoted by $M, u \models_{IS-\lambda} F(x)$.

# 5. Λ-SATISFIABILITY OF ROUGH LOGICAL FORMULAE

## Definition 3

The λ-satisfiability of rough logical formulae $F_1, F_2 \in RL_{IS}$ with respect to logical connectives $\neg, \vee, \wedge, \rightarrow, \leftrightarrow$ and quantifier $\forall$ is defined recursively as follows:

(1)  $M, u \models_{IS-\lambda} P(x_1, \cdots, x_n) = T_{Iu}(P(u(x_1), \cdots, P(u(x_n)) = \lambda$, where $\lambda \in [0,1]$ is real number, $P(x_1, \cdots, x_n)$ is λ-satisfiable to degree at least $\lambda$ on $IS$:

(2)  $M, u \models_{IS-\lambda} \neg F_1 = 1 - M, u \models_{IS-\lambda} F_1$

(3)  $M, u \models_{IS-\lambda} (F_1 \vee F_2) = M, u \models_{IS-\lambda} F_1 \vee M, u \models_{IS-\lambda} F_2$

(4)  $M, u \models_{IS-\lambda} (F_1 \wedge F_2) = M, u \models_{IS-\lambda} F_1 \wedge M, u \models_{IS-\lambda} F_2$

(5)  $M, u \models_{IS-\lambda} (F_1 \rightarrow F_2) = M, u \models_{IS-\lambda} \neg F_1 \vee M, u \models_{IS-\lambda} F_2$

(6)  $M, u \models_{IS-\lambda} (F_1 \leftrightarrow F_2) = (M, u \models_{IS-\lambda} \neg F_1 \vee M, u \models_{IS-\lambda} F_2)$
    $\wedge (M, u \models_{IS-\lambda} \neg F_2 \vee M, u \models_{IS-\lambda} F_1)$

(7)  $M, u \models_{IS-\lambda} (\forall x) F_1(x) = M, u \models_{IS-\lambda} F_1(x) \wedge \cdots \wedge M, u \models_{IS-\lambda} F_1(x_n)$

In (7) $U$ is limited to be a finite universe of objects[34], $x$ is an individual variable on $U$. $e_i$ is a value of $x$ on $U$.

## 6. RELATED OPERATIONS OF SEMANTICS BASED ON THE ROUGH LOGIC

Let $F$, $F_1$, $F_2$, $F_3$ be the formulae in $RL_{IS}$. The operation rules of meaning based on rough logical formulae are defined as follows recursively:

### Definition 4

Let $m(F_1)$ and $m(F_2)$ correspond to meaning of $F_1$ and $F_2$ respectively. Operations of them on usual connectives $\neg, \vee, \wedge, \rightarrow$ and $\leftrightarrow$ are defined as follows[4,21]:

(1) $m(\neg F_1) = U - m(F_1)$;

(2) $m(F_1 \vee F_2) = m(F_1) \cup m(F_2)$;

(3) $m(F_1 \wedge F_2) = m(F_1) \cap m(F_2)$;

(4) $m(F_1 \rightarrow F_2) = \neg m(F_1) \cup m(F_2)$;

(5) $m(F_1 \leftrightarrow F_2) = (m(\neg F_1) \cup m(F_2)) \cap (m(\neg F_2) \cup m(F_1))$

### Example 1

Let $IS = (U, A)$ be an information system, as shows in Table 1. $F = a_3 \wedge c_0$ be a rough logical formula on $IS$. By the definition above, we may compute the meaning of formula as follows:

$$m(F) = m(a_3 \wedge c_0) = m(a_3 \cap m(c_0) = \{2, 3, 5\} \cap \{1, 2, 3, 4, 6\} = \{2, 3\}$$

Operations of meanings of form $m(F)$ have two special operation symbols except for usual union $(\cup)$, intersection $(\cap)$ and complementation $(\neg)$ of sets. That is, inclusion operation symbol $\propto_\lambda$ to degree at least $\lambda$ and closeness operation symbol $\infty_\lambda$ to degree at least $\lambda$, where $\lambda \in [0,1]$. $\propto_\lambda$ is simplified the denotation of $\propto$ if $\lambda = 0$ or $\lambda = 1$, and $\infty_\lambda$ is simplified the denotation of $\infty$ when $\lambda = 0$ or $\lambda = 1$.

### 6.1. $\lambda$-Inclusion Operation

Let $F_1$, $F_2 \in RL_{IS}$ be rough logical formulae defined in $IS$. $m(F_1)$ is included in $m(F_2)$ to degree at least $\lambda$. The operation symbol $\propto$ is defined as follows[26-37].

$$K(m(F_1) \cap m(F_2)) / K(m(F_1))m(F_1) \neq \varnothing$$

$$\propto_\lambda (m(F_1), m(F_2)) =$$

$$1 \ m(F_1) = \varnothing$$

where $\propto_\lambda$ is an inclusion symbol to degree at least $\lambda$, $K(\bullet)$ is the total number of elements in set $\bullet$.

## 6.2. $\lambda$-Closeness Operation

Let $F_1$, $F_2 \in RL_{IS}$ be rough logical formulae defined in a given information system on $IS$, $m(F)$ is close to $m(F_2)$ to degree at least $\lambda$. In formally, it is defined as follows[19,32,36,39]:

$$\infty_\lambda (m(F_1, m(F_2))$$

iff

$$|T_{I_u}(F_1) - T_{I_u}(F_2)|$$

$$<1\text{-}\lambda \wedge m(F_1) \propto_\lambda m(F_2) \wedge m(F_2) \propto_\lambda m(F_1)$$

where $\infty_\lambda$ is a closeness relation symbol to degree at least $\lambda$. $T_{I_u}$ is a united assignment symbol to rough logical formula. It is defined as follows:

$$T_{I_u}(\bullet) = \lambda$$

where $\lambda \in [0,1]$ is a real number. $I$ is an interpretation symbol. $u$ is an assignment symbol.

## 7. RELATED PROPERTIES OF SEMANTICS OF ROUGH LOGIC

The properties of $\lambda$-degree closeness relation $\infty_\lambda$ are listed as follows:

## Property 1

By definition, a assertion or rough logical formula $F$ is taken truth value to degree at least $\lambda$ then the meaning set $m(F)$ corresponding to $F$ closes to the universe $U$ to degree at least $\lambda$, denoted by $\infty_\lambda(m(F), U)$ or $m(F)\infty_\lambda U$.

## Property 2

Let $F$ be a rough logical formula defined on information system $IS = (U, A)$, $\alpha$ and $\beta$ be the term [26,28-30,33], if $\forall x \in U$, $\infty_\lambda(\alpha(x), \beta(x))$, then $\infty_\lambda((m(F(\alpha)), m(F(\beta))))$.

## Property 3

Let $F_1$ and $F_2$ be rough logical formulae defined on information system $IS = (U, A)$, $F_1$ and $F_2$ is equivalent with respect to $\lambda$ iff meaning set $m(F_1)$ is close to meaning set $m(F_2)$ to degree at least $\lambda$. In formally, denoted by

$$|-|-_{IS} F_1 \leftrightarrow_\lambda F_2 \text{ iff } |-_{IS} \infty_\lambda(m(F_1), m(F_2))$$

where $|-_{IS}$ is to take true symbol on *IS* for formula.

## Property 4

Let $F_1$ and $F_2$ be rough logical formulae defined on information system $IS = (U, A)$.

if $\infty_\lambda(m(F_1), m(F_2))$ then $\infty_\lambda(m_*(F_1), m_*(F_2))$

where $m_*(\bullet)$ is lower approximation of $m(\bullet)$.

## Property 5

Let $F_1$ and $F_2$ be rough logical formulae defined on information system $IS = (U, A)$,

if $|-_{IS} \infty_\lambda(m(F_1), m(F_2)$ then $|-_{IS} \infty_\lambda(m^*(F_1), m^*(F_2))$

where $m^*(\bullet)$ is upper approximation of $m(\bullet)$.

## Property 6

Let $F_1$, $F_2$ and $F_3$ be rough logical formulae defined on information system $IS = (U, A)$,

if $|-_{IS} \infty_\lambda(m(F_1), m(F_2))$ then $|-_{IS} \infty_\lambda(m(F_1 \wedge F_3), m(F_2 \wedge F_3))$.

## Property 7

Let $F_1$ and $F_2$ be rough logical formulae defined on information system $IS = (U, A)$,

if $\vdash_{IS} \infty_\lambda(m(F_1), m(F_2))$ then $\vdash_{IS} \infty_\lambda(\neg m(F_1), \neg m(F_2))$.

## Property 8

Let $F_1$ and $F_2$ be rough logical formulae defined on information system $IS = (U, A)$,

if $\vdash_{IS} \infty_\lambda(m(F_1), m(F_2)) \wedge \vdash_{IS} \infty_\lambda(m(F_1), U)$ then $\vdash_{IS} \infty_\lambda(m(F_2), U)$.

## Property 9

Let $F_1$ and $F_2$ be rough logical formulae defined on information system $IS = (U, A)$,

if $\vdash_{IS} \infty_\lambda(m(F_1), m(F_2))$ then $\vdash_{IS} \infty_\lambda(U - m(F_1), U - m(F_2))$.

## Property 10

Let $F_1$ and $F_2$ be rough logical formulae defined on information system $IS = (U, A)$, If $F_1$ implicates $F_2$ to degree at least $\lambda$ then meaning set $m(F_1)$ of $F_1$ is included in meaning set $m(F_2)$ of $F_2$ to degree at least $\lambda$, denoted by

if $\vdash_{IS} F_1 \rightarrow_\lambda F_2$ then $\vdash_{IS} \propto_\lambda (m(F_1), m(F_2))$.

## Property 11

$\forall F_1, F_2, F_3 \in RL_{IS}$, the absorbance laws corresponding to their meaning $m(F_1), m(F_2)$ and $m(F_3)$ are satisfied, denoted by

$\infty_\lambda(m(F_1) \cup (m(F_1) \cap m(F_2)), m(F_1))$

and

$\infty_\lambda(m(F_1) \cap (m(F_1) \cup m(F_2)), m(F_1))$.

## Property 12

Some special properties of meaning based on rough logical formulae defined on $IS$ are listed as follows:

(i)   $m(a_v) \cap m(a_u) = \varnothing$, where $a \in A$ is an attribute in $A$. $u, v \in V_a$ are a attribute value in set of attribute values, and $u \neq v$. $\varnothing$ is an empty set symbol.

(ii)  $\bigcup_{v \in V_a} m(a_v) = U$, where $a \in A$ is an arbitrary attribute in $A$. $U$ is a universe.

(iii) $m(\neg a_u) = \bigcup_{v \in V_a} m(a_v)$, for each $a \in A$, $u \neq v$.

The proof of the properties is straight according to the definitions in the above. For example, the proof of Property 6 may be denoted in the following.

## Proof

$$m(F_1 \wedge F_3) = \{ x \in U : x \models_{IS_\lambda} F_1 \wedge F_3 \} = \{ x \in U : x \models_{IS_\lambda} F_1 \wedge x \models_{IS_\lambda} F_3 \} = \{ x$$

$$\in U : x \models_{IS_\lambda} F_1 \} \cap \{ x \in U : x \models_{IS_\lambda} F_3 \} = m(F_1) \cap m(F_3) \}$$

For the same reason,

$$m(F_2 \wedge F_3) = m(F_2) \cap m(F_3).$$

Now suppose, $m(F_1 \wedge F_3) \neq m(F_2 \wedge F_3)$, then $\exists x \in U$, $\in$ and $\wedge \neg$. Namely, $\phi$, but $\propto_\lambda$. Because $m$, so $m$ and $[x] \propto_\lambda m(F_3)$. Because $[x] \neg \propto_\lambda (m(F_2) \cap m(F_3))$, so $[x] \neg \propto_\lambda m(F_2)$, that is, $x \notin_\lambda m(F_2)$, but $[x] \propto_\lambda m(F_1)$, so $x \in_\lambda m(F_1)$. So $m(F_1) \neq m(F_2)$, this is contrary to $m(F_1) = m(F_2)$. The proof is finished.

## 8. NORMAL FORMS BASED ON MEANING OF ROUGH LOGICAL FORMULAE

### 8.1. Disjunction Normal Form

Let $F = (A_{1_1} \wedge \cdots \wedge A_{1_r}) \vee \cdots \vee (A_{n_1} \wedge \cdots \wedge A_{n_t})$ be a disjunction normal form of rough logical formula in a given information system, disjunction normal form of meaning $m(F)$ corresponding to $F$ is denoted by

$$m(F) = (m(A_{1_1}) \cap \cdots \cap m(A_{1_r})) \cup \cdots \cup (m(A_{n_1}) \cap \cdots \cap m(A_{n_t}))$$

## 8.2. Conjunction Normal Form

Let $F = (A_{1_1} \vee \cdots \vee A_{1_r}) \wedge \cdots \wedge (A_{n_1} \vee \cdots \vee A_{n_t})$ be a conjunction normal form of rough logical formula in a given information system, conjunction normal form of meaning $m(F)$ corresponding to $F$ is denoted by

$$m(F) = (m(A_{1_1}) \cup \cdots \cup m(A_{1_r})) \cap \cdots \cap (m(A_{n_1}) \cup \cdots \cup (m(A_{n_t}))$$

where $A_{i_j}$ is propositional variable or their negation.

## 8.3. Skolem Clause Form

In first-order logic, all quantifiers are moved to the front of formula, and each existent quantifier is eliminated from the prefixal form by using Skolem's method. Thus, original logical formula is equally transformed into the prefix form of containing only full quantifiers. To eliminate all full quantifiers, the prefix form is equally transformed into the Skolem clause form. Let $F$ be a rough logical formula in a given information system, which could equally be transformed into following Skolem normal form according to Skolem ways,

$$F = C_1 \wedge \cdots \wedge C_n$$

where each $C_i$ is a disjunction of atoms or their negation. By the definition of meaning operation in above, we could get the meaning to correspond to $F$ as follows:

$$m(F) = m(C_1) \cap \cdots \cap m(C_n)$$

each $m(C_i) = m(L_{i_1}) \cup \cdots \cup m(L_{i_k})$, i=1,$\cdots$,n, $L_{i_j}$ is a propositional variable or their negation or predicate without any quantifier or their negation, called as literal. $m(C_i)$ is called semantic clause, $m(L_{i_j})$ is called semantic literal, $m(F)$ is called Skolem's semantic clause form.

## 9. SEMANTIC REASONING OF ROUGH LOGIC

For any rough logical formula $\phi \in RL_{IS}$, there exists a set $m(\phi)$ corresponding to this formula $\phi$. We call it meaning of rough logical formulae defined in a given information system. Because it is generated by rough logical formula, so the properties of the meaning depend on the rough logical formulae. Thus, we will transform the reasoning based on logic into the reasoning of semantics based on rough logical formulae. Here we will prove that the related properties of semantics based on rough logical formulae. Such as, we may prove $b_4 \rightarrow c_0$ is true[40] in information Table 1.

## Proof

By semantic analysis of rough logic, we could compute the truth value as follows:

$$T_{I_u}(b_4 \rightarrow c_0) = K(m(b_4 \rightarrow c_0)) / K(U) = K(m(\neg b_4 \vee c_0)) / K(U)$$
$$= K(\{4,5,6\} \cup \{1,2,3,4\}) / (U) = 1$$

## 9.1. Deductive Reasoning of Semantics

We will illustrate the deductive reasoning of semantics with real example.

## Example 2

It shows that $m$ (LH$\varphi$) is to equal roughly $m$ (H$\phi$)$^{[12,13,19,21,34,40,43,44]}$ in semantic analysis, namely, we prove

$$m (\text{LH}\phi) =_R m (\text{H}\phi)$$

where L and H is lower and upper approximate operators respectively[1,5,19,21]. Rough equality may also be called as closeness to degree at least $\lambda$, thus we need only to prove:

$$m (\text{LH}\phi) \infty_\lambda m (\text{H}\phi)$$

which is equivalent to prove following two forms:

$$B_* (m (\text{LH}\phi)) \infty_\lambda B_* (m (\text{H}\phi)$$

and

$$B^* (m (\text{H}\phi) \infty_\lambda B^* (m (\text{LH}\phi))$$

*Table 2. Information System IS=(U,A)*

| Patient | Sex | Age | TV | ... |
|---------|--------|-----|-----|-----|
| Wang | Male | 65 | 3.5 | ... |
| Li | Female | 43 | 5.1 | ... |
| Liu | Female | 70 | 8.2 | ... |
| Wan | Male | 33 | 6.0 | ... |

where $LH\phi$ and $H\phi$ are operator rough logical formula[1,5,6,13,19,25,35], $B_*(\bullet)$ and $B^*(\bullet)$ denote the lower and upper approximations of indiscernibility relation $B$ with respect to set $\bullet$ respectively. Closeness form of the lower approximation is proved as follows:

**Proof**

(1)   $L\neg\phi \rightarrow \neg\phi$ Definition of operator $L$[1,5,38]

(2)   $m(L\neg\phi) \propto m(\neg\phi)$ (1) and Property 10[1,5,38]

(3)   $B_*(m(L\neg\phi)) \propto_\lambda B_*(m(\neg\phi))$ (2) and the properties of rough sets[1,5]

(4)   $B_*(m(\phi)) \propto_\lambda B_*(m(H\phi))$ Exchange position of logical formulae in (3)[34] and dual of L and H [1,5]

(5)   $B_*(m(L\phi)) \propto_\lambda B_*(m(HL\phi))$ Replace $\phi$ by $L\phi$ in (4)

(6)   $B_*(m(HL\phi)) \propto_\lambda B_*(m(L\phi))$ Definition of L and H and properties of rough sets[1,5]

(7)   $B_*(m(L\phi)) \infty_\lambda B_*(m(HL\phi))$ (5),(6) and $\lambda$-closeness definition

(8)   $B_*(m(LH\phi)) \infty_\lambda B_*(m(HLH\phi))$ Replace by $H\phi$ in (7)

(9)   $B_*(m(LH\phi)) \infty_\lambda B_*(m(HH\phi))$ Properties of rough sets[1,5]

(10)  $B_*(m(HH\phi)) \infty_\lambda B_*(m(H\phi))$ Properties of rough sets[1,5]

(11)  $B_*(m(LH\phi)) \infty_\lambda B_*(m(H\phi))$ The "hypothetical syllogism" in (9) and (10)[1,5]

Similarly, we may prove the closeness form of the upper approximation. We will also show that

$$m(((P \vee Q) \wedge \neg(\neg P \wedge (\neg Q \wedge R)))) \vee \neg(P \vee Q) \wedge \neg(P \vee R)) \infty_\lambda U$$

where $P, Q, R \in RL_{IS}$, $\lambda \in [0,1]$ is real number, $U$ is a universe of objects.

## 9.2. $\lambda$-Precision Reasoning of Semantics

We try to study $\lambda$-precision reasoning of the semantics. Let $C$ be a clause in rough logic defined in a given information system $IS=(U,A)$, then $m(C)$ is a semantic clause corresponding to $C$; If $L$ is a literal in rough logic, then $m(L)$ is a semantic literal corresponding to $L$. Let $m(L_1)$ and $m(L_2)$ be two semantic literals, if $(m(L_1), U)=1$ and $(m(L_2), U)=0$ or $(m(L_1), U)=0$ and $(m(L_2), U)=1$, then $m(L_1)$ and $m(L_2)$ are called as complementary semantic literal pair[19,23−25,36].

## Theorem

For $\forall F \in RL_{IS}$, meaning $m(F)$ to correspond to $F$ could be transformed equivalently into semantic clause form

$$m(C_1) \cap \cdots \cap m(C_n)$$

where each $m(C_i)$ is the union of form $m(a)$ or negation of its, $a \in A$ is an attribute on $A$.

## Definition 13

Let $m(L_1)$ and $m(L_2)$ be semantic literal, where $m(L_1)$ is close to $U$ to degree at least $\lambda$, $m(L_2)$ is close to $U$ to degree at most $1-\lambda$, if $\lambda \geq 0.5$,

$T_{I_u}(m(L_1)) > \lambda$ and $T_{I_u}(m(L_2)) < 1-\lambda$; Or $m(L_1)$ is close to $U$ to degree at most $\lambda$, $m(L_2)$ is close to $U$ to degree at least $1-\lambda$, if $\lambda < 0.5$, $T_{I_u}(m(L_1)) < \lambda$ and $T_{I_u}(m(L_2)) \geq 1-\lambda$, where $L_1$ and $L_2$ are $\lambda$-complement literal pair in rough logic on *IS*, then $m(L_1)$ and $m(L_2)$ is called as $\lambda$-complement semantic literal pair[23–25,36].

## Definition 14

Let $m(C_1)$ and $m(C_2)$ be without common variable semantic clause. $m(L_1)$ in $m(C_1)$ and $m(L_2)$ in $m(C_2)$ are $\lambda$-complement semantic literal pair, then $\lambda$-precision reasoning of semantics $m(C_1)$ and $m(C_2)$ is defined as follows:

$$SR_\lambda(m(C_1), m(C_2)) = (m(C_1) \backslash m(L_1)) \cup$$

$$(m(C_2) \backslash m(L_2)) = m(C'_1) \cup m(C'_2)$$

where $\backslash$ is a subtraction sign of sets, $m(C'_1) = m(C_1) \backslash m(L_1)$, $m(C'_2) = m(C\_2) \backslash m(L_2)$.

## Example 3

Let *IS*=$(U,A,V,f)$ be an information system, as show on information Table 1 in the above. We may get a semantic form based on the meaning of rough logical formula on $IS^{[6,7,21-25,34,36]}$. We extract the formula $F \in RL_{IS}$ as follows:

$$F(a_5, b_2, b_4, c_0, \neg e_0) = (a_5 \vee b_4)$$

$$\wedge b_2 \wedge_0 (c_0 \vee \neg e_0) \tag{1}$$

Formula (1) may be written as the following semantic form:

$$m(F(a_5, b_2, b_4, c_0, \neg e_0))$$
$$= (m(a_5) \cup m(b_4)) \cap m(b_2) \cap (m(c_0) \cup m(\neg e_0)) \tag{2}$$

This is a semantic clause form, where each intersection item is a semantic clause. The ground semantic clause form is defined as follows:

$$m(F(a_5, b_2, b_4, c_0, \neg e_0)) = (a_5^{\{1,6\}} \cup b_4^{\{1,2,3\}}) \cap b_2^{\{4,5,6\}} \cap (c_0^{\{1,2,3,4\}} \cup \neg e_0^{\{2,3,4,5\}}) \tag{3}$$

This shows that ground clause is the clause of containing no variable. In (3), each item is a ground semantic clause. When $\lambda$ is defined as 0.6, obviously, $a_5^{\{1,6\}}$ and $c_0^{\{1,2,3,4\}}$ is a $\lambda$-complement ground semantic literal pair. So, the reasoning form $SR_\lambda(m(C_1), m(C_2))$ is defined as follows:

$$SR_\lambda(m(C_1), m(C_2)) = (a_5^{\{1,6\}} \cup b_4^{\{1,2,3\}} \backslash a_5^{\{1,6\}}) \cup (c_0^{\{1,2,3,4\}} \cup \neg e_0^{\{2,3,4,5\}} \backslash e_0^{[1,2,3,4]}) \tag{4}$$

Hence, the semantic form (3) could be rewritten as follows:

$$m(F(a_5, b_2, b_4, c_0, \neg e_0)) = (b_4^{\{1,2,3\}} \cup \neg e_0^{\{2,3,4,5\}}) \cap b_2^{\{4,5,6\}} \tag{5}$$

In face, when $\lambda = 0.6$, $a_5^{\{1,6\}}$ and $\neg e_0^{\{2,3,4,5\}}$ is also a $\lambda$-complement ground semantic literal pair, hence the reasoning form $SR_\lambda(m(C_1), m(C_2))$ could be obtained as follows:

$$m(F(a_5, b_2, b_4, c_0, \neg e_0)) = (b_4^{\{1,2,3\}} \cup c_0^{\{1,2,3,4\}}) \cap b_2^{\{4,5,6\}} \tag{6}$$

## 9.3. Lock Reasoning of Semantics

Let $\Delta$ be a set of lock semantic clauses, that is, the semantic literals in each semantic clause in $\Delta$ is indexed with an integer, such as, $m(C)$: $_r m(L_1) \cup _k m(L_2)$, here $r$ and $k$ are a lock on semantic literals $m(L_1)$ and $m(L_2)$ respectively. Reasoning of two lock semantic clauses in $\Delta$ is always to delete two complementary lowest lock semantic literals in two lock semantic clauses respectively. Obtained reasoning form is the union of the remnants after deleting two lowest lock semantic literals in two lock semantic clauses respectively. If there are more than one lock for the same semantic literal, then we keep only a lowest lock semantic literal, and delete the other to obtain a new clause, which is added in $\Delta$. The procedure is illustrated as follows with real example:

(1)   $_1 m(L_1) \cup _2 m(L_2)$

(2)  $_3m(L_3) \cup_4 m(L_2)$

If semantic reasoning of (1) and (2) is done, because lowest lock semantic literal $_1m(L_1)$ in (1) and lowest lock semantic literal $_3m(L_3)$ in (2) are complementary lock semantic literal pair, so the two lowest lock semantic literals are deleted from (1) and (2) respectively. We have the following lock semantic clause:

(3)  $_2m\ (L_2) \cup_4 m\ (L_2)$.

In (3), lock semantic literals $_2m\ (L_2)$ and $_4m\ (L_2)$ are the same semantic literal $m(L_2)$, and 2 and 4 are different lock. Thus we keep only lowest lock semantic literal $_2m(L_2)$, another is deleted. To have

(4)  $_2m(L_2)$.

The (4) is called as lock semantic reasoning form of lock semantic clauses (1) and (2). Note that if the literals of lock semantic clause (2) are indexed differently, such as (2'). $_4m\ (L_3) \cup_3 m(L_2)$.

Then the semantic literal $_4m\ (L_3)$ in (2') is no permitted to do semantic reasoning, because the lock of semantic literal $m\ (L_3)$ in (2') is 4, to be not the lowest lock semantic literal in (2'). The lowest lock semantic literal $_3m(L_2)$ in (2') is not complementary to lowest lock semantic literal $_1m\ (L_1)$ in (1). So, semantic literals in each clause are indexed with an integer, which will be a guarantee to increase efficiency of semantic reasoning. Lock semantic reasoning is defined as follows [6,7,23–25,36,37]:

## Definition 15

Let $m(C_1)$ and $m(C_2)$ be two ground semantic clauses [6,7,23–25,36,37], and each semantic literal in them is indexed with an integer. Again, let $_rm(L_1)$ and $_km(L_2)$ be lowest lock semantic literals to occur in $m(C_1)$ and $m(C_2)$ respectively. If $m(C)$ is the clause obtained removing $_rm(L_1)$ and $_km(L_2)$ from $m(C_1)$ and $m(C_2)$ respectively and keeping only lowest lock semantic literal, deleting the other same semantic literal, then $m(C)$ is called as binary lock semantic reasoning form of $m(C_1)$ and $m(C_2)$.

## Example 4

Consider the following two lock semantic clauses from Table 2:

(1)  $m(C_1) =_1 m(a_5) \cup_2 m(b_4) \cup_3 m(d_1)\ )$

(2)  $m(C_2) =_4 m(C_3) \cup_5 m(b_4)\ )$

Their ground semantic clauses are the following (3) and (4) respectively.

(3)  $m(C_1) =_1 a_5^{\{1,2,3,4,5,6\}} \cup_2 b_4^{\{1,2,3\}} \cup_3 d_1^{\{1,4,6\}}$ .

(4)  $m(C_2) =_4 c_3^{\{\}} \cup_5 b_4^{\{1,2,3\}}$ .

Lock semantic literal $_1 a_5^{\{1,2,3,4,5,6\}}$ is the lowest lock semantic literal in (3). Again $_4 c_3^{\{\}}$ is the lowest lock semantic literal in (4). $_1 a_5^{\{1,2,3,4,5,6\}}$ and $_4 c_3^{\{\}}$ are exactly complementary lock semantic literal pair. So $_1 a_5^{\{1,2,3,4,5,6\}}$ and $_4 c_3^{\{\}}$ are deleted from (3) and (4) respectively, to have

(5)  $_2 b_4^{\{1,2,3\}} \cup_3 d_1^{\{1,4,6\}} \cup_5 b_4^{\{1,2,3\}}$ .

In (5), there are different locks in the same semantic literal, integers 2 and 5. Therefore, the lowest lock semantic literal $_2 b_4^{\{1,2,3\}}$ is kept, and to delete another $_5 b_4^{\{1,2,3\}}$, to have

(6)  $m(C) = {}_2 b_4^{\{1,2,3\}} \cup_3 d_1^{\{1,4,6\}}$ .

$m(C)$ is a lock semantic reasoning form of $m(C_1)$ and $m(C_2)$ .

Let $\Delta = m(C_1), \cdots, m(C_n)$ be semantic clause set of rough logical formulae. If there is $\lambda$-precision semantic reasoning of the semantic clause $m(C)$ from $\Delta$, then the $\Delta$ is included in $m(C)$ to degree at least $\lambda$, that is,

$$m(C_1) \cap \cdots \cap m(C_n) \alpha_\lambda m(C)$$

is true[19,36,40] on $IS$ .

## 10. APPLICATIONS OF SEMANTICS OF ROUGH LOGIC

The solving problem in $AI$ is an idea of collapsing a complex problem into simple, solvable sub-problems[19,30,33,36]. And then the answers of the local problems could be amalgamated into the answer of the original whole problem. Hence we study the knowledge representation, namely representing the practical problem by a rough logical formula. And the original whole logical formula is decomposed into sub-formulae, till predicates or propositions. The sub-formulae, predicates or propositions are solved by semantics of rough logic, and then the local answers of sub-formulae are amalgamated into the solution of the whole logical formula. The solving problem procedure based on semantics of the rough logic is listed as follows:

(1)  Gathering a group of data related with solving problem in the situation;

(2)   The group of data is constructed as a rough logical formula $F$ defined on a given information system, and then to do semantic analysis for the rough logical formula $F$, find out the meaning set $m(F)$ corresponding to $F$;

(3)   By Skolem way, the rough logical formula $F$ is equivalently transformed into the following clause form CNF:

$$C_1 \wedge \cdots \wedge C_n$$

where each clause $C_i = L_{i_1} \vee L_{i_2} \vee \cdots \vee L_{i_k}$ is a disjunction of literals. Literal $L_{i_j}$ is the predicate, proposition or negative of them.

(4)   By semantic analysis we find out the meaning set $m(C_i)$ corresponding to $C_i$, $i = 1, \cdots, n$, that is, $m(C_i) = \{x \in U : x \models_{IS} C_i\}$. The symbol $\models_{IS}$ is a satisfiability symbol for rough logical formulae [19,21–25,36].

(5)   The meaning set corresponding to the clause form $C_1 \wedge \cdots \wedge C_n$ is written by $m(C_1) \cap \ldots \cap m(C_n)$.

## Example 5

By semantic analysis we developed a system of diagnosis and treating in Chinese Traditional Medicine in 2003, denoted by $IS = (U, A)$, where $U$ is a set of the patients, $A$ is a set of symptoms (attributes) for the patients. The system possesses the function to test blood viscosity concentration for patients [26,30,33]. The data set of the patient gathered in clinic is denoted by $P = \{Name, Sex, Age, Testing - Value\}$. Such as, $P = \{Wang, Male, 65, 3.5\}$, where Wang is a value of attribute Name, Male is a value of attribute Sex, 65 is a value of attribute Age, and 3.5 is blood viscosity concentration of the patient tested via testing instruments. We represent the solving problem with the rough logical formula.

By the data set of the patient gathered in clinic we may construct an information system as follows: We could extract the rough logical formula as follows from the Table 2.:

$$F = Name_{Wang} \wedge Sex_{Male} \wedge Age_{65} \wedge TV_{3.5}.$$

Now we do semantic analysis for the rough logical formula and collapse this formula into some sub-formulae or predicates, and then to solve these sub-formulae or predicates with semantic analysis in the given information system [27,30,33]. Final we amalgamate the answers of the sub-formulae into an answer of the whole formula. More description may find in the references [30,33]

In this developed system, by semantic analysis we need compute 18 index values of testing blood viscosity concentration via clinic, the 9 levels of sub-types (Concentration-ConL, Viscosity-VL, Aggregation-AL, Coagulation-CoaL, Hematocrit-HL, Erythrocyte Aggregation-EAL, Red Cell Rigidity-RCRL,

Blood Plasma Viscosity-BPVL, Platelet Aggregation-BPAL), the 4 levels of blood viscosity concentration (BHVS,BLVS,BHLVS and BLHVS) are computed [27,30,33].

## 11. PERSPECTIVE OF STUDYING SEMANTICS OF ROUGH LOGIC

Kripks studied related properties and related reasoning of modal logic through Semantic Analysis of Modal Logic [6], Luis defined meaning of Modal Logical formula as a subset of state space, and studied the resolution of Modal Logic by semantics of modal logic [7]. Zadeh defined meaning of fuzzy propositional logical formula as a granulation, to try studying approximate reasoning of Fuzzy Logic by it in 1979 [8,9,10]. Pawlak proposed Rough Sets based on the semantics of indiscernibility relation, and defined upper and lower approximations of undefinable set by it [1,2], implementing the computing problem of elements on boundary by Frege in 1914 [10]. From problem solving in artificial intelligence, Hobbs defined indiscernibility relation based on semantic analysis of predicates in logical formula [11].

In this Chapter we study related properties and related reasoning through semantic analysis of the rough logic. It will inspire what we study the applications of rough logic to various specialities by semantic analysis. Besides, meaning of rough logical formula could be decomposed and amalgamated according to equivalent transformation of rough logical formula. Which will offer new theory and methodology for granular computing, and will also offer new idea of applications for classical logic and other nonstandard logic. So, we will further study the theoretical significance and practice value of studying semantic analysis of classical logic and other nonstandard logic.

## REFERENCES

[1] Pawlak, Z. (1991). *Rough sets-theoretical aspects of reasoning about data*. Dordrecht, The Netherlands: Kluwer Academic Publishers.

[2] Pawlak, Z. (1982). Rough Sets. International Journal of Information and Computer Sciences, 11,1982,341-356.

[3] Liu, Q., Liu, S. H., & Zheng, F. (2001). Rough Logic and Its Applications in Data Mining. *Journal of Software, 12*(3), 415-419. (In Chinese).

[4] Pawlak, Z. (1987). Rough Logic.*Bull. Polish Acad. Aci. Tech., 35*(5-6), 253-258.

[5] Lin, T. Y., & Liu, Q. (1996). First-order rough logic I: Approximate reasoning via rough sets. *Fundamenta Informaticae, 27*(2-3), 137-154.

[6] Kripke, S. (1963). Semantic Analysis of Modal Logic. *Zeitxchrift für Mathematische Logik und Grundlagen der Mathematik*, 67-96.

[7] Farinas-del-Cerro, L. (n.d.). Resolution of Modal Logic. In *Proceedings of the Eightth International Conference on Atomata Deduction* (LNCS 170,pp. 153-171).

[8] Zadeh, L. A. (1979).Fuzzy Sets and Information Granularity. In M. Gupta, R. Ragade, and R. Yager (eds.), *Advances in Fuzzy Set Theory and Applications* (pp. 3-18). Amsterdam.

[9] Zadeh, L. A. (1998). *Some reflections on soft computing, granular computing and their roles in the conception, design and utilization of information/intelligent systems.* Berlin, Germany: Springer.

[10] Pawlak, Z. (1996, July 1-5)). Rough Sets: Present State and Perspectives. In *Proceedings of the Sixth International Conference onInformation Processing and Management of Uncertainty in Knowledge-Based Systems* (IPMU'96), (pp. 1137-1146). Granda, Spain.

[11] Hobbs, J. R. (1985).Granularity. InProceedings of IJCAI (pp. 432-435). Los Angeles.

[12] Orlowska, E. (1985). A logic of indiscernibility relation. In A. Skowron (ed), *Computation Theory*, (Lecture Notes in Computer Science 208, pp. 177-186).

[13] Liu, Q. (1998). Operator Rough Logic and its Resolution Principle. *Chinese Journal of Computer*,5(21), 476-480. (In Chinese).

[14] Nakamura, A. (1996). A rough logic based on incomplete information and its applications. *International Journal of Approximate Reasoning, 15*, 367-378.Liu, Q., & Wang, Q. Y. (2005, September). Granular Logic with Closeness Relation and Its Reasoning, (LNAI 3641, pp. 709-711). Berlin, Germany: Springer

[15] Yao, Y. Y., & Liu, Q. (1999, September 11). *A Generalized Decision Logic in Interval-Set-Valued Information table*, (LNAI 1711, pp. 285-294). Berlin, Germany: Springer.

[16] Banerjee, M., & Khan, A. (2007). *Propositional Logic from Rough Set Theory, Transactions on Rough Sets VI*, (LNCS 4374, pp. 1-25). Berlin Heidelberg: Spring Verlag.

[17] Chakraborty, M. K., & Banerjee, M. (1993). Rough logic with rough quantifiers. Warsaw University of Technology. *ICS Research Report, 49*(93).

[18] Liu, Q., & Huang, Z. H. (2004). G-Logic and Resolution Reseaning. *Chinese Journal of Computer,27*(7), 865-873.(In Chinese).

[19] Rasiowa, H., & Skowron, A. (1985). Rough concepts logic. In A.Skowron (ed), *Computation Theory* (Lecture Notes in Comp.Sci.208, pp. 288-297).Liu, Q. (2005). *Rough Sets and Rough Reseaning* (Third). Beijing, China: Science Press. (In Chinese).Hamilton, A. G. (1980). *Logic for Mathematicans*. Cambridge, UK: Cambridge University Press.

[20] Chang, C. L., & Lee, R. C. T. (1973). *Symbolic logic and machine theorem proving.* New York: Academic Press.Liu, X. H. (1989). *Fuzzy Logic and Fuzzy Reseaning*. Jilin, China: Press. Of Jilin University.

[21] Liu, Q. (1998). The OI-resolution of operator rough logic. In L. Polkowski and A. Skowron (eds), *Lecture Notes in Artificial Intelligence* (1424, pp. 432-435). Berlin, Germany: Springer.

[22] Liu, Q. (2003, June). Granules and Reasoning Based on Granular Computing. In *Proceedings of the 16th International Conference on Industrial and Engineering Applications of Artificial Intelligence and Expert Systems* (IEA/AIE 2003), (LNAI 2718, pp. 516-526).

[23] Polkowski, L. (2006, July 20-22). A Calculus on Granules from Rough inclusions in Information Systems. In Proceedings of International Forum on Theory of GrC from Rough Set Perspective, *Journal of Nanchang Institute of Technology, 25*(2), 22-27. Nanchang, China.

[24] Skowron, A., & Stepaniuk, J. (2001). Extracting patterns using information granules. In Proceedings of International workshop on Rough Set Theory and Granular Computing (RSTGC-2001), *Bulleting of International Rough Set Society, 5*(1/2), 135-142.

[25] Skowron, A. (2001). Toward intelligent systems: calculi of information granules. In Proceedings of International Workshop on Rough Set Theory and Granular Computing (RSTGC- 2001), *Bulleting of International Rough Set Society, 5*(1/2), 9-30.

[26] Liu, Q. (2004, April). Granules and Applications of Granular Computing in Logical Reseaning. *Research and Development of Computer, 41*(4), 546-551. (In Chinese).

[27] Liu, Q. (2002, November 4-6). Approximate Reasoning Based on Granular Computing in Granular Logic. In *Proceedings of ICMLS2002* (pp. 1258-1262).

[28] Lin, T. Y. (1998). Granular Computing on Binary Relations II: Rough Set Representations and Belief Functions. In A. Skowron and L. Polkowski (eds), *Rough Sets in Knowledge Discovery* (pp. 121-140). Berlin, Germany: Physica Verlag.

[29] Liu, Q., Jiang, F., & Deng, D. Y. (2003). *Design and Implement for the Diagnosis Software of Blood Viscosity Syndrome Based on Hemorheology on GrC* (Lecture Notes in AI 2639, pp. 413-420). Berlin, Germany: Springer-Verlag.

[30] Wang, X. J. (1982). *Introduction for mathematical logic.* Beijing, China: Beijing, Press.

[31] Liu, Q. (1996). Accuracy Operator Rough Logic and Its Reasoning. In *Proceedings of RSFD '96 International Conference* (pp. 55-60). Tokyo, Japan: The University of Tokyo.

[32] Liu, Q., & Sun, H. (2006, July). Theoretical Study of Granular Computing. In *Proceedings of RSKT2006* (LNAI 4062, pp. 93-102). Hong Kong, China: Springer.

[33] Liu, Q., & Wang, J. Y. (2006, May). Semantic Analysis of Rough Logical Formulas Based on Granular Computing. In *Proceedings of IEEE GrC2005* (pp. 393-396). Washington, DC: IEEE Press.

[34] Lin, T. Y. (2006, July 20-22). Granular Computing on Partitions, Coverings Neighborhood Systems. In Proceedings of International Forum on Theory of GrC from Rough Set Perspective. *Journal of Nanchang Institute of Technology, 25*(2), 22-27.

[35] Skowron, A. (2006, July 20-22). Rough-Granular Computing. In Proceedings of International Forum on Theory of GrC from Rough Set Perspective. *Journal of Nanchang Institute of Technology, 25*(2), 22-27.

[36] Liu, Q. (2001). Neighborhood Logic and Its Data Reasoning on Neighborhood-Valued Information Table. *Chinese Journal of Computers, 24*(4), 405-410. (In Chinese).

[37] Yao, Y. Y. (2006, July 20-22). Three Perspectives of Granular Computing. In Proceedings of International Forum on Theory of GrC from Rough Set Perspective. *Journal of Nanchang Institute of Technology, 25*(2), 22-27.

[38] Zhang, B., & Zhang, L. (1990). *Theory and Applications for Problem Solving*. Tsinghua, China: Publisher of Tsinghua University. (In Chinese).

[39] Yao, J. T., & Yao, Y. Y. (2002). Induction of classification rules by granular computing. In *Proceedings of the International Conference on Rough Sets and Current Trends in Computing* (pp. 331-338). Berlin, Germany: Springer.

[40] Liu, G. L. (2005, July 25-27). The Topological Structure of Rough Sets over Fuzzy Lattices. In *Proceedings of the IEEE International Conference on Granular Computing* (vol. 1, pp. 535-538). Beijing, China.

[41] Pei, D. W. (2004). Rough Set Models on Two Universes. *Int. J. General Systems 33*(5), 569-581.

[42] Wu, W. Z. (2006, May 10-12). Rough Set Approximations vs. Measurable Space. In *Proceedings of the 2005 IEEE International Conference on Granular Computing* (pp. 329-332). Atlanta, GA.

[43] Miao, D. Q. (2005, August-September). Rough Group, Rough Subgroup and their Properties. In *Proceedings of the 10th International Conference* (RSFDGrC2005), (LNAI 3641, Vol. 1, pp. 104-113). Regina, Canada.

[44] Dai, J. H. (2004). Structure of Rough Approximations Based on Molecular Lattices In *Proceedings of 4th International Conference on Rough Sets and Current Trends in Computing* (RSCTC2004), (pp. 1197-1204). Uppsala, Sweden.

# Chapter 12
# Rough Entropy Clustering Algorithm in Image Segmentation

**Dariusz Małyszko**
*Bialystok University of Technology, Poland*

**Jarosław Stepaniuk**
*Bialystok University of Technology, Poland*

## ABSTRACT

*Clustering understood as a data grouping technique represents fundamental procedures in image processing. The present chapter's concerns are combining the concept of rough sets and entropy measures in the area of image segmentation. In this context, comprehensive investigations into rough set entropy based clustering image segmentation techniques have been performed. Segmentation presents low-level image transformation routines concerned with image partitioning into distinct disjoint and homogenous regions. In the area of segmentation routines, threshold based algorithms and clustering algorithms most often are applied in practical solutions when there is a pressing need for simplicity and robustness. Rough entropy threshold based segmentation algorithms simultaneously combine optimal threshold determination with rough region approximations and region entropy measures. In the present chapter, new algorithmic schemes RECA in the area of rough entropy based partitioning routines have been proposed. Rough entropy clustering incorporates the notion of rough entropy into clustering models, taking advantage of dealing with some degree of uncertainty in analyzed data. RECA algorithmic schemes performed usually equally robust compared to standard k-means algorithms. At the same time, in many runs they yielded slightly better performances making possible future implementation in clustering applications.*

## 1. INTRODUCTION

During last decades, constantly growing research attention has been focused on data clustering as fundamental technique in data analysis. Clustering or data grouping describes important method of unsupervised classification that arranges pattern data, most often vectors in multidimensional space, in the clusters or

DOI: 10.4018/978-1-60566-324-1.ch012

groups. Patterns or vectors in the same cluster are similar according to predefined criteria, in contrast to distinct patterns from different clusters (Jain, 1989) (Xu, Wunsch, 2005). Clustering algorithms are widely recognized as robust, high quality techniques of data analysis. Possible areas of application of clustering algorithms include data mining, statistical data analysis, compression, vector quantization and pattern recognition (Jain, 1989). Image analysis is the area where grouping data into meaningful regions (referred to as image segmentation) presents the first step into more detailed problem specific routines and procedures in computer vision and image understanding.

There is a growing need for effective segmentation routines capable of handling emerging different types of novel imagery suitable particularly for their distinct characteristics and taking into account their area of application. High quality of image segmentation requires incorporating reasonably as much information of an image as possible to retrieve. This kind of combining diverse information in a segmentation understood as a means of improving algorithm performance has been widely recognized and acknowledged in the literature of the subject.

In practical applications, most often image regions do not depict well-defined homogeneous characteristics, so it seems naturally appropriate to use techniques that additionally incorporate the ambiguity in information for performing the thresholding operation. In recent years (Pawlak, Skowron, 2007) (Pawlak, 1991) the theory of rough sets has gained considerable importance with numerous applications in diverse areas of research, especially in data mining, knowledge discovery, artificial intelligence and information systems analysis. Combination of thresholding methods with rough set theory has been introduced in (Pal, Shankar, Mitra, 2005). The authors minimize the roughness value in order to perform image thresholding by optimizing an entropy measure, which they refer to as the "rough entropy of image". Rough entropy measure calculation of the cluster centers is based on lower and upper approximation generated by assignments data objects to the cluster centers. Roughness of the cluster center is calculated from lower and upper approximations of each cluster center. In the next step, rough entropy is calculated as the sum of all entropies of cluster center roughness values. Higher roughness measure value describes the cluster model with more uncertainty at the border. Uncertainty of the class border should be possibly high as opposed to the class lower approximation. For each selected cluster centers, rough entropy measure determines quality measure or fitness value of this cluster centers. In this way, combining clustering schemes with uncertainty and entropy handling by means of rough entropy in the area of image segmentation should take best advantages of all described techniques.

## 1.1. Motivation

The present study proposes and thoroughly investigates new granular rough entropy method in the area of image clustering that extends and supplements algorithm proposed in (Pal, Shankar, Mitra, 2005), one-dimensional 1D GMRET thresholding algorithm proposed in (Malyszko, Stepaniuk, n.d.) and two-dimensional 2D GMRET thresholding algorithm in (Malyszko, Stepaniuk, 2008). Maximization of rough entropy of the image results in maximization of roughness in multiple clustering areas - providing the optimal threshold value of partitioning. The present study contribution consists in extension of rough entropy based threshold calculation schemes, which from definition are confined to low dimensional data into clustering schemes capable of handling high dimensional data. Clustering routines are more sophisticated and robust techniques that generally better describe underlying data structure compared to threshold based segmentation procedures.

## 1.2. Nomenclature

In the present study, research matter is primarily concerned with the following notions and definitions:

- $(x_1, x_2, \ldots)$: objects representing analyzed data
- $U$: universe of all data objects
- $X$: subset of the set of all data objects $U$
- $x_i$: one data object from the universe $U$
- $A$: attribute or feature set of data objects
- $B$: nonempty subset of $A$ (B $A$)
- $LOW(AS_B, X)$: lower approximation of $X$ relative to attribute set in $B$
- $UPP(AS_B, X)$: upper approximation of $X$ relative to attribute set in $B$
- $AS_B$: standard approximation space
- $(C_1, C_2, \ldots, C_k)$: clusters
- $Card(X)$: cardinality of the set $X$

Detailed description of rough set notions has been given in (Pawlak, 1991) (Pedrycz, Skowron, Kreinovich, 2008).

## 1.3. Paper Organization

In Section 2, review of existing segmentation techniques has been provided. Selected rough set concepts are explained in Section 3. In Section 4 evolutionary algorithms are described. Rough entropy based segmentation algorithms together with proposed RECA algorithm are outlined in Section 5. Experimental setup and results are given in Section 6. Conclusions, discussion and further research are finally shortly outlined.

## 2. IMAGE SEGMENTATION AND CLUSTERING

### 2.1. Overview of Segmentation Methods

Segmentation operation is essential and extremely important preprocessing step in the majority of image analysis based routines such as computer vision with practical applications ranging from object extraction and detection, change detection, monitoring and identification tasks. After preprocessing stage of image handling routines, with for example noise removal, smoothing, and sharpening of image contrast, follows image segmentation step, and subsequently more specific, high-level analysis is performed such as depicting objects and regions, and final interpretation of the image or scene. In almost all areas, the quality of segmentation step determines the quality of the final image analysis output. Segmentation process is defined as an operation of image partitioning into some non-overlapped regions such that each region exhibits homogeneous properties and no two adjacent regions are homogeneous. Segmentation routines present exact partitioning of input image into distinct, homogenous regions (by means of intensity, color, texture or other relevant features). Segmentation is the standard image partitioning process that results in determining and creation of disjoint and homogeneous image regions. Regions resulting from the image segmentation according to (Fu, Mui, 1981), (Haralick, Shapiro, 1985) should be uniform and homogeneous with respect to some characteristics, regions interiors should be simple and without many small holes, adjacent regions should be significantly different with respect to the uniformity characteristics and each segment boundary should be comparatively simple and spatially accurate.

Unsupervised segmentation and supervised segmentation routines start by creating partition of the image data into groups by means of defining similarity measure, which values for image data are then compared and on that basis image data partitioning follows. Image segmentation routines are divided into: histogram based routines, edge-based routines, region merge routines, clustering routines and some combination of the above routines. Exhaustive overview of the segmentation methods is available in(Fu, Mui, 1981), (Haralick, Shapiro, 1985). Edge detection approaches to image segmentation deal with discovering image locations where distinct changes in grey level or color are detected. The most difficult task in this type of algorithms is maintenance of the continuity of detected edges. Segments have always to be enclosed by continuous edges. However, usually disconnected or isolated edges within areas with more details have to be combined by using specialized heuristics. Region growing or merging presents an approach for image segmentation where large continuous regions or segments are detected first and afterwards, small regions are subjected to merging operation by use of homogeneity criteria. Region growing and merging routines are sequential in nature, dependent upon the order in which regions grow or merge. Furthermore, algorithms based on combining edge-based and region-based techniques are capable to exploit the complementary nature of edge and region information. Additionally, many segmentation techniques make use of particular data analysis approaches such as neural networks, fuzzy computing, evolutionary computing, multiscale resolution based techniques and morphological analysis. Some of segmentation methods are based on unique frameworks, such as active contour models, active shape models, watersheds etc. Into this framework-based segmentation approaches falls thresholding and clustering with rough entropy based segmentation quality measure that is the subject of this paper.

## 2.2. Image Types and Attributes

Currently acquired imagery materials present many types of images starting from light intensity images, range images through magnetic resonance images, thermal images to SAR images, aerial images and satellite images. Depending on method of acquisition, each kind of imagery exhibits specific properties such as data dimensionality, data spatial resolution, temporal data resolution. In contrast to monochrome images, color images have the information of brightness, hue and saturation for each pixel. The color perceived by human is a combination of three color stimuli such as red (R), green (G), and blue (B), which forms a color space. From RGB representation, many other kinds of color representation or spaces are derived by means of linear or nonlinear transformations. In practical applications, color models that are used to represent the colors in various representations such as RGB (red, green, blue), CMY (cyan, magenta, yellow), HSV (hue, saturation, intensity), HSI, CIE L u v. Image attributes most frequently used in image processing are intensity, color, texture, statistical measures such as mean value or variance. In image analysis routines, computer vision many other attributes are used such as spatial relationship, object topology. Some introductory information on image types and representation is provided in(Jain, 1989).

## 2.3. Clustering Techniques

A comprehensive review of different clustering techniques is provided in (Jain, 1989). Clustering refers to and describes the process of data partitioning into groups of similar objects. The resultant data groups are depicted as objects clumps, classes or clusters. Data representation based on less numerous data clusters unavoidably leads to losses of certain finer details, but results in data model simplification. Data modeling roots take its origin in mathematics, statistics, and numerical analysis. In a machine learning perspective clusters correspond to hidden patterns, the search for clusters is unsupervised learning, and the resulting system represents a data concept. In practical applications clustering outstands in data mining routines such as scientific and business data exploration, information retrieval and text mining, spatial database applications, Web analysis, CRM, marketing, medical diagnostics, computational biology, and many others. Clustering routines are divided into hierarchical and partitioning procedures. Hierarchical clustering algorithms are divided in agglomerative and divisive methods. In divisive setting, hierarchy of data object partitions is created, starting from one cluster and performed consecutive splitting of clusters until predefined quality of clustering is reached. In agglomerative methods, merging operations start from all data objects assigned to separate clusters and merging operations are performed until all data objects are assigned to only one cluster. Partitioning routines perform assignment to data objects to cluster prototypes and iteratively recalculate cluster prototypes by means of averaged data objects assigned to the given cluster. Additional group of clustering routines compose algorithms for high dimensional data. In this setting, the main division of clustering depends on subspace clustering, projection techniques and co-clustering techniques.

## 3. ROUGH SETS AND ROUGH ENTROPY

### 3.1. Rough Set Theory Essentials

Information granules (Zadeh, 1979), (Zadeh, 1996), (Zadeh, 1997), (Yao, 2007) are viewed as linked collections of objects (data points, in particular) drawn together by the criteria of indistinguishability, similarity or functionality. Information granules and the ensuing process of information granulation is a vehicle of abstraction leading to the emergence of high-level concepts.

A granule is most often defined as a closely coupled group or clump of objects (for example pixels in image processing setting), in the examined space that are interpreted as an indivisible entity because of its indistinguishable character, similarity, proximity or functionality. Granulation process basically depends on and subsequently results in compression and summarization of information. In the last decades, rough set theory has been attracted growing attention as a robust mathematical framework for granular computing. Rough set theoryRough set theory has been introduced by (Pawlak, 1991) in the 1980's creating a comprehensive platform for discovering hidden patterns in data with extensive applications in data mining. It has recently emerged as a important mathematical tool for managing uncertainty that arises from granularity in the domain of discourse - that is, from the indiscernibility between objects in a set.

Rough set theoryhas been applied in many practical areas including decision analysis, information retrieval, system modeling, voice recognition, software engineering, character recognition, concurrent systems, signal processing, image processing, classification and clustering. The intention is to approximate a rough (imprecise) concept in the domain of discourse by a pair of exact concepts, called the lower and upper approximations. These exact concepts are determined by an indiscernibility relation on the domain, which, in turn, may be induced by a given set of attributes ascribed to the objects of the domain. The lower approximation is the set of objects definitely belonging to the vague concept, whereas the upper approximation is the set of object possibly belonging to the same. An information system is a pair where U represents a non-empty finite set called the universe and A a nonempty finite set of attributes. Let B $\subseteq$ A and X $\subseteq$ U. Taking into account these two sets, it is possible to approximate the set X making only the use of the information contained in B by the process of construction of the lower and upper approximations of X.

Let IND(B) $\subseteq$ U $\times$ U be defined by

(x, y) $\in$ IND(B) if and only if, for all a $\in$ B a(x) = a(y)

An approximation space $AS_B = (U, IND(B))$.

For X $\subseteq$ U, let $[x]_B$ denotes the equivalence class of the object x relative to B (the equivalence relation IND(B)), the sets

$$LOW(AS_B, X) = \{x \in U : [x]_B \subseteq X\}$$

and

$$UPP(AS_B, X) = \{x \in U : [x]_B \cap X \neq \varnothing\}$$

are called the B-lower and B-upper approximations of X in U. It is possible to express numerically the roughness R(AS$_B$,X) of a set X with respect to B (Pawlak, 1991), by assignment

$$R(AS_B, X) = 1 - \frac{Card(LOW(AS_B, X))}{Card(UPP(AS_B, X))}$$

In this way, the value of the roughness of the set X equal 0 means that X is crisp with respect to B, and conversely if $R(AS_B, X) > 0$ then X is rough (i.e., X is vague with respect to B). Detailed information on rough set theory has been provided in (Pawlak, 1991), (Stepaniuk, 2008). Essentials and research background of granular computing has been provided in (Pedrycz, Skowron, Kreinovich, 2008).

## 3.2. Entropy Measure

Entropy is a concept introduced and primarily used in the Second Law of Thermodynamics. Entropy measures the spontaneous dispersion of energy as a function of temperature. It was introduced into communications theory by (Cover, Thomas, 1991) following the rapid development of communications. In this context, most often entropy measures the efficiency of the information transferred through a noisy communication channel. Additionally, in data compression, the concept of entropy has been extensively used as a measure of information content generated by information source. The mathematical definition of the entropy by (Cover, Thomas, 1991) is:

$$H = -\sum_{i=0}^{n} p_i \log(p_i)$$

where H is an entropy, $p_i$ is the statistical probability density of an event *i*. Many different measures of entropies have been proposed in the literature to generalize Shannon's entropy, e.g. Renyi's entropy, Kapur's entropy, and Havrda-Charvat's structural-entropy.

## 3.3. Rough Entropy Measure

Rough entropy measure presents extension of notion of entropy into the domain of rough sets. Rough entropy is measured on the base of determination of lower and upper approximations of created image segments. Each prototyped segment has connected lower and upper approximations that contain objects that are assigned to these segments according to some predefined criteria as has been further explained in Section 5. For each segment, segment roughness is calculated and further, rough entropy of all segments is calculated and summed up resulting in rough entropy of the segmented image. Rough entropy for one-threshold calculation has been proposed by (Pal, Shankar, Mitra, 2005). In (Shankar, 2007) detailed investigation in entropy and rough entropy measure has been provided.

## 4. EVOLUTIONARY ALGORITHMS

## 4.1. General Remarks

Evolutionary algorithms are classified as population based optimization techniques, that make extensive use of the mechanisms met in evolution and natura genetics. Several techniques have been developed inside evolutionary area such as genetic algorithms, evolutionary algorithms, genetic programming, evolution strategies. These algorithms are finding optimal solutions in solution spaces. For this reason combining clustering techniques with genetic algorithms robustness in optimization should yield high quality performance and results (Hall, Barak, Bezdek, 1999), (Maulik, Bandyopadhyay, 2000). Evolutionary algorithms have proved their usefulness and exhibited robust improved performance in a great deal of combinatorial problems compared to other soft computing techniques. Evolutionary algorithms (Goldberg, 1989) as heuristic approaches, play an important role in many areas of artificial intelligence, optimization problems, machine learning. Evolutionary algorithms present a family of computational models inspired by evolution. For genetic *k*-means and its harmonic and fuzzy variants, selection of cluster number and other algorithm specific parameter values is required. Next, the population should be initialized with randomly created cluster centers. From the initial population by subsequent iterations are created new populations by operations of selection, cross-over and mutation. For every solution in population, fitness value is calculated according to the specific fitness function, determined by particular solution problem. Solutions with high fitness values come into mating pool. The process is repeated until termination criteria are met.

## 4.2. Evolutionary Algorithm Performance

Investigation into application of evolutionary algorithms in $k$-means clustering based image segmentation routines is given in (Malyszko, Wierzchon, 2007). Chromosomes represent solutions consisting of centers of $k$ clusters - each cluster center is a $d$-dimensional vector of values in the range between 0 and 255 representing intensity of gray or color components. Selection operation tries to choose the best suited chromosomes from parent population that come into mating pool and after crossover and mutation operation create child chromosomes of child population. Most frequently genetic algorithms make use of tournament selection that selects into mating pool the best individual from predefined number of randomly chosen population chromosomes. This process is repeated for each parental chromosome. The crossover operation presents probabilistic process exchanging information between two parent chromosomes during formation of two child chromosomes. Typically, one-point or two-point crossover operation is used. According to (Pawlak, 1991), crossover rate 0.9 - 1.0 yields the best results. Mutation operation is applied to each created child chromosome with a given probability pm. After crossover operation, children chromosomes that undergo mutation operation flip the value of the chosen bit or change the value of the chosen byte to other in the range from 0 to 255. Typically mutation probability rate is set in the range 0.05 - 0.1 by (Pawlak, 1991),. Termination criterion determines when algorithm completes execution and final results are presented to the user. Termination criterion should take into account specific requirements. Most often termination criterion is that algorithm terminates after predefined number of iterations. Other possible conditions for termination of the $k$-means algorithms depend on degree of population diversity or situation when no further cluster reassignment takes place. In the present research, apart from rough entropy measure for evaluation of population solutions three additional measures are taken into account, $\beta$-index, $k$-means based partition measure and within cluster variance measure.

### Quantitative Measure $\beta$-Index

The $\beta$–index measure refers to the ratio of the total variation and within-class variation. Let define $n_i$ as the number of pixels in the $i$-th ($i = 1, 2,...,K$) region form segmented image. Then, let define $X_{ij}$ as the gray value of $j$-th pixel ($j = 1,...,n_i$) in the region $i$ and $X_i$ the mean of $n_i$ values of the $i$-th region.

The $\beta$-index is defined in the following way

$$\beta = \frac{\sum_{i=1}^{k} \sum_{j=1}^{n_i} (X_{ij} - \overline{X})^2}{\sum_{i=1}^{k} \sum_{j=1}^{n_i} (X_{ij} - \overline{X_i})^2}$$

where $n$ is the size of the image and X represents the mean value of the image pixel attributes. This index defines the ratio of the total variation and the within-class variation. In this context, important notice is the fact that $\beta$–index value increases as the increase of the number of clusters.

## Quantitative Measure *KM*: *k*-Means Partition Measure

In case of *k*-means clustering schemes, the quality of clustering partitions is evaluated by calculating the sum of squares of distances of all points from their nearest cluster centers. This type of measure is a good quantitative measure describing quantitatively clustering model. In this research, this sum of squares of distances from cluster centers is further referred to as *KM* measure and applied in the assessment of RECA and k-means experimental results. During optimalization routines, the values of *KM* measure should be minimized.

## Quantitative Measure wV: Within Class Variance Measure

Within-variance measure presents comparatively not complicated measure calculated by summing up within-variances of all clusters. This measure values are presented in two experiments carried out on two images: building image and nature image from Berkeley image database. Within class variance should be as low as possible and during optimalization this value should be minimized.

## 5. ROUGH ENTROPY CLUSTERING ALGORITHM

### 5.1. Granular Rough Entropy Thresholding

Rough entropy has been for the first time introduced and applied in the area of image thresholding routine in (Pal, Shankar, Mitra, 2005). The authors propose application of rough entropy during determination of optimal threshold value in one-level thresholding algorithm. Threshold value is selected on the base of calculation separately rough entropy for each possible attribute value. In (Pal, Shankar, Mitra, 2005) the threshold algorithm is confined to the gray-level image thresholding with one-dimensional attribute values in the range from 0 to 255. In this context, separate calculation of all 256 possible threshold values is performed. From calculated rough entropy values, the highest rough entropy value is determined and attribute value for this maximal rough entropy measure is selected as optimal threshold value that is further used during image segmentation. Rough entropy for the given threshold requires prior partition of the image into granules, and minimal and maximal attribute values in the granule create attribute interval <min, max>. Processed threshold value *N*, also creates two intervals <*0, N*), <*N, 255*> in case of attribute values in the range from 0 to 255.

For the given granule, if granule <min, max> interval is contained completely in one of the threshold intervals, then lower and upper approximation for this interval is increased by one. Otherwise upper approximation is increased by one for two attribute intervals. Presented solution is designed for thresholding routines with one threshold. In publication (Malyszko, Stepaniuk, n.d.) an extension of this approach has been given in the area of multilevel one-dimensional thresholding. Further investigation has given a way to two dimensional rough entropy thresholding proposed in (Malyszko, Stepaniuk, 2008). In this paper, an clustering extension of rough entropy based segmentation algorithm has been presented.

## 5.2. 1D GMRET Algorithm

In this Subsection, originally proposed in publication (Malyszko, Stepaniuk, n.d.) extension of one dimensional iterative splitting Rough Entropy Algorithm is presented in the form of Multilevel Rough Entropy Thresholding Routine - 1D GMRET. The 1D GMRET algorithm, as a threshold based segmentation technique, in the successive iterative steps, tries to find optimal solutions, it means predefined number of thresholds - that after segmentation maximize roughness measure that leads to minimal roughness of segmentation and exhibits high quality homogenous segments. After assigning values for N attribute thresholds, attribute space is divided into (N + 1) segments or separate attribute ranges. In the algorithm run, not separate image cells but granules or clumps of neighboring pixels are processed. Each processed image granule, after computation of granule minimal and maximal attribute values, contributes to the lower and upper approximation of each attribute segment or attribute range. Lower and upper approximations are further taken into account by calculation of segment roughness and roughness entropy. In the 1D GMRET algorithm, initial population of Size solutions is created. Each solution or chromosome consists of N randomly created threshold values sorted in ascending order. Additionally, for each chromosome, its fitness value is calculated according to Rough Entropy Measure given in Algorithm 1. Next, standard evolutionary populations are created with consecutive selection, crossover and mutation operations. Procedure is iteratively repeated until selected termination condition is met, for example until given number of populations has been created. Finally, algorithm presents the pool of solutions in the form of N threshold values each. From these solutions, the best should be selected as threshold values for threshold based segmentation. The way of calculation of rough entropy measure is presented briefly in Algorithm 1. Detailed algorithm description is given in publication (Haralick, Shapiro, 1985). Algorithm as an input takes image that is to be segmented, threshold number and granule parameters: GX, GY, SGX and SGY. Parameters GX and GY determine granule Sites, for example GX = 2 and GY = 2 determines granule sizes as 2 x 2 and means that each granule comprises of four pixels or image cells extending in X and Y directions. Parameters SGX and SGY determine shift between adjacent granules. Taking as an example parameters SGX and SGY set to value 1 leads to the creation of adjacent granules that are shifted by 1 in X and Y image directions.

In Algorithm 1 procedure for calculating Rough Entropy Measure for given input intervals sorted in ascending order is given. In case of 1D GMRET algorithm, chromosomes consist of N threshold values from attribute space, most often from 0 to 255 in case of 8-bit features. In case of standard $k$-means clustering, the clusters centers are initialized randomly to $k$ $d$-dimensional points with values in the range from 0 to 255. Fitness value is calculated for each chromosome in the population according to the rules given further in this Section. In case of 1D GMRET algorithm, chromosomes are randomly initialized to N threshold values in the range from 0 to 255. Fitness value is calculated according to formula given in Algorithm 1 description. The Set G of all granules is created from granules with sizes GX and GY, that are spread over the entire image (each granule shifted by GSX and GSY in X and Y directions).

## 5.3. 2D GMRET Algorithm

In case of standard 1D GMRET algorithm as thoroughly has been described in (Malyszko, Stepaniuk, 2008), the main aim of the algorithm is targeted into finding predefined number of N optimal thresholds for further threshold based segmentation operation that finally creates segmentations of input images. The 1D GMRET algorithm has been devised for and investigated in the area of one dimensional thresh-

*Algorithm 1. 1D granular rough entropy calculation rough entropy measure*

```
Data:
Input Image, granule parameters: GX,GY,GSX,GSY ;
T0, T1,..., Tn−1, n Input Thresholds ;
1. Create the set Int of intervals generated according to Input Thresholds
T(1) =< 0, T0), T(2) =< T0 + 1, T1)... T(n) =< Tn−1 + 1, 255 >
2. Create the Set G of all granules
3. Initialize arrays Upper(0..n) and Lower(0..n) for each generated interval T to zero values
for i = 1 to total no granule do
  max(i) = maximum gray value of pixels in granule(i);
  min(i) = minimum gray value of pixels in granule(i);
  foreach Interval T(i) of Int do
    if < min(i), max(i) > contained completely in T(i) then
      Lower(i)++;
      Upper(i)++;
    end
    else if < min(i), max(i) > contained partially in T(i) then
      Upper(i)++;
    end
  end
end
Rough_entropy = 0;
for l = 1 to n do
  roughness(l) = 1 - [ L(l) / U(l)];
end
for l = 1 to n do
  Rough_entropy = Rough_entropy −[ e2 ] × [roughness(l) × log(roughness(l));
end
```

old based segmentation, meaning that thresholded image consists of one-dimensional data, for example pixels values in the range from 0 to 255. However, taking into account more processed image features with different attributes of the same image scene should improve segmentation quality. Solutions of this kind are frequently met during segmentation of satellite imagery, when images with several bands are available. The information contained in this section describes extension of granular 1D GMRET algorithm into segmentation of simultaneous two images referred to as 2D – dimensional thresholding. Two-dimensional 2D GMRET algorithm takes as an input two separate 1D dimensional images or image bands. In this setting, each image band represents one feature or attribute related to the analyzed scene. The 2D GMRET algorithm has been described in (Malyszko, Stepaniuk, 2008).

In Algorithm 2, 3, 4, 5 procedures for calculating Rough Entropy Measure for given input intervals sorted in ascending order are given together with managing iterative evolutionary population in search of optimal solutions. In this regard, population of S separate solutions in the form of two threshold series each is created, and procedure given in Algorithm 2 is performed until termination criteria are met. In each iteration, data structures initialization proceeds as described in Algorithm 3. For the given two thresholds series in each dimension, two-dimensional ranges are created. Two two-dimensional arrays for storing lower and upper approximations Lower, Upper are zeroed. Next, for each granule two-dimensional mean value and standard deviation value is computed. Further, depending whether mean value (1) + standard deviation (1) is contained in given range assignment to appropriate Lower and Upper approximation is performed. If calculated value is completely contained in given 2D range T, both approximations are incremented, otherwise only Upper approximation is incremented. Consequently, three further calculations are performed in the same way for: mean value (1) + standard

*Algorithm 2. Rough entropy based grouping schemes for 1d GMRET, 2D GMRET and RECA algorithm*

**Data**: Input Image
**Result**: Optimal rough entropy solutions
Create X population with Size random N-level solutions (chromosomes)
**repeat**
  **forall** chromosomes of X **do**
    calculate their rough entropy measure values
Rough Entropy Measure;
  **end**
  create mating pool Y from parental X population ;
  apply selection, cross-over and mutation operators to Y population;
  replace X population with Y population ;
**until** until termination criteria ;

*Algorithm 3. 2D granular rough entropy calculation–initialization routines*

**Data**: Input Image, granule parameters: GX,GY,GSX,GSY ;
$T_{10}, T_{11}, ..., T_{1n-1}$, n Input first dimension thresholds ;
$T_{20}, T_{21}, ..., T_{2n-1}$, n Input second dimension thresholds ;
**Result**: 2D Rough Entropy Measure
1. Create two dimensional set INT of intervals generated according to
Input Thresholds
$T(1, 1) = < 0 - T_{10}, 0 - T_{20} >, ..., T(n, 1) = < T_{1n-1} - 255, 0 - T_{20}) >$
$T(1, 2) = < 0 - T_{10}, T_{20} - T_{21} >, ..., T(n, 2) = < T_{1n-1} - 255, T_{20} - T_{21} >$
...
$T(1, n) = < 0 - T_{10}, T_{2n-1} - 255 >, .., T(n, n) = < T_{1n-1} - 255, T_{2n-1} - 255 >$
2. Create the Set G of all granules
3. Initialize arrays Upper(0..n, 0..n) and Lower(0..n, 0..n) for each generated interval T(.,.) to zero values

deviation (1), mean value (2) - standard deviation (2), mean value (2) + standard deviation (2). In the calculations, mean value (1) represents mean value in the first dimension, mean value (2) represents mean value in the second dimension. The same naming convention applies for standard deviation values. After all granules have been processed, rough entropy measure is calculated according to routine given in Algorithm 5. On the base of calculated rough entropy measure, each solution undergoes selection, cross-over, mutation operation and elite solutions are additionally retained in the population with the best β-index values. Next, further iterative evolutionary steps as described in Algorithm 2 are performed until termination criteria are met.

## 5.4. RECA Algorithm

In Rough Entropy Clustering, similar to other divisive clustering algorithmic schemes, initial cluster centers are selected. The main aim of the algorithm is to find in the successive steps optimal cluster centers. The number of clusters is given as input parameter. Algorithm does not impose any constraints on data dimensionality. For each cluster center, two approximations are maintained, lower and upper approximations that describe the region connected with this cluster. For each object in universe (namely pixel data in image segmentation setting) as described in Algorithm 7, the closest cluster center is determined, and lower and upper approximations for that cluster are incremented by 1. Additionally, upper approximation of the clusters that are located within the distance not greater less distance form the closest cluster is incremented also by 1 value. After all data objects (image pixels) are processed,

*Algorithm 4. 2D granular rough entropy-calculation of lower and upper approximations*

```
foreach granule do
  mean(1..2) = mean gray value of pixels in granule;
  std(1..2) = standard deviation of gray values of pixels in granule
  separately for first and second image;
  Find Interval T(i, j) that contains granule center
    if < mean(1), mean(1) − std(1) > contained completely in T(i, j) then
    Lower(i, j)++; Upper(i, j)++;
    end
    else Upper(i -1, j)++;
    if < mean(1), mean(1) + std(1) > contained completely in T(i, j) then
    Lower(i, j)++;Upper(i, j)++;
    end else Upper(i+1,j)++;
    if < mean(2), mean(2) - std(2) > contained completely in T(i, j) then
    Lower(i, j)++; Upper(i, j)++;
    end else Upper(i, j − 1)++;
    if < mean(2), mean(2) + std(2) > contained completely in T(i, j) then
    Lower(i, j)++; Upper(i, j)++;
    end else Upper(i, j + 1)++;
end
```

*Algorithm 5. 2D rough entropy-roughness and rough entropy*

```
n – number of thresholds in each of two dimensions
Rough_entropy = 0;
for k = 1 to n do
  for l = 1 to n do
    roughness(k,l) = 1 - [ Lower(k,l) / Upper(k,l)];
for k = 1 to n do
  for l = 1 to n do
    Rough_entropy = Rough_entropy −[ e / 2 ] × [roughness(k,l) × log(roughness(k,l));
```

and lower and upper approximation for each cluster are determined, roughness value for each cluster is determined as described in Algorithm 7.

Rough Entropy clustering incorporates the notion of rough entropy into clustering model. Rough entropy measure calculation of the cluster centers is based on lower and upper approximation generated by assignments data objects to the cluster centers. Roughness of the cluster center is calculated from lower and upper approximations of each cluster center. In the next step, rough entropy is calculated as sum of all entropies of cluster center roughness values. Higher roughness measure value describes the cluster model with more uncertainty at the border. Uncertainty of the class border should be possibly high as opposed to the class lower approximation. For each selected cluster centers, rough entropy measure determines quality measure or fitness value of this cluster centers. In order to search thoroughly space of all possible class assignments for predefined number of cluster centers, evolutionary algorithm has been employed. Each solution in the evolutionary population, represented by chromosome, consists of N cluster centers. After calculation of rough entropy measure for this class centers, new mating pool of solution is selected from parental population, based on the rough entropy measure as fitness measure. Higher fitness measure makes selection of the solution into mating pool more probable. From the parental mating pool a new child population is created by means of selection, cross-over, mutation operations. The procedure is repeated predefined number of times or stops when some other predefined criteria are met. Detailed algorithm flow with evolutionary processing is described in Algorithm 6.

*Algorithm 6. RECA Algorithm Flow*

```
Data: Input Image
Result: Optimal Cluster Centers
Create X population with Size random N-level solutions (chromosomes)
repeat
  forall chromosomes of X do
calculate their rough entropy measure values RECA
Rough Entropy Measure;
  end
  create mating pool Y from parental X population ;
  apply selection, cross-over and mutation operators to Y population;
  replace X population with Y population ;
until until termination criteria ;
```

*Algorithm 7. RECA - calculation of cluster Lower and Upper Approximations, Roughness and Entropy Roughness*

```
Rough_entropy = 0;
foreach Data object D do
  Determine the closest cluster center Ci for D
  Increment Lower(Ci)++ Increment Upper(Ci)++
  foreach Cluster Ck not further then EPS from D do
    Increment Upper(Ck)++
  end
end
for l = 1 to N(number of data objects) do
  roughness(l) = 1 - [ Lower(l) / Upper(l)];
for l = 1 to N(number of data objects) do
  Rough_entropy = Rough_entropy −[ e / 2 ] × [roughness(l) × log(roughness(l));
```

## 6. EXPERIMENTS

## 6.1. Experimental Setup

In order to perform proper assessment of rough entropy algorithmic schemes, experiments have been carried out for four images sets: Lenna images, IKONOS images, building images and nature images. The set of Lenna images consisted of four images standard image, and three convoluted images with the window 3x3 with operations: min, max and mean operation.

The set of IKONOS images consisted from four images in Red, Green, Blue and Infra Red bands. The nature image as a color RGB image consisted from three bands R, G and B. The building image is a gray level image. In the experiments two additional bands have been created by convolution with the window 3x3 operations as min and max image.

Images in the experiments were combined by two single 1D bands. In the experiments three bands combinations R-G, R-G and R-B of this image have been created and put as an input to 2D RECA algorithm and k-means algorithm. In this way, for Lenna images, six separate 2D images were created by creating pairs: Lenna Std − Max, Std − Min, Std − Mean, Max − Min Max − Mean and Min − Mean. For IKONOS imagery 2D pairs of images have been created: Red − Green, Red−Blue, Red−Infrared, Green−Blue, Green−Infrared, Blue−Infrared. For the nature image three 2D pairs have been created:

*Figure 1. Lenna gray 1D image - standard image and its min, max, mean windowed versions*

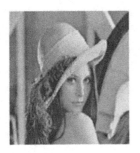 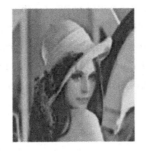 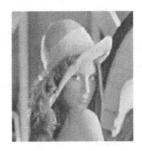 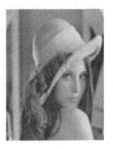

*Figure 2. Satellite imagery in four bands - red, green, blue and Infrared images*

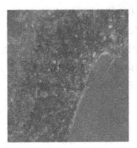 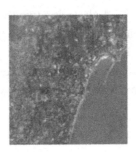 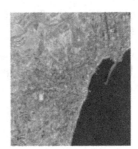 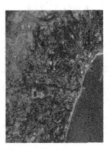

*Figure 3. Two further images explored in experiments: (a) nature image and (b) building image*

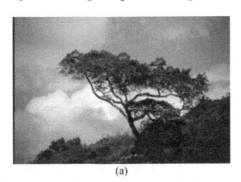 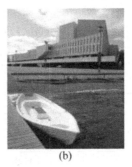

(a)　　　　　　　　　　　　　　　　　(b)

R–G, R–B and B–G. For the building image three 2D images have been created as Std–Min, Std–Max and Min–Max image.

In the experiments *k*-means algorithmic clustering schemes are compared against RECA clustering solutions. In the first experiment, six 2D Lenna images were taken as input. For each 2D image pair, two independent 2D RECA algorithms have been performed and compared to results with two independent standard 2D *k*-means algorithm results. In case of 2D RECA algorithm, in each algorithm run, population of 40 solutions has been created and successively iterated through 50 generations, according to rules given in Algorithms 2 and 7. After evolutionary algorithm iteration has been completed, five best solutions relative to β-index have been retained in the population, creating population elite. During selection operation tournament selection has been applied with tournament rank equal three. After iteration completions, three measures are presented in order to assess the quality of generated partitions: β-index value, *KM* partition measure and within class variance measure as described in Section 4. The measures are presented independently for 2D *k*-means algorithm clusterings and 2D RECA algorithm clusterings. In case of two first experiments with Lenna and IKONOS images, additional measure in the form of KM measure has been presented. In case of nature and building images the additional measure is within class variance *wV*.

## 6.2. Experimental Results

### Lenna Images

In Table 1 index-values of the solutions from 2D RECA algorithm two runs for R = 5 cluster centers are presented together with *k*-means clusterings. For each experiment, independently measures β-index and KM are given separately for 2D *k*-means and 2D RECA. Solutions that yielded better results than 2D standard *k*-means algorithm based segmentations are bolded. In each experiment as input images pairs of images Std −Min, Std −Max, Std −Mean, Min −Max, Min −Mean, Max −Mean have been taken as input.

### IKONOS Images

In Table 2 β-index values of the solutions from 2D RECA algorithm two runs for R = 5 cluster centers are presented together with *k*-means clusterings. For each experiment, independently measures β-index and KM are given separately for 2D k-means and 2D RECA. Solutions that yielded better results than 2D

*Table 1. Quality Indices for 1D-1D Images Lenna for 2D RECA*

| Image Lenna | KM *k*-means | β *k*-means | KM RECA | β RECA |
|---|---|---|---|---|
| Std-Max | 654471 | 10.32 | 661310 | **10.33** |
| Std-Min | 679808 | 11.48 | 658499 | 11.45 |
| Std-Mean | 512745 | 19.18 | 505791 | 19.16 |
| Max-Min | 828134 | 7.64 | 826195 | 7.49 |
| Max-Mean | 629493 | 11.93 | 549895 | **11.95** |
| Min-Mean | 606263 | 14.02 | 690796 | 13.30 |

*Table 2. Quality indices for 1D-1D images IKONOS for 2D RECA*

| Image IKONOS | WV *k*-means | β*k*-means | WV RECA | β RECA |
|---|---|---|---|---|
| R-G | 651299 | 10.08 | 644974 | 10.07 |
| R-B | 1169170 | 8.35 | 1188696 | 8.34 |
| R-IR | 802402 | 9.34 | 824512 | 9.30 |
| G-B | 1385100 | 6.88 | 1395058 | 6.88 |
| G-IR | 825952 | 10.68 | 831808 | **10.69** |
| B-IR | 1561344 | 6.53 | 162340 | 6.53 |

standard k-means algorithm based segmentations are bolded. In each experiment as input images pairs of images Red − Green, Red − Blue, Red − Infrared, Green − Blue, Green −Infrared, Blue − Infrared have been taken as input.

## Nature Image

Segmentation evaluation in the form of $\beta$-index and within class variance has been presented in Table 3, independently for $k$-means and RECA algorithm. The number of clusters has been chosen to 6 clusters for both algorithms.

## Building Image

Segmentation evaluation in the form of $\beta$-index and within class variance has been presented in the Table 4 and 5, independently for $k$-means and RECA algorithm. The number of clusters has been chosen to 4 and 6 clusters for both algorithms and results are presented in Table 4 (4 clusters) and Table 5 (6 clusters).

## DISCUSSION AND CONCLUSION

In the present study, detailed research investigation into rough entropy based image segmentation has been performed. Rough entropy based clustering scheme presents extension of rough entropy based

*Table 3. Quality indices for nature images IKONOS for 2D RECA*

| Image | wV $k$-means | $\beta$ $k$-means | wV RECA | $\beta$ RECA |
|---|---|---|---|---|
| R-G | 241 | 8.08 | 241 | 8.08 |
| R-B | 411 | 7.79 | 451 | 7.682 |
| G-B | 253 | 13.46 | 252 | 13.40 |

*Table 4. Quality indices for building image with 2D RECA for 4 clusters*

| Image | wV $k$-means | $\beta$ $k$-means | wV RECA | $\beta$ RECA |
|---|---|---|---|---|
| STD-MIN | 611 | 11.46 | 610 | 11.46 |
| STD-MAX | 638 | 10.70 | 638 | 10.70 |
| MIN-MAX | 798 | 8.59 | 799 | 8.59 |

*Table 5. Quality indices for building image with 2D RECA for 6 clusters*

| Image | wV $k$-means | $\beta$ $k$-means | wV RECA | $\beta$ RECA |
|---|---|---|---|---|
| STD-MIN | 361 | 19.38 | 379 | 18.70 |
| STD-MAX | 371 | 18.38 | 373 | 18.31 |
| MIN-MAX | 519 | 13.23 | 526 | 12.94 |

thresholding algorithm that results in more robust, completely new approach into rough entropy computation. Proposed algorithm addresses the problem of extension of rough entropy thresholding into rough entropy based clustering scheme RECA. The suitable metric for rough entropy is presented and assessed as described in Section 5.4. In the present paper, new algorithmic scheme in the area of rough entropy based partitioning routines has been proposed. RECA clustering algorithm is based on the notion of rough entropy measure of object space partitioning or universe. Rough entropy of data partitioning quantifies the measure of uncertainty generated by the clustering scheme, and this rough entropy relates to the border of the partitioning, so rough entropy measure should be as high as it is possible. Experiments on two different types of 2D images are performed and compared to standard 2D $k$-means algorithm. Results proved comparably equal or better performance of RECA algorithmic schemes. In this way, future research in the area of rough entropy based clustering schemes is possible with prospect of practical robust and improved clustering performance. Fuzzy version of RECA algorithm has been explored and detailed in (Malyszko, Stepaniuk, 2008). Rough entropy measure determines how uniformly sets or segments are constructed. The rough entropy measure after the evaluation gives rise to the optimalization step that constructs the other set of prototype solutions. For this reason, generic evolutionary algorithm has been applied. The experimental results suggest that data complexity impacts the generated clustering solutions. The best performance has been obtained for the number of clusters up to 5 clusters. Higher number of cluster centers adds up to more optimalization complexity and final results quality. The same dependency is coupled with data dimensionality and further research should lead to better understanding of this type of interrelation.

Proposed algorithmic schemes that are based primarily on the notion of rough sets are directly applicable into the clustering routines that are aimed at creating and determining data groups, clumps or granules of data that are similar to each other within the cluster. This approach requires prior determining the metric between each pair of object that describe how much these object are similar to each other. In this way, there is possible to extend proposed algorithmic scheme into hierarchical clustering schemes.

Rough entropy clustering algorithms need not to be limited to the image analysis and are suitable to all attributed data, provided that proper distance measure has been defined. Additionally, the notion of rough entropy measure is straightforwardly extensible into other granulation computing area where it is possible to construct and compute lower and upper approximations. Presented in this publication material may become starting point for further rough entropy exploration.

## ACKNOWLEDGMENT

The research was supported by the grant N N516 069235 from Ministry of Science and Higher Education of the Republic of Poland and by the grant N N516 377436 from Ministry of Science and Higher Education of the Republic of Poland. The present publication was also supported by the Bialystok Technical University Rector's Grant.

## REFERENCES

Cover, T., & Thomas, J. (1991). *Elements of Information theory*. New York: JohnWiley & Sons, Inc.Fu, S. K., & Mui, J. K. (1981). A survey on image segmentation. *Pattern Recognition, 13*, 3–16.

Goldberg, D. (1989). *Genetic Algorithms in Search, Optimization and Machine Learning*. Reading, MA: Addison-Wesley.

Hall, O., Barak, I., & Bezdek, J. C. (1999). Clustering with a genetically optimized approach. *IEEE Transactions on Evolutionary Computation, 3*, 103–112. doi:10.1109/4235.771164

Haralick, R. M., & Shapiro, L. G. (1985). Image segmentation techniques. *Computer Vision Graphics and Image Processing, 29*, 100–132. doi:10.1016/S0734-189X(85)90153-7

Jain, A. K. (1989). *Fundamentals of Digital Image Processing*. Upper Saddle River, NJ: Prentice Hall.

Malyszko, D., & Stepaniuk, J. (2008, June 16-18). Granular Multilevel Rough Entropy Thresholding in 2D Domain. IIS 2008. In *Proceedings of the 16ᵗʰ International Conference Intelligent Information Systems* (pp. 151-160). Zakopane, Poland.

Malyszko, D., & Stepaniuk, J. (2008, October 23-25). Standard and Fuzzy Rough Entropy Clustering Algorithm in image segmentation. In [Akron, Ohio.]. *Proceedings of RSCTC, 2008*, 409–418.

Malyszko, D., & Stepaniuk, J. (n.d.). [In Press]. *Granular Multilevel Rough Entropy Thresholding*. Rough Entropy

Malyszko, D., & Wierzchon, S. T. (2007). Standard and genetic *k*-means clustering techniques in Image Segmentation. In *Proceedings of CISIM* (pp.299–304).

Maulik, U., & Bandyopadhyay, V. (2000). Genetic algorithm-based clustering technique. *Pattern Recognition, 33*, 1455–1465. doi:10.1016/S0031-3203(99)00137-5

Pal, S., K., Shankar, B. U., & Mitra, P. (2005). Granular computing, rough entropy and object extraction. *Pattern Recognition Letters, 26*(16), 2509–2517. doi:10.1016/j.patrec.2005.05.007

Pawlak, Z. (1991). *Rough sets: theoretical aspects of reasoning about data*. Dordrecht, The Netherlands: Kluwer Academic.

Pawlak, Z., & Skowron, A. (2007). Rudiments of rough sets. *Information Sciences, 177*(1), 3–27. doi:10.1016/j.ins.2006.06.003

Pedrycz, W., Skowron, A., & Kreinovich, V. (Eds.). (2008). *Handbook of Granular Computing*. New York: Wiley. doi:10.1002/9780470724163

Shankar, U. (2007). Novel Classification and segmentation techniques with application to remotely sensed images. *T. Rough Sets, 7*, 295–380.

Stepaniuk, J. (2008). *Rough - Granular Computing in Knowledge Discovery and Data Mining, Series: Studies in Computational Intelligence*. Berlin, Germany: Springer.

Xu, R., & Wunsch, D. (2005). Survey of clustering algorithms. *IEEE Transactions on Neural Networks, 16*, 645–678. doi:10.1109/TNN.2005.845141

Yao, J. T. (2007, November 2-4). A Ten-Year Review of Granular Computing. In *Proceedings of 2007 IEEE International Conference on Granular Computing* (pp. 734-739). Sillicon Valley, CA.

Zadeh, L. A. (1979). Fuzzy sets and information granularity. In Gupta, M. M., Ragade, R. K., & Yager, R. R. (Eds.), *Advances in Fuzzy Set Theory and Applications* (pp. 3–18). Amsterdam.

Zadeh, L. A. (1996). Fuzzy logic computing with words. *IEEE Transactions on Fuzzy Systems*, *4*(2), 103–111. doi:10.1109/91.493904

Zadeh, L. A. (1997). Toward a theory of fuzzy information granulation and its centrality in human reasoning and fuzzy logic. *Fuzzy Sets and Systems*, *90*, 111–117. doi:10.1016/S0165-0114(97)00077-8

# Chapter 13
# Modelling Classification by Granular Computing

**Yan Zhao**
*University of Regina, Canada*

## ABSTRACT

*A granular structure includes granules, levels, hierarchies and multiple hierarchies. Classification can be modelled by granular computing regarding these components. More specifically, classification tasks can be understood as a search in a certain search space represented by a granule network. This chapter discusses the basic components of a granular structure, followed by the modelling of classification in terms of these components. The top-down, bottom-up strategies for searching classification solutions within different granule networks are discussed.*

## 1. INTRODUCTION

Granular Computing (GrC), as a newly developed computing paradigm, is studied by researchers in computational intelligence to explore varying levels of granularity in problem solving and information management (Bargiela & Pedrycz, 2002; Bargiela & Pedrycz, 2007; Lin, 2003; Lin *et al.*, 2002, Inuiguchi *et al.*, 2003; Polkowski & Artiemjew, 2007; Yao, 2007; Yao, 2006; Yao, 2007; Yao & Zhou, 2007; Zadeh, 1997; Zadeh, 1998). A granule is a collection of entities that can represent basic knowledge and concepts of human intelligence, and thus is regarded as the primitive notion of granular computing. A family of granules forms a granulated view at a certain level of resolution or scale. Granules at different levels are linked together by an order relation to compose a hierarchical structure, which provides a structured description of a system or an application under consideration. For a problem, one may need to construct multiple hierarchies for various descriptions and interpretations. Granular computing provides

DOI: 10.4018/978-1-60566-324-1.ch013

a systematic and effective means for building conceptual models, organizing and discovering knowledge, as well as solving real-world problems by practical heuristics and strategies.

Based on granular computing, a concept can be described by a granule directly or be defined by a logical formula. Once the basic granules and formulas are properly identified, one is able to investigate the relations among concepts and define computational operations upon concepts (Yao, 2006). The relationships, such as sub- and super-concepts, along with disjointed and overlapping concepts, can be conveniently expressed in forms of rules, with quantitative measures to indicate the strength. Rule mining, therefore, can be viewed as a process of forming concepts and finding relationships between concepts in terms of granules and their formulas (Yao & Yao, 2002).

Classification, also known as supervised learning, is a common method used in data mining, machine learning and pattern recognition (Breiman *et al.*, 1984; Cendrowska, 1987; Cestnik *et al.*, 1987; Clark & Niblett, 1989; Grzymala-Busse, 1992; Brzymala-Busse, 2005; Michalski & Larson, 1980; Mitchell, 1987; Pal, 2004; Quinlan, 1983; Quinlan, 1992; Zhong *et al.*, 2001). For classification tasks, concept formation involves the identification of granules and the description of granules regarding their classes, and concept relationship identification involves the connections of granules regarding their classes. The classification problem can be properly modelled by granular computing theory.

This chapter investigates classification tasks with respect to the basic components of granular computing, and discusses the classification of a granule, a granulation, in addition to the construction of a set of classification rules within a granule network. Two searching strategies, the top-down approach and the bottom-up approach, are studied to cope with two granule networks, a formula-based network and a granule-based network, respectively.

## 2. GRANULAR STRUCTURES

Granular computing exploits structures in terms of granules, granulations and hierarchies based on multilevel and multiview representations. In this section, we use an information table to demonstrate a concrete granular structure.

### 2.1 Information Tables and a Logic Language

An information table provides a convenient way to describe a finite set of objects, called a universe, by a finite set of attributes (Pawlak, 1982). It represents all available information and knowledge.

### Definition 1

An information table is the following tuple:

$$S = (U, At, \{V_a \mid a \in At\}, \{I_a \mid a \in At\}),$$

*where U is a finite nonempty set of objects, At is a finite nonempty set of attributes, $V_a$ is a nonempty set of values of $a \in At$, $I_a : U \rightarrow V_a$ is an information function.*

The mapping $I_a(x) = v$ means that the value of object $x$ on attribute $a$ is $v$, where $v \in V_a$. An information table can be conveniently represented in a tabular form, where the rows correspond to the set of objects of the universe, the columns correspond to the set of attributes, and each cell is the value of an object with respect to an attribute.

In order to describe information in an information table, a logic language $L$ can be used by adopting and modifying the decision logic language used in rough set theory (Pawlak, 1991; Yao & Zhou, 2007).

## Definition 2

A logic language L consists of a set of formulas, which are defined by the following two rules:

(1) *An atomic formula of L is a descriptor* $(aR_a v)$ *where* $a \in At$, $v \in V_a$ *and* $R_a$ *is a relation defined on* $V_a$.

(2) *The well-formed formulas (wff) of L is the smallest set of formulas containing the atomic formulas and closed under* $\neg$, $\wedge$, $\vee$, $\rightarrow$ *and* $\leftrightarrow$.

Language $L$ is used to define relationships between an attribute and its possible values. The standard rough set theory uses the trivial equality relation on attribute values (Pawlak, 1991). An atomic formula in such a setting is defined in the form of $a = v$. The equality relation is a special case of $R_a$. Generally, $R_a$ can represent similarity, dissimilarity or ordering of values in the domain $V_a$.

Given a formula $\phi \in L$, if an object $x \in U$ satisfies $\phi$, we write $x \models_S \phi$, or $x \models \phi$ if the information table $S$ is understood. A formula $\phi$ is valid in $S$ if it is satisfied by all objects in the universe; $\phi$ is invalid in $S$ if it is not satisfied by any object in the universe. The set $m_S(\phi) = \{x \in U \mid x \models \phi\}$ is called the meaning of the formula $\phi$ in the information table $S$. If $S$ is understood, we simply write $m_S(\phi)$ as $m(\phi)$

## 2.2 Granules

As the primitive notion of granular computing, a granule plays two distinctive roles. It may be an element of another granule and is considered to be a part forming that granule. It also may consist of a family of granules and is considered to be a whole (Yao, 2007).

The concept of definability is essential to data analysis. In fact, definable granules are the basic units that can be described and discussed, upon which other concepts can be developed.

## Definition 3

*A granule* $X \subseteq U$ *is definable in an information table* $S$ *if it is associated with at least one formula* $\phi \in L$, i.e., $X = m_S(\phi)$.

A formula $\phi \in L$ can be viewed as the description of a granule $m(\phi)$; a definable granule $X = m(\phi)$ contains the set of objects having the property expressed by $\phi$. A connection between formulas of $L$ and subsets of $U$ is thus established. This formulation enables us to study concepts in a logic setting in terms of formulas, and also in a set-theoretic setting in terms of granules.

In the context of an information table $S$, for any two formulas $\phi_1$, $\phi_2 \in L$, we can say $\phi_1$ is a refinement of $\phi_2$, or equivalently, $\phi_2$ is a coarsening of $\phi_1$, denoted as $\phi_1 \preceq \phi_2$, if and only if $m(\phi_1) \subseteq m(\phi_2)$. The refinement relation of formulas is reflexive and transitive. Given two formulas $\phi_1$ and $\phi_2$, their meet $\phi_1 \wedge \phi_2$ defines the largest intersection of the object sets $m(\phi_1)$ and $m(\phi_2)$, and their join $\phi_1 \vee \phi_2$ defines the smallest union of the object sets $m(\phi_1)$ and $m(\phi_2)$. Under the refinement relation, all formulas form an ordered set.

In many data mining applications, one is only interested in formulas of a certain form. Suppose we restrict the connectives of language $L$ to only the conjunction connective $\wedge$, which means that each formula is a conjunction of atomic formulas. Such a formula is referred to as a conjunctor. A granule $X \subseteq U$ is a conjunctively definable granule in an information table $S$ if there exists a conjunctor $\phi \in L$ such that $m(\phi) = X$. Similarly, we can define disjunctive definable granules.

*Support* is a commonly used measure for evaluating the generality of a granule $X \subseteq U$:

$$support(X) = \frac{|X|}{|U|},$$

where $|.|$ is the cardinality of the set. The support also is called the generality of a granule. If the granule is defined by a formula $\phi$, then $support(m(\phi))$ may be interpreted as a measure of the degree of truth of the formula $\phi$ in the information table. A formula is more general if it has a higher support and thus covers more objects of the universe.

The distance between two granules $X_1, X_2 \subseteq U$ can be defined as follows:

$$dis(X_1, X_2) = \begin{cases} 1 - \dfrac{|X_1 \cap X_2|}{|X_1 \cup X_2|}, & \text{if } X_1 \cup X_2 \neq \varnothing; \\ 0, & \text{otherwise.} \end{cases}$$

The measure $dis(X_1, X_2)$ reaches the minimum value 0 if the two granules are equivalent, and reaches the maximum value 1 if the two granules are disjointed. If $0 < dis(X_1, X_2) < 1$, then the two granules are overlapping.

## 2.3 Levels and Granulations

A family of granules collectively characterizes a level of description and understanding, and forms a granulated view, called a granulation. Different levels of descriptions focus on different resolutions. A granule at a higher level can be decomposed into many granules at a lower level, and conversely, some granules at a lower level can be combined into a granule at a higher level. A granule at a lower level provides a more detailed description than that of a parent granule at a higher level, and a granule at a higher level has a more abstract description than a child granule at a lower level. Granules at the same level can be pairwise disjointed or overlapping with each other. It should be noted that although granules in the same level form a granulation, granules in a granulation are not necessarily arranged in a level. Granules in a granulation share the same syntactic properties. For example, they are all defined by conjunctors of the same number of atomic formulas, or they all reside as the leaf nodes of a hierarchical structure.

Partitions and coverings are two commonly used granulations.

### Definition 4

*A partition of a granule* $X$, denoted as $\pi(X)$, is a collection of non-empty and pairwise disjointed granules of $X$ whose union is $X$. A covering of a granule $X$ $_{\text{, denoted as}}$ $\tau(X)$, is a collection of non-empty granules of $X$ whose union is $X$.

According to the definition, a partition consists of disjointed granules of the universe, and a covering consists of possibly overlapping granules. Partitions are a special case of coverings.

In the context of an information table $S$, for any two granulations $\vartheta_1$ and $\vartheta_2$, we can say $\vartheta_1$ is a refinement of $\vartheta_2$, or equivalently, $\vartheta_2$ is a coarsening of $\vartheta_1$, denoted by $\vartheta_1 \sqsubseteq \vartheta_2$, if and only if every granule of $\vartheta_1$ is contained in some granule of $\vartheta_2$. Given two granulations $\vartheta_1$ and $\vartheta_2$, their meet $\vartheta_1 \wedge \vartheta_2$ is the finest granulation of $\vartheta_1$ and $\vartheta_2$ containing all nonempty intersections of a granule from $\vartheta_1$ and a granule from $\vartheta_2$, and their join $\vartheta_1 \vee \vartheta_2$ is the coarsest granulation of $\vartheta_1$ and $\vartheta_2$ containing all non-empty unions of a granule from $\vartheta_1$ and a granule from $\vartheta_2$. The refinement relation of granulations is a partial ordering.

A granulation is called a definable granulation in an information table $S$ if every granule is a definable granule. A granulation is called a conjunctively/disjunctively definable granulation if each granule is defined by a conjunction/disjunction of atomic formulas.

A granulation may not be a partition or a covering of the universe. This is because we often do not have the possibility to consider or manage all the subsets to form a covering. In such a case, the completeness condition of a partition or a covering is not satisfied. The support measure can be extended for evaluating the generality of a granulation $\vartheta$:

$$support(\vartheta) = \frac{|\bigcup\{X \in \vartheta \mid X \subseteq U\}|}{|U|}.$$

If the granulation is a partition or a covering of the universe, then the support equals to one, that is, $support(\pi(U)) = 1$ and $support(\tau(U)) = 1$.

Given two granulations $\vartheta_1$ and $\vartheta_2$ of the same universe, the distance between them can be defined as:

$$dis(\vartheta_1, \vartheta_2) = (1 - \frac{a}{|\cup\{X_1 \in \vartheta_1\}|}) + (1 - \frac{b}{|\cup\{X_2 \in \vartheta_2\}|})$$
$$= 2 - \frac{a}{|\cup\{X_1 \in \vartheta_1\}|} - \frac{b}{|\cup\{X_2 \in \vartheta_2\}|},$$

where $a = |\cup\{X_1 \in \vartheta_1 \mid \exists X_2 \in \vartheta_2 (X_1 \subseteq X_2)\}|$ is the number of granules of $\vartheta_1$ that each is contained in some granule of $\vartheta_2$, and $b = |\cup\{X_2 \in \vartheta_2 \mid \exists X_1 \in \vartheta_1 (X_2 \subseteq X_1)\}|$ is the number of granules of $\vartheta_2$ that each is contained in some granule of $\vartheta_1$. The measure $dis(\vartheta_1, \vartheta_2)$ reaches the minimum value 0 when the two granulations are the same, and reaches the maximum value 2 when every granule of one granulation neither contains nor is contained in some granule of the other. If the distance is equal to or smaller than 1, then one granulation is a refinement of the other.

If the granulation is a covering or a partition of the universe, then the above equation can be rewritten as follows:

$$dis(\vartheta_1, \vartheta_2) = (1 - \frac{a}{|U|}) + (1 - \frac{b}{|U|}) = 2 - \frac{a+b}{|U|}.$$

Chakraborty and Samanta suggest a consistent measure for two knowledges, which also can be used to measure a pair of granulations (2007).

## 2.4 Hierarchies

A hierarchy can be viewed as a family of interacting and interrelated granules, or, a structure of partially ordered granulations, with each level being made up of a family of granules (Yao, 2007). Trees and lattices are typical examples of hierarchical structures that systematically represent problems to be solved. A hierarchy not only makes a complex problem more easily understandable, but also leads to efficient, although perhaps approximate, solutions.

We can construct a hierarchy based on the refinement relation of granulations. Yao *et al.* summarize some hierarchies and their sub-hierarchies (Yao *et al.*, 2005). A definable hierarchy, containing a family of definable granulations, is a sub-hierarchy of a hierarchy. A conjunctively definable hierarchy, containing a family of conjunctively definable granulations, is a sub-hierarchy of a definable hierarchy. Furthermore, a granulation is called an attribute set definable granulation if all granules are conjunctively defined by the same subset of attributes. The family of such granulations forms an attribute set definable hierarchy, which is a sub-hierarchy of a conjunctively definable hierarchy. A granulation is called a tree definable granulation if all granules are conjunctively definable and can form a tree structure. The family of such granulations forms a tree definable hierarchy, which also is a sub-hierarchy of a conjunctively definable hierarchy. It can be proved that when the atomic formulas are defined by the equality relation, both an attribute set definable hierarchy and a tree definable hierarchy also are partition hierarchies. A granulation in the lower level is a finer partition of the granulation in the higher level. The relationships of these hierarchies are illustrated in Figure 1.

The support measure can be extended for evaluating the generality of a hierarchy $H$ :

$$support(H) = \frac{| \bigcup \{X \in \vartheta_l\} |}{|U|},$$

where the granulation $\vartheta_l$ is composed by all the leaf granules of the hierarchy. If the granulation $\vartheta_l$ is a partition or a covering of the universe, then the support equals to one.

## 2.5 Granule Networks

A hierarchy represents a problem from one particular angle or point of view. Some useful information may be lost with a hierarchy instead of a web or a network. For the same problem, many interpretations and descriptions may co-exist. It may be necessary to construct and compare multiple hierarchies. Describing a granule network can facilitate the search for a desired hierarchy or hierarchies.

Many structures have been proposed to describe a granule network of a given universe (Wille, 1992; Yao & Zhou, 2007; Zhao & Yao, 2005; Zhao & Yao, 2007). Generally, each node is a definable non-empty granule, and is labeled by its corresponding formula or formulas. A path from a coarse granule to a fine granule indicates a refinement relation of formulas or a subset relation of granules. Here, we consider two networks, a formula-based network and a granule-based network.

A formula-based network contains all the distinctive formulas, and defines a granulation in terms of the refinement relation of formulas. Suppose only conjunctors are considered, according to a hierarchical structure, the root node is the universe, the biggest granule, defined by the formula $\varnothing$. The second level contains all the granules defined by 1-conjunctors consisting of only one atomic formula; the third level contains all the granules defined by 2-conjunctors consisting of two atomic formulas, and so on. By indicating the level of a granulation, one is able to know the number of atomic formulas in each formula.

*Figure 1. The relationships of different hierarchies*

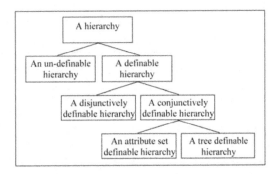

Complementary to a formula-based network, a granule-based network contains all the distinctive definable granules, and defines a granulation in terms of the subset relation of granules. Since the granules are generated from a particular information table, some logical formulas may be invalid, and different formulas may indicate the same granule. For a granule-based network, if two granules $m(\phi) = m(\psi)$ and $\phi$ consists of less atomic formulas than $\psi$ does, then only the shorter formula $\phi$ is used to label the granule. Consequently, all the granules in the granule-based network are defined by their shortest formula.

Let us use a simple example to illustrate the difference between a conjunctor-based network in the logical setting and a granule-based network in the set-theoretic setting. Suppose we have Table 1 with six objects. Each object is defined by three attributes $A$, $B$ and $C$. A conjunctor-based network is illustrated in Figure 2, with all the non-empty granules being shown. The top level is the universe; the second level is the family of 1-conjunctor granules, and so on. The paths coming from the root to the 1-conjunctor granules indicate the refinement relation of formulas. The network has four levels in total. All the distinctive conjunctors are showed in the network. One can use a partition-based method or a covering based method to discover one particular hierarchy.

Figure 3 shows a granule-based network, with all the non-empty granules being shown. The top level is the largest granule, the universe; the second level contains the definable granules $\{2, 3, 4, 5\}$, labeled by the formula $C = c_2$, $\{1, 2, 3\}$ labeled by $B = b_1$, and $\{4, 5, 6\}$ labeled by $B = b_2$. The paths coming from the root to these granules indicate the subset relation of granules. Referring to the conjunctor-based network shown in Figure 2, we can see that the granule $\{4, 5, 6\}$ can be defined by the conjunctors $A = a_3$, $B = b_2$ and $A = a_3 \land B = b_2$. Since the atomic formulas $A = a_3$ and $B = b_2$ are shorter than the conjunctor $A = a_3 \land B = b_2$, thus they both are preserved. The third level contains four definable granules, and they form a finer granulation over the second level. The fourth level contains three definable granules, and they form a finer granulation over the third level.

*Table 1. An information table*

|  | $A$ | $B$ | $C$ |
|---|---|---|---|
| 1 | $a_1$ | $b_1$ | $c_1$ |
| 2 | $a_1$ | $b_1$ | $c_2$ |
| 3 | $a_2$ | $b_1$ | $c_2$ |
| 4 | $a_3$ | $b_2$ | $c_2$ |
| 5 | $a_3$ | $b_2$ | $c_2$ |
| 6 | $a_3$ | $b_2$ | $c_3$ |

## 3. MODELLING CLASSIFICATION

For classification tasks, it is assumed that each object of the universe is associated with a unique class. Without loss of generality, we denote $At = C \cup \{\mathbb{D}\}$, where $C$ is the set of condition attributes that describe the objects, and $\mathbb{D}$ is a decision attribute that indicates the class labels of the objects. Such an information table is also called a decision table. A table with multiple decision attributes can be easily transformed into a table with a single decision attribute by considering the Cartesian product of the original decision attributes.

Suppose the decision attribute $\mathbb{D}$ has $m$ possible values, and thus partitions the universe into $m$ granules, i.e., $\pi_{\mathbb{D}}(U) = \{D_1, D_2, ..., D_m\}$. For any $d_i \in V_{\mathbb{D}}$, $1 \le i \le m$, we denote the definable granule as $D_i = m(\mathbb{D} = d_i)$. A classification task studies the relationship between the granules defined by the decision attribute $\mathbb{D}$ and the granules defined by a subset of condition attributes. We study the classifi-

*Figure 2. A conjunctor-based network*

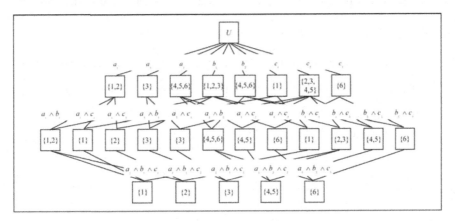

*Figure 3. A granule-based network*

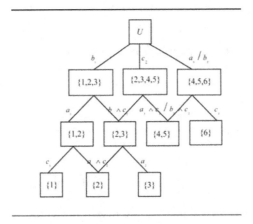

cation of a granule, a granulation containing a family of granules, a hierarchy containing multilevel granulations, and a network containing multiple hierarchies.

## 3.1 Classifying a Granule

## Definition 5

*A granule* $X$ *is consistently classified if* $X \subseteq D_i$ *for some* $D_i \in \pi_{\mathbb{D}}(U)$, *otherwise,* $X$ *is inconsistently classified.*

A consistently classified granule is not necessarily definable. On the other hand, a definable granule is not necessarily consistently classified. If a granule $X$ is consistently classified and defined by a formula $\phi \in L$, then a certain classification rule is in the from of $\phi \rightarrow \mathbb{D} = d_i$, and $X$ is said to be a certain solution to $d_i$. If $X$ is inconsistently classified, then denote $d_{i(X)} \in V_{\mathbb{D}}$ as the class satisfying the majority of $X$, an approximate classification rule is defined as $\phi \rightarrow \mathbb{D} = d_{i(X)}$. The granule $X$ is said to be an approximate solution to the class $d_{i(X)}$. Intuitively, only the objects in the set $X \cap D_{i(X)}$ arc correctly classified, where $D_{i(X)} = m(\mathbb{D} = d_{i(X)})$

Let $\rho : 2^U \rightarrow \Re^+$ be a function to measure the degree of consistency between two granules $X$ and $D_i$, where $\Re^+$ are non-negative real numbers. Two of such measures are discussed below to capture various aspects of classification.

The *sure classification* measure of a granule $X$ is given by:

$$\rho_1(X) = \begin{cases} 1, & X \subseteq D_{i(X)}; \\ 0, & \text{otherwise.} \end{cases}$$

Sure classification represents the degree of objects that can be classified by $d_{i(X)}$ without any uncertainty. The measure $\rho_1(X)$ reaches the maximum value 1 if $X$ is consistently classified, and reaches the minimum value 0 if $X$ is inconsistently classified.

The *accuracy of classification* of a granule $X$ is defined by:

$$\rho_2(X) = \begin{cases} \dfrac{|X \cap D_{i(X)}|}{|X|}, & X \neq \varnothing; \\ 1, & \text{otherwise.} \end{cases}$$

The accuracy of classification of $X$, in fact, is the confidence of the rule $\phi \rightarrow \mathbb{D} = d_{i(X)}$ where $\phi$ defines the set $X$. The measure $\rho_2(X)$ reaches the maximum value 1 if $X$ is consistently classified.

When $\rho_2(X) < 1$, $X$ is inconsistently classified. Given a threshold for the accuracy of classification $\rho_2(X)$, we can prune some of the approximate solutions, and keep only the satisfactory solutions to the classification task. For two granules with $X_1 \subseteq X_2$, we have $\rho_2(X_1) \geq \rho_2(X_2)$. A certain solution is a special case of an approximate solution with $\rho_1(X) = \rho_2(X) = 1$.

## 3.2 Classifying a Granulation

### Definition 6

Granulation $\vartheta$ is consistently cla*ssified if each granule is consistently classified, otherwise,* $\vartheta$ is inconsistently classified.

The condition of each granule being consistently classified requires that each granule $X \in \vartheta$ belongs to some granule of $\pi_\mathbb{D}(U)$. Therefore, a granulation $\vartheta$ is consistently classified if and only if $\vartheta$ is a refinement of $\pi_\mathbb{D}(U)$.

Let $\rho : \Pi \rightarrow \Re^+$ be a function to measure the degree of consistency between the granulation $\vartheta$ and the partition $\pi_\mathbb{D}(U)$. Some of such measures are discussed below.

*Sure classificatio*n of a granulation $\vartheta$ is given by:

$$\rho_1(\vartheta) = \begin{cases} 1, & \vartheta \sqsubseteq \pi_\mathbb{D}; \\ 0, & \text{otherwise.} \end{cases}$$

The measure $\rho_1(\vartheta)$ reaches the maximum value 1 if $\vartheta$ is consistently classified, and reaches the minimum value 0 if $\vartheta$ is inconsistently classified.

Accuracy of classifying a granulation can be defined in two different forms:

$$\rho_2(\vartheta) = \frac{|\bigcup\{X \in \vartheta \mid X \subseteq D_{i(X)}\}|}{|U|};$$

$$\rho_3(\vartheta) = \frac{|\bigcup\{X \cap D_{i(X)} \mid X \in \vartheta\}|}{|U|}.$$

The measure $\rho_2(\vartheta)$ is the ratio of all the objects in the consistently classified granules. It reaches 1 if all the granules are consistently classified. There exist inconsistently classified granules when $\rho_2(\vartheta) < 1$. For two granulations with $\vartheta_1 \sqsubseteq \vartheta_2$, we have $\rho_2(\vartheta_2) \geq \rho_2(\vartheta_1)$. The measure $\rho_3(\vartheta)$ is the ratio of the correctly classified objects in all granules. For two granulations with $\vartheta_1 \sqsubseteq \vartheta_2$, we have $\rho_3(\vartheta_2) \geq \rho_3(\vartheta_1)$. Given thresholds for $\rho_2(\vartheta)$ or $\rho_3(\vartheta)$, we can obtain satisfactory solutions to the classification task.

When the granulation $\vartheta_l$ is considered, we actually evaluate the accuracy of classification of the whole hierarchy. A hierarchy is classified if the granulation $\vartheta_l$ is consistently or satisfactorily classified.

## 3.3 Modelling Classification as a Search in a Granule Network

Given a classification problem, the classification task can be modelled as a search for certain or satisfactory solutions in a search space. Generally, there are two basic search strategies, top-down and bottom-up.

### 3.3.1 Top-Down Algorithms

A top-down algorithm for classification starts the search from the biggest granule and searches down for finer and consistently classified granules. It can search for an attribute that partitions the universe and defines a set of granules, or, search for an attribute-value that covers a portion of the universe and defines one granule. Both a partition-based method and a covering-based method can restrict the searching granules, and facilitate the search for classification solutions.

A partition-based algorithm aims to result in a partition of the universe with each granule being consistently classified or satisfyingly classified by some decision class. The algorithm looks for the most promising attribute to split an examined granule in each round. Each child granule is labeled by one of the possible values of the selected attribute. The child granules naturally cover their parent granule, and pairwise disjoint with each other. A general partition-based algorithm, an ID3-liked algorithm, is illustrated in Algorithm 1.

**Algorithm 1. A general partition-based classification algorithm**

```
Input: an information table S = (U, At = C ∪ {D}, {Vₐ | a ∈ At}, {Iₐ | a ∈ At})
Output: a set of classification rules
While the universe U is not a consistently classified granule and a
finer partition can be induced, do the following:
1. Choose an inconsistently classified granule based on a specific
search strategy.
2. For all attributes in C, choose an attribute a based on a cer-
tain criterion.
3. Partition the inconsistently classified granule based on a. La-
bel each arc coming out from the granule by an atomic formula de-
fined by a and one possible value of a.
4. Repeat Steps 1-3 until all the leaf granules are consistently
classified, or no finer partition can be induced.
5. For each consistently classified leaf granule, construct a rule
in the form of φ → D = d_{i(X)}, where φ is a conjunctor defined by all
atomic formulas along the path from the root to the leaf.
6. Output the rules.
```

The specific search strategy for choosing an inconsistently classified granule can be depth-first, breadth-first or best-first. The standard ID3 algorithm applies the depth-first approach (Quinlan, 1983). A breadth-first approach can be easily simulated (Yao, Zhao & Yao, 2004).

Various measures can be applied in order to find the most promising attribute for partition. For example, Quinlan's ID3 (1983) and C4.5 (1993), as well as Cestnik *et al.*'s ASSISTANT (1987) use information entropy measurements. Breiman and Friedman's CART (1984) uses the *Gini* index. Some measures used for partition-based algorithms are listed below.

$$NumberOfAttribute(a) = |V_a|;$$

$$ConditionalEntropy(a, \mathbb{D}) = -\sum_{v \in V_a} p(a = v) \sum_{d_i \in \mathbb{D}} p(\mathbb{D} = d_i \mid a = v) \log p(\mathbb{D} = d_i \mid a = v)$$

$$= -\sum_{v \in V_a} \sum_{d_i \in \mathbb{D}} p(\mathbb{D} = d_i, a = v) \log p(\mathbb{D} = d_i \mid a = v);$$

$$JointEntropy(a, \mathbb{D}) = -\sum_{v \in V_a} \sum_{d_i \in \mathbb{D}} p(\mathbb{D} = d_i, a = v) \log p(\mathbb{D} = d_i, a = v);$$

$$Gini(a, \mathbb{D}) = 1 - \sum_{v \in V_a} p(a = v) \sum_{d_i \in \mathbb{D}} p^2(\mathbb{D} = d_i \mid a = v).$$

A covering-based algorithm aims to result in a covering of the granule, which is defined by a particular decision class. Each granule of the covering being consistently classified or satisfyingly classified. The algorithm looks for the most promising atomic formulas (attribute-value pairs) that conjunctively classify the decision class. It is possible that the granules being searched overlap. It is easy to understand that covering-based algorithms search a bigger space than partition-based algorithms, and therefore covering-based rules tend to be larger in quantity and more general in quality than partition-based rules. A general covering-based algorithm, a PRISM-liked algorithm, is illustrated in Algorithm 2.

### Algorithm 2. A general covering-based classification algorithm

```
Input: an information table  S = (U, At = C ∪ {𝔻}, {V_a | a ∈ At}, {I_a | a ∈ At})

Output: a set of classification rules
For each  d_i ∈ V_𝔻,  do the following:

1. Choose an atomic formula  φ ∈ L based on a certain criterion;

2. Label the arc towards the granule  m(φ) by  φ;

3. Repeat Steps 1-2 by conjuncting a newly chosen atomic formula
φ' ∈ L to  φ, i.e.,  φ = φ ∧ φ', until  m(φ) is consistently classified

by  d_i or no more atomic formula can be conjuncted.

4. Construct a rule in the form of  φ → 𝔻 = d_i, and remove  m(φ) from

U.

5. Repeat Steps 1-4 until all objects satisfying  𝔻 = d_i have been

removed from U.

6. Output the rules.
```

Many measures can be applied when looking for the most promising attribute-value pairs for composing a covering granule. For example, Cendrowska's PRISM (1987) uses the confidence measure, and Clark and Niblett's CN2 (1989) uses the information entropy. We also can apply the support measure and the distance measure we have previously defined. Some measures used for covering-based algorithms are listed below.

$$confidence(\mathbb{D} = d_i \mid a = v) = p(\mathbb{D} = d_i \mid a = v);$$
$$coverage(\mathbb{D} = d_i \mid a = v) = p(a = v \mid \mathbb{D} = d_i);$$
$$Entropy(a = v) = \sum_{d_i \in \mathbb{D}} p(\mathbb{D} = d_i \mid a = v) \log p(\mathbb{D} = d_i \mid a = v);$$
$$support(m(a = v)) = p(a = v);$$
$$dis(m(\mathbb{D} = d_i), m(a = v)) = 1 - \frac{\mid m(\mathbb{D} = d_i \wedge a = v) \mid}{\mid m(\mathbb{D} = d_i \vee a = v) \mid}.$$

### 3.3.2 Bottom-Up Algorithms

A bottom-up algorithm for classification starts the search from the $\mid C \mid$-conjunctor definable granules, i.e., the individual objects in the information table, and searches up for coarsened and definable granules. The idea of bottom-up algorithms is that if all the child granules are certain solutions, then they are trivial solutions and can be described by their parent granule inductively.

Mitchell (1978) suggests three bottom-up search algorithms implemented in a *version space*. They are the general-to-specific approach, the specific-to-general approach, and a two-way search combining both the directions from general to specific and from specific to general. They are described as Algorithms 3-5.

**Algorithm 3. A bottom-up classification algorithm from specific to general**

```
Input: an information table  S = (U, At = C ∪ {D}, {Vₐ | a ∈ At}, {Iₐ | a ∈ At})
Output: a set of classification rules
For each  dᵢ ∈ V_D,  do the following:

1. Convert all objects in m(D= dᵢ) into positive, and the rest into
negative.
2. Set Φ to be the set of formulas defining all the positive ob-
jects. Let Φ = ∅.
Set N to be the set of all negative objects. Let N = ∅.
3. For each new training object x, do the following:
If x is positive, then
P1. Add the |C|-conjunctor defining x to Φ;

P2. Update Φ so as to ensure that it still contains the set of maxi-
mally specific and satisfactory conjunctors;
P3. Delete all φ ∈ Φ that match a previously observed negative ob-
```

ject $n \in N$.

If $x$ is negative, then

N1. Add $x$ to $N$;

N2. Delete all $\phi \in \Phi$ that match $x$.

4. For each $\phi \in \Phi$, construct a rule in the form of $\phi \Rightarrow \mathbb{D} = d_i$.

5. Output the rules.

## Algorithm 4. A bottom-up classification algorithm from general to specific

Input: an information table $S = (U, At = C \cup \{\mathbb{D}\}, \{V_a \mid a \in At\}, \{I_a \mid a \in At\})$

Output: a set of classification rules

For each $d_i \in V_{\mathbb{D}}$, do the following:

1. Convert all objects in $m(\mathbb{D} = d_i)$ into positive, and the rest into negative.

2. Set $\Phi$ to be the set of formulas defining all the positive objects. Let $\Phi = \varnothing$.

Set $P$ to be the set of all positive objects. Let $P = \varnothing$.

3. For each new training object $x$, do the following:

If $x$ is negative, then

N1. Update $\Phi$ so as to ensure that it still contains the set of maximally general and satisfactory conjunctors;

N2. Delete all $\phi \in \Phi$ that fail to match a previously observed positive object $p \in P$.

If $x$ is positive, then

P1. Add $x$ to $P$;

P2. Delete all $\phi \in \Phi$ that fail to match $x$.

4. For each $\phi \in \Phi$, construct a rule in the form of $\phi \Rightarrow \mathbb{D} = d_i$.

5. Output the rules.

## Algorithm 5. A bottom-up classification algorithm by using a two-way search

Input: an information table $S = (U, At = C \cup \{\mathbb{D}\}, \{V_a \mid a \in At\}, \{I_a \mid a \in At\})$

Output: a set of classification rules

For each $d_i \in V_{\mathbb{D}}$, do the following:

1. Convert all objects in $m(\mathbb{D} = d_i)$ into positive, and the rest into negative.

2. Set $G$ to be the set containing the most general conjunctor, the 0-conjunctor. Set $S$ to be the set containing the most specific conjunctors, the $|C|$-conjunctors.

3. For each new training object, do the following:
If it is positive, then update $S$ so as to ensure that it still contains the set of maximally specific, satisfactory conjunctors;
If it is negative, then update $G$ so as to ensure that it still contains the set of maximally general, satisfactory conjunctors;
4. If $S = G$ then construct a rule in the form of $\phi \rightarrow \mathbb{D} = d_i$.

5. Output the rules.

Algorithm 5 also is termed as an AQ algorithm, which is characterized by Michalski and Larson's AQ11 (1980).

We can compare the top-down and bottom-up strategies from the following two aspects. Firstly, based on the search direction, the top-down strategy starts from the most general granule, and then heuristically searches down for the most promising solutions, while the bottom-up strategy starts from the most specific granules, and consecutively searches up. The names of the two strategies directly come from the search directions they follow.

We then investigate the operations. The top-down strategy starts with the most general formulas and then refines the formulas if the defined granules are not consistently or satisfactorily classified. The bottom-up strategy, on the other hand, starts with finest consistently classified granules regarding a selected decision class, and then try to find more general formulas that can describe all of them but no granules classified by other decision classes. Consequently, the rules produced by top-down algorithms will vary depending on the order in which the atomic formulas are conjuncted. On the other hand, the rules produced by bottom-up algorithms will vary depending on the order in which the training objects present, or say, the order that larger granules are formed. This is computationally more expensive than the rules produced by top-down algorithms. It is prone to disruption by noisy data and inconsistent decision tables. Different operations decide the two strategies looking for different search spaces. The top-down strategy searches consistent granules in a definable search space. More specifically, we can use a conjunctor-based network as the search space. The bottom-up strategy searches logical formulas within consistently classified granules. We thus can search in a granule-based network.

## 4. INTERACTIVE TOP-DOWN CLASSIFICATION AND EXHAUSTIVE BOTTOM-UP CLASSIFICATION

An interactive approach (Zhao & Yao, 2005; Zhao & Yao, 2007) is suggested for searching solutions of classification using a top-down strategy. It not only provides a feasible way for searching in a large and complex search space, but also provides freedom of choices regarding heuristics and measures based on users' needs. It overcomes the limitation of most of the existing automatic classification algorithms that fix on one heuristic to decide where to classify and how to classify.

ICS, using a conjunctor-based network as the search space, is such an interactive classification system (Zhao, Yao & Yan, 2007). The graphical user interface of ICS is shown in Figure 4. The result of the search is a granule tree on the upper left frame. The name of a granule tree is derived from the fact that the classification results are searched in a granule network, and can be arranged as multilevel granulations and organized as a hierarchy.

Users require these three types of information to make a decision for classification.

- First, the user needs to know the classification accuracy of the hierarchy, i.e., the constructed granule tree. At the initial stage, the granule tree only has a root, the entire universe, the biggest granule. If it is not consistently classified by any class, the user starts the classification process, and the granule tree grows branches. The classification accuracy of the hierarchy is the evaluation of the granulation consisted by all the leaf granules.

- Second, the user needs to know the classification accuracy of a selected granulation. Initially, the only granule is the root. If an atomic formula is conjuncted to the root, then the user obtains a 1-conjunctor associated with a subset of the universe. The user can choose any one of the granules to investigate. As a result, he/she can alternatively create a 2-conjunctor granule based on this 1-conjunctor granule, or originate another 1-conjunctor granule based on the root. The classification accuracy of a selected granulation decides either to continue or to cease the classification task.

- Third, the user needs to know the classification accuracy of a selected granule. When a granule is consistently classified, the finer granules of it are all consistently classified, and thus do not need to further classified. When a granule is not yet consistently classified, the user needs to decide which atomic formula can be further conjuncted.

*Figure 4. The graphic user interface of ICS*

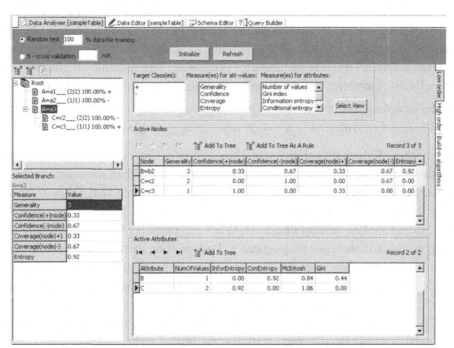

We can use the information Table 1 as an example. Suppose there are two decision classes $\mathbb{D} = +$ and $\mathbb{D} = -$ that induce the partition $\pi_{\mathbb{D}}(U) = \{\{1, 2, 6\}, \{3, 4, 5\}\}$.

To describe and classify both the classes, a partition-based granule tree is required. All attributes and the corresponding measures are of concern. As shown in Figure 4, the table "Active Attributes" contains all the available attributes that can be conjuncted to the selected node $A = a_3$ in the granule tree. The selected measures that are associated to attributes are NumOfValues, InforEntropy, ConEntropy, McIntosh and Gini. Whenever an attribute is selected based on one of these measures, the granules defined by all of its possible values are added to the granule tree, and they are pairwise disjointed. In this example, $C = c_2$ and $C = c_3$ are added to form two conjunctors. The partition-based approach ensures that no portion will be missed for classification. The constructed granule tree is in fact a tree-definable hierarchy, or an attribute set definable hierarchy. For our example, according to the conditional entropy measure, a partition-based granule tree can generate the following four rules as shown in Figure 4:

$$A = a_1 \rightarrow \mathbb{D} = +, \; A = a_2 \rightarrow \mathbb{D} = -, \; A = a_3 \wedge C = c_2 \rightarrow \mathbb{D} = -$$

and $A = a_3 \wedge C = c_3 \rightarrow \mathbb{D} = +$.

If one needs to achieve a partial success, namely, to describe and classify one particular decision class, then a covering-based granule tree is more suitable. In this case, all attribute-value pairs and the corresponding measures are of concern. As shown in Figure 4, the table "Active Nodes" contains all the available attribute value pairs that can be conjuncted to the selected node $A = a_3$ in the granule tree.

The selected measures that are associated to attributes are Generality, Confidence, Coverage and Entropy. Whenever an attribute-value pair is selected according to one of these measures, the granule defined by it is added to the granule tree, and it covers a part of the decision class in concern. It is the user's responsibility to ensure that the decision class is covered by the learned granules. One can apply the depth-first method to explore each granule sequentially, or apply the breath-first method to explore the granules at the same level. A mixture method also is allowed. The constructed granule tree is in fact a conjunctively definable hierarchy. For the running example, suppose the decision class $\mathbb{D} = +$ needs to be classified. According to the conditional probability measure, a covering-based granule tree can generate the following three rules: $A = a_1 \rightarrow \mathbb{D} = +$, $C = c_1 \rightarrow \mathbb{D} = +$ and $C = c_3 \rightarrow \mathbb{D} = +$.

Instead of searching for certain solutions, one sometimes can search for satisfactory solutions. Pre-pruning methods are used by top-down algorithms that prematurely halt the search when a predefined threshold is met. For example, ASSISTANT (Cestnik *et al.*, 1987) and *k*LR (Yao, Zhao & Yao, 2004) use an accuracy threshold as a cut-off criterion, while CN2 (Clark & Niblett, 1989) uses the Laplacian function. One also can apply a support threshold. When the support of a certain granule is too small to be significant as a good solution, one may ignore it. Post-pruning methods consist of three parts. First, grow a decision tree or decision rules for the data. Second, prune from the tree/rules a sequence of subtrees/sub-rules. Finally, try to select from the sequence of subtree/sub-rules which estimates the true regression function as best as possible. The examples of post-pruning algorithms are CART (Breiman *et al.*, 1984) and C4.5 (Quinlan, 1993). According to the three steps, the space complexity for constructing the tree is not saved, but only the rule presentation is simplified and coarsened.

An exhaustive approach is suggested for searching solutions of classification using a bottom-up strategy. A granule-based network is suitable for this task. The search for certain classification solutions can be roughly described as follows. For each $d_i \in V_{\mathbb{D}}$, we do the following. First, label all the leaf nodes that are consistent solutions of the class $d_i$. Then, the process moves upwards. Label a granule as consistently classified if all of its child granules are consistently classified, and unlabel the child granules. Keep moving upwards until it cannot be carried out further. We thus can construct a rule in the form of $\phi \rightarrow \mathbb{D} = d_i$ for each labeled granule, where the formula $\phi$ is the shortest conjunctor defining the granule. An efficient Apriori-liked algorithm can be applied for speeding up the search in a complex search space. This method can be modified to search for both certain and satisfactory solutions of classification, when some evaluation measures are applied in the search process. For our running example, suppose the decision class $\mathbb{D} = +$ needs to be classified. According to the exhaustive bottom-up search algorithm, the smallest leaf granules $\{1\}, \{2\}$ and $\{6\}$ in the granule-based network (Figure 3) are first labeled. By moving upwards, the larger granule $\{1, 2\}$ is labeled instead of its child granules $\{1\}$ and $\{2\}$. As a result, two decision rules can be learned: $A = a_1 \rightarrow \mathbb{D} = +$ and $C = c_3 \rightarrow \mathbb{D} = +$.

## 5. CONCLUSION

Granular computing exploits multilevel and multiview representations in problem solving. A hierarchy represents one view of a problem with multiple levels of granulations. Different hierarchies can be constructed in order to achieve various descriptions and interpretations of the problem. The structure of granular computing, including granules, granulations, hierarchies and multiple hierarchies, can be used for modelling classification tasks ideally. The structure also enables us to study concepts in a logic setting in terms of formulas, and in a set-theoretic setting in terms of granules.

The top-down classification algorithms can be modelled as a search in a formula-based granule network for all consistently or satisfactorily classified granules. An interactive approach has been implemented for the top-down search in a conjunctor-based network. On the other hand, the bottom-up classification algorithms can be modelled as a search in a granule-based network for the formulas that can describe all the consistently classified granules regarding a particular decision class. The heuristics and measures of this approach can be further studied.

## REFERENCES

Bargiela, A., & Pedrycz, W. (2002). *Granular Computing: An Introduction*. Boston: Kluwer Academic Publishers.

Bargiela, A., & Pedrycz, W. (2008). Toward a theory of Granular Computing for human-centered information processing. *IEEE Transactions on Fuzzy Systems*, *16*, 320–330. doi:10.1109/TFUZZ.2007.905912

Breiman, L., Friedman, J. H., Olshen, R. A., & Stone, P. J. (1984). *Classification and regression trees*. Belmont, CA: Wadsworth International Group.

Cendrowska, J. (1987). PRISM: An algorithm for inducing modular rules. *International Journal of Man-Machine Studies, 27,* 349–370. doi:10.1016/S0020-7373(87)80003-2

Cestnik, B., Kononenko, I., & Bratko, I. (1987). ASSISTANT 86: a knowledge-elicitation tool for sophisticated users. In *Proceedings of the 2nd European Working Session on Learning* (pp. 31-45).

Chakraborty, M. K., & Samanta, P. (2007). Consistency-degree between knowledges. In Proceedings of Rough Sets and Intelligent Systems Paradigms (pp.133-142).

Clark, P., & Niblett, T. (1989). The CN2 induction algorithm. *Machine Learning, 3*(4), 261–283. doi:10.1007/BF00116835

Grzymala-Busse, J. W. (1992). LERS:A system for learning from examples based on rough sets. In Slowinski, R. (Ed.), *Intelligent Decision Support* (pp. 3–18). Boston: Kluwer Academic Publishers.

Grzymala-Busse, J. W. (2005). LERS:A data mining system. In *The Data Mining and Knowledge Discovery Handbook* (pp. 1347–1351). Boston: Kluwer Academic Publishers. doi:10.1007/0-387-25465-X_65

Inuiguchi, M., Hirano, S., & Tsumoto, S. (Eds.). (2003). *Rough Set Theory and Granular Computing.* Berlin, Germany: Springer.

Lin, T. Y. (2003). Granular computing. In *Proceedings of the 9th International Conference of Rough Sets, Fuzzy Sets, Data Mining, and Granular Computing* (LNCS 2639, pp. 16-24).

Lin, T. Y., Yao, Y. Y., & Zadeh, L. A. (Eds.). (2002). *Data Mining, Rough Sets and Granular Computing.* Heidelberg: Physica-Verlag.

Michalski, R., & Larson, J. (1980). *Incremental generation of vl1 hypotheses: the underlying methodology and the description of program AQ11 (Technical Report ISG 83-5).* Urbana-Champaign, IL: Computer Science Department, University of Illinois.

Mitchell, T. M. (1978). *Version Spaces: An Approach to Concept Learning* (Ph.D. Thesis). Stanford, CA: Computer Science Department, Stanford University.

Pal, S. K. (2004). Soft data mining, computational theory of perceptions, and rough-fuzzy approach. *Information Sciences, 163,* 5–12. doi:10.1016/j.ins.2003.03.014

Pawlak, Z. (1982). Rough sets. *International Journal of Computer and Information Sciences, 11*(5), 341–356. doi:10.1007/BF01001956

Pawlak, Z. (1991). *Rough Sets:Theoretical Aspects of Reasoning about Data.* Boston: Kluwer Publishers.

Polkowski, L., & Artiemjew, P. (2007). On granular rough computing: factoring classifiers through granulated decision systems. In *Proceedings of the International Conference on Rough Sets and Emerging Intelligent Systems Paradigms* (LNAI 4585, pp. 280–289).

Quinlan, J. R. (1983). Learning efficient classification procedures and their application to chess endgames. In Michalski, J. S., Carbonell, J. G., & Mitchell, T. M. (Eds.), *Machine Learning: An Artificial Intelligence Approach* (pp. 463–482). San Francisco: Morgan Kaufmann.

Quinlan, J. R. (1993). *C4.5: Programs for Machine Learning.* San Francisco: Morgan Kaufmann.

Wille, R. (1992). Concept lattices and conceptual knowledge systems. *Computers & Mathematics with Applications (Oxford, England)*, *23*, 493–515. doi:10.1016/0898-1221(92)90120-7

Yao, J. T. (2007). A ten-year review of granular computing. In *Proceedings of the 3rd IEEE International Conference on Granular Computing* (pp. 734-739).

Yao, J. T., Yao, Y. Y., & Zhao, Y. (2005). Foundations of classification. In Lin, T. Y., Ohsuga, S., Liau, C. J., & Hu, X. (Eds.), *Foundations and Novel Approaches in Data Mining* (pp. 75–97). Berlin, Germany: Springer. doi:10.1007/11539827_5

Yao, Y. Y. (2006). Three perspectives of granular computing. *Journal of Nanchang Institute of Technology*, *25*(2), 16–21.

Yao, Y. Y. (2007). The art of granular computing. In *Proceeding of the International Conference on Rough Sets and Emerging Intelligent Systems Paradigms* (LNAI 4585, pp. 101-112).

Yao, Y. Y., & Yao, J. T. (2002). Granular computing as a basis for consistent classification problems. In *Proceedings of PAKDD Workshop on Toward the Foundation of Data Mining, 5*(2), 101-106.

Yao, Y. Y., Zhao, Y., & Yao, J. T. (2004). Level construction of decision trees in a partition-based framework for classification. In Proceedings of Software Engineering and Knowledge Engineering (pp. 199-205).

Yao, Y. Y., & Zhou, B. (2007). A logic language of granular computing. In *Proceedings of the 6th IEEE International Conference on Cognitive Informatics* (pp. 178-185).

Zadeh, L. A. (1997). Towards a theory of fuzzy information granulation and, its centrality in human reasoning and fuzzy logic. *Fuzzy Sets and Systems*, *19*, 111–127. doi:10.1016/S0165-0114(97)00077-8

Zadeh, L. A. (1998). Some reflections on soft computing, granular computing, and their roles in the conception, design and utilization of information/intelligent systems. *Soft Computing, 2*, 23–25. doi:10.1007/s005000050030

Zhao, Y., & Yao, Y. Y. (2005). Interactive user-driven classification using a granule network. In *Proceedings of the Fifth International Conference of Cognitive Informatics* (pp. 250-259).

Zhao, Y., & Yao, Y. Y. (2007). Interactive classification using a granule network. In Wang, Y. X. (Ed.). International Journal of Cognitive Informatics and Natural Intelligence, 1(4), 87-97.

Zhao, Y., Yao, Y. Y., & Yan, M. W. (2007). ICS: an interactive classification system. In *Proceedings of the 20th Canadian Conference on Artificial Intelligence* (pp. 134-145).

Zhong, N., Dong, J. Z., Liu, C. N., & Ohsuga, S. (2001). A hybrid model for the discovery in data. *Knowledge-Based Systems*, *14*, 397–412. doi:10.1016/S0950-7051(01)00153-8

# Chapter 14
# Discovering Perceptually Near Granules

**James F. Peters**
*University of Manitoba, Canada*

## ABSTRACT

*The problem considered in this chapter is how to discover perceptual granules that are in some sense near each other. One approach to the solution to the problem of discovering perceptual granules close to each other comes from near set theory. This is made clear in this chapter by considering various nearness relations that define coverings of sets of perceptual objects that are near each other. A perceptual granule is something that is graspable by the senses or by the mind. Every perceptual granule is represented by a set of perceptual objects that have their origin in the physical world. This means that a perceptual granule does not include the empty set. Hence, each family of perceptual granules is a dual chopped lattice. Both perceptual near sets and tolerance near sets are presented in this chapter. Both the theory and applications of perceptually near granules are presented in this chapter.*

## 1. INTRODUCTION

*The better theory is the more precise description of the [object] it provides. –Ewa Orlowska, Studia Logica, 1990.*

The main problem considered in this chapter is how to discover perceptual granules that are in some sense close to each other. An approach to the solution to this problem comes from near set theory (see, e.g., Peters (2007c, 2007d), Peters and Wasilewski (2009), Peters (2010)). Perceptual objects that have similar appearance are considered perceptually near each other, i.e., perceived objects that have matching or, at least, similar descriptions. A description is a tuple of values of functions representing perceptual object features.

DOI: 10.4018/978-1-60566-324-1.ch014

Near set theory provides a basis for observation, comparison and classification of perceptual granules. That is, this article considers relations between perceptual granules that are near sets. A *perceptual granule* is a set of perceptual objects originating from observations of objects in the physical world. Near sets are disjoint sets that resemble each other. Sets of perceptual objects where two or more of the elements objects have similar descriptions are penultimate near sets. Work on a basis fornear sets began in 2002, motivated by image analysis and inspired by a study of the perception of the nearness of physical objects carried out in cooperation with Zdzisław Pawlak in (Pawlak and Peters, 2002). This initial work led to the introduction of near sets (Peters, 2007b), elaborated in (Peters, 2007c), (Peters and Wasilewski, 2008), including tolerance near sets (Peters, 2009a), (Peters, 2010), (Pal & Peters (2010) having strong affinities with proximity space theory (Naimpally & Warrack (1970)),. Perceptual granules are markedly different from classical information granules. Basically, a perceptual granual is extracted from a physical continuum based on perception. By contrast, a classical information granule (at least in the rough set approach to information granulation) is extracted from an information table. The main idea for perceptual granules and perceptually near granules comes from Henri Poincaré (Poincare, 1905). The physical continuum (*with elements that are sets of sensations such as light intensities in a visual space*) are contrasted with the mathematical continuum (real numbers) where almost solutions are common and given equations have no exact solutions. An *almost solution* of an equation (or a system of equations) is an object which, when substituted into the equation, transforms it into a numerical 'almost identity', i.e., a relation between numbers which is true only approximately (within a prescribed tolerance) (Sossinsky, 1986). The idea of an almost solution leads to the creation of tolerance perceptually near granules that are introduced in this article. A perception-based approach to discovering resemblances between disjoint sets of perceptual objects such as digital images leads to a tolerance space form of near sets that models human perception in a physical continuum (Peters, 2009a, 2010).

Near set theory begins with the selection of probe functions that provide a basis for describing and discerning affinities between objects in distinct perceptual granules (see, *e.g.*, Peters (2007a, 2007b, 2007c, 2007d), Peters (2008a, 2008b), Skowron and Peters (2008)). Probe functions are real-valued functions representing features of physical objects such as image patches in digital images or behaviours of individual biological organisms or swarms of organisms or collections of artificial organisms such as robot societies (Henry and Peters (2007), Pavel (1993), Peters (2007a, 2007b)). It is also the case that various nearness relations define coverings of sample perceptual granules. A catalogue of a wide spectrum of perceptual granules that result from such coverings is included in this chapter. By way of illustration of the basic approach to the granulation of perceptual objects, sample near images and communicating systems designs, are considered in this chapter. Comparisons across coverings of different perceptual granules (*i.e.*, comparison of descriptions of classes of perceptual objects in such partitions) defined by nearness relations facilitate observation and classification of perceptual granules.

Robert Hooke (1665) provides a good paradigm for the discovery of perceptual granules. For Hooke, one either observes with the senses objects that can be described sufficiently for understanding (if one were to tell some else what has been observed). Or one observes with the help sensors or scientific instruments such as a microscope, binoculars, magnifying glass or hearing aid (if sound is of interest). In the first case, the senses usually are sufficient for observing the behaviour of organisms (this is the ethological approach to discovering perceptual granules). In the second case, there many features of physical objects that escape the senses. In that case, the features of granules can be discovered by some form of magnification.

Another means of discovering perceptual granules was suggested by Charles Darwin (1859), who called attention to affinities that one can observe between different members of the same species (see, *e.g.*, Figure 1). The basic idea is start with a set of sample perceptual objects O, partitioning O provisionally, and either adding new objects similar to ones in existing classes in the partition of O or by beginning a new partition of O with classes containing newly discovered objects with distinguishing features. This is analogous to what Charles Darwin did during the voyage of the H.M.S. Beagle during the 1830s, starting in 1831 and ending in 1836. That is, Darwin (1845) kept adding to his collection of specimens (Keynes, 2000) and eventually, in some cases, found affinities between a set of specimens of interest and his expanding set of specimens found during the voyage of the Beagle. There are 3 smaller mollusc snail shells (class Gastropoda) grouped together on the lefthand side of Figure 1 (the affinities of these shells can be gauged by their colour, shape and size). Similarly, the 2 snail shells on the righthand side of Figure 1 have obvious affinities. It also possible to find parallels between the original approach to approximation introduced by Zdzisław Pawlak (1981) and Darwin's classification method during his search for the origin of selected species during the voyage of the H.M.S. Beagle, Darwin (1845).

A lattice structure for families of perceptual granules is considered in this chapter. First, observe that each perceptual granule is defined by a set of perceptual objects that have their origin in the physical world. This means that a perceptual granule does not include the empty set. This leads to the observation that each family of perceptual granules is a dual chopped lattice. In effect, lattice theory (Grätzer (1978, 2006), Grätzer and Lasker (1968)) provides a foundation for perceptual granule theory. The dual chopped lattice structure of families of perceptual granules is directly related to a recent result in near set theory, namely, each family of near sets is a dual chopped lattice (Peters and Wasilewski (2009)).

This chapter is organized as follows. Perceptual objects, perceptual granules, and perceptual systems are defined in Section 2. In Section 3, nearness relations are briefly considered. Near perceptual granules are considered in Section 4. Perceptual near sets are defined in Section 5. Probabilistically near communicating systems are briefly introduced in Section 6. Rough sets as near perceptual granules are briefly considered in Section 7.

## 2. PERCEPTUAL OBJECTS, PERCEPTUAL GRANULES, AND PERCEPTUAL SYSTEMS

Perceptual objects are known by their descriptions. A *perceptual object* is something presented to the senses or knowable by the mind OED (1933). Examples of perceptual objects include observable organism

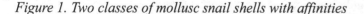

*Figure 1. Two classes of mollusc snail shells with affinities*

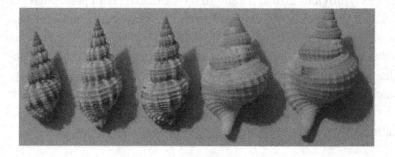

behaviour, growth rates, soil erosion, events containing the outcomes of experiments such as energizing a network, testing digital camera functions, microscope images, MRI scans, and the results of searches for relevant web pages. In keeping with the approach to pattern recognition suggested by Pavel (1993), the features of a perceptual object are represented by probe functions or, simply, by probes. Examples of probes are functions that measure such things as conditional probability, contour, colour, shape, texture, and bilateral symmetry. In general, a probe function can be thought of as a sensor. The introduction of probe functions opens the door to a study of feature extraction and object recognition (see, *e.g.*, Henry and Peters (2007)) normally carried out in science and pattern recognition. A probe makes it possible to determine if two objects are associated with the same pattern without necessarily specifying which pattern (classification). A detailed explanation about probe functions vs. attributes in the classification of objects is given in Peters (2007a, 2007b).

An *object description* is defined by means of a tuple of function values $\varphi(x)$ associated with a perceptual object $x \in X$ (see Table 1). The important thing to notice is the choice of functions $\varphi_i \in B$ used to describe an object of interest. Assume that $B \subseteq F$ (see Table 1) is a given set of functions representing features of sample objects O. Let $X \subseteq O$ and let $\varphi_i \in B$, where $\varphi_i: O \rightarrow R$. In combination, the functions representing object features provide a basis for an *object description* $\varphi: O \rightarrow R^L$, a vector containing measurements (returned values) associated with each functional value $\varphi_i(x)$ for $x \in X$, where $|\varphi| = L$, i.e. the description length is L. In general, an object description has the form shown in (1).

$$\varphi_B(x) = (\varphi_1(x), \ldots, \varphi_i(x), \ldots, \varphi_L(x)). \tag{1}$$

The intuition underlying a description $\varphi_B(x)$ is a recording of measurements from sensors, where each sensor is modeled by a function $\varphi_i$.

*Table 1. Description symbols*

| Symbol | Interpretation |
|---|---|
| R | Set of real numbers, |
| O | Set of perceptual objects, |
| X | $X \subseteq O$, a perceptual granule, |
| x | $x \in X$, sample object in perceptual granule X, |
| F | Set of functions representing object features, |
| $B$ | $B \subseteq F$, set of sample functions representing object features, |
| $\varphi$ | $\varphi: O \rightarrow R^L$, object description, |
| L | Description length, |
| $\varphi_i$ | $\varphi_i \in B$, where $\varphi_i: O \rightarrow R$, probe function, |
| $\varphi_B(x)$ | $\varphi_B(x) = (\varphi_1(x), \ldots, \varphi_i(x), \ldots, \varphi_L(x))$, description of x, |
| <O, F > | perceptual system, |
| $PG_F(O)$ | Family of perceptual granules, i.e. collection of all subsets of O. |

*Figure 2. Sample finite lattices*

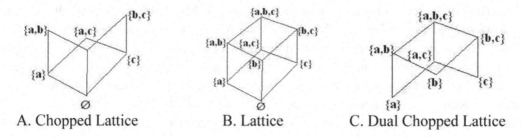

A. Chopped Lattice       B. Lattice       C. Dual Chopped Lattice

## Definition 2.1: Perceptual Granule

A perceptual granule is a finite, non-empty set $O_F$ (for simplicity, O is an abbreviation for $O_F$) containing sample perceptual objects with common descriptions. The empty set $\varnothing$ is not a perceptual granule, since it contains no objects. Hence, the empty set is not contained in $O_F$.

Let $PG_F(O)$ denote the family of finite, non-empty perceptual granules (i.e., collection of all subsets of $O_F$, not including the empty set). That is, $PG_F(O) = \{X \mid X \subseteq O_F, X \neq \varnothing\}$.

## 2.1 Perceptual Granules as Dual Chopped Lattices

It can be shown that $PG_F(O)$ is a particular form of finite lattice called a dual chopped lattice (see Figure 2C) described by Grätzer (2006). This can be explained with a proof-by-picture approach.

Let $O = \{a, b, c\}$ be a non-empty set of perceptual objects. The subsets of O such as $\{a, b\}$ are examples of perceptual granules. The family of perceptual granules $PG_F(O)$ is an example of particular form of lattice (see Figure 2B).

Briefly, a binary relation $\leq$ is a *partial order* of X when it is reflexive, transitive, and antisymmetric, Birkhoff and MacLane (1967), for example, $PG_F(O)$ is a partially ordered set (poset) under the inclusion relation $\subseteq$. The relation $\subseteq$ is *antisymmetric*, since $A \subseteq B$ and $B \subseteq A$ implies that $A = B$ for A, $B \subseteq PG_F(O)$. An element $U \subseteq PG_F(O)$ is an upper bound if for A, $B \subseteq PG_F(O)$ when both $A \subseteq U$ and $B \subseteq U$. An element $L \subseteq PG_F(O)$ is a *join* (i.e., least upper bound) of A, $B \subseteq PG_F(O)$ when it is an upper bound contained in all other upper bounds of A and B, i.e., $A \subseteq L$ and $B \subseteq L$. Union $\cup$ is the *join operation* defined on $PG_F(O)$. The *meet* of A, $B \subseteq PG_F(O)$ is the greatest lower bound of A and B. Intersection $\cap$ is the meet operation defined on $PG_F(O)$.

A *lattice* is a poset in which any two elements have both a meet and a join. For example, $< PG_F(O)$, $\cup, \cap>$ is a lattice (see, e.g., Figure 2B). An algebra $< PG_F(O), \cap>$ is an example of a meet-semilattice if and only if $\cap$ is a binary operation of $PG_F(O)$ that is idempotent, commutative and associative.

For simplicity, only a particular chopped lattice is defined, here. Briefly, an (n-ary) partial operation on a non-empty set X is a mapping from a subset of $X^n$ to X. A *chopped lattice*, Grätzer and Lasker (1968), Grätzer (1978) is a partial algebra such as $< PG_F(O), \cup, \cap>$, where $< PG_F(O), \cap>$ is a semilattice and $\cup$ is a partial operation on $PG_F(O)$. A more general view of chopped lattices is given in Grätzer (2006) and not included, here. A chopped lattice is easily obtained from a lattice by removing unit, e.g., the set O from $PG_F(O)$. An example of a finite chopped lattice for a 3-element set is shown in Figure 4A. A *dual chopped lattice* is obtained by removing the empty set from a finite lattice.

An algebra $< PG_F(O), \cup, \cap >$ is a dual chopped lattice if and only if the algebra $< PG_F(O), \cap >$ is a join semilattice and $\cap PG_F(O) \times PG_F(O) \to PG_F(O)$ is a partial function such that $A \cap B$ is the greatest lower bound of two perceptual granules $A, B \subseteq PG_F(O)$ provided $A \cap B \subseteq PG_F(O)$, which is the case with the family of perceptual granules. From Definition 2.1, the empty set $\notin PG_F(O)$. Hence, informally, the following observation can be made.

## Observation 2.1

The family of perceptual granules $PG_F(O)$ is a dual chopped lattice.

This observation is a direct result of recent work on near set theory, since it can be proved that each family of near sets from a finite, non-empty set of perceptual granules is a dual chopped lattice, Peters and Wasilewski (2008). Let $Near_F(O)$ denote a family of near sets. Notice that the empty set is not included in merology, Wolenski (2001). This also means that each family of perceptual granules $(PG_F(O))$, family of near sets $(Near_F(O))$ and mereology have something in common, i.e., perceptual granules, near sets and mereology have no empty set.

## 2.2 Perceptual Systems

Let $X, Y \subseteq O$ denote sets of perceptual objects. Sets $X, Y$ are considered near each other if, and only if $X$ and $Y$ contain perceptual objects with at least partial matching descriptions.

### Definition 2.1: Perceptual System (Peters (2007b), Peters and Wasilewski (2009), Peters (2010))

A *perceptual system* (is denoted by $<O, F>$, where $O$ is a set of perceptual objects and $F$ is a set of probe functions.

Let $x_1, ..., x_r \in O$ and $\varphi_1, ..., \varphi_c \in F$. A perceptual system $<O, F>$ is can be represented in table form as shown in Figure 4.

In Figure 3, the general form of a description in (1) is instantiated by using particular probe functions $\varphi_1, ..., \varphi_i, ..., \varphi_L \in F$ where $\varphi_i: O \to R$ in an object description $\varphi: O \to R^L$ for a particular perceptual object such as $x_r$ in the sample description in (2).

$$\phi_B(x_r) = \phi_1(x_r), \ ... \ , \phi_L(x_r). \tag{2}$$

In effect, the object description $\phi(x_r)$ in (2) is a point in $R^L$ with coordinates represented by probe function values. The descriptions represented in the table in Figure 4 each have length $L = c$, where $c$ is the number of columns (not including column X) in Figure 3.

The notion of a perceptual system was introduced by Peters (2007a, 2007b) and elaborated in Peters and Wasilewski (2009), Peters (2010). The idea of a perceptual system has its origins in earlier work on granulation by Peters, Skowron, Synak and Ramanna (2003) and in the study of rough set-based ethology by Peters, Henry and Ramanna (2005a) and by Peters (2005b). Such a system is a new perception-based interpretation of the traditional notion of a deterministic information system (Pawlak (1981)) as a real-

*Figure 3. Representation of a perceptual system*

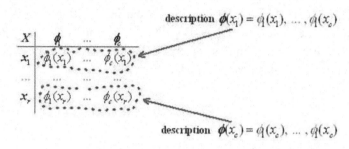

*Figure 4. Satellite images of North Basin, Lake Winnipeg from McCullough (2007)*

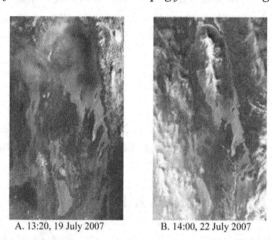

A. 13:20, 19 July 2007     B. 14:00, 22 July 2007

valued, total, deterministic information system. Non-deterministic information systems were introduced by Lipski (1981) and elaborated by Pawlak and Orłowska (1984); see, also, Sakai and Okuma (2004). Deterministic information systems were introduced independently by Pawlak (1981) and elaborated by Orlowska (1998); see, also, Polkowski (2002). It was also Orłowska (1982, 1985) who originally suggested that an approximation space provides a formal basis for perception or observation. This view of approximation spaces captures the kernel of near set theory, where perception is viewed at the level of classes in coverings of perceptual granules rather than at the level of individual objects (see, e.g., Peters (2007a, 2007b, 2007c, 2007d, 2008a, 2009a, 2010), Peters, Skowron and Stepaniuk (2007)).

## 3. NEARNESS RELATIONS

**Approximate**, *a [L. approximat-us to draw near to.]***A.** *adj.***1.** *Very near, in position or in character; closely situated; nearly resembling.*

*–Oxford English Dictionary, 1933.*

*Table 2. Nearness relation symbols*

| Symbol | Interpretation |
|---|---|
| $\sim_{\mathrm{F}}$ | $\left\{\left(x,y\right) \in O \times O \mid \forall \phi_i \in \mathcal{F}.\phi_i(x) = \phi_i(y)\right\}$, indiscernibility relation, |
| $\cong_{\mathcal{F}}$ | weak indiscernibility (wi) relation, |
| $\cong_{\mathcal{F},\varepsilon}$ | weak tolerance nearness relation (wt), |
| $\rhd\lhd_{\mathcal{F}}$ | nearness relation symbol, |
| $\underline{\rhd\lhd}_{\mathcal{F}}$ | weak nearness relation symbol, |
| $\underline{\underline{\rhd\lhd}}_{\mathcal{F}}$ | weak tolerance nearness relation symbol. |

The basic idea in the perceptual near set approach to object recognition is to compare object descriptions. Sample perceptual objects are perceptually near each other if and only if the objects have similar descriptions. Recall that each set of functions representing perceptual object features defines a description of an object (see Table 1). To establish a nearness relation, we first consider the traditional indiscernibility relation. Let $B \subseteq F$ be a set of functions representing object features. The *indiscernibility* relation $\sim_B$ introduced by Zdzisław Pawlak (1981) is distinguished from the *weak indiscernibility* relation $\cong_{\mathcal{F}}$ introduced by Ewa Orłowska (1982). In keeping, with the original indiscernibility relation symbol $\sim_F$ introduced by Pawlak (1981), the symbol $\cong_{\mathcal{F}}$ is used instead of the original weak indiscernibility relation *wind* symbol proposed by Orłowska (1998).

## Definition 3.1: Indiscernibility Relation (Pawlak, 1981)

Let <O, F > be a perceptual system. The indiscernibility relation $\sim_F$ is defined as follows:

$$\sim_{\mathcal{F}} = \left\{\left(x,y\right) \in O \times O \mid \forall \phi_i \in \mathcal{F}.\phi_i(x) = \phi_i(y)\right\}$$

## Definition 3.2: Weak Indiscernibility Relation (Orłowska, 1998)

Let <O, F > be a perceptual system. The weak indiscernibility relation $\cong_F$ is defined as follows:

$$\cong_{\mathcal{F}} = \left\{\left(x,y\right) \in O \times O \mid \exists \phi_i \in \mathcal{F}.|\ (x) = \phi_i(y)\ |= 0\right\}$$

## Definition 3.2: Weak Tolerance Relation

Let $<O, F>$ be a perceptual system. For $\varepsilon \in [0, 1]$, $B \in F$, the weak tolerance relation $\underset{B,\varepsilon}{\simeq}$ is defined as follows:

$$\underset{B,\varepsilon}{\simeq} = \left\{ (x,y) \in O \times O \mid \left| \phi_B(x) - \phi_B(y) \right| \le \varepsilon \right\}.$$

That is, in general, the relation $\underset{B,\varepsilon}{\simeq}$ is reflexive and symmetric but not transitive.

## Definition 3.3: Nearness Relation (Peters and Wasilewski (2009))

Let $<O, F>$ be a perceptual system and let $X, Y \subseteq O$. The set X is perceptually near to the set Y ($X \bowtie_{F} Y$), if and only if there are $x \in X$ and $y \in Y$ such that $x \sim_F y$.

## Definition 3.4: Weak Nearness Relation (Peters and Wasilewski (2009))

Let $<O, F>$ be a perceptual system and let $X, Y \subseteq O$. The set X is perceptually near to the set Y ($X \bowtie_{F} Y$), if and only if there exists $\varphi_i \in F$, $x \in X$ and $y \in Y$ such that $x \simeq_{\phi_i} y$.

## Definition 3.4: Weak Tolerance Nearness Relation

Let $<O, F>$ be a perceptual system and let $X, Y \subseteq O$, $\varepsilon \in [0, 1]$. The set X is perceptually near to the set Y ($X \bowtie_{F} Y$), if and only if there exists $\varphi_i \in F$, $x \in X$ and $y \in Y$ such that $x \simeq_{\phi_i,\varepsilon} y$.

The weak nearness relation $\bowtie_{F}$ is useful in cases where comparisons of object descriptions depend on fine-grained (i.e., matching) feature values. For example, in comparing human DNA samples and fingerprints, exact matches of feature values are often required. The weak tolerance nearness relation $\bowtie_{F}$ is a direct result of work on weak nearness relations by Peters and Wasilewski (2009) and Peters (2009a, 2010). This form of a nearness relation is particularly useful in discovering perceptual granules containing classes of objects with approximately the same description. Such granules commonly occur in cases where exact matches between probe function values in object descriptions are not necessary or are less likely. For example, in comparing segmented satellite images, areas of the segmentations can be compared using the weak tolerance nearness relation in partitioning segmented images into regions containing pixel windows with approximately the same descriptions. In this case, a perceptual granule consists of a class of objects with similar descriptions within some $\varepsilon$ (Peters (2009a, 2010), Pal & Peters (2010)). A brief summary of some of the perceptual granules* that result from the relations introduced in this chapter is given in Table 3.

*Table 3. Perceptual granules from near set theory*

| Symbol | Interpretation |
|---|---|
| $O/\sim_{\mathcal{F}}$ | $\{x/\sim_{\mathcal{F}} \mid x \in O\}$, set of equivalence classes, |
| $O/\simeq_{\mathcal{F}}$ | $\{x/\simeq_{\mathcal{F}} \mid x \in O\}$, set of wi classes, |
| $O/\simeq_{\mathcal{F},\mathcal{E}}$ | $\{x/\simeq_{\mathcal{B},\mathcal{E}} \mid x \in O\}$, set of wt classes, |
| $x/\sim_{\mathcal{F}}$ | $x/\sim_{\mathcal{F}} = \{y \in X \mid y \sim_{\mathcal{F}} x\}$, equivalence class, |
| $x/\simeq_{\mathcal{F}}$ | $x/\simeq_{\mathcal{F}} = \{y \in X \mid y \simeq_{\mathcal{F}} x\}$, weak indiscernibililty (wi) class, |
| $x/\simeq_{\mathcal{F},\mathcal{E}}$ | $x/\simeq_{\mathcal{F},\mathcal{E}} = \{y \in X \mid y \simeq_{\mathcal{F},\mathcal{E}} x\}$, weak tolerance (wt) class, |
| $x/\sim_{\mathcal{F}}$ | $x/\sim_{\mathcal{F}} = \{y \in X \mid y \sim_{\mathcal{F}} x\}$, perceptual granule (equivalence class), |
| $x/\simeq_{\mathcal{F}}$ | $x/\simeq_{\mathcal{F}} = \{y \in X \mid y \simeq_{\mathcal{F}} x\}$, perceptual granule (wi class), |
| $x/\simeq_{\mathcal{F},\mathcal{E}}$ | $x/\simeq_{\mathcal{F},\mathcal{E}} = \{y \in X \mid y \simeq_{\mathcal{F},\mathcal{E}} x\}$, perceptual granule (wt class), |
| $O/\sim_{\mathcal{F}}$ | $O/\sim_{\mathcal{F}} = \{x/\sim_{\mathcal{F}} \mid x \in O\}$, quotient set (set of classes), |
| $O/\simeq_{\mathcal{F}}$ | $O/\simeq_{\mathcal{F}} = \{x/\simeq_{\mathcal{F}} \mid x \in O\}$, quotient set (set of classes), |
| $O/\simeq_{\mathcal{F},\mathcal{E}}$ | $O/\simeq_{\mathcal{F},\mathcal{E}} = \{x/\simeq_{\mathcal{F},\mathcal{E}} \mid x \in O\}$, quotient set (set of classes), |
| $\Pi(O, \mathcal{F}, \sim_{\mathcal{F}})$ | $\bigcup\{O/\sim_{\mathcal{B}} \mid \mathcal{B} \subseteq \mathcal{F}\}$, family of all quotient sets defined by $\sim_{\mathcal{F}}$, |
| $\Pi(O, \mathcal{F}, \simeq_{\mathcal{F}})$ | $\bigcup\{O/\simeq_{\mathcal{B}} \mid \mathcal{B} \subseteq \mathcal{F}\}$, family of all quotient sets defined by $\simeq_{\mathcal{F}}$, |
| $\Pi(O, \mathcal{F}, \simeq_{\mathcal{F},\mathcal{E}})$ | $\bigcup\{O/\simeq_{\mathcal{B},\mathcal{E}} \mid \mathcal{B} \subseteq \mathcal{F}\}$, family of all quotient sets defined by $\simeq_{\mathcal{F},\mathcal{E}}$, |
| $\sim_{\mathcal{F}}$ | indiscernibility relation, |
| $\bowtie_{\mathcal{F}}$ | nearness relation, |
| $\underline{\bowtie}_{\mathcal{F}}$ | weak nearness relation, |
| $\underline{\underline{\bowtie}}_{\mathcal{F}}$ | weak tolerance nearness relation, |
| $PG_{\mathcal{F}}(O)$ | $PG_{\mathcal{F}}(O) = \{X \mid X \subseteq O_{\mathcal{F}}, X \neq \varnothing\}$, family of perceptual granules, |
| $Near_{\mathcal{F}}(O)$ | family of near sets introduced by Peters and Wasilewski (2008) |

## 4. NEAR PERCEPTUAL GRANULES

Examples of perceptual granules that are near each other are briefly described in this section. Extensive coverage of perceptually near digital images, both theory and numerous applications, are given in (Pal & Peters (2010)). Near set theory was originally inspired by a comparison of pairs of digital images that are perceptually but not necessarily spatially near each other. This is the basic idea in Example 4.1. A practical application of the weak tolerance nearness relation is given in terms of a comparison of satellite images in Example 4.2.

## Example 4.1 Near Images

Let <Im, F> be a perceptual system for a sample space Im containing images and a set of probe functions F representing image features. Each image is a composite of n × n pixel windows. Let x ∈ X, y ∈ Y denote pixel windows in images X and Y. Let $\bar{g}$ : Im → $\Re$ denote a function that maps each pixel window to the average grey level of the pixels in the window. Image X is weakly near image Y (X $\underset{\overset{\unlhd}{=}}{\unrhd}$, Y) if and only if there exists x ∈ X, y ∈ Y such that $x \underset{\bar{g},\varepsilon}{\simeq} y$, i.e., $\left| \bar{g}(x) - \bar{g}(y) \right| \leq \varepsilon$.

## Example 4.2 Near Satellite Images

This example suggests an approach to comparing satellite images useful in geographic information systems. Let <Im, F> be a perceptual system for sample space Im containing satellite images and a set of probe functions F = { $\bar{g}$ } defined in Example 4.1. The discovery of perceptual granules in satellite images is illustrated in terms of the images in Figure 4. For example, Figure 4A shows a satellite image taken of the North Basis, south of Long Point, Lake Winnipeg, Manitoba in the early afternoon of 19 July 2007. In Figure 4B, a satellite image for the same Lake Winnipeg location taken 3 days later from McCullough (2007). There is interest in assessing the closeness (weak nearness) of satellite images by way of investigating such things as changing terrain, environment, algae growth, and soil erosion. To discover perceptual granules in satellite images that are near each other, consider first the segmentation of the images (see Figure 5 and Algorithm 1).

**Algorithm 1: Image Segmentation Method**

```
Input: Digital image X containing n pixel windows, threshold th
Output: Segmented image
```

*Figure 5. Segmented satellite images of North Basin, Lake Winnipeg*

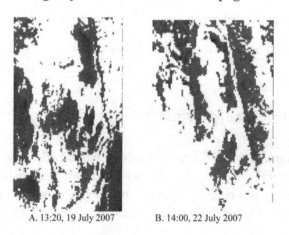

A. 13:20, 19 July 2007      B. 14:00, 22 July 2007

```
Partition X into n pixel widows, p = pixel, w = {p | p ∈ X }, w is a
pixel window
while n ≠ 0 {
read window w ∈ X;
if g̅ (w) ≥ th
p ← g̅ (w) for each pixel p ∈ w;
else p ← 255 (white) for each pixel p ∈ w;
n ← n - 1;
}
```

The method used to obtain the segmentations in Figure 4A and Figure 4B is given in Algorithm 1. Let w denote a pixel window defined by a set of k pixels, $|w| = k^2$. Basically, the pixels in all pixel windows with an average grey level $\overline{g}$ greater than or equal to some threshold *th* (i.e., $\overline{g}(w) \geq$ th) are coloured with the average value $\overline{g}(w)$. Otherwise, the pixels in all of the rest windows where $\overline{g}(w) <$ th are coloured white.

Notice that there is quite a separation (i.e., change) in the segmentations in Figure 5A and Figure 5B for the satellite images in Figure 4A and Figure 4B, respectively. For simplicity, we consider a comparison of the average grey level of the pixel windows in the same location in the two satellite images. Let x ∈ X, y ∈ Y be pixel windows in segmented satellite images X and Y, respectively (see Figure 6).

Let $x/\simeq_{\overline{g},\varepsilon}$ and $y/\simeq_{\overline{g},\varepsilon}$ denote perceptual granules (classes) containing x and y, respectively (see Figure 6). In effect, the union of these perceptual granules constitutes a new perceptual system <$O_w$, F> such that

$$\left\langle O_w, \mathcal{F} \right\rangle = \left\langle x/\simeq_{\overline{g},\varepsilon} \cup y/\simeq_{\overline{g},\varepsilon}, \{\overline{g}\} \right\rangle, \tag{2}$$

where there are pixel window x∈ $x/\simeq_{\overline{g},\varepsilon}$ (Figure 6A), pixel window y ∈ $y/\simeq_{\overline{g},\varepsilon}$, probe function $\overline{g} \in$ F, ε ∈ [0, 1] such that $\left|\overline{g}(x) - \overline{g}(y)\right| \leq \varepsilon$.

*Figure 6. Sample perceptual granule from segmented satellite images*

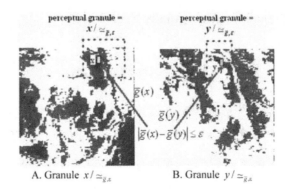

A. Granule $x/\simeq_{\overline{g},\varepsilon}$          B. Granule $y/\simeq_{\overline{g},\varepsilon}$

## 5. PERCEPTUAL NEAR SETS

Near set theory originally was inspired by a comparison of images (see, e.g., Peters, Skowron, Stepaniuk (2006), Peters (2007c)). This has led to the introduction of perceptual near sets.

### Definition 5.1: Perceptual Near Sets (Peters and Wasilewski (2009))

Let <O, F> be a perceptual system and let X, Y $\subseteq$ O, X $\neq$ Y. Let F denote a set of functions representing features of objects in O. Set X is perceptually near Y if, and only if X $\rhd\lhd_{\digamma}$ Y, i.e., there are objects in

X and Y have similar descriptions defined by the functions in F.

   Let Near$_F$(O) denote the family of near sets associated with <O, F>. Since Near$_F$(O) is a collection of perceptual granules that are near each other, from Definition 2.1 we know that the empty set is not included in Near$_F$(O). Hence, by Theorem 2.1,

### Theorem 5.1 (Peters and Wasilewski (2009))

The family of near sets Near$_F$(O) is a dual chopped lattice.

### Remark 5.1

Let X, Y $\subseteq$ O, X $\neq$ Y in the perceptual system <O, F>. X $\rhd\lhd_{\digamma}$ Y means that X/$\sim_F$ and Y/$\sim_F$ are examples

perceptual granules such that there are classes x/$\sim_F$ $\in$ X/$\sim_F$ and y/$\sim_F$ $\in$ Y/$\sim_F$ that are perceptually near each other, i.e., the description of objects in x/$\sim_F$ is similar to the description of objects in y/$\sim_F$ with respect to all features represented by functions in F.

### Example 5.1

Let O be a set of sample segmented images like those in Figure 4. Let X, Y $\subseteq$ O, X $\neq$ Y (i.e., a pair of different images) in the perceptual system <O, F>, where B $\subseteq$ F is a set of functions representing features of segmented images. Assume x/$\sim_B$ $\in$ X/$\sim_B$ and y/$\sim_B$ $\in$ Y/$\sim_B$ contain pixel windows with similar descriptions. Then the images in Figure 6A and Figure 6B contain perceptually near sets.

   Let $\| \varphi_B(x_r) - \varphi_B(x_r) \|_2$ denote the L$_2$ norm of a vector of description differences.

**Algorithm 2. Discovery Method for Perceptually Near Sets**

**Input:** Sets X, Y containing sample perceptual objects, set F containing functions representing object features. Assume |X| = |Y| indexed from 1 to n;
**Output:** Perceptual Near sets or nil.
Construct description $\pmb{\phi}_B(x_r) = \phi_1(x_r), \dots, \phi_L(x_r)$ for each $\varphi_i$ in B, $x_r$ in X;
Construct description $\pmb{\phi}_B(y_r) = \phi_1(y_r), \dots, \phi_L(y_r)$ for each $\varphi_i$ in B, $y_r$ in Y;

```
Similarity = False; r = 1; i = 1;
repeat
repeat
if || φ(x ) - φ(x ) || = 0 {Similarity = True};
        r        r
r = r + 1;
until (Similarity) or (r = n);
i = i + 1;
until (Similarity) or (i = n);
if Similarity {output X, Y} else {nil};
}
```

## Definition 5.2: Weak Perceptual Near Sets (Peters and Wasilewski (2009))

Let <O, F> be a perceptual system and let X, Y $\subseteq$ O, X $\neq$ Y. Let F denote a set of functions representing features of objects in O. Set X is weakly perceptually near Y if, and only if X $\underset{\neg}{\bowtie}$ Y, i.e., if there exists

$\varphi_i \in F$, x $\in$ X and y $\in$ Y such that $x \simeq_{\phi_i} y$, then X is weakly perceptually near Y.

## Example 5.2

Let X, Y $\subseteq$ O, X $\neq$ Y in the perceptual system <O, F>, where O is a set of sample segmented images and F = { $\bar{g}$ }. Consider a set of pixel windows X in Figure 4A and a set of pixel windows Y in Figure 4A and use $\bar{g}$ defined in Example 4.1. If we can identify at least one pixel window x $\in$ X and y $\in$ Y with similar average grey level, i.e., $\bar{g}$ (x) = $\bar{g}$ (y), then, X and Y are weakly perceptually near sets.

## Definition 5.3: Tolerance Near Sets (Peters (2009a), Peters (2010)).

Let <O, F> be a perceptual system and let X, Y $\subseteq$ O, X $\neq$ Y. Sets X and Y are tolerance near sets if, and only if X $\underset{\neg}{\bowtie\!\!\!=}$ Y, i.e., if there exists $\varphi_i \in F$, x $\in$ X, y $\in$ Y, ε $\in$ [0, 1] such that $x \simeq_{\phi_i, \varepsilon} y$, then X is near Y.

## Example 5.2

Let <O, F> be a perceptual system as defined in Example 5.2 and let X, Y $\subseteq$ O, X $\neq$ Y. Consider a set of pixel windows X in Figure 6A and a set of pixel windows Y in Figure 6A. Let ε $\in$ [0, 1]. If we can identify at least one pixel window x $\in$ X and y $\in$ Y such that $\left| \bar{g}(x) - \bar{g}(y) \right| \leq \varepsilon$, then, X and Y are tolerance near sets. This is the case in Figure 6.

### Algorithm 3. Discovery Method for Weak Tolerance Perceptually Near Sets

**Input:** Sets X, Y containing sample perceptual objects, set F containing functions representing object features. Assume |X| = |Y|

```
indexed from 1 to n. Let ε denote a tolerance.
Output: Tolerance Near sets.
Construct description 𝜙_B(x_r) = 𝜙_1(x_r), ... , 𝜙_L(x_r) for each φ_i in B, x_r in X;

Construct description 𝜙_B(y_r) = 𝜙_1(y_r), ... , 𝜙_L(y_r) for each φ_i in B, y_r in Y;

Similarity = False; r = 1; i = 1;
repeat
repeat
if || φ_B(x_r) - φ_B(x_r) ||_2 ≤ ε {Similarity = True};
r = r + 1;
until (Similarity) or (r = n);
i = i + 1;
until (Similarity) or (i = n);
if Similarity {output X, Y} else {nil};
}
```

A degree-of-nearness measure is given in Henry and Peters (2008b) and Pal & Peters (2010). Classification of perceptual objects using the near set approach compared with various forms of support vector machines has been reported in Henry and Peters (2008). Both of these topics are outside the scope of this article.

## 6. PROBABILISTICALLY NEAR COMMUNICATING SYSTEMS

This section illustrates an approach to discovering probabilistically near system events based on a directed graph (digraph) representation of a real-time embedded system (Peters (2009b)). In this case, a probability function *Pr* will be used as a probe function to measure the likelihood of a behaviour in communicating systems represented by digraphs. Before we show this, we first explain the basic approach using the probabilistic method.

### 6.1 Basic Approach: Probabilistic Method

In the context of engineering systems, the basic goal of the probabilistic method (PM) is to investigate properties (regularities) of observed outcomes of experiments with a real-time embedded system. Let $\Omega$ denote a sample space that is the set of all possible outcomes of a random process and let $\wp(\Omega)$ denote the family of sets representing allowable events. Also, let $\varnothing$, R denote the empty sets and the set of reals, respectively. Before we give the steps in the PM, we first define a probability space $(\Omega, \wp(\Omega), Pr)$.

### Definition 6.1: Probability Space (Mitzenmacher, Upfal (2005))

A *probability space* (Mitzenmacher, Upfal (2005)) consists of

- Sample space $\Omega$,

- Family of sets $\wp(\Omega)$,
- Probability function Pr: $\wp(\Omega) \to [0, 1]$, i.e., for any event $A \subseteq \Omega$, $0 \le \Pr(A) \le 1$, $\Pr(\varnothing) = 0$, and $\Pr(\Omega) = 1$.

The assumption made here is that values of Pr are uniformly distributed, i.e., for event $A \in \Omega$,

$$\Pr(A) = \frac{|A|}{|\Omega|}.$$

## Definition 6.2: Probabilistic Method

The *probabilistic method* (PM) is a way of proving that a structure with desired properties exists, Alon and Spencer (2000), Spencer (1994). To do this, it is necessary to define an appropriate probability space of structures and then show that the desired properties hold in the specified space with positive probability. Specifically, do the following:

1. Identify a sample space $\Omega$ that is a set of all possible outcomes of a system experiment, e.g., sending a message over a given network.
2. Description of the outcomes for each possible event, i.e., describe particular system experimental outcomes of interest for testing purposes, e.g., in Figure 7B, event $A_1$ consists of outcomes where a message is sent to either node 1 or 3.
3. Events, i.e., each event $A \in \Omega$ consist of experimental outcomes.
4. Probability function Pr, i.e., use Pr to measure the likelihood of occurrence of A.

By way of comparison of events in different communicating systems, we consider the conditional probability of a specific event B given the occurrence of an event A.

## Definition 6.3: Conditional Probability

Let A, B $\in \Omega$ and $\Pr(A) > 0$. The *conditional probability* (Grimmet and Stirzaker (2001) that event B occurs given that event B occurs is defined to be

$$\Pr(B \mid A) = \frac{\Pr(B \cap A)}{\Pr(A)}.$$

## 6.2 Probability Space for a Communicating System

The probability space for a communicating system results from modeling the system with a digraph (see, e.g., Figure 7A). A node in a system digraph represents a message-source. An arc in a system digraph models a path followed by a message. For a finite communicating system, the sample space $\Omega$ consists of outcomes of sending a message over a network. Let Pr: $\wp(\Omega) \to [0, 1]$ denote a probability function define on the family of sets $\wp(\Omega)$. A directed graph (digraph) like the one in Figure 7A is used to model a communication (message-passing) system. The assumption made here is that when the system represented by the diagraph is "energized" (i.e., a message is sent of over the network represented by the digraph), there is some uncertainty about which transition will fire at a particular instant in time. Let $1 \rightarrow 1$ denote a transition from node 1 to node 1 (i.e., node 1 sends itself a message) and let $1 \rightarrow (1, 3)$ denote the occurrence that $1 \rightarrow 1$ followed by $1 \rightarrow 3$ when a message is sent at node 1. The assumption here is that occurrences of transitions tend to be random and a random experiment with a communicating system results from sending a message over a network. It is also assumed that no more than one node can send a message at any one time. Hence,

## Proposition 6.1

There is a probability space associated with the digraph representing a finite communicating system.
This gives us the sample space

- $\Omega_1 = \{1 \rightarrow 1, 1 \rightarrow 2, 1 \rightarrow 3,$
- $1 \rightarrow (1, 2), 1 \rightarrow (1, 3), 1 \rightarrow (2, 3), (2)$
- $1 \rightarrow (1, 2, 3), 2 \rightarrow 3\}.$

Figure 7B shows five system events, where

- $A_1 = \{1 \rightarrow 1, 1 \rightarrow 3\}, A_2 = \{1 \rightarrow (1, 2), 1 \rightarrow (1, 3)\},$
- $A_3 = \{1 \rightarrow 2, 2 \rightarrow 3\}, A_4 = \{1 \rightarrow (2, 3), 1 \rightarrow (1, 2, 3)\},$
- $B_1 = \{1 \rightarrow 3, 1 \rightarrow (1, 3), 1 \rightarrow 2, 1 \rightarrow (2, 3)\}.$

Consider, now, events $A_1$ and $B_1$ in Figure 7 (see Figure 8). The shaded area of Figure 8A represents event $A_1$. The interaction between events $A_1$ and $B_1$ are represented by the shaded areas in Figure 8B. There is interest in the conditional probability $\Pr(B_1 \mid A_1)$ that provides a basis of comparison with other systems (see (3)).

$$\Pr(B_1 \mid A_1) = \frac{\Pr(B_1 \cap A_1)}{\Pr(A_1)} = \frac{\frac{1}{8}}{\frac{2}{8}} = \frac{1}{2}. \tag{3}$$

*Figure 7. Sample space derived from a system digraph*

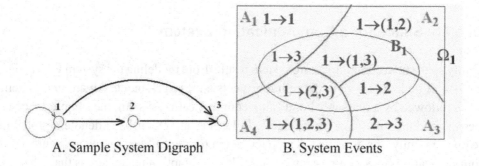

A. Sample System Digraph          B. System Events

## 6.3 Affinities Between Communicating Systems

It is possible to discover affinities between communicating systems by comparing conditional probabilities for seemingly quite different systems. To see, consider a specialization of Definition 3.4 (weak nearness relation). A sample space $\Omega$ is defined to be the set of possible outcomes of experiments with a communicating system. The elements of the sample space O are sample spaces derived from behavioural representations of communicating systems as digraphs. Let $Pr \in F$ be a probe function defined on the probability space $(\Omega, \wp(\Omega), Pr)$. Then Definition 3.4 is specialized in the following way.

## Definition 6.4: Probabilistic Nearness Relation

Let $\Omega_1, \Omega_2$ denote distinct sample spaces. Let O denote a non-empty set of sample spaces. Let $< O, F >$ be a perceptual system where $\Omega_1, \Omega_2 \in O$ and $B \subseteq F$. Then $\Omega_1$ is probabilistically near $\Omega_2$, i.e., $\Omega_1 \bowtie$ $\Omega_2$, if and only if there exists $Pr \in B$, X, $B_1 \in \Omega_1$ and Y, $B_2 \in \Omega_2$ such that $\Omega_1 \simeq_{Pr} \Omega_2$, i.e.,

$$Pr(B_1 | X) = Pr(B_2 | Y).$$

In effect, probability space $(\Omega_1, \wp(\Omega_1), Pr)$ is near space $(\Omega_2, \wp(\Omega_2), Pr)$ in the case where $Pr(B_1 | X) = Pr(B_2 | Y)$ for $B_1, X \in \Omega_1$, $B_2, Y \in \Omega_2$. Let sys1, sys2 denote communicating systems used to derive sample spaces $\Omega_1, \Omega_2$, respectively. A sample space derived from the possible outcomes of experimenting with a system represent the set of system behaviours. A *system behaviour* is an observable transition sequence that defines a path over which a signal (message) travels. A *communicating system* sys is defined by a set of behaviours that constitute a sample space. Then, for example, the behaviours in systems sys1, sys2 are represented by samples spaces $\Omega_{sys1}, \Omega_{sys2}$, respectively. Further, let $O_{sys}$ denote a set of communicating systems, where each system is represented by a set of behaviours. It is also assumed that the family of sets $PG_F(O_{sys})$ consists of events (sets of outcomes of system experiments) in a sample space $\Omega_{sys}$. Let $<O_{sys}, F>$ be a perceptual system, where O is a set of sample spaces. Let $\Omega_{sys1}, \Omega_{sys2} \in O_{sys}$. Further, let $B_1, A_i \in \Omega_{sys1}$ denote events in $\Omega_{sys1}$ and let $B_2, A_j \in \Omega_{sys2}$ denote events in $\Omega_{sys2}$. Then $\Omega_{sys1}$ and $\Omega_{sys2}$ (in effect, sys1 and sys2) are perceptually near each other, i.e., $\Omega_{sys1} \bowtie_F \Omega_{sys2}$, if and only if there exists $Pr \in F$, $B_1, A_i \in \Omega_{sys1}$ and $B_2, A_j \in \Omega_{sys2}$ such that $\{B_1, A_i\} \simeq_{Pr} \{B_2, A_j\}$, i.e., $Pr(B_1 | A_i) = Pr(B_2 | A_j)$. Hence, from Definition 3.4 and Definition 5.4, we obtain

*Figure 8. Selected system events*

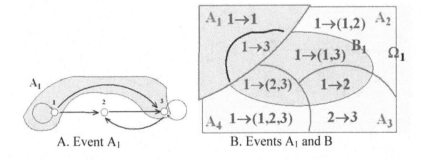

A. Event $A_1$        B. Events $A_1$ and B

## Proposition 6.2

Communicating systems are perceptually near each other if and only if the corresponding sample spaces are probabilistically near each other.

### Example 6.1: Near Communicating Systems

By way of illustration of affinities between communicating systems, consider the system in Figure 9 and the publisher system design in Figure 8. Let [c], [pub], [co] denote client, publisher, and collaborator, respectively.

Let $\Omega_1$, $\Omega_2$ denote sample spaces in Figure 7B and Figure 9B, respectively. It can shown that the probability space $(\Omega_1, \wp(\Omega_1), Pr)$ represented in Figure 7 is perceptually near space $(\Omega_2, \wp(\Omega_2), Pr)$ represented by Figure 9, i.e., $\Omega_1 \bowtie_{\bar\triangleleft_\Phi} \Omega_2$.

Let $3^n$ denote $3 \rightarrow 3 \rightarrow \ldots \rightarrow 3$ (i.e., n countable cyclic transitions on node 3). Similarly, $1^n$ denotes n countable cyclic transitions on node 1. From Figure 9A, we obtain the sample space

- $\Omega_2 = \{1 \rightarrow 1^n, 1 \rightarrow 2, 1 \rightarrow 3, 1 \rightarrow 4,$
- $1 \rightarrow (1^n, 2), 1 \rightarrow (1^n, 3), 1 \rightarrow (2, 3), 1 \rightarrow (1^n, 2, 3), 1 \rightarrow (1^n, 4, 2, 3), (4)$
- $2 \rightarrow 3, 4 \rightarrow 2, 4 \rightarrow (2, 3) \}$.

Figure 9B shows five system events that includes event B2 represented with a torus shape, i.e.,

- $A_1 = \{1 \rightarrow 1^n, 1 \rightarrow 3, 1 \rightarrow (1^n, 2)\}$,
- $A_2 = \{1 \rightarrow (1^n, 3), 1 \rightarrow (1^n, 4, 2, 3), 4 \rightarrow 2\}$,
- $A_3 = \{1 \rightarrow 2, 1 \rightarrow 4, 1 \rightarrow (2, 3), 1 \rightarrow (1^n, 2, 3)\}$,
- $A_4 = \{1 \rightarrow 2, 1 \rightarrow 4, 2 \rightarrow 3, 4 \rightarrow (2, 3), 1 \rightarrow (1^n, 2)\}$,
- $B_2 = \{1 \rightarrow 3, 1 \rightarrow 4, 1 \rightarrow (1^n, 2), 1 \rightarrow (2, 3), 2 \rightarrow 3, 4 \rightarrow 2\}$.

Consider, now, events $A_3$ and $B_2$ in Figure 8 (see Figure 10). The shaded area of Figure 10A represents event $A_3$. The interaction between events $A_3$ and $B_2$ is represented by the shaded areas in Figure 10B. There is interest in the conditional probability $Pr(B_2 \mid A_3)$ inasmuch as it provides a basis of comparison with events in the system represented by Figure 8. systems (see (5)).

*Figure 9. 4-node communicating system*

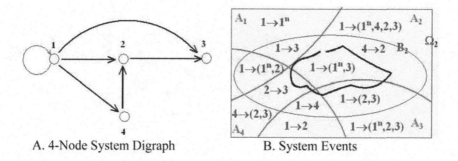

A. 4-Node System Digraph          B. System Events

$$\Pr(B_2 \mid A_3) = \frac{\Pr\left(B_2 \cap A_3\right)}{\Pr(A_3)} = \frac{\frac{2}{12}}{\frac{4}{12}} = \frac{2}{4} = \frac{1}{2}$$

(5)

This means that $\Omega_1 \bowtie \Omega_2$ for sample space $\Omega_1$ defined in (2) and sample space $\Omega_2$ defined in (4). In effect, from Prop. 5.2, the 3-node communicating system in Figure 7A and the 4-node system in Figure 9A are probabilistically near each other.

## 7. ROUGH SETS AS NEAR PERCEPTUAL GRANULES

This section briefly presents some fundamental concepts in rough set theory resulting form the seminal work by Zdzisław Pawlak (for an overview, see, *e.g.*, Peters and Skowron (2006, 2007)). The rough set approach introduced by Zdzisław Pawlak (1981a, 1981b, 1982) and Pawlak and Skowron (2007a, 2007b, 2007c). An overview of rough set theory and applications is given by Polkowski (2002). Let O denote a set of perceptual objects and let F denote as set of functions representing features of the objects in O. Let <O, F> denote a perceptual system, where $f: O \to R$ for every $f \in$ F.

Let $O/\sim_B$ denote the set of all classes in the partition of O defined by $\sim_B$. For $x \in$ O, the notation $x/\sim_B$ denotes an equivalence class containing x. For $X \subseteq O$, $B \subseteq F$, the sample perceptual granule $X$ can be approximated with a B-lower and B-upper approximation denoted by $B_*X$ and $B^*X$, respectively, where

$$\mathcal{B}_*X = \bigcup_{x/\sim_B \subseteq X} x/\sim_B \text{ and } \mathcal{B}^*X = \bigcup_{x/\sim_B \cap X \neq \varnothing} x/\sim_B .$$

Whenever $B_*X$ is a proper subset of $B^*X$, i.e., $B_*X \subset B^*X$, i.e., $\mathcal{B}^*X - \mathcal{B}_*X \neq \varnothing$, the sample $X$ has been classified imperfectly, and the set X is considered a rough set. Notice, from Definition 5.1, $B_*X \bowtie_{\overline{?}} X$ and $B^*X \bowtie_{\overline{?}} X$, since the classes in an approximation of X contain objects with descriptions that match the description of at least one perceptual object in X. Hence, the pairs $B_*X, X$ and $B^*X, X$ are examples of near perceptual granules. In general,

*Figure 10. Selected events in a sample space for a 4-node system*

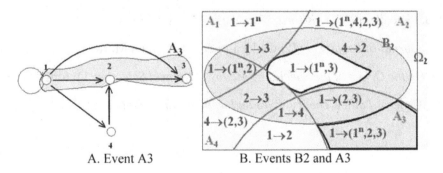

A. Event A3          B. Events B2 and A3

**Proposition 7.1** (Peters (2007d))

The pairs $B_*X, X$ and $B^*X, X$ are near sets.

**Proposition 7.2** (Peters (2007d))

Any equivalence class $x/\sim_{\mathfrak{F}}$, $|x| \geq 2$, is a near set.


## 8. CONCLUSION

This article considers relations between perceptual granules that are near sets. The discovery of new perceptual granules begins with the selection of probe functions that provide a basis for comparing objects in distinct perceptual granules. An important result is this paper is that every family of perceptual granules is a dual chopped lattice. This result is a generalization concerning lattices of families of near sets introduced by Peters and Wasilewski (2009), namely, every family of near sets is a dual chopped lattice. The results of the join operation $\cup$ (union) in a chopped lattice point to the fact that the join of perceptual granules results in a new perceptual granule (dually, the join of near sets results in a new near set).


## ACKNOWLEDGMENT

It was Piotr Wasilewski who pointed out that each family of near sets is a dual chopped lattice. Many thanks, also, to Som Naimpally, Piotr Wasilewski, Homa Fashandi, Christopher Henry, Amir H. Meghdadi, Andrzej Skowron, Jarosław Stepaniuk, Mihir Chakraborty, and Sheela Ramanna for their insights concerning topics in this paper. This research has been supported by the Natural Sciences and Engineering Research Council of Canada (NSERC) grant 185986, Manitoba Centre of Excellence Fund (MCEF) grant, and Canadian Arthritis Network (CAN) grant SRI-BIO-05.


## REFERENCES

Alon, N., & Spencer, J. H. (2000). *The Probabilistic Method* (2nd ed.). New York: John Wiley & Sons, Inc.doi:10.1002/0471722154

Birkhoff, G., & MacLane, S. (1967). *Algebra*. New York: The Macmillan Co.

Darwin, C. (1845). *Journal of Rsearchers* (2nd ed.). London, UK: John Murray.

Darwin, C. (1859). *On the Origin of the Species by Means of Natural Selection*. Oxford, UK: J. Murray.

Grätzer, G. (1978). *General Lattice Theory. Pure and Applied Mathematics, 75*. New York: Academic Press, Inc.

Grätzer, G. (2006). *The Congruences of a Finite Lattice. A Proof-by-Picture Approach*. Boston: Birkhäuser.

Grätzer, G., & Lasker, H. (1968). Extension theorems on congruences of partial lattices. *Notices of the American Mathematical Society, 15*, 732–785.

Grimmett, G. R., & Stirzaker, D. R. (2001). *Probability and Random Processes*. Oxford, UK: Oxford University Press.

Henry, C., & Peters, J. F. (2007). Image pattern recognition using approximation spaces and near sets. In *Proceedings of Eleventh Int. Conf. on Rough Sets, Fuzzy Sets, Data Mining and Granular Computing* (RSFDGrC 2007, Joint Symposium JRS 2007), (Springer Lecture Notes in Artificial Intelligence, vol. 4482, pp. 475-482).

Henry, C., & Peters, J. F. (2008). Near set index in an objective image segmentation evaluation framework. In Geobia 2008, Pixels, Objects, Intelligence: GEOgraphic Object Based Information Analysis for the 21st Century. Alberta, Canada: University of Calgary.

Hooke, R. (1665). *Micrographia or Some Physiological Descriptions of Minute Bodies*. New York: Cosimo, Inc.

Hooke, R. (1665). *Micrographia or Some Physiological Descriptions of Minute Bodies*. NY: Cosimo Classics.

Keynes, R. (Ed.). (2000). *Charles Darwin's Zoology Notes & Specimen Lists from H.M.S. Beagle*. Cambridge, UK: Cambridge University Press.

Lipski, W. (1981). On databases with incomplete information. *Journal of the ACM, 28*, 41–70. doi:10.1145/322234.322239

McCullough, G. (2007). Manitoba North Basis, south of Long Point, Lake Winnipeg. Retrieved from http://home.cc.umanitoba.ca/%7Egmccullo/LWsat.htm

Mitzenmacher, M., & Upfal, E. (2005). *Probability and Computing. Randomized Algorithms and Probabilistic Analysis*. Cambridge, UK: Cambridge University Press.

Naimpally, S. A., & Warrack, B. D. (1970). *Proximity Spaces. Cambridge Tract in Mathematics No. 59*. Cambridge, UK: Cambridge University Press.

National Geographic. (2008). *National Geographic, Penguins, Mar.* Retrieved from http://animals.nationalgeographic.com/animals/photos/penguins/adelie-penguin_image.html

Orłowska, E. (1982). *Semantics of Vague Concepts. Applications of Rough Sets (Report 469)*. Warsaw, Poland: Polish Academy of Sciences Institute for Computer Science.

Orlowska, E. (1985). Semantics of Vague Concepts. In Dorn, G., & Weingartner, P. (Eds.), *Foundations of Logic and Linguistics. Problems and Solutions* (pp. 465–482). London: Plenum Press.

Orłowska, E. (1998). Incomplete Information: Rough Set Analysis. *Studies in Fuzziness and Soft Computing, 13*, 1–22.

Orłowska, E., & Pawlak, E. (1984). Representation of nondeterministic information. *Theoretical Computer Science, 29*, 27–39. doi:10.1016/0304-3975(84)90010-0

Pal, S. K., & Peters, J. F. (Eds.). (2010). Rough Fuzzy Image Analysis. Foundations and Methodologies. Boca Raton, FL: CRC Press, Taylor & Francis Group, ISBN 13: 9781439803295.

Pavel, M. (1993). *Fundamentals of Pattern Recognition* (2nd ed.). New York: Marcel Dekker, Inc.

Pawlak, Z. (1981a). *Classification of Objects by Means of Attributes. (Report 429)*. Warsaw, Poland: Institute for Computer Science, Polish Academy of Sciences.

Pawlak, Z. (1981b). *Rough Sets. (Report 431)*. Warsaw, Poland: Institute for Computer Science, Polish Academy of Sciences.

Pawlak, Z. (1982). Rough sets. *International J. Comp. Inform. Science, 11*, 341–356. doi:10.1007/BF01001956

Pawlak, Z., & Skowron, A. (2007a). Rudiments of rough sets. *Information Sciences, 177*, 3–27. doi:10.1016/j.ins.2006.06.003

Pawlak, Z., & Skowron, A. (2007b). Rough sets: Some extensions. *Information Sciences, 177*, 28–40. doi:10.1016/j.ins.2006.06.006

Peters, J. F. (2005b). Rough ethology: Towards a Biologically-Inspired Study of Collective Behavior in Intelligent Systems with Approximation Spaces. *Transactions on Rough Sets, III*, (. *LNCS, 3400*, 153–174.

Peters, J. F. (2007a). Classification of objects by means of features. In *Proceedings of the IEEE Symposium Series on Foundations of Computational Intelligence* (IEEE SCCI 2007), (pp. 1-8). Honolulu, HI.

Peters, J. F. (2007b). (in press). Classification of perceptual objects by means of feature. *Int. J. of Info. Technology & Intelligent Computing*.

Peters, J. F. (2007c). Near sets. Special theory about nearness of objects. *Fundamenta Informaticae, 75*(1-4), 407–433.

Peters, J. F. (2007d). Near sets. General theory about nearness of objects. *Applied Mathematical Sciences, 1*(53), 2609–2029.

Peters, J. F. (2008a). Approximation and perception in ethology-based reinforcement learning. In Pedrycz, W., Skowron, A., & Kreinovich, V. (Eds.), *Handbook on Granular Computing*. New York: Wiley. doi:10.1002/9780470724163.ch30

Peters, J. F. (2008b). Affinities between perceptual granules: Foundations and perspectives. In Bargiela, A., & Pedrycz, W. (Eds.), *Human-Centric Information Processing Through Granular Modelling* (pp. 49–66). Berlin-Heidelberg, Germany: Springer.

Peters, J. F. (2009a). Tolerance near sets and image correspondence. *Int. J. of Bio-Inspired Computation, 1*(4), 239–245. doi:10.1504/IJBIC.2009.024722

Peters, J. F. (2009b). Analyzing system behaviour with Bayesian analysis of system patterns. Int. J. of Computer Science. *Systems Engineering and Information Technology, 2*(1), 17–23.

Peters, J. F. (2010). (in press). Corrigenda and addenda: Tolerance near sets and image correspondence. Int. *J. of Bio-Inspired Computation, 2*(5).

Peters, J. F., Henry, C., & Ramanna, S. (2005a). Rough Ethograms: Study of Intelligent System Behavior. In Kłopotek, M. A., Wierzchoń, S., & Trojanowski, K. (Eds.), *New Trends in Intelligent Information Processing and Web Mining (IIS05)* (pp. 117–126). Gdańsk, Poland. doi:10.1007/3-540-32392-9_13

Peters, J. F., & Pawlak, Z. (2007). Zdzisław Pawlak life and work (1906-2006). *Information Sciences, 177*, 1–2. doi:10.1016/j.ins.2006.06.004

Peters, J. F., & Skowron, A. (2006). Zdzislaw Pawlak: Life and Work. *Transactions on Rough Sets, 5*, 1–24. doi:10.1007/11847465_1

Peters, J. F., Skowron, A., & Stepaniuk, J. (2006). Nearness in approximation spaces. In G. Lindemann, H. Schlilngloff et al. (Eds.), Proc. Concurrency, Specification \& Programming (CS & P'2006), (pp. 434-445). Berlin, Germany: Informatik-Berichte Nr. 206, Humboldt-Universität zu Berlin.

Peters, J. F., Skowron, A., & Stepaniuk, J. (2007). Nearness of objects: Extension of approximation space model. *Fundamenta Informaticae, 79*, 1–16.

Peters, J. F., Skowron, A., Synak, P., & Ramanna, S. (2003). Rough sets and information granulation. In Bilgic, T., Baets, D., Kaynak, O. (Eds.), *Tenth Int. Fuzzy Systems Assoc. World Congress IFSA*, (Lecture Notes in Artificial Intelligence 2715, 370-377). Instanbul, Turkey. Berlin, Germany: Springer Verlag.

Peters, J. F., & Wasilewski, P. (2009). Foundations of near set theory, Information Sciences. *International Journal (Toronto, Ont.), 179*(18), 3091–3109.

Poincare, H. (1905). *Science and Hypothesis, trans. By J. Lamor.* London, UK: Walter Scott Publishing.

Polkowski, L. (2002). *Rough Sets. Mathematical Foundations.* Berlin Heidelberg, Germany: Springer-Verlag.

Sakai, H., & Okuma, A. (2004). Basic algorithms and tools for rough non-deterministic information analysis. *Transactions on Rough Sets I,* (. *Springer LNCS, 3100*, 209–231.

Skowron, A., & Peters, J. F. (2008). Rough-granular computing. In Pedrycz, W., Skowron, A., & Kreinovich, V. (Eds.), *Handbook on Granular Computing* (pp. 285–329). New York: Wiley. doi:10.1002/9780470724163.ch13

Sossinsky, A. B. (1986). Tolerance space theory and some applications. *Acta Applicandae Mathematicae: An International Survey Journal on Applying Mathematics and Mathematical Applications, 5*(2), 137–167.

Spencer, J. (1994). Ten Lectures on the Probabilistic Method, 2nd Ed. Society for Industrial and Applied Mathematics (SIAM), Philadelphia.

Woleński, J. (2001). Review of S. Leśniewski, Collected Works, Vols. 1-II. *Modern Logic, 8*(3 & 4), 195–201.

## ENDNOTE

*     The perceptual granule $\Pi(O, F, \sim_F)$ was suggested by Piotr Wasilewski (see Peters and Wasilewski (2009)).

# Chapter 15
# Granular Computing in Object-Oriented Software Development Process

**Jianchao Han**
*California State University, USA*

## ABSTRACT

*Granular computing as a methodology of problem solving has been extensively applied in a variety of fields for a long history, but the special research interest in granular computing has only been developed in past decades. So far most granular computing researchers address the mathematical foundation and/ or the computation model of granular computing. However, granular computing is not only a computing model for computer-centered problem solving, but also a thinking model for human-centered problem solving. Fortunately, some authors have presented the structures of such kind models and investigated various perspectives of granular computing from different application points of views. In this paper we present the principles, models, components, strategies, and applications of granular computing. Our focus will be on the applications of granular computing in various aspects and phases of the object-oriented software development process, including user requirement specification and analysis, software system analysis and design, algorithm design, structured programming, software testing, and system deployment design. Our objective is to reveal the importance and usefulness of granular computing as a human-centered problem solving strategy in object-oriented software development process.*

## 1. INTRODUCTION

The basic principles of granular computing involve granularity, granulation and computations with granules and relationships among them. The idea has been studied extensively in various research communities and application domains for a long time in a variety of ways, either implicitly or explicitly (Bargiela & Pedrycz 2002). However, as a general computing paradigm of problem solving, granular computing has

DOI: 10.4018/978-1-60566-324-1.ch015

only been investigated for decades, but has received much attention in computing intelligence society in recent years. The following is a brief history of modern granular computing development:

- Zadeh (1979) first introduced the notion of information granulation in 1979 and suggested that fuzzy set theory may find potential applications in this respect, which pioneers the explicit study of granular computing. With the concept of his information granulation, Zadeh further presented granular mathematics (Zadeh, 1997).
- Pawlak (1982) proposed the rough set theory to deal with inexact information by using rough sets to approximate a crisp set in 1982, and investigated the granularity of knowledge from the point of view of rough set theory (Pawlak, 1998).
- Hobbes (1985) presented a theory of granularity as the base of knowledge representation, abstraction, heuristic search, and reasoning in 1985. In his theory the problem world is represented as various grains and only interesting ones are abstracted to learn concepts.
- Giunchigalia and Walsh (1992) presented a theory of abstraction to improve the conceptualization of granularities in 1992, where the conceptualization of the world can be performed at different granularities and switched between granularities.
- Lin (1997B) suggested the term "granular computing" to label this growing research field in 1997. Lin also proposed a theoretical model of granular computing with neighbor system based on binary relations (Lin, 1979; Lin, 1997A).
- Yao, Y. (2005) investigated the trinity model of granular computing from three perspectives: philosophy, methodology, and computation, and discussed a hierarchical architecture of granular computing.
- In the past decade, different granular computing models have been conducted in various aspects and applied in various application domains, including machine learning, data mining, bioinformatics, e-Business, network security, high-performance computing and wireless mobile computing, etc. The essence of these models has been addressed by researchers to build efficient computational algorithms for handling huge amounts of data, information and knowledge. The objectives of these computation models are computer-centered and mainly concern the efficiency, effectiveness, and robustness of using granules such as classes, clusters, subsets, groups and intervals in problem solving. In recent years, some researchers have investigated the granular computing paradigm from perspectives of philosophy, cognitive science, and human thinking (Yao, Y., 2004; Yao, Y., 2005) as well as the general strategies of interactions between granules (Yao, J., 2006) and operations on granule coverings (Wu & Yang, 2005). Yao, J. (2007) summarizes and reviews the development of granular computing in the past ten years.

So far most granular computing researcher address the mathematical foundation and/or the computation model of granular computing, while neglect the research of its importance and usefulness in our human beings daily problem solving. Granular computing is not only a computing model for computer-centered problem solving, but also a thinking model for human-centered problem solving. Actually the basic concept of granular computing has been extensively applied in many problem solving disciplines with different formats either consciously or unconsciously by human beings. Recently, some authors have presented the structures of such kind models and investigated various perspectives of granular computing from different application points of views. For instance, Yao, Y. (2003) scrutinizes the structured writing with granular computing strategies and demonstrates that by consciously using granular computing strategies and heuristics of granular computing, a scientist has a better chance to produce a clear, structured, and comprehensible document.

A software development process is an integral part of any software development project and is defined as being a series of actions conducted to design and manufacture complex software. Developing complex software needs extensive human creative thinking and effort. This is a very typical human-centered problem solving domain. Object-oriented software development process usually consists of user requirement specification and analysis, software system analysis, system design and detail design, system implementation, testing, and deployment, although different software process models may vary and iterate. Han and Dong (2007) discuss the applications of granular computing in software engineering, which will be extended to the applications of granular computing in various phases of the object-oriented software development process in this paper. By investigating these strategies of granular computing in various phrases of software process, we expect that software developers can consciously apply them in the process of software development and gain benefit of high-quality software products.

The rest of this paper is organized as follows. In Section 2, the basic concepts and components of granular computing are reviewed. In Section 3, the object-oriented software development process is briefly summarized. In Section 4, the perspective and application of granular computing in various phases of object-oriented process are investigated, including user requirement analysis, system analysis, system design, system implementation, software testing, and system deployment design. Section 5 is the concluding remark.

## 2. PRINCIPLES OF GRANULAR COMPUTING

Although there does not exist a formal, precise and uncontroversial definition and a framework of granular computing, it has been generally understood as a paradigm of problem solving with granules as the basic elements and granulation as the primary operation. Besides granules and granulation, relationships among granules and computations with granules constitute the main ingredients of granular computing. In this section, we summarize these concepts and components.

Basically, granules are used to represent the elementary units of a complex system that is considered, and collectively provide a representation of the unit with respect to a particular level of granularity. Each granule may reflect a specific aspect of the problem or form a portion of the system domain. In the real-world problem solving, we may need to consider the levels of detail of a system. On the different levels, granules may represent different units. Using object-oriented software as an example, one can see that the software system is considered as a whole, its ingredients are a collection of classes. However, when a class is developed, its granules are instance fields, methods, and constructors/destructors. All granules form a hierarchy structure. The hierarchy structure consists of multiple levels and granules are located at different levels. Varieties of hierarchy structures reflect different granulation criteria and granular views.

Granulation is to granulate a complex problem into granules, including the construction, representation, and interpreation of granules. It concerns the procedures for constructing granules. Granulation is a very natural concept and appears almost everywhere in different names. Granulation includes two important aspects (Yao, Y. 2004; Yao, Y., 2005).

Granulation methods deal with how a problem or a set of elements is granulated into granules. Top-down method starts from the problem space as a whole and partitions the problem into sub-spaces, which, in turn, are partitioned again, to construct desired granules; while bottom-up methods attempts to put individual elements together to form blocks, which, in turn, are united to build granules at expected levels.

Granulation criteria determines whether a granule should be granulated into smaller granules for top-down construction, or whether different elements/granules should be put together to form a larger granule for bottom-up construction. Partition vs. covering should be distinguished. A partition of the universe is a collection of pair-wise disjoint nonempty granules, and the union of these granules forms the whole universe. However, a granular covering of the universe is a collection of granules that cover the whole universe, where those granules may overlap. Operations on partitions and coverings have been investigated in literature (Wu & Yang, 2005; Yao, J., 2006; Yao, Y., 2005).

Granular relationships between granules can be interpreted mathematically as set relations or philosophically as concept relations. From another point of view, each granule may be interpreted as an implication rule or a set of attribute-value pairs, e.g., in classification and clustering analysis. Relationships between granules can also be represented as binary relations and interpreted as dependency, inheritance, etc. (Yao, J., 2007) Generally speaking, there are two types of relationships among granules: interrelationship and intra-relationship. The former is the basis of grouping small objects together to construct a larger granule based on similarity, indistinguishability, and functionality, while the latter concerns the decomposition of a large granule into smaller units and the interactions between components of a granule as well. A granule is a refinement of another granule if it is contained in the latter. Similarly, the latter is called a coarsening of the former. This relationship functions like set-containment in the set-based domains.

Computation with Granules: Computation with granules is to compute and reason the granular entities in terms of their relationships. Different operations can be performed on granules for various computation and reasoning tasks and purposes. These operations can be categorized as either computations within granules or computations between granules. Computations within granules are usually performed on the intra-relationships of granules. Typical computations in this category include finding characterization of granules, e.g. membership functions of fuzzy granules (Zadeh, 1979; Zadeh, 1997); inducing rules from granules, e.g. classification rules that characterize the classes of objects; forming concepts that granules entail. On the other hand, computations between granules usually operate on the interrelations between granules, transformations from one granule to another, clustering granules, and dividing granules.

## 3. OBJECT-ORIENTED SOFTWARE ENGINEERING PROCESS

There are many different methodologies for software engineering (Reifer, 2006). Traditional methodologies include the waterfall methodology, the spiral methodology, the iterative methodology, and the incremental methodology. Some new methodologies such as the object-oriented methodology, the agile (extreme) methodology, the aspect-oriented methodology have been explored recently. Even for the object-oriented methodology, there exist different versions, e.g. UML (the Unified Modeling Language) and RUP (Rational Unified Process) (O'Docherty, 2005). All these methodologies share some common engineering process activities, which are classically divided into the following phrases:

- **Requirements** describe what the software product is going to achieve, and capture two aspects: the business model for understanding the context of the software product, and the system requirements model or functional specification for specifying the capabilities of the expected product.

- **Analysis** identifies what can be done and clears about the relevant entities, their properties and their inter-relationships. Analysis also verifies the understanding of the requirements.
- **Architecture Design** works out how to implement the requirements by breaking the system down into logical processes and physical subsystems, deciding the internal and external communications, and choosing the right technologies.
- **Detailed Design** is to design subsystems by specifying a clear, unambiguous description of the way the components of the software should be used and how they will behave if used properly.
- **Implementation** is writing pieces of code that work together to form subsystems, which in turn collaborate to form the whole system to meet the specification.
- **Testing** tests the software product against the system requirements to see if it fits the original goals.
- **Deployment** delivers the software product, including hardware and software, to the end user, along with manuals and training materials.
- **Maintenance** is a long term job to ensure the software system works properly by solving problems, updating the start-of-art technologies, adding functionalities, improving the performance of the system, etc.

The object-oriented software engineering process covers all above phases. The tasks of these phases and the tools that are used to achieve the goal have been developed. Granular computing technology can be applied in the activities of these phases of the object-oriented software process. In the rest of this section, we'll describe the tasks and tools for each phase, and the application of the granular computing technology will be discussed in next section.

- *Object-oriented requirement analysis* is to transfer the customer's requirements document or mission statement into a complete, unambiguous description of the system to be developed. The use case model has been extensively applied in the object-oriented requirement analysis. A use case starts with an actor, then descends into the business or the system, and eventually returns to the actor. Use cases define the way in which part of a business or a system is used by documenting our understanding of the business operations (business requirements) and specifying what the software should be able to do (system requirements). The tasks of requirement analysts include identifying business actors, writing the project glossary, developing use cases, and illustrating use cases on a communication diagram and on an activity diagram. The outcome of this phrase includes an actor list, a use case list, a use case diagram, use case details and survey.
- *Object-oriented system analysis* is to discover what the software system is going to handle and decompose the complex user requirements into the essential elements and their relationships. The object-oriented system analysis model has both static and dynamic parts. The goal of the static analysis is to conclude a class diagram. The activities of the static analysis involve finding classes, exploring class relationships, drawing class and object diagrams, drawing relationships between classes and objects, and identifying attributes of classes. On the other hand, the goal of dynamic analysis is to extract a communication diagram to demonstrate that the static model (class diagram) is feasible.
- *Object-oriented system design* is to invent a solution to the problem that arises from the requirement analysis and investigate how the software will be implemented by proposing the software architecture. The activities of this system architecture design include choosing a system topology,

making technology choices, designing a concurrency policy and a security policy, partitioning the system into subsystems and layers of subsystems, and deciding how machines, subsystems and layers will communicate. The network architecture of the software system could be one-tier vs. multi-tier architecture, and client-server vs. distributed architecture. The network topology is depicted by a basic deployment diagram.

- ***Object-oriented subsystem design*** is to design the implementation details of subsystems and their layers and finalize the user interfaces. The activities of detailed design include mapping classes, operations and variables, as well as compositions and associations between classes, handling persistence, designing a relational database, designing the business services, and determining the layout and look of the user interfaces.

- ***Object-oriented system implementation*** is to convert the system design and specification into programs written in computer programming languages. The implementation can be either top-down or bottom-up, where the former codes the framework of the system first and then adds components incrementally, while the latter starts the implementation of essential components and integrates these components into complex components, subsystems and the whole system.

- ***Object-oriented system testing*** is to test the implemented components, subsystems, and the system against the system design and user requirements. Various software testing techniques have been developed and applied, such as white-box testing, black-box testing, alpha testing, beta testing, regression testing, unit testing, partitioning testing, integration test, use-case testing.

- ***Object-oriented system deployment plan*** is to specify how the system will be delivered to the end user and installed in the working context. The outcome of the system deployment plan is a deployment diagram that shows machines, processors and deployed artifacts for the software product. It also determines the environments of the software product and interactions between the environments, the system and the system components. For a tiered software system, the deployment diagram demonstrates tiers, communications between tiers, and relationships between components in each tier.

## 4. GRANULAR COMPUTING IN OBJECT-ORIENTED SOFTWARE ENGINEERING PROCESS

Granular computing as a machine-centered computation model has been extensively studied in machine learning, data mining, fuzzy set theory, rough set theory, but not paid enough attention as a human-centered thinking paradigm, although some research on this line has been conducted. From the previous section, one may see that basic components and concepts of granular computing, such as granules, partitions, hierarchies, are actually applied in problem solving process in our daily life. Granular computing provides the infrastructure for data, information and knowledge engineering as well as uncertainty management. In software engineering, the strategies of granular computing are also broadly used in all phases. Granulate-and-conquer is a softer version of classical divide-and-conquer strategy. A very common technique used in the classical "non-partitioning" recursive call is dynamic programming. Functional decomposition is to partition user requirement into granules (functions). Structured programming is to organize the computer programs as a collection of modules (procedures, functions, routines). The intra-relationships among these granules are based on their ingredients such as input parameters, output results, executable statements, whereas the interrelationships involve the module interfaces and procedure calls. In object-oriented programming, granules are classes, intra-relationships are the interactions between components of classes such as instance fields, methods and constructors in the Java language; and the interrelationships are class inheritance, aggregation, association, delegation, dependency, etc.

In this section, we scrutinize the different phases of the software development process based on object-oriented technologies, including user requirement analysis, system analysis, system design, system implementation, software testing, and system deployment design.

## 4.1. Granular Computing in Object-Oriented Requirement Analysis

In the object-oriented methodology, user requirements analysis involves two main aspects: identifying business actors and use cases. Both aspects can be conducted with granular computing paradigm. However, only identifying use cases will be investigated in this subsection.

Basically, each use case is a snippet of the business and may involve two-way communication between actors. Consider the business requirement as the problem domain, and the use cases will be the granules. Although there's no set rule for deciding how to granulate the business into use cases and most analysts partition the business process into use cases based on common sense, business logic, and their experience. The basic thinking lines of granular computing can be followed.

- Granules: Use cases.
- Granulation method: top-down decomposition for complete covering and bottom-up combination to form a hierarchy of use cases.
- Granular relationships: *inheritance* (specialization and generalization) in which a large case is decomposed into small cases or a set of small cases are combined to constitute a large case; *inclusion* where the source case has some of its steps provided by the target case; and *extension* where the source case adds steps to the target case.
- Granular computation: identifying the process of use cases, including input data, output data and business logic, as well as the communication with actors.

Consider the following example of the user requirement from a car rental company (O'Docherty, 2005):

*Since we automated the tracking of cars at our stores – using bar codes, counter-top terminals and laser readers – we have seen many benefits: the productivity of our rental assistants has increased 20%, cars rarely go missing and our customer base has grown strongly (according to our market research, this is at least partly due to the improved perception of professionalism and efficiency).*

*The management feels that the Internet offers further exciting opportunities for increasing efficiency and reducing costs. For example, rather than printing catalogs of available cars, we could make the catalog available to every Internet surfer for browsing on-line. For privileged customers, we could provide extra services, such as reservations, at the click of a button. Our target saving in this area is a reduction of 15% in the cost of running each store.*

*Within two years, using the full power of e-commerce, we aim to offer all of our services via a Web browser, with delivery and pick-up at the customers' home, thus achieving our ultimate goal of the virtual rental company, with minimal running costs relative to walk-in stores.*

From above requirement, we can identify some use cases (granules) as follows (O'Docherty, 2005):

- U1: Browse index: A customer browses the index of car models;
- U2: View Result: A customer is shown the subset of car models that was retrieved;
- U3: View Car Model Details: A customer is shown the details of a retrieved car model, such as description and advert;
- U4: Search: A customer searches for car models by specifying categories, makes and engine sizes;
- U5: Log On: A member logs on to the system using his/her membership number and current password;
- U6: View Member Details: A member views some of the details stored by the system, such as name, address and credit card details;
- U7: Make Reservation: A member reverses a car model when viewing its details;
- U8: View Rentals: A member views a summary of the cars they are currently renting;
- U9: Change Password: A member changes the password that they use to log on;
- U10: View Reservation: A member views summaries of their unconcluded reservations, such as data, time, car model;
- U11: Cancel Reservation: A member cancels an unconcluded reservation;
- U12: Log Off: A member logs off from the system;
- U13: Look for Car Models: A customer retrieves a subset of car models from the catalog.

One can find out all the use cases to cover the business requirements, although some of them may overlap. Some relationships among these use cases can be also identified as follows:

- U1 specializes U13 and includes U2;
- U2 is included by U1 and U4, and extended by U3;
- U3 extends U2 but is extended by U7;
- U4 specializes U13 and included U2;
- U5 is extended by U6, U8, U9, U10 and U12;
- U6 extends U5;
- U7 extends U3;
- U8 extends U5;
- U9 extends U5;
- U10 extends U5 and is extended by U11;
- U11 extends U10;
- U12 extends U5;
- U13 is an abstract use case and is generalized by U1 and U4.

## 4.2. Granular Computing in Object-Oriented System Analysis

The basic goal of system analysis is to find candidate classes that describe the objects that might be relevant to the system, relationships between the classes, as well as attributes for the classes. With granular computing terminology, classes are granules that all together should cover the system requirement and satisfy the needs of use cases that have been identified before.

Granulation method in system analysis is to identify classes. Candidate classes are often indicated by nouns in the use cases except those that represent the system, actors, boundaries, and trivial types. Two basic rules should be followed to identify classes: high cohesion inside classes and low coupling between classes. Class identification might be top-down and/or bottom-up, but the general complete coverage is necessary.

Granular relationships in the system analysis correspond to class relationships, which can include the following types: inheritance (is-a relationship) where a subclass inherits all of the attributes and behavior of its super-class(es); association, where objects of one class are associated with objects of another class; aggregation (strong association), where an instance of one class is made up of instances of another class; composition (strong aggregation) where the composed object can't be shared by other objects and dies with its composer; and others as well.

Computation with granules is two-fold. First, determine the internal structure and behaviors of objects of classes, including the instance fields and method/constructor prototypes; and second, interface the connections between classes. Associating classes often affects the design of internal structures of classes.

Going back to the example in the previous subsection, one can design the following classes for the car rental online system (O'Docherty, 2005).

- C1: Customer
- C2: Member
- C3: NonMember
- C4: Rental
- C5: CarModel
- C6: Car
- C7: CarDetails
- C8: InternetAccount
- C9: CreditCard
- C10: Address

Some relationships between above classes can be extracted. For example, *A Car can be rented under a Rental; A Member is-a Customer; A NonMember is-a Customer; A Member is guaranteed by a CreditCad; A Car is an example of a CarModel; etc.*

Granular computing strategy has been extensively used in software system analysis, especially in designing classes in object-oriented analysis. The followings are two typical examples in Java-based systems. First, we consider *AbstractCollection*, an abstract class in JDK. The architecture of *AbstractCollection* in Java is illustrated as follows (Sun Microsystems, 2005):

```
AbstractCollection
    AbstractList
        AbstractSequentialList
            LinkedList
        ArrayList
            AttributeList
            RoleList
            RoleUnresolvedList
```

```
    Vector
            Stack
AbstractSet
    HashSet
            LinkedHashSet
            JobStateReasons
    TreeSet
    EnumSet
    CopyOnWriteArraySet
AbstractQueue
    AbstractQueue
    ArrayBlockingQueue
    ConcurrentLinkedQueue
    DelayQueue
    LinkedBlockingQueue
    LinkedList
    PriorityBlockingQueue
    PriorityQueue
    SynchronousQueue
```

In this architecture, the class *AbstractCollection* has three sub-classes: *AbstractList, AbstractSet* and *AbstractQueue. AbstractList* has three sub-classes: *AbstractSequentialList*, which has in turn a subclass *LinkedList, ArrayList*, which has three sub-classes *AttributeList, RoleList* and *RoleUnresolvedList*, and *Vector*, which has a single sub-class *Stack. AbstractSet* has four sub-classes: *HashSet*, which is inherited by two sub-classes *LinkedHashSet* and *JobStateReasons, TreeSet, EnumSet*, and *CopyOnWriteArraySet*. Finally, *AbstractQueue* is granulated into nine sub-classes.

The second example that is considered in Java is the class *Throwable*, where *Throwable* is granulated into two sub-classes: *Error* and *Exception. Error* is in turn granulated into *AnnotationFormatError, AssertionError*, etc., while *Exception* is in turn granulated into *IOException, ClassNotFoundException*, etc. Some classes are granulated further into sub-classes. Part of various *Throwables* (*Errors* and *Exceptions*) and their (inheritance) relationships is shown as follows (Watt & Brown, 2001; Sun Microsystems, 2005):

```
Throwable
    Error
        AnnotationFormatError
        AssertionError
        AWTError
        CoderMalfunctionError
        FactoryConfigurationError
        LinkageError
            ClassCircularityError
            ClassFormatError
            ExceptionInInitializerError
            IncompatibleClassChangeError
```

```
            NoClassDefFoundError
            UnsatisfiedLinkError
            VerifyError
        ThreadDeath
        TransformerFactoryConfigurationError
        VirtualMachineError
    Exception
        IOException
            EOFException
            FileNotFoundException
            MalformedURLException
            UnknownHostException
        ClassNotFoundException
        CloneNotSupportedException
        RuntimeException
            ArithemeticException
            ClassCastException
            IllegalArgumentException
                NumberFormatException
                IllegalFormatException
                InvalidParameterException
                InvalidKeyException
                ......
            IllegalStateException
            IndexOutOfBoundsException
                ArrayIndexOutOfBoundsException
                StringIndexOutOfBoundsException
            NoSuchElementException
                InputMismatchException
            NullPointerException
            ......

    ......
```

## 4.3. Granular Computing in Object-Oriented System Design

Basically the software system design is to decompose a system into physical and logical components, and determine the technologies to be used to implement the system. Traditional system design focuses on the system functional partitioning, while modern software system design is based on object-oriented technology. In this subsection, object-oriented system architecture design and technology are discussed from the perspective of granular computing.

System design involves multiple steps, including system topology, software partitioning, concurrency and security policies as well as communications between components. Our discussion will concentrate in the topology design and system partitioning.

The first task of the system design is normally to determine the topology of a networked system. One popular system topology is the three-tier architecture to separate user interfaces, program logic and data in the system. In this architecture, the client tier presents the user interface to the user so that he/she can enter data and view results; the middle tier – also known as the business logic tier or server tier – runs multi-thread program code using large processors and lots of memory; and the data tier stores the data and provides safe concurrent access to it, typically with the help of a database management system. Thus, the system is granulated into three components. Besides the design of these three tiers, the protocols between tiers are also important. Existing technologies can be chosen to implement each of them, and shown below (O'Docherty, 2005).

- Client tier technologies in Web-based systems
    - HTML forms
    - JavaScript
    - ActiveX controls
    - Java applets
- Client tier to middle tier protocols
    - IMAP (email)
    - HTTP/CGI
    - FTP / Telnet
    - TCP/IP
    - JRMP / IIOP
- Middle tier technologies in Web- based systems
    - JSP for building Web pages on-the-fly
    - ASP for Microsoft technology
    - CGI scripts written in languages/ PERL
    - Servlets accessible by Java applets or JSPs
- Middle tier to data tier protocols
    - JDBC net with Java-based system
    - EJBs
    - JRMP
    - TCP/IP
    - IIOP
- Data tier technologies
    - DBMS
    - JDBC net server
    - Database client
    - EJB data source

Considering the example of the car rental company system, with the object-oriented system design partitioning, one can granulate the software system components into the following layers (O'Docherty, 2005):

- User Interface Layer
    - HTMLLayer

- ○   SwingLayer
- ○   MicroLayer
- Control Layer
  - ○   HTTPCGILayer
  - ○   RMIControlLayer
- Network Layer
  - ○   ServletsLayer
  - ○   RMILayer
- Server Layer
- Business Layer
- JDBC Layer
  - ○   DBMS
  - ○   PersistenceLayer

In the above layers, the JDBC Layer provides data persistence using the standard JDBC library to access a relational database that serves the needs for the lifetime of the system. The Business Layer implements the entity objects that contain JDBC code for shipping data to and from the database. The Server Layer translates the objects and messages in the Business Layer into business services. Objects in this layer are EJB session objects. The Network Layer consists of the ServletsLayer and the RMILayer to provide remote access and communication between the application and the server. The ServletsLayer translates objects in the Server Layer into simple commands and questions from the client, performs necessary actions, and then passes the next HTML page back to the client. On the other hand, the RMILayer contains the EJB session objects in the ServerLayer. When communicating with the Contrl Layer, the RMILayer uses the same protocol objects that the ServletsLayer uses. The Control Layer sits between the User Interface Layer and the Network Layer, and provides the network communication for the HTML Layer by the standard HTTPCGILayer and simplifies interaction with the server objects and hides the details of RMI by the RMIControlLayer. Finally, the User Interface Layer provides various graphical user interfaces.

## 4.4. Granular Computing in Object-Oriented System Implementation

Granular computing strategies have also been broadly used in software system implementation. The typical object-oriented program structure is actually a granular structure. Consider a Java-based software system, which can be characterized as follows (Horstmann, 2007):

Software system

- Packages
  - ○   Classes
    - ▪   Instance fields
    - ▪   Constructors
    - ▪   Methods
  - ○   Interfaces
    - ▪   Method prototypes

In this structure, a software system is designed as a set of packages, which may be installed in different physical devices. Each package contains a set of interfaces and a set of classes which are partitioned into three types of components.

Using the object-oriented methodology, the car rental company software system can be granulated into the following packages:

- The Car Rental System
  - Swing
    - Swing Interface Classes
  - Micro
    - Micro Interface Classes
  - Control
    - Control Classes
  - Protocol
    - Protocol Classes
  - RMI
    - RMI Classes
  - Servlets
    - Servlet Classes
  - Server
    - Server Classes
  - Business
    - Business Classes

During the design of classes, algorithms are one of designer's main concerns. Granular computing is also an important strategy for this purpose. Let's consider divide-and-conquer technique that is frequently used in algorithm design. The general paradigm of divide-and-conquer is described as below (Goodrich & Tamassia, 2004):

- Divide: divide the problem **S** in two or more disjoint subsets **S**1, **S**2, ...
- Recur: solve the sub-problems recursively
- Conquer: combine the solutions for **S**1, **S**2, ..., into a solution for **S**
- The base cases for the recursion are sub-problems of constant size

In the above paradigm, each sub-problem is a granule, which can be granulated further into smaller sub-problems. Granulation process usually follows the top-down method and the obtained granules should completely cover the parent problem. The granularity constitutes a hierarchy, where the top is the problem originally given, while at the bottom are all base cases. The computing with granules consists of not only dividing of a non-base problem or solving a base problem but also the combining solutions to sub-problems to form a solution to the parent problem.

Another important general algorithm design paradigm is dynamic programming, which is actually a special case of divide-and-conquer, and thus a granular computing strategy. The main difference between them is: divide-and-conquer solves each sub-problem individually, while dynamic programming stores solutions to all sub-problems so that when a sub-problem is reencountered, the solution can be obtained directly without resolving it (Levitin, 2002).

## 4.5. Granular Computing in Object-Oriented Software Testing

Granular computing strategy can also be applied in object-oriented software testing. Software testing for object-oriented system can be divided in to four levels (Binder, 1999), which form a granular structure. This object-oriented software testing granular structure is illustrated as follows.

Testing the object-oriented system

- Testing clusters of objects
  - Testing individual object classes
    - Testing the individual operations associated with objects

In this granular structure, testing the object-oriented system is the objective of the system testing, and can be conducted by verifying and validating against the system requirement specification. To this end, the object-oriented system can be granulated into clusters of objects. Groups of objects which act in combination to provide a set of services should be integrated and tested together (Binder, 1999). However, object-oriented systems have neither obvious top-down nor bottom-up structures, and clusters of objects must be grouped using associations between objects and knowledge of their operations, as well as the features of the system that are implemented by these objects. Three possible approaches to integrating objects to form clusters could be user-case or scenario based, thread based, and object interaction based (Sommerville, 2007).

- Use-case or scenario based approach is to integrate all objects that support the same use-case or scenario. The testing in approached can be based on the description of the use-case or scenario and the mode of use of the system specified by the use-case or scenario.
- Thread based approach is to cluster all objects that are explored in the same threads. The corresponding testing is to test the system's response to a particular input or set of input events. In this approach, events and event threads as well as their processing must be identified.
- Object interaction based is, on the other hand, to group objects that interact. For example, interacting objects can be identified by following the method-message paths to trace through a sequence of object interactions which stop when an object operation does not call on the services of any other objects.

When testing individual object classes, the following testing coverage should be included:

- The testing in isolation of all operations associated with the object;
- The testing and implementation of all attributes (instance fields) associated with the object;
- The exercise of the object in all possible states to simulate all events that cause a state change in the object.

Operations that should be tested and threads that will be executed in this use-case can be identified through this sequence.

There are many strategies of software testing (Binder, 1999), which may or may not be appropriate to object-oriented system, but these testing strategies can be viewed from the perspective of granular computing. Consider the partition testing, where the input data and output results of a system are usually divided into a number of different groups that have common characteristics such as a sequence of integer intervals or menu selections. The partitions can be identified by using the system specification or user requirement. Once a set of partitions is obtained, test cases from each partition can be chosen. For detailed testing, each partition can be partitioned further into finer cases.

In object-oriented methodology, unit testing is to test individual classes, including class methods and constructors. JUnit is a unit testing framework for the Java programming language. This frame granulates a class to be tested into methods and constructors, and for each constructor and method, it granulates further into a number of test cases with different parameters. With JUnit, Test Driven Development (TDD) becomes very easy to organize and implement.

Another popular software testing strategy is called integration testing. System integration involves building a system from its components and testing the resultant system for problems that arise from components interactions. This integration process can be accomplished either top-down, where the overall skeleton of the system is developed first and components are added second, or bottom-up, where clusters of components that deliver some system functionality are identified and integrated by adding interactions between clusters to make them work together. The component can be divided into or constructed from finer components. The integration testing is usually incremental. It first integrates a minimal system configuration and tests this system, and then adds components to this minimal system configuration and tests after each added increment.

## 4.6. Granular Computing in Object-Oriented System Deployment Design

The system deployment diagram is an outcome of the system design that shows the horizontal partitions of the software product. It can include all sorts of features such as machines, processes, files, folders, and dependencies. The object-oriented system deployment can be designed using granular computing. The basic idea is to granulate the system into tiers according to the tiered architecture of the system, and then granulate each tier into components. The relationships between components of each tier as well as the relationships between tiers should also be discovered and identified.

Consider the car rental company system in the previous example. The deployment design can be granulated as follows (O'Docherty, 2005):

The car rental system
Client Tier

- HTML Client
  - Web Browser
- GUI Client
  - Middle Tier
- Middle Server 1
  - Web Server
  - Business Server
    - Servlets
    - Protocol

- ▪ Business
  - ◦ Middle Server 2
  - ◦ ......
- Data Tier
  - ◦ Database Server 1
    - ▪ DBMS 1
  - ◦ Database Server 2
    - ▪ DBMS 2

The system is of three-tier architecture to separate user interfaces, program logic and data in the networked system. In this system, any one program involves at least three machines: the client tier presents the user interface for the user to enter data and view results; the middle tier (also known as the business logic tier or server tier) runs multi-threaded program code using large processors and lots of memory; and the data tier stores the data and provides safe concurrent access to it.

In the above deployment design, the data tier comprises two database servers each of which hosts a DBMS process for managing access to data so that the system throughput and reliability can be improved. The DBMSs running on these database servers may or may not be the same. The middle tier communicates with the data tier and consists of two server machines for the same reason. Each middle server hosts a business server for handling business requests and a web server for handling static HTML content and forwarding business requests to the business server. In the client tier, the HTML client hosts a web browser for the user to access the system, while the GUI client provides a specific graphical user interface for the user to use the system.

The granular relationships between tiers and components in each tier need also be discovered. For example, in the above deployment design, the data access to the data server for the business server is provided by the DBMS using a specific protocol, the web server passes business requests to the business server and receives the reply from the business server, and the web browser in the HTML server accesses the web server using HTTP, while the GUI client accesses the business server using JRMP.

## 5. CONCLUDING REMARKS

Object-oriented software development is both a thinking process and a problem solving process. The principle of granular computing was presented and the object-oriented software development process was reviewed in this paper. We especially examined different phases of object-oriented software development process from the perspectives of granular computing, including user requirement analysis, system analysis, system design, system implementation, software testing, and system deployment design. It evidences that granular computing as a human thinking model plays an essential role in the object-oriented software process, although software analysts, designers and developers have been unconsciously applying the granular computing strategies in these phases in their routine work. We conclude that consciously using granular computing methodology in the object-oriented software process will improve the quality of software products.

## REFERENCES

Bargiela, A., & Pedrycz, W. (2002). *Granular Computing: an Introduction*. Boston: Kluwer Academic Publishers.

Binder, R. V. (1999). *Testing Object-oriented Systems: Models, Patterns and Tools*. Reading, MA: Addison Wesley Longman.

Giunchglia, F., & Walsh, T. (1992). A theory of abstraction. *Artificial Intelligence, 56*, 323–390. doi:10.1016/0004-3702(92)90021-O

Goodrich, M., & Tamassia, R. (2004). *Algorithm Design: Foundations, Analysis, and Internet Examples* (2nd ed.). New York: John Wiley & Sons, Inc.

Han, J., & Dong, J. (2007). Perspectives of Granular Computing in Software Engineering. In Lin, T. Y., Hu, X., Han, J. (Ed.), *Proceedings of IEEE International Conference on Granular Computing* (pp. 66-071). San Jose, CA: IEEE Press.

Hobbs, J. R. (1985). Granularity, In Joshi, A. K. (Ed.), *Proceedings. of the 9th International Joint Conference on Artificial Intelligence* (pp. 432-435). San Francisco: Morgan Kaufmann.

Horstmann, C. (2007). *Big Java* (3rd ed.). New York: John Wiley & Sons, Inc.

Levitin, A. V. (2002). *Introduction to the Design & Analysis of Algorithms*. Reading, MA: Addison Wesley.

Lin, T. Y. (1989). Neighborhood Systems and Approximation in Database and Knowledge Base Systems In Ras, Z. W. & Saitta (Eds.), *Proceedings of the Fourth International Symposium on Methodologies of Intelligent Systems* (pp. 75-86). Amsterdam: Elsevier.

Lin, T. Y. (1997A). Neighborhood Systems - A Qualitative Theory for Fuzzy and Rough Sets. In Wang, P. (Ed.), *Advances in Machine Intelligence and Soft Computing* (*Vol. IV*, pp. 132–155). Durham, NC: Duke University Press.

Lin, T. Y. (1997B). Granular computing: From rough sets and neighborhood systems to information granulation and computing in words. In [Aachen, Germany.]. *Proceedings of European Congress on Intelligent Techniques and Soft Computing, II*, 1602–1606.

O'Docherty, M. (2005). *Object-Oriented Analysis & Design*. New York: John Wiley & Sons, Ltd.

Pawlak, Z. (1982). Rough sets. *International Journal of Computer and Information Sciences, 11*, 341–356. doi:10.1007/BF01001956

Pawlak, Z. (1998). Granularity of knowledge, indiscernibility and rough sets. In [Anchorage, AK.]. *Proceedings of IEEE International Conference on Fuzzy Systems, 1*, 106–110.

Reifer, R. J. (2006). *Software Management* (7th ed.). New York: Wiley-Interscience.

Sommerville, I. (2007). *Software Engineering* (7th ed.). Reading, MA: Addison-Wesley.

Sun Microsystems. (2005). *Sun Microsystems*. Retrieved from http://java.sun.com/j2se/1.5.0/docs/api/

Watt, D., & Brown, D. (2001). *Java Collections*. New York: John Wiley & Sons, Inc.

Wu, C., & Yang, X. (2005). Information Granules in General and Complete Coverings. In Hu, X., Liu, Q., Skowron, A., Lin, T. Y., Yager, R. R., & Zhang, B., (Eds.), Proceedings of IEEE International Conference on Granular Computing (pp. 675-678). Beijing, China, IEEE Press.

Yao, J. T. (2006). Information Granulation and Granular Relationships. In Zhang, Y. & Lin, T. Y. (Eds.), *Proceedings of IEEE International Conference on Granular Computing* (pp. 326-329), Atlanta, GA: IEEE Press.

Yao, J. T. (2007). A Ten-Year Review of Granular Computing, In Lin, T. Y., Hu, X., Han, J. (Eds.), *Proceedings of IEEE International Conference on Granular Computing* (pp. 734-739), San Jose, CA IEEE Press.

Yao, Y. Y. (2004). A partition model of granular computing. *LNCS Transactions on Rough Sets, 1*, 232–253.

Yao, Y. Y. (2005). Perspectives of Granular Computing. In Hu, X., Liu, Q., Skowron, A., Lin, T. Y., Yager, R. R., & Zhang, B., (Eds.). In*Proceedings of IEEE International Conference on Granular Computing* (pp. 85-90), Beijing, China: IEEE Press.

Yao, Y. Y. (2007). Structured Writing with Granular Computing Strategies. In Lin, T. Y., Hu, X., Han, J. (Eds.), *Proceedings of IEEE International Conference on Granular Computing* (pp. 72-77). San Jose, CA, IEEE Press.

Zadeh, L. A. (1979). Fuzzy sets and information granularity. In Gupta, M., Ragade, R., & Yager, R. (Eds.), *Advances in Fuzzy Set Theory and Applications* (pp. 3–18). Amsterdam: North-Holland Publishing Co.

Zadeh, L. A. (1997). Towards a theory of fuzzy information granulation and its centrality in human reasoning and fuzzy logic. *Fuzzy Sets and Systems, 19*, 111–127. doi:10.1016/S0165-0114(97)00077-8

# Chapter 16
# Granular Computing in Formal Concept

**Yuan Ma**
*University of Science and Technology Liaoning, China*

**Zhangang Liu**
*University of Science and Technology Liaoning, China*

**Xuedong Zhang**
*University of Science and Technology Liaoning, China*

## ABSTRACT

*Granular computing has permeated through the field of formal concept; it is another new and rapid developmental aspect of formal concept. In this chapter, we'll regard supremum semisublattice, infimum semisublattice and sublattice as "granule". When a set of granules covers the lattice, "granular space" is called on the concept lattice. We study mainly granular spaces generated by ideal-filter☐congruence relations and tolerance relations. We emphasize properties of these granular spaces and generating methods of these granular spaces. By our viewpoint to study granular computing in formal concept, we find out that it shows profound relation and essence of various sublattices.*

## BACKGROUND

Granular computing and formal concept as new ideas of the field of knowledge discovery have been received more attention about their relation. Granular computing was first proposed by L.A. Zadeh in 1998. Much affection had been generated in various scientific fields in recent decade. Formal concept analysis was firstly proposed by Rudolf Wille, a German professor, in 1982. The most basic elements of human thinking—concept and their hierarchy was explored, analyzed and researched with mathematical method by this theory. It is a branch of lattice theory. In recent years, granular computing has permeated through the field of formal concept as well. The granules and their hierarchy which were generated by equivalence relations in formal concept were researched by Y.Y. Yao & J.T. Yao in 2002 by Du W.L & Miao D.Q in 2005 and by Z. Zheng, H. Hu, Z. Shi. The properties of granules generated by equivalence

DOI: 10.4018/978-1-60566-324-1.ch016

relations in concept lattice were researched profoundly. Some further works were done by us on granular computing in formal concept, too. The speech was given which is titled by "Granular Spaces Generated by Congruence Relations in Concept Lattice" in the Assembly Discussions on "granular computing" of the 5th Chinese Conference on Rough Set and Software Computation in 2005. It aroused many echoes. Under such background, we more expand the research about granular spaces generated by congruence relations, and promote the research about granular spaces generated by ideal-filter and also advance the research about granular spaces generated by tolerance relation.

## 1. BASIC DEFINITION

### Definition 1.1

Let $U$ be a set of objects, $M$ is a set of attributes, and $I \subseteq U \times M$ is a relation between $U$ and $M$. $\theta$ is called a **formal context** (**context** for short). Let $A$ is a subset of $U$ and $B$ is a subset of $M$, we define two functions $f(A)$ and $g(B)$ as:

$$f(A) = \{m \in M \mid \forall u \in A , (u, m) \in I\} \quad g(B) = \{ u \in U \mid \forall m \in B , (u, m) \in I \}$$

then, $(A, B)$ is called a **formal concept** (**concept** for short) on context $(U, M, I)$ with $f(A) = B$ and $g(B) = A$, where $[a]^\theta = [(a^\theta)_\theta, a^\theta]$, $B \subseteq M$. $A$ is called **extent** of the concept, $B$ is called **intent** of the concept. The set of all concepts on $(U, M, I)$ is denoted by $\mathfrak{B}(U, M, I)$

If $A, A_1, A_2 \subseteq U$, $B, B_1, B_2 \subseteq M$, there are some properties, which will be used in this chapter, as follows:

1)$A_1 \subseteq A_2 \Rightarrow f(A_2) \subseteq f(A_1)$ 1')$B_1 \subseteq B_2 \Rightarrow g(B_2) \subseteq g(B_1)$

$\theta$ 2')$B \subseteq f(g(B))$

3)$f(A) = f(g(f(A)))$ 3')$g(B) = g(f(g(B)))$

4)$f(A_1 \cup A_2) = f(A_1) \cap f(A_2)$ 4')$g(B_1 \cup B_2) = g(B_1) \cap g(B_2)$

Note that 4) and 4') can be extended as follows: given by an index set $T$, if for each $t \in T$, $A_t \subseteq U$ and $B_t \subseteq M$, then

$$f(\bigcup_{t \in T} A_t) = \bigcap_{t \in T} f(A_t) , \quad g(\bigcup_{t \in T} B_t) = \bigcap_{t \in T} g(B_t) .$$

On the other hand, by 2) and 2'), for any subset $A$ of $U$, $\left(g\big(f(A)\big), f(A)\right)$ must be a concept and for any subset $B$ of $M$, $\left(g(B), f\big(g(B)\big)\right)$ must be a concept as well. Especially, for an object $u$, $\left(g\big(f(u)\big), f(u)\right)$

is called **object concept** and is denoted by $\gamma u$, for a attribute $m$, $\big(f\big(g(m)\big), g(m)\big)$ is called **attribute concept** and is denoted by $\mu m$.

## Definition 1.2

$(A_1, B_1)$ is called the **child concept** of $(A_2, B_2)$, and $(A_2, B_2)$ is called the **parent concept** of $(A_1, B_1)$, If $(A_1, B_1)$ and $(A_2, B_2)$ are two concepts on a context and $A_1 \subseteq A_2$ (equivalent to $B_2 \subseteq B_1$), It was denoted by $(A_1, B_1) \leq (A_2, B_2)$. Apparently, the relation $\leq$ is reflexive, antisymmetric and transitive, thus $\leq$ is a partial order on the concept set.

Let $S \subseteq \mathfrak{B}(U, M, I)$. If for all $(A, B) \in S$, $(X, Y) \leq (A, B)$, then $(X, Y)$ is called a **lower bound** of $S$. If for all $(A, B) \in S$, $(A, B) \leq (X, Y)$, then, $(X, Y)$ is called a **upper bound** of $S$. If there exists a maximum element in the set of all lower bounds of $S$, it is called the **infimum** of $S$ and write $\wedge S$. Dually, If there exists a minimum element in the set of all upper bounds of $S$, it is called the **supremum** of $S$ and write $\vee S$. Especially, if $S$ includes only two elements $(A, B)$ and $(C, D)$, the infimum of $S$ is denoted by $(A, B) \wedge (C, D)$ and the supremum is denoted by $(A, B) \vee (C, D)$. If $\{(A_t, B_t) | t \in T\}$ is a set of concepts, it has been proved that the infimum and the supremum of the set is must exist. They are $\left( \underset{t \in T}{\cap} A_t, f(\underset{t \in T}{\cap} A_t) \right)$ and $\left( g(\underset{t \in T}{\cap})B_t, \underset{t \in T}{\cap} B_t \right)$, respectively.

Thus the partial ordered set ( $\mathfrak{B}(U, M, I), \leq$ ) is a complete lattice, the **concept lattice** is called on the context $(U, M, I)$ and denoted by $\underline{\mathfrak{B}}(U, M, I)$ (Add a short line under $\mathfrak{B}$. The elements of $\underline{\mathfrak{B}}(U, M, I)$ will inherit the relation $\leq$ in $\underline{\mathfrak{B}}(U, M, I)$).

## Definition 1.3

The granules in $\underline{\mathfrak{B}}(U, M, I)$ contain the infimum granules, the supremum granules and the regular granules.

If $[a]_\theta = [a_\theta, (a_\theta)^\theta]$ and the infimum operation is closed, that is, $\forall S' \subseteq S$, $\wedge S' \in S$, then $S$ is called an **infimum semisublattice** on $\underline{\mathfrak{B}}(U, M, I)$ or an **infimum granule**.

If $S \subseteq \underline{\mathfrak{B}}(U, M, I)$ and the supremum operation is closed, that is $\forall S' \subseteq S$, $\vee S' \in S$, then $S$ is called an **supremum semisublattice** on $\underline{\mathfrak{B}}(U, M, I)$ or a **supremum granule**.

If $S \subseteq \underline{\mathfrak{B}}(U, M, I)$ is an infimum semisublattice as well as a supremum semisublattice on $\underline{\mathfrak{B}}(U, M, I)$ then $S$ is called a **sublattice** on $\underline{\mathfrak{B}}(U, M, I)$ or a **regular granule**.

Apparently regular granule is infimum granule as well as supremum granule.

Let $\mathfrak{S}$ be the set of granules on

$(34, be), (13, bc), (134, bce), (123, abcd),$
$(1235, abcdf), (1234, abcde), (1345, bcef), (12345, abcdef).$

and

$$\cup \mathfrak{S} = \frac{(34, be), (13, bc), (134, bce), (123, abcd), (1235, abcdf),.}{(1234, abcde), (1345, bcef), (12345, abcdef)}$$

then $\mathfrak{S}$ is called a **granular space** on

$(34, be), (13, bc), (134, bce), (123, abcd), (1235, abcdf),$
$(1234, abcde), (1345, bcef), (12345, abcdef).$

If any two granules in $\mathfrak{S}$ do not have common elements, that is, $a^\theta = \vee \{x \in \mathscr{V} \mid a\theta x\}$ is a partition

of

$(34, be), (13, bc), (134, bce), (123, abcd), (1235, abcdf),$
$(1234, abcde), (1345, bcef), (12345, abcdef).$

then $\mathfrak{S}$ is called a granular space of **partition type** on

$(34, be), (13, bc), (134, bce), (123, abcd),$
$(1235, abcdf), (1234, abcde), (1345, bcef), (12345, abcdef).$

otherwise $\mathfrak{S}$ is called a granular space of **overlapping type** on

$(34, be), (13, bc), (134, bce), (123, abcd),$
$(1235, abcdf), (1234, abcde), (1345, bcef), (12345, abcdef).$

## Example 1.1

As Figure 1 illustrates, (a) is a regular granular space (all the granules are sublattices). (b) is a infimum granular space (The bottommost granule is infimum semisublattice, other granules are sublattices. Because sublattice is also the infimum semisublattice, so this is a infimum granular space). (c) is a supremum granular space (The most right side granule is supremum semisublattice, other granules are sublattices. Because sublattice is also the supremum semisublattice, so this is a supremum granular space). They are all granular spaces of partition type. (d) is a regular granular space. It is the overlapping type.

## Definition 1.4

Assume that $S \subseteq \mathfrak{B}(U, M, I)$. If $(A, B) \in S$ and $(C, D) \leq (A, B)$ implies $(C, D) \in S$, then $S$ is called an **order ideal** of $\mathfrak{B}(U, M, I)$. If $S' = \{(A_t, B_t) \mid t \in T\} \subseteq S$, with $T$ is an index set, then

*Figure 1. Granular space on* $\mathfrak{B}(U, M, I)$

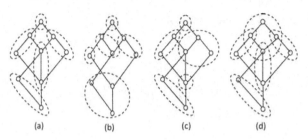

(a)       (b)       (c)       (d)

$\wedge S' = (\underset{t \in T}{\cap} A_t, f(\underset{t \in T}{\cap} A_t))$. Since $(A_1, B_1) \in S$ and $(\underset{t \in T}{\cap} A_t, f(\underset{t \in T}{\cap} A_t)) \leq (A_1, B_1)$, $(\underset{t \in T}{\cap} A_t, f(\underset{t \in T}{\cap} A_t)) \in S$, that is, $\wedge S' \in S$. This indicates that each order ideal is an infimum granule of

$(34, be), (13, bc), (134, bce), (123, abcd),$

$(1235, abcdf), (1234, abcde), (1345, bcef), (12345, abcdef).$

Let $S \subseteq \mathfrak{B}(U, M, I)$. If $(A, B) \in S$ and $(C, D) \geq (A, B)$ implies $(C, D) \in S$, then $S$ is called an **order filter** of $a_\theta = \wedge \{x \in \mathscr{V} \mid a\theta x\}$. Similarly, each order filter is a supremum granule of $\mathfrak{B}(U, M, I)$.

If $(A, B) \in \mathfrak{B}(U, M, I)$ then, the set $S = \{(C, D) \mid (C, D) \leq (A, B)\}$ is denoted by $((A, B)]$ and is called a **principal ideal** of $\mathfrak{B}(U, M, I)$. If $S' = \{(A_t, B_t) \mid t \in T\} \subseteq S$, which $T$ is a index set, then $\forall t \in T, A_t \subseteq A$ and $B_t \supseteq B$, that is, $\underset{t \in T}{\cap} A_t \subseteq A$ and $\underset{t \in T}{\cap} B_t \supseteq B$. We have that $\wedge S' = (\underset{t \in T}{\cap} A_t, f(\underset{t \in T}{\cap} A_t)) \leq (A, B)$ and $\theta$, hence, we can draw a conclusion that $\wedge S' \in S$ and $\vee S' \in S$. Thus every principal ideal is a regular granule of $\mathfrak{B}(U, M, I)$.

If $(A, B) \in \mathfrak{B}(U, M, I)$ then the set $\{(C, D) \mid (C, D) \geq (A, B)\}$ is denoted by $[(A, B))$ and is called the **principal filter** of $\mathfrak{B}(U, M, I)$. Similarly, each principal filter is a regular granule of $\mathfrak{B}(U, M, I)$.

If $S \subseteq \mathfrak{B}(U, M, I)$ such that (1) $S$ is an order ideal, (2) every pair of elements in $\theta$ has common upper bound, then $S$ is called an **ideal**. As ideal is special case of order ideal, each ideal is an infimum granule on $\mathfrak{B}(U, M, I)$.

If $S \subseteq \mathfrak{B}(U, M, I)$ such that (1) $S$ is an order filter, (2) every pair of elements in $S$ has common lower bound, then $S$ is called a **filter**. As filter is a special case of order filter, each filter is a supremum granule of $\mathfrak{B}(U, M, I)$.

If, $(A, B) \leq (C, D)$, the **interval** which begins at $(A, B)$ and ends in $(C, D)$ is the set $\{(E, F) \mid (A, B) \leq (E, F) \leq (C, D)\}$ and denoted by $[(A, B), (C, D)]$. Apparently, for $\theta \subseteq \mathscr{V} \times \mathscr{V}$ we have that $A \subseteq A_t \subseteq C$, with $T$ is an index set, that is, $(A, B) \leq (\underset{t \in T}{\cap} A_t, f(\underset{t \in T}{\cap} A_t)) \leq (C, D)$ Hence, their infimum belongs to $[(A, B), (C, D)]$

On the other hand, we have that $\forall t \in T$,, $(A,B) \leq (g(\underset{t \in T}{\cap} B_t), \underset{t \in T}{\cap} B_t) \leq (C,D)$ and their supremum

$(g(\underset{t \in T}{\cap} B_t), \underset{t \in T}{\cap} B_t)$ belongs to $[(A,B),(C,D)]$, too. It indicates that all the intervals are regular granules

of $\mathfrak{B}(U,M,I)$.

Although infimum semisublattice,supremum semisublattice and sublattice are all granules, but order ideal, order filter, principal ideal, principal filter, ideal, filter and interval are the most general granules. In the later parts we will research some granular spaces that are formed from them.

In this section, we have defined the supremum granules, the infimum granules, the regular granules, the granular spaces of partition type and the granular spaces of overlapping type and showed the order ideals, the order filters, the principal ideals, the principal filters, the ideals, the filters and the intervals are most familiar granules.

## 2. IDEAL-FILTER GRANULE

Firstly, we present a simple granular space, It consists of only two granules. it is called the ideal-filter granular space.

### Definition 2.1

If $\mathscr{V}$ is a concept lattice. The ideal-filter granular space of $\mathscr{V}$ is a granular space $\mathfrak{S}$ that consists of only two granules. One is the principal ideal of a certain concept $(A,B)$, $G_1 = \{(X,Y) \mid (X,Y) \leq (A,B)\}$, the other is the principal filter of the other certain concept $(C,D)$ $G_2 = \{(X,Y) \mid (X,Y) \geq (C,D)\}$.

Since $\mathfrak{S} = \{G_1, G_2\}$ is a granular space, $G_1$ and $G_2$ such that $G_1 \cup G_2 = \mathscr{V}$. This means that any concept of $\mathscr{V}$ is either the child concept of $(A,B)$ or the parent concept of $(C,D)$ and by Definition 1.4, the principal filter and the principal ideal must be granule, hence, Definition 2.1 is rational.

### Example 2.1

A concept lattice $\mathscr{V}$ is shown in Figure 2. Four ideal-filter granular spaces of $\mathscr{V}$ is shown in Figure 3. The concept $(A,B)$ and $(C,D)$ are denoted by black solid round. (a), (b),(c) are the granular spaces of partition type. (d) is the granular space of overlapping type.

### Definition 2.2

Concepts $(A,B)$ and $(C,D)$ in Definition 2.1 is called a pair of **characteristic concepts** on $\mathscr{V}$, $G_1$ is the ideal granule and

$(34, be), (13, bc), (134, bce), (123, abcd),$

$(1235, abcdf), (1234, abcde), (1345, bcef), (12345, abcdef).$

is the filter granule.

With respect to the pair of characteristic concepts, we have the theorems, as follows:

## Theorem 2.1

Let the context of concept lattice $\mathscr{V}$ be $(U, M, I)$ $(A, B)$ and $(C, D)$ are a pair of characteristic concepts in $\mathscr{V}$, if and only if $U \times D \cup A \times M \supseteq I$ (The sketch map is shown in Figure 4).

## Proof

Firstly, we prove an Affirmation: If $u \notin A$ and $U \times D \cup A \times M \supseteq I$, then $f(u) \subseteq D$.

For any $m$ such that $(u, m) \in I$, since $u \notin A$, $(u, m) \notin A \times M$. Then, $(u, m) \in U \times D$, that is, $m \in D$. Hence $f(u) = \{m \mid (u, m) \in I\}$ is a subset of $D$.

*Figure 2. A concept lattice $\mathscr{V}$*

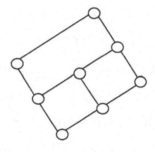

*Figure 3. Four ideal-filter granular space of concept lattice $\mathscr{V}$*

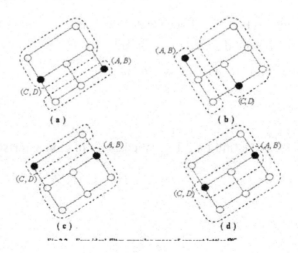

(If) If $(A, B), (C, D)$ such that $U \times D \cup A \times M \supseteq I$, we prove that any concept of

$(\varnothing, \varnothing), (5, f), (4, e), (1, c), (3, b), (145, cef),$
$(45, ef), (15, cf), (35, bf), (135, bcf), (14, ce), (345, bef),$

is either the child concept of $(A, B)$ or the parent concept of $(C, D)$.

If $X \subseteq A$, then $(X, Y)$ is the children concept of $(A, B)$. If $X \nsubseteq A$, then there exists $u \in X$, but $u \notin A$. Hence by the above Affirmation, $f(u) \subseteq D$. On the other hand, $f(X) \subseteq f(u)$, so $f(X) = Y \subseteq D$ and then, $(X, Y)$ is the parent concept of $(C, D)$.

(Only if) If each concept $(X, Y)$ of $\mathscr{V}$ is either the child concept of $(A, B)$ or the parent concept of $(C, D)$ then we prove $U \times D \cup A \times M \supseteq I$.

For an arbitrary $(u, m) \in I$, if $u \in A$ then, $(u, m) \in A \times M$. If $u \notin A$ then $(g(f(u)), f(u))$ is not the child concept of $(A, B)$, since if $(g(f(u)), f(u)) \leq (A, B)$ then, $g(f(u)) \subseteq A$, at the same time, $u \in g(f(u))$. It contradicts with the fact that $u \notin A$), Hence, $(g(f(u)), f(u))$ is a parent concept of $(C, D)$, that is, $f(u) \subseteq D$. Since $(u, m) \in I$, then, $m \in f(u)$ and $m \in D$, $(u, m) \in U \times D$. Since $(u, m)$ is an arbitrary element of $I$ then, $U \times D \cup A \times M \supseteq I$.

## Example 2.2

The concept lattice $\mathscr{V}$ shown in Figure 2, The context of $\mathscr{V}$ is shown in Table 1. The extents and the intents of concepts of $\mathscr{V}$ are shown in Figure 5, where we use a notion, which is an order pair consisted of number and alphabet in concept lattice, to denote a concept, i.e. Concept $(\{1, 2\}, \{b, d\})$ is denoted by (12, bd). Corresponding with Figure 3 (a), (b), (c), (d), the various situation of $U \times D \cup A \times M \supseteq I$ are shown in Figure 6 (a), (b), (c), (d).

For these ideal-filter granular spaces, people are more interested in those of partition type. Hence, we have the following theorem and a method to get all ideal-filter granular spaces of partition type of concept lattice $\mathscr{V}$ with double concept in anti-context.

*Figure 4. Sketch map of $U \times D \cup A \times M \supseteq I$*

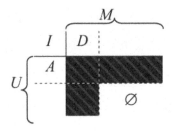

## Theorem 2.2

The ideal-filter granular space with a pair of characteristic concepts $(A, B), (C, D)$ is partition type, if and only if $C \nsubseteq A$ and $B \nsubseteq D$.

## Proof

We first prove that if $C \nsubseteq A$, then $B \nsubseteq D$ (by the same way, if $B \nsubseteq D$, then $C \nsubseteq A$). If $C \nsubseteq A$ but $B \subseteq D$, then $g(B) \supseteq g(D)$. Since $C \nsubseteq A$, there exists $u \in C$ and $u \notin A$. However $u \in C = g(D) \subseteq g(B) = A$ contradicts with the fact $u \notin A$, then, we have that $B \nsubseteq D$. It means that if $U \times D \cup A \times M \supseteq I$, then either $C \subseteq A$ and $B \subseteq D$ or $C \nsubseteq A$ and $B \nsubseteq D$.

If $C \subseteq A$ and $B \subseteq D$, then $(C, D) \leq (A, B)$ Thus

$$(C, D) \in \{(X, Y) \mid (X, Y) \leq (A, B)\} = G_1 \text{ and}$$

$$(A, B) \in \{(X, Y) \mid (X, Y) \geq (C, D)\} = G_2.$$

*Table 1. A context*

| $I$ | $a$ | $b$ | $c$ | $d$ |
|---|---|---|---|---|
| 1 | X | X |   | X |
| 2 |   | X | X | X |
| 3 |   |   | X |   |
| 4 | X | X |   |   |

*Figure 5. Concepts of $\mathscr{V}$*

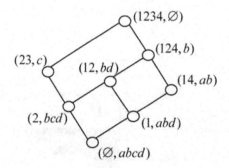

In this case, $G_1$ and $G_2$ overlap each other.

If $C \not\subseteq A$ and $B \not\subseteq D$, then $(C, D) \not\leq (A, B)$. And considering the other fact: if

$$(E, F) \in \{(X, Y) \mid (X, Y) \leq (A, B)\} \cap \{(X, Y) \mid (X, Y) \geq (C, D)\}$$

then, we have that $(C, D) \leq (E, F) \leq (A, B)$. Which is contradicts with the fact that $(C, D) \not\leq (A, B)$. It means that $G_1 = \{(X, Y) \mid (X, Y) \leq (A, B)\}$ and $G_2 = \{(X, Y) \mid (X, Y) \geq (C, D)\}$ do not have common elements, that is, $\{G_1, G_2\}$ is a partition of $\mathscr{V}$.

By theorem 2.2, We have that a method to get all ideal-filter granular spaces of partition type of a concept lattice $\mathscr{V}$.

## Definition 2.3

The concept $\left[(A, B)\right]_\theta$ is **double concept** if it is both an object concept and an attribute concept. $(U, M, U \times M - I)$ is called anti-context of $(U, M, I)$ and $U \times M - I$ is denote by $\overline{I}$.

## Example 2.3

The anti-context of the context in Table 1 is shown in Table 2. The concept lattice of this anti-context is shown in Figure 7. Among these concepts, concept $(23, a)$ is both the object concept of $2$ and the attribute concept of $a$. Hence it is a double concept. Concept $(3, abd)$ is both the object concept of $3$ and the attribute concept of $b$. It is also a double concept. Concept $\left[(A, B)\right]_\theta$ is both the object concept of $1$ and the attribute concept of $c$. It is a double concept as well.

*Figure 6. Some instants of $U \times D \cup A \times M \supseteq I$ in $\mathscr{V}$*

|   | b | c | d | a |
|---|---|---|---|---|
| 1 | × |   | × | × |
| 4 | × |   |   | × |
| 2 | × | × | × | ∅ |
| 3 |   | × |   |   |

(a)

|   | a | b | d | c |
|---|---|---|---|---|
| 2 |   | × | × | × |
| 3 |   |   |   | × |
| 1 | × | × | × | ∅ |
| 4 | × | × |   |   |

(b)

|   | c | a | b | d |
|---|---|---|---|---|
| 1 |   | × | × | × |
| 2 | × |   | × | × |
| 4 |   | × | × |   |
| 3 | × |   | ∅ |   |

(c)

|   | b | c | d | a |
|---|---|---|---|---|
| 1 | × |   | × | × |
| 2 | × | × | × |   |
| 4 | × |   |   | × |
| 3 |   | × |   | ∅ |

(d)

*Figure 7. The concept lattice of anti-context*

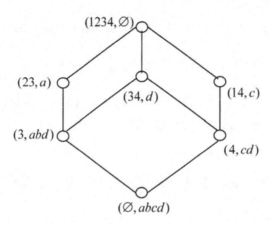

*Table 2. An anti-context*

| I | a | b | c | d |
|---|---|---|---|---|
| 1 |   |   | X |   |
| 2 | X |   |   |   |
| 3 | X | X |   | X |
| 4 |   |   | X | X |

## Theorem 2.3

A pair of characteristic concepts $(A, B), (C, D)$ of context $(U, M, I)$ such that $C \nsubseteq A$, $B \nsubseteq D$, if and only if there exists a double concept of object $u$ and attribute $m$, $(g_{\bar{I}}(m), f_{\bar{I}}(u))$, in anti-context $(U, M, \bar{I})$ and $A = g(m)$, $\big[(A, B)\big]_\theta$.

### Proof

Firstly, we still use $f$ and $g$ to denote $f$ and $g$ in the context $(U, M, I)$, respectively, whereas use $f_{\bar{I}}$ and $g_{\bar{I}}$ to denote $f$ and $g$ in anti-context $(U, M, \bar{I})$, respectively.

(If) If $U \times D \cup A \times M \supseteq I$ and $\mathscr{V} / \theta$, $B \nsubseteq D$, we prove there exists $u, m$ such that $A = g(m)$, $D = f(u)$ and object concept of $u$ equals to attribute concept of $m$ in anti-context.

Since $C \nsubseteq A$, there exists $u \in C$ and $u \notin A$. Because $u \notin A$, by the Affirmation in Theorem 2.1, we must have that ①$\big[(A, B)\big]_\theta$. On the other hand, by $u \in C$ we have that ② $f(u) \supseteq f(C)$. By ①②, $f(u) = f(C) = D$, and then, ⓐ$f_{\bar{I}}(u) = M - D$. Since $u \notin A$, it means that $u \in U - A$ and then,ⓑ

$f_{\bar{I}}(u) \supseteq f_{\bar{I}}(U - A)$. Note we have that $U \times D \cup A \times M \supseteq I$ is equivalent to $(U - A) \times (M - D) \subseteq \bar{I}$, then, ⓒ $f_{\bar{I}}(U - A) \supseteq M - D$.

In such case, by ⓐⓑⓒ, we have that $M - D = f_{\bar{I}}(u) \supseteq f_{\bar{I}}(U - A) \supseteq M - D$. Hence $\mathscr{V} / \theta$. In a similar way, we can also have that $g_{\bar{I}}(m) = g_{\bar{I}}(M - D) = U - A$. Hence $(U - A, M - D)$ is a concept in the anti-context, and it is both object concept of $u$ and attribute concept of $m$. It also holds that $f(u) = D$ and dually, $g(m) = A$.

(Only if)Assume that $(E, F)$ is the object concept of $u$ and the attribute concept of $m$ in the anti-context. Let $A = U - E$, $D = M - F$, we prove that $U \times D \cup A \times M \supseteq I$ and $f(u) = D, g(m) = A$. Let $g(D) = C$ and $f(A) = B$, we also prove that $C \not\subseteq A$, $B \not\subseteq D$.

Since $\left[(A, B)\right]_\theta$ is a concept of the anti-context, $E \times F \subseteq \bar{I}$. Let arbitrary of $(v, n) \in I$, then $(v, n) \notin E \times F$. There exists either $v \notin E$ or $n \notin F$, that is, either $v \in A$ or $n \in D$, and that is too, either $(v, n) \in A \times M$ or $(v, n) \in U \times D$. Then, it means that $(v, n)$ must belongs to $U \times D \cup A \times M$. Since the arbitrary of$(v, n)$ on $I$, $U \times D \cup A \times M \supseteq I$ and $(E, F)$ is the object concept of $u$ of the anti-context, that means that it holds that $f_{\bar{I}}(u) = F$, $u \in g_{\bar{I}}(f_{\bar{I}}(u)) = g_{\bar{I}}(F) = E = U - A$, then, $u \notin A$. On the other hand $f(u) = M - F = D$, it means that $u \in g(f(u)) = g(D) = C$, Hence $A \not\supseteq C$. By the same reason, we have that $g(m) = A$ and $D \not\supseteq B$.

By Theorem 2.2 and Theorem 2.3, we have that a method to get all idea-filter granular spaces of partition type with double concept in anti-context.

## Example 2.4

Context $(U, M, I)$ and anti-context $(U, M, \bar{I})$ are shown in Figure 8(a),(b), respectively. Concept lattice of $(U, M, I)$ and concept lattice of $(U, M, \bar{I})$ are shown in Figure 9(a),(b), respectively. The object concepts and attribute concepts are indicated in the figures. There are three double concepts in the anti-context. One is *of* 1 and *of* $d$, the other is *of* 3 and *of* $b$, still other is *of* 4 and *of* $c$. There are three ideal-filter granular space of partition type in $\mathfrak{B}(U, M, I)$. The first one determined by double concept of 1 and of $d$ is shown in Figure 10(a). The second one determined by double concept of 3 and of $b$ is as shown in Figure 10(b), The last one determined by double concept of 4 and of $c$ is as shown in Figure 10(c).

In this section we researched the ideal-filter granular space. It is the granular space which only contains two granules. We studied its properties and proved that the ideal-filter granular spaces of partition type can be gotten from double concept in the anti-context.

*Figure 8. A context and its anti-context*

| $I$ | $a$ | $b$ | $c$ | $d$ | $e$ |
|---|---|---|---|---|---|
| 1 | × | × | × |   | × |
| 2 |   | × | × |   |   |
| 3 | × |   | × | × | × |
| 4 |   | × |   | × |   |
| 5 |   |   | × | × | × |

| $\overline{I}$ | $a$ | $b$ | $c$ | $d$ | $e$ |
|---|---|---|---|---|---|
| 1 |   |   |   | × |   |
| 2 | × |   |   | × | × |
| 3 |   | × |   |   |   |
| 4 | × |   | × |   | × |
| 5 | × | × |   |   |   |

(a)                            (b)

*Figure 9. A concept lattice of the context and anti-concept*

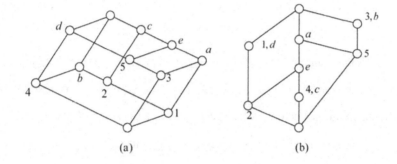

(a)                            (b)

## 3.CONGRUENCE GRANULE

We will study a more complex granular space in this section. These granular spaces are generated by congruence relation. Each of granules in such granular space is an interval and all of them must form a partition of the whole concept lattice. So this is a kind of the granular space of partition type.

### Definition 3.1

Assume that $\mathscr{V}$ is a concept lattice, $\theta$ is an equivalence relation on $\mathscr{V}$ and **infimum and supremum compatible** (infimum and supremum compatible is that for an index set $T$, for any of t such that $\forall t \in T, (A_t, B_t), (C_t, D_t) \in \mathscr{V}$ and $[J, D]$, then $(12345, \varnothing)$ and $\left( \bigwedge_{t \in T}(A_t, B_t) \right) \theta \left( \bigwedge_{t \in T}(C_t, D_t) \right)$), then $\theta$ is called the **congruence relation** on $\mathscr{V}$.

### Theorem 3.1

Assume that $\mathscr{V} / \theta$ is a concept lattice and $\theta$ is a congruence relation on $\mathscr{V}$, $L$ is an $D$-equivalence class containing $(A, B)$, then $F$ is called **congruence granule**. Let $(a_\theta)^\theta$ then the congruence granule $[(A, B)]_\theta$ must be the interval $[\,(\underline{A}, \underline{B}), (\overline{A}, \overline{B})\,]$.

*Figure 10. All ideal-filter granular spaces of partition type in a concept lattice*

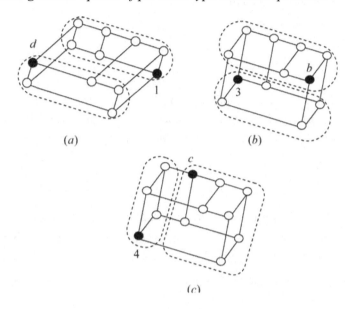

(a)          (b)

(c)

## Proof

For a given concept $(A, B)$, we define an index set $T$ such that $[(A, B)]_\theta = \{(C_t, D_t) \mid t \in T\}$, then $\underset{t \in T}{\vee}(C_t, D_t) = \vee [(A, B)]_\theta = (\bar{A}, \bar{B})$. On the other hand, for all $t \in T$, let $(A_t, B_t)$ be $(A, B)$, then $\underset{t \in T}{\vee}(A_t, B_t) = (A, B)$. Since $n$ is the congruence relation, that is, $v \in V$, then $m \in M - N$. Thus $u \in V$.

Similarly, we have that $\nearrow$, then each element $(X, Y)$ of $u$ such that $(\underline{A}, \underline{B}) \leq (X, Y) \leq (\bar{A}, \bar{B})$. Conversely, assume that there is an element $(X, Y)$ such that $(\underline{A}, \underline{B}) \leq (X, Y) \leq (\bar{A}, \bar{B})$. Since both $(\underline{A}, \underline{B})$ and $(\underline{X}, \underline{Y})$ are the smallest elements of some equivalence class, respectively, and both $(\bar{A}, \bar{B})$ and $(\bar{X}, \bar{Y})$ are the biggest elements of an equivalence class, respectively, considering the other fact that the two equivalence classes are either not intersecting or just the same one. Now,

$$(\underline{A}, \underline{B}) \leq (X, Y) \leq (\bar{A}, \bar{B}) \text{ and } (\underline{X}, \underline{Y}) \leq (X, Y) \leq (\bar{X}, \bar{Y})$$

are intersection. Then, we have that $l_4$ and $C = A \times B$ are just the same one equivalence class. It means that $l_k = \underbrace{R \times S^T \times R \times S^T \times \cdots}_{k \text{ factors}}$. $u$ contains all the elements which is greater than or equal to $(\underline{A}, \underline{B})$ and smaller than or equal to $(\bar{A}, \bar{B})$. So $|M|$ is the interval $[(\underline{A}, \underline{B}), (\bar{A}, \bar{B})]$.

By Theorem 3.1 and Definition 1.4, we have that every equivalence class of the congruence relation of $\mathscr{V}$ is a regular granule. All the $u_1, u_2, \cdots, u_k \in U$ -equivalence class of $\mathscr{V}$ is denoted by $u$, Because

$(V, N, I \cap V \times N)$ must be a partitions of $\mathscr{V}$, $C \subseteq V$ is a regular granular space of partition type. it is called the **congruence granular space**.

## Example 3.1

A context is shown in Table 3. The concept lattice of it is shown in Figure 11.

Some congruence granular spaces of the concept lattice are shown in Figure 12. The close curves in Figure 12 are the equivalence classes of the congruence relation, that is, the congruence granules.

## Theorem 3.2

Assume that $\mathscr{V} = \mathfrak{B}(U, M, I)$ is a concept lattices. A equivalence relation $\theta$ on $\mathscr{V}$ is a congruence relation, If and only if there exists $V \subseteq U, N \subseteq M$ such that for every equivalence class, $[(A,B)]_\theta$, $(X,Y) \in [(A,B)]_\theta$ equivalents to $X \cap V = A \cap V$ and $Y \cap N = B \cap N$ $(V, N)$ is called a **characteristic value of congruence granular space** $\mathscr{V} / \theta$ and $(A \cap V, B \cap N)$ is called characteristic value of granule $\left[(A, B)\right]_\theta$.

## Example 3.2

The characteristic values $(V, N)$ of the five congruence granular spaces in Figure 12 are shown as follows:

a)  $V = \{3, 4, 5\}, N = \{b, e, f\}$;

b)  $V = \{1, 3, 4, 5\}, N = \{b, c, e, f\}$

c)  $V = \{1, 4, 5\}, N = \{c, e, f\}$;

d)  $V = \{1, 2, 3, 5\}, N = \{a, b, c, d, f\}$

e)  $V = \{1, 2, 3, 4\}, N = \{a, b, c, d, e\}$ (see Figure 11 and Figure 12 for reference).

*Figure 11. A concept lattice*

*Table 3. A context*

| I | a | b | c | d | e | f |
|---|---|---|---|---|---|---|
| 1 | X | X |   |   | X | X |
| 2 |   | X | X |   |   | X |
| 3 |   |   | X | X |   | X |
| 4 | X | X | X | X |   | X |

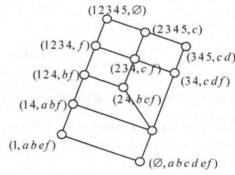

# Theorem 3.3

Assume that $\mathscr{V}$ is a concept lattice of a context $(U, M, I)$, $\theta$ is a congruence relation on $\mathscr{V}$, $(V, N)$ is the characteristic value of granular space $\mathscr{V}/\theta$. Then characteristic values $(A \cap V, B \cap N)$ of each granule $[(A, B)]_\theta$ in $\mathscr{V}/\theta$ is a concept of subcontext $(V, N, I \cap V \times N)$.

## Proof

For an arbitrary granule $[(A, B)]_\theta$ from $\mathscr{V}/\theta$ and let its characteristic value be $A \cap V = C$, $B \cap N = D$. By Theorem 3.2, we have that every concept $(X, Y)$ in granule $[(A, B)]_\theta$ satisfies that $X \cap V = C$ and $Y \cap N = D$, that is, every concept in $[(A, B)]_\theta$ satisfies that the intersection of its extent and $V$ is C and the intersection of its intent and $N$ is D. By Theorem 3.1, we have that $[(A, B)]_\theta$ is the interval of $[(\underline{A}, \underline{B}), (\overline{A}, \overline{B})]$. Hence, $(\underline{A}, \underline{B})$ and $(\overline{A}, \overline{B})$ respectively are the smallest and the greatest concept which satisfies that the intersection of extent and V is C and the intersection of intent and N is D.

That is, $(\underline{A}, \underline{B}) = \left(g\left(f(C)\right), f(C)\right)$ and $(\overline{A}, \overline{B}) = \left(g(D), f\left(g(D)\right)\right)$.

Let $f_1$ and $g_1$ be $f$ and $g$ in context $(V, N, I \cap V \times N)$, respectively. It means that for

$$P \subseteq V, \quad f_1(P) = \left\{m \in N \mid \forall u \in P, (u, m) \in I \cap V \times N\right\}$$

for

*Figure 12. Some space of congruence granule of a concept lattice*

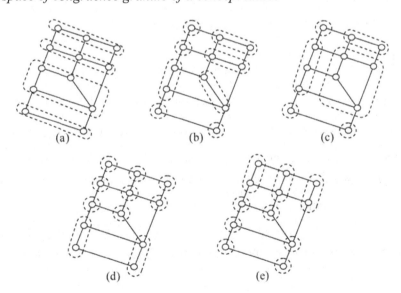

$$Q \subseteq N, \quad g_1(Q) = \left\{ u \in V \mid \forall m \in Q, (u,m) \in I \cap V \times N \right\}$$

Apparently, for $P \subseteq V$, we have that $f_1(P) = f(P) \cap N$ and for $Q \subseteq N$, we have that $g_1(Q) = g(Q) \cap V$. Since $C \subseteq V$, $f_1(C) = f(C) \cap N = \underline{B} \cap N = D$ and since $D \subseteq N$, $g_1(D) = g(D) \cap V = \overline{A} \cap V = C$. Then, $f_1(C) = D, g_1(D) = C$. Hence, $(C, D)$ is a concept of subcontext $(V, N, I \cap V \times N)$.

Since every concept in $\mathscr{V}$ belongs to a granule, $(X \cap V, Y \cap N)$ of any concept $(X, Y)$ in $\mathscr{V}$ is the characteristic value of a granule. So $(X \cap V, Y \cap N)$ must be a concept of $(V, N, I \cap V \times N)$.

Then, we will give the method to generate all congruence granular spaces of a concept lattice.

## Definition 3.2

Assume that $(U, M, I)$ is a context, $u \in U$ and $m \in M$, then

$$u \swarrow m \Leftrightarrow u \cancel{X} m \text{ and } f(u) \subset f(v) \Rightarrow v I m$$

$$u \nearrow m \Leftrightarrow u \cancel{X} m \text{ and } g(m) \subset g(n) \Rightarrow u I n$$

$$u \swarrow\!\!\nearrow m \Leftrightarrow u \swarrow m \text{ and } u \nearrow m$$

## Example 3.3

The relation $\swarrow$, $\nearrow$ and $\swarrow\!\!\nearrow$ of the context in Table 3 are shown as Figure 13. Since $\swarrow$, $\nearrow$ and $\swarrow\!\!\nearrow$ appears only if $u \cancel{X} m$, we can put them in the blank of the cross table of context accordingly. In section 4, we will denote the entry of row $u$ and column $m$ in the table of context by $< u, m >$ for convenience. For instance, in Figure 13, $\langle 1, a \rangle = \times$, $\langle 1, d \rangle = \swarrow$, $\langle 2, e \rangle = \varnothing$.

## Definition 3.3

Let $u_1, u_2, \cdots, u_k \in U$ and $m_1, m_2, \cdots, m_k \in M$ such that $u_i \swarrow m_i, i = 1, \cdots, k$ and $u_i \nearrow m_{i-1} = 2, \ldots, k$, then denote it by $u_1 \swarrow\!\!\swarrow m_k$. The complement of $\swarrow\!\!\swarrow$ is denoted by $\cancel{\swarrow\!\!\swarrow}$, i.e. $u \cancel{\swarrow\!\!\swarrow} m \Leftrightarrow not(u \swarrow\!\!\swarrow m)$.

Apparently, the relation $\swarrow\!\!\swarrow$ between $u$ and $m$ could be found in the following way. Let $R$ and $S$ be matrixes with $|U|$ rows and $|M|$ columns, where $|U|$ is the number of the elements in set $U$ and $|M|$ is the number of the elements in set $M$.

In these matrixes, every row corresponds to an object $u$ and every column corresponds to an attribute $m$. If $u \swarrow m$, then the entry of row $u$ and column $m$ in $R$ is 1 else is 0. If $u \nearrow m$, then the entry of

*Figure 13. Relation of ↗↙⤢ in a context*

| | $a$ | $b$ | $c$ | $d$ | $e$ | $f$ |
|---|---|---|---|---|---|---|
| 1 | × | × | ⤢ | ↙ | × | × |
| 2 | ⤢ | × | × | ⤢ | | × |
| 3 | ↙ | ⤢ | × | × | | |
| 4 | × | × | × | × | ⤢ | × |
| 5 | | | × | × | | ⤢ |

row $u$ and column $m$ in $S$ is 1 else is 0. For example, the matrixes $R$ and $S$ of the context in Figure 13 are shown in Figure 14 as follows.

Let $l_1 = R, l_2 = R \times S^T, \cdots, l_k = \underbrace{R \times S^T \times R \times S^T \times \cdots}_{k \text{ factors}}$.

When $l_{2t+1} = l_{3t+3}$ first appear, if the entry of the row $u$ and column $m$ is 1 in the $l_{2t+1}$ ,then $u \swarrow\swarrow m$, otherwise $u \not\swarrow\!\!\swarrow m$ ,where multiplication operation of matrix shown in Figure 15 as below arithmetic:

- $A$ is a $r \times p$ matrix,
- $B$ is a $p \times s$ matrix and
- $C = A \times B$, then $C_{ij} = \bigoplus_{t=1}^{p}(A_{it} \otimes B_{tj})$
- $1 \le i \le r, 1 \le j \le s$ where $0 \otimes 0 = 0, 0 \otimes 1 = 0, 1 \otimes 0 = 0, 1 \otimes 1 = 1$ and $0 \oplus 0 = 0$, $0 \oplus 1 = 1$, and Figure 16.
- $1 \oplus 0 = 1$, $1 \oplus 1 = 1$. For the above $R$ and $S$, we have that $l_1 = R$

*Figure 14.*

$$R = \begin{array}{c} \\ 1 \\ 2 \\ 3 \\ 4 \\ 5 \end{array} \begin{array}{c} a\ b\ c\ d\ e\ f \\ \begin{pmatrix} 0 & 0 & 1 & 1 & 0 & 0 \\ 1 & 0 & 0 & 1 & 0 & 0 \\ 1 & 1 & 0 & 0 & 0 & 0 \\ 0 & 0 & 0 & 0 & 1 & 0 \\ 0 & 0 & 0 & 0 & 0 & 1 \end{pmatrix} \end{array} \qquad S = \begin{array}{c} \\ 1 \\ 2 \\ 3 \\ 4 \\ 5 \end{array} \begin{array}{c} a\ b\ c\ d\ e\ f \\ \begin{pmatrix} 0 & 0 & 1 & 0 & 0 & 0 \\ 1 & 0 & 0 & 1 & 0 & 0 \\ 0 & 1 & 0 & 0 & 0 & 0 \\ 0 & 0 & 0 & 0 & 1 & 0 \\ 0 & 0 & 0 & 0 & 0 & 1 \end{pmatrix} \end{array}$$

*Figure 15.* $\not\swarrow\!\!\swarrow$ *relation*

| $\not\swarrow\!\!\swarrow$ | $a$ | $b$ | $c$ | $d$ | $e$ | $f$ |
|---|---|---|---|---|---|---|
| 1 | | × | | | × | × |
| 2 | | × | × | | × | × |
| 3 | | | × | | × | × |
| 4 | × | × | × | × | | × |
| 5 | × | × | × | × | × | |

- $l_1 \neq l_3$, then, continue to calculate $l_4$ and $l_5$ with Figure 17.

Since $l_3 = l_5$, we have that the relation $\diagup\diagup$ and the relation $\diagup\!\!\!\diagdown$. The relation $\diagup\!\!\!\diagdown$ is shown as the Figure 15.

## Theorem 3.4

If $(V, N)$ is a characteristic value of a congruence granular space of the concept lattice $\mathscr{V}$ of the context $(U, M, I)$, then the arrows on $(V, N)$ are closed, it means that for an arbitrary $v \in V$, if $v \nearrow m$, then $m \in N$, for an arbitrary $n \in N$, if $u \swarrow n$, then $u \in V$.

## Theorem 3.5

$(V, N)$ is a characteristic value of a congruence granular space of the reduced context $(U, M, I)$, if and only if $(U - V, N)$ is a concept of the context $(U, M, \diagup\!\!\!\diagdown)$.

## Proof

(If) Let $(V, N)$ be a characteristic value of a congruence granular space. Then the arrows are closed on $(V, N)$. If $u \in V$ and $(U, M, I)$ is reduced, then there exists $m$ such that $u \nearrow m$ and $m \in N$. Con-

*Figure 16.*

$$
l_2 = R \times S^T = 
\begin{array}{c}
 \\
1 \\
2 \\
3 \\
4 \\
5
\end{array}
\begin{array}{c}
1\ 2\ 3\ 4\ 5 \\
\begin{pmatrix}
1 & 1 & 0 & 0 & 0 \\
0 & 1 & 0 & 0 & 0 \\
0 & 1 & 1 & 0 & 0 \\
0 & 0 & 0 & 1 & 0 \\
0 & 0 & 0 & 0 & 1
\end{pmatrix}
\end{array}
\qquad
l_3 = R \times S^T \times R = 
\begin{array}{c}
 \\
1 \\
2 \\
3 \\
4 \\
5
\end{array}
\begin{array}{c}
a\ b\ c\ d\ e\ f \\
\begin{pmatrix}
1 & 0 & 1 & 1 & 0 & 0 \\
1 & 0 & 0 & 1 & 0 & 0 \\
1 & 1 & 0 & 1 & 0 & 0 \\
0 & 0 & 0 & 0 & 1 & 0 \\
0 & 0 & 0 & 0 & 0 & 1
\end{pmatrix}
\end{array}
$$

*Figure 17.*

$$
l_4 = R \times S^T \times R \times S^T = 
\begin{array}{c}
 \\
1 \\
2 \\
3 \\
4 \\
5
\end{array}
\begin{array}{c}
1\ 2\ 3\ 4\ 5 \\
\begin{pmatrix}
1 & 1 & 0 & 0 & 0 \\
0 & 1 & 0 & 0 & 0 \\
0 & 1 & 1 & 0 & 0 \\
0 & 0 & 0 & 1 & 0 \\
0 & 0 & 0 & 0 & 1
\end{pmatrix}
\end{array}
\qquad
l_5 = R \times S^T \times R \times S^T \times R = 
\begin{array}{c}
 \\
1 \\
2 \\
3 \\
4 \\
5
\end{array}
\begin{array}{c}
a\ b\ c\ d\ e\ f \\
\begin{pmatrix}
1 & 0 & 1 & 1 & 0 & 0 \\
1 & 0 & 0 & 1 & 0 & 0 \\
1 & 1 & 0 & 1 & 0 & 0 \\
0 & 0 & 0 & 0 & 1 & 0 \\
0 & 0 & 0 & 0 & 0 & 1
\end{pmatrix}
\end{array}
$$

versely, if $n \in N$ made $u \mathbin{\diagup\diagup} n$, then $u$ must belong to $V$ by the definition of $\diagup\diagup$ and arrows close on $(V, N)$. That is, $u \in V$, if and only if $\exists n \in N$ make $u \mathbin{\diagup\diagup} n$, and $u \in U - V$, if and only if $\forall n \in N$, $u \mathbin{\diagup\kern-0.6em\times} n$, it means that If and only if $U - V = g_1(N)$, where $g_1$ is the $g$ operation on $\diagup\kern-0.6em\times$. Now, assume that $m \in M - N$ and $u \mathbin{\diagup} m$. By arrows closed on $(V, N)$, since $u \in U - V$, then, $u \mathbin{\diagup\diagup} m$, hence, $m \notin f_1(U - V)$. It means that $f_1(U - V) \subseteq N$. In order to prove $f_1(U - V) = N$, we also need to prove $f_1(U - V) \supseteq N$. Taking an arbitrary $m \notin f_1(U - V)$ then $\exists\ u \in U - V$, $u \mathbin{\diagup\diagup} m$, and then $m \in M - N$. Hence $f_1(U - V) \supseteq N$, then, $f_1(U - V) = N$. That is, $(U - V, N)$ is a concept of $(U, M, \diagup\kern-0.6em\times)$.

(Only if) Let $(U - V, N)$ be a concept of $(U, M, \diagup\kern-0.6em\times)$. Since $u \mathbin{\diagdown} n$ and $n \in N$, $u \in V$. Now, we prove if $u \mathbin{\diagup} m$ and $v \in H$, then $m \in N$. By contradiction, let $m \notin N$ then there exists $u \in U - V$ such that $u \mathbin{\diagup\diagup} m$. Since $v \in V (v \notin U - V)$, there is a $n \in N$ such that $v \mathbin{\diagup\diagup} n$. By $u \mathbin{\diagup\diagup} m$, $v \mathbin{\diagup} m$ and $v \mathbin{\diagup\diagup} n$, we have that $u \mathbin{\diagup\diagup} n$. It is contradicts to the fact that $u \mathbin{\diagup\kern-0.6em\times} n$. Then, arrows are closed on $(V, N)$

Above all, $(V, N)$ is a characteristic value of a congruence granular space of the reduced context $(U, M, I)$, iff $(U - V, N)$ is a concept of the context $(U, M, \diagup\kern-0.6em\times)$.

## Example 3.4

The concepts decided by $\diagup\kern-0.6em\times$ relation in Figure 15 are shown as follows:

$(12345, \varnothing), (1234, f), (1235, e), (2345, c),$
$(1245, b), (23, cef), (123, ef), (234, cf), (124, bf),$
$(24, bcf), (235, ce), (12, bef), (125, be),$
$(245, bc), (25, bce), (45, abcd), (4, abcdf), (5, abcde),$
$(2, bcef), (\varnothing, abcdef).$

The characteristic value of the congruence granular spaces deduced by them as follows:

$(\varnothing, \varnothing), (5, f), (4, e), (1, c), (3, b), (145, cef),$
$(45, ef), (15, cf), (35, bf), (135, bcf), (14, ce), (345, bef),$
$(34, be), (13, bc), (134, bce), (123, abcd),$
$(1235, abcdf), (1234, abcde), (1345, bcef), (12345, abcdef).$

The congruence granular spaces generated by the characteristic values are shown in Figure 18.
In this section we studied various properties of the granular spaces which are generated by the con-

gruence relations, and showed the method to get all congruence granular spaces in a concept lattice by matrix obtaining characteristic values of congruence spaces.

## 4. TOLERANCE GRANULE

In this part, we'll study a granular space that is more complex than the one studied in previous sections. The granules in this kind of granular spaces can overlap each other. Such granular spaces are generated by tolerance relation, so they are called as tolerance granular space.

*Figure 18. All the space of congruence granule of a concept lattice*

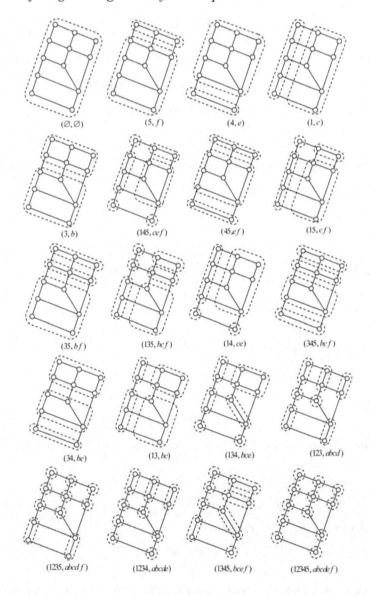

## Definition 4.1

Let $\mathscr{V}$ is a concept lattice. If $\theta \subseteq \mathscr{V} \times \mathscr{V}$ and $\theta$ is reflexive, symmetric, infimum compatible and supremum compatible (the meaning of infimum compatible and supremum compatible was shown in Definition 3.1), then call $\theta$ as a **tolerance relation**. For any element $a$ of $\mathscr{V}$, let $a_\theta = \wedge\{x \in \mathscr{V} \mid a\theta x\}$ and $a^\theta = \vee\{x \in \mathscr{V} \mid a\theta x\}$.

Then the interval $[a]_\theta = [a_\theta, (a_\theta)^\theta]$ is called a **tolerance granule** of $\theta$. Dually, the interval $[a]^\theta = [(a^\theta)_\theta, a^\theta]$ is a tolerance granule of $\theta$ as well.

## Example 4.1

A concept lattice $\mathscr{V}$ is shown by Figure 19. A tolerance relations $\theta$ of $\mathscr{V}$ is shown by Table 4. For the tolerance relations $\theta$ and each $a$ in $\mathscr{V}$, the $a_\theta$, $a^\theta$, $(a_\theta)^\theta$ and $(a^\theta)_\theta$ are shown by Table 5, the interval $[a]_\theta$ and $[a]^\theta$ (tolerance granule of $\theta$) are shown by Table 6. These tolerance granules of $\theta$ are drawn with broken line in Figure 20.

By Definition 3.1, we have that the congruence relation is a special equivalence relation that is supremum compatible and infimum compatible. It means that it is reflexive, symmetric, transitive, supremum compatible and infimum compatible. And then, by Definition 4.1, the difference between tolerance relation and congruence relation is only that the former doesn't need to be transitive. Hence, the congruence relation is a special case of the tolerance relation. Then, we can get all tolerance relations of a concept lattice using disturbance and response.

## Definition 4.2

Assume that $\mathbb{K} = (U, M, I)$ is a context, $I \subseteq J_0 \subseteq U \times M$, then $J_0$ is called a **disturbance of the context** $\mathbb{K}$ (or a disturbance of the relation $I$). Replace every row in table of $J_0$ by $\mathbb{K}'s$ the smallest

*Figure 19. A complete lattice*

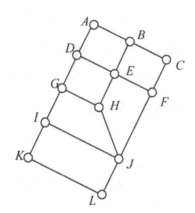

*Table 4. A tolerance relation*

| θ | A | B | C | D | E | F | G | H | I | J | K | L |
|---|---|---|---|---|---|---|---|---|---|---|---|---|
| A | X | X | X | X | X | X | | | | | | |
| B | X | X | X | X | X | X | | | | | | |
| C | X | X | X | X | X | X | | | | | | |
| D | X | X | X | X | X | X | X | X | X | X | | |
| E | X | X | X | X | X | X | X | X | X | X | | |
| F | X | X | X | X | X | X | X | X | X | X | | |
| G | | | | X | X | X | X | X | X | X | X | X |
| H | | | | X | X | X | X | X | X | X | X | X |
| I | | | | X | X | X | X | X | X | X | X | X |
| J | | | | X | X | X | X | X | X | X | X | X |
| K | | | | | | | X | X | X | X | X | X |
| L | | | | | | | X | X | X | X | X | X |

*Figure 20. A tolerance granular space*

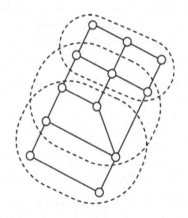

intent containing the row itself, (it means that $f_{J_1}(u) = f(g(f_{J_0}(u)))$) to get table of $J_1$. Replace every column in table of $J_1$ by $\mathbb{K}'s$ the smallest extent containing the column itself(it means that $g_{J_2}(m) = g(f(g_{J_1}(m)))$) to get table of $J_2$. Replace every row in table of $J_2$ by $\mathbb{K}'s$ the smallest intent containing the row to gettable of $J_3$. Keep on replacing in this way until $J_{i+1} = J_i$ appear firstly. Denote the $J_i$ by $J$ and $J$ is called by **response** for disturbance $J_0$. $D$

## Example 4.2

A context $\mathbb{K} = (U, M, I)$ is shown by Figure 19, the concept lattice of it is shown by Table 7.

*Table 5.* $a_\theta$, $a^\theta$, *and* $(a_\theta)^\theta$, $(a^\theta)_\theta$

|   | $a_\theta$ | $a^\theta$ | $(a_\theta)^\theta$ | $(a^\theta)_\theta$ |
|---|---|---|---|---|
| $A$ | $F$ | $A$ | $A$ | $F$ |
| $B$ | $F$ | $A$ | $A$ | $F$ |
| $C$ | $F$ | $A$ | $A$ | $F$ |
| $D$ | $J$ | $A$ | $D$ | $F$ |
| $E$ | $J$ | $A$ | $D$ | $F$ |
| $F$ | $J$ | $A$ | $D$ | $F$ |
| $G$ | $L$ | $D$ | $G$ | $J$ |
| $H$ | $L$ | $D$ | $G$ | $J$ |
| $I$ | $L$ |  | $G$ | $J$ |
| $J$ | $L$ | $D$ | $G$ | $J$ |
| $K$ | $L$ | $G$ | $G$ | $L$ |
| $L$ | $L$ | $G$ | $G$ | $L$ |

*Table 6. and* $[a]^\theta$

|   | $[a]_\theta$ | $[a]^\theta$ |
|---|---|---|
| $A$ | $[F, A]$ | $[F, A]$ |
| $B$ | $[F, A]$ | $[F, A]$ |
| $C$ | $[F, A]$ | $[F, A]$ |
| $D$ | $[J, D]$ | $[F, A]$ |
| $E$ | $[J, D]$ | $[F, A]$ |
| $F$ | $[J, D]$ | $[F, A]$ |
| $G$ | $[L, G]$ | $[J, D]$ |
| $H$ | $[L, G]$ | $[J, D]$ |
| $I$ | $[L, G]$ | $[J, D]$ |
| $J$ | $[L, G]$ | $[J, D]$ |
| $K$ | $[L, G]$ | $[L, G]$ |
| $L$ | $[L, G]$ | $[L, G]$ |

Its concepts are $(12345, \varnothing)$, $(1234, f)$, $(2345, c)$, $(124, bf)$, $(234, cf)$, $(345, cd)$, $(14, abf)$, $(24, bcf)$, $(34, cdf)$, $(4, abcdf)$, $(1, abef)$, and $(\varnothing, abcdef)$. They are shown in Figure 21. We can add "×" at some blank positions in Table 7 in order to get a disturbance of $I$. For example, let $\langle 1, c \rangle = \times$ to form $J_0$. $J_0$ is shown by Figure 22(a) (about notion $\langle u, m \rangle$, see Example 3.3). Replace every row in table of $J_0$ by $\mathbb{K}'s$ the smallest intent, which is containing the row itself, to get $J_1$. $J_1$ is shown by Figure 22(b). Replace every column in table of $J_1$ by $\mathbb{K}'s$ the smallest extent, which is containing the column itself, to get $J_2$. $J_2$ is shown by Figure 22(c). Replace every row in table of $J_2$ by $\mathbb{K}'s$ the smallest intent containing the row to get $J_3$. $J_3$ is shown by Figure 22(d). Replace every column in table of $J_3$ by $\mathbb{K}'s$ the smallest extent containing the column to get $J_4$. We find $J_4 = J_3$, hence denote $J_3$ by $J$ and $J$ is just response of $J_0$.

If $J \supseteq I$ is a response, then by Definition 4.2, its every row and every column is intent and extent of $\mathscr{C}$, respectively. Conversely, if $J \supseteq I$ and every row and every column of $J$ respectively is intent

*Table 7. A context*

| I | a | b | c | d | e | f |
|---|---|---|---|---|---|---|
| 1 | X | X |   |   | X | X |
| 2 |   | X | X |   |   | X |
| 3 |   |   | X | X |   | X |
| 4 | X | X | X | X |   | X |
| 5 |   |   | X | X |   |   |

*Figure 21. The intent, extend, and their code name in a lattice*

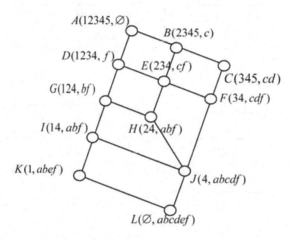

*Figure 22. A process producing response*

| $J_0$ | a | b | c | d | e | f |
|---|---|---|---|---|---|---|
| 1 | × | × | × |   | × | × |
| 2 |   | × | × |   |   | × |
| 3 |   |   | × | × |   |   |
| 4 | × | × | × | × |   | × |
| 5 |   |   | × | × |   |   |

(a)

| $J_1$ | a | b | c | d | e | f |
|---|---|---|---|---|---|---|
| 1 | × | × | × | × | × | × |
| 2 |   | × | × |   |   | × |
| 3 |   |   | × | × |   |   |
| 4 | × | × | × | × |   | × |
| 5 |   |   | × | × |   |   |

(b)

| $J_2$ | a | b | c | d | e | f |
|---|---|---|---|---|---|---|
| 1 | × | × | × | × | × | × |
| 2 |   | × | × | × |   | × |
| 3 |   |   | × | × |   |   |
| 4 | × | × | × | × |   | × |
| 5 |   |   | × | × |   |   |

(c)

| $J_3$ | a | b | c | d | e | f |
|---|---|---|---|---|---|---|
| 1 | × | × | × | × | × | × |
| 2 | × | × | × | × |   | × |
| 3 |   |   | × | × |   |   |
| 4 | × | × | × | × |   | × |
| 5 |   |   | × | × |   |   |

(d)

and extent of $\mathscr{V}$, then $J$ is just its own response. Thus $J \supseteq I$ is a response, if and only if its every rows and every columns is intent and extent of $\mathscr{V}$, respectively.

## Theorem 4.1

Given by a context $(U, M, I)$ and a tolerance relation $\theta$, then $J$ defined as a response:

$$(u, m) \in J \Leftrightarrow \gamma u \theta(\gamma u \wedge \mu m) \quad \left( \Leftrightarrow (\gamma u \vee \mu m)\theta\mu m \right)$$

Conversely, if $J$ is a response, then $\theta$ defined as a tolerance relation:

$$(A, B)\theta(C, D) \Leftrightarrow A \times D \cup C \times B \subseteq J.$$

## Example 4.3

The relation $\theta$ is shown by Table 4, concept lattice of $\theta$ is shown in Figure 19. The object concepts and the attribute concepts in the concept lattice are shown in Fig 7. In this case, we have that $\gamma 1$ and $\mu d$ satisfy $\gamma 1 \theta(\gamma 1 \wedge \mu d)$, then $(1, d) \in J$. $\gamma 3$ and $\mu b$ satisfy $\gamma 3 \theta(\gamma 3 \wedge \mu b)$ then $(3, b) \in J$. Whereas $\gamma 3 \theta(\gamma 3 \wedge \mu e)$ doesn't hold, then $(3, e) \notin J$. $\gamma 5 \theta(\gamma 5 \wedge \mu a)$ doesn't hold, then $(5, a) \notin J$, etc.

The last result of $J$ is shown by Table 8. Conversely, for the relation $J$ is shown by Table 8, the extents and intents of concepts of the concept lattice in Figure 19 are shown by Figure 21. Concept $G$ $(124, bf)$ and concept $E$ $(234, cf)$ such that $\{1, 2, 4\} \times \{c, f\} \cup \{2, 3, 4\} \times \{b, f\} \subseteq J$, it means that $G\theta E$. Concept $G$ $(124, bf)$ and concept $C$ $(345, cd)$ don't satisfy that $\{1, 2, 4\} \times \{c, d\} \cup \{3, 4, 5\} \times \{b, f\} \subseteq J$ (because $(5, b) \notin J$), then $G$ and $C$ doesn't haverelation $\theta$. Step by step, we obtain a tolerance relation $\theta$ shown as Table 4.

By Theorem 4.1, we have that a method to find out all of the tolerance granules through disturbances and responses mechanism.

*Table 8. A relation J*

| J | a | b | c | d | e | f |
|---|---|---|---|---|---|---|
| 1 | X | X | X | X | X | X |
| 2 | X | X | X | X | X | X |
| 3 | X | X | X | X |   | X |
| 4 | X | X | X | X | X | X |
| 5 |   |   | X | X |   | X |

*Figure 23. Object concepts and attribute concepts of the lattice*

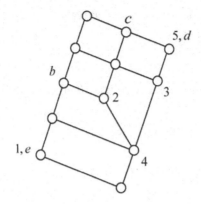

## Theorem 4.2

Assume that $\mathbb{K} = (U, M, I)$ is a context, $J$ is a response of a disturbance $J_0$, a tolerance relations generated by $J$ is $\theta$, $(A, B) \in \mathfrak{B}(\mathbb{K})$, then two tolerance granules containing $(A, B)$ are intervals (note that sometimes they may be equal):

$[(g(f_J(A)), f_J(A)), (g_J(f_J(A)), f(g_J(f_J(A))))]$ and

$[(g(f_J(g_J(B))), f_J(g_J(B))), (g_J(B), f(g_J(B)))]$

where $f, g$ are operations on $I$ and $f_J, g_J$ are operations on $J$.

## Proof

By Theorem 4.1, each concept $(C, D)$ that has the relation $\theta$ with $(A, B)$ must satisfy that $A \times D \cup C \times B \subseteq J$. Hence, $(A, B)_\theta$ and $(A, B)^\theta$ in Definition 4.1 are as follows:

$$(A, B)_\theta = \wedge \{(C, D) \in \mathfrak{B}(\mathbb{K}) \mid A \times D \cup C \times B \subseteq J\} \tag{1}$$

$$(A, B)^\theta = \vee \{(C, D) \in \mathfrak{B}(\mathbb{K}) \mid A \times D \cup C \times B \subseteq J\} \tag{2}$$

Note that $A \times D \subseteq J \Leftrightarrow D \subseteq f_J(A)$ $C \times B \subseteq J \Leftrightarrow C \subseteq g_J(B)$; then

$(A, B)_\theta = (g(f_J(A)), f_J(A))$ $(A, B)^\theta = (g_J(B), f(g_J(B)))$

and then

$((A, B)_\theta)^\theta = (g_J(f_J(A)), f(g_J(f_J(A))))$ $((A, B)^\theta)_\theta = (g(f_J(g_J(B))), f_J(g_J(B)))$

*Table 9. Some's data about concept (A,B)*

| $(A, B)$ | $(A, B)_\theta$ | $(A, B)^\theta$ | $(AB)^\theta$ | $\left((AB)^\theta\right)_\theta$ |
|---|---|---|---|---|
| $(12345, \varnothing)$ | $(345, cd)$ | $(12345, \varnothing)$ | $(12345, \varnothing)$ | $(345, cd)$ |
| $(1234, f)$ | $(34, cdf)$ | $(1234, f)$ | $(1234, f)$ | $(34, cdf)$ |
| $(2345, c)$ | $(345, cd)$ | $(12345, \varnothing)$ | $(12345, \varnothing)$ | $(345, cd)$ |
| $(124, bf)$ | $(4, abcdf)$ | $(124, bf)$ | $(124, bf)$ | $(4, abcdf)$ |
| $(234, cf)$ | $(34, cdf)$ | $(1234, f)$ | $(1234, f)$ | $(34, cdf)$ |
| $(345, cd)$ | $(345, cd)$ | $(12345, \varnothing)$ | $(12345, \varnothing)$ | $(345, cd)$ |
| $(124, bf)$ | $(4, abcdf)$ | $(124, bf)$ | $(124, bf)$ | $(4, abcdf)$ |
| $(24, bcf)$ | $(4, abcdf)$ | $(124, bf)$ | $(124, bf)$ | $(4, abcdf)$ |
| $(34, cdf)$ | $(34, cdf)$ | $(1234, f)$ | $(1234, f)$ | $(34, cdf)$ |
| $(14, abf)$ | $(4, abcdf)$ | $(124, bf)$ | $(124, bf)$ | $(4, abcdf)$ |
| $(4, abcdf)$ | $(4, abcdf)$ | $(124, bf)$ | $(124, bf)$ | $(4, abcdf)$ |
| $(1, abef)$ | $(\varnothing, abcdef)$ | $(1, abef)$ | $(1, abef)$ | $(\varnothing, abcdef)$ |
| $(\varnothing, abcdef)$ | $(\varnothing, abcdef)$ | $(1, abef)$ | $(1, abef)$ | $. (\varnothing, abcdef) .$ |

In such case, by Definition 4.1, tolerance granules are

$$[(A, B)]_\theta = [(g(f_J(A)), f_J(A)), (g_J(f_J(A)), f(g_J(f_J(A))))] \tag{3}$$

$$[(A, B)]^\theta = [(g(f_J(g_J(B))), f_J(g_J(B))), (g_J(B), f(g_J(B)))] \tag{4}$$

## Example 4.5

A Context $\mathbb{K} = (U, M, I)$ is shown by Table 7. Disturbance $J_0$ and response $J(= J_3)$ are shown by Figure 22(a) and (d), respectively. By (1)(2)(3)(4) $(A, B)_\theta$, $(A, B)^\theta$, $((A, B)_\theta)^\theta$, $((A, B)^\theta)_\theta$ of each concept $(A, B)$ in $\mathfrak{B}(\mathbb{K})$ are shown in Table 9. Thus there are 4 tolerance granules, they are $[(345, cd), (12345, \varnothing)]$, $[(34, cdf), (1234, f)]$, $[(4, abcdf), (124, bf)]$ and $[(\varnothing, abcdef), (1, abef)]$ These tolerance granules are shown in Figure 24.

In fact, we are conscious of that this tolerance relation is still a congruence relation. Therefore the granular space shown in Figure 24 is still congruence granular space. How to get "real" incongruence tolerance relation? For this, we have the following results.

*Figure 24. A tolerance granular space*

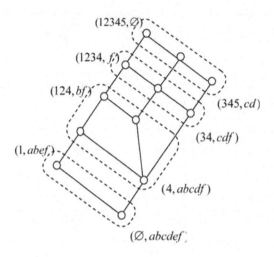

## Definition 4.3

Let $\mathbb{K} = (U, M, I)$ be a context, $J_0$ be a disturbance of $I$, $J$ is its response. If $\langle u, m \rangle \in \{\swarrow, \nearrow, \swarrow\nearrow\}$ in the table of $I$, while $\langle u, m \rangle$ in the table of $J$ is "$\times$",then we say that $\langle u, m \rangle$ is covered by "$\times$" in the table of $J$. If all $\swarrow$, $\nearrow$ and $\swarrow\nearrow$ on object $u$ in the table of $J$ are not covered, then we say that $u$ is an **inactive object of disturbance** $J_0$. If all $\swarrow$, $\nearrow$ and $\swarrow\nearrow$ on attribute $m$ in the table of $J$ are not covered, then we say that $m$ is an **inactive attribute of disturbance** $J_0$.

## Example 4.6

Assume that a context is shown by Table 7. Its arrow relation is shown by Table 10. A disturbance $J_0$ of the context is shown by Figure 22(a), Its response $J(=J_3)$ is shown by Figure 22(d). Its covers are

*Table 10. Arrow relation*

|   | a | b | c | d | e | f |
|---|---|---|---|---|---|---|
| 1 | X | X | ☐ | ✓ | X | X |
| 2 | ☐ | X | X | ☐ |   | X |
| 3 | ✓ | ☐ | X | X |   | X |
| 4 | X | X | X | X | ☐ | X |
| 5 |   |   | X | X |   | ☐ |

*Table 11. Covered occasions of response*

|   | a | b | c | d | e | f |
|---|---|---|---|---|---|---|
| 1 | X | X | X | X | X | X |
| 2 | X | X | X | X |   | X |
| 3 | ✓ | ☐ | X | X |   |   |
| 4 | X | X | X | X | ☐ | X |
| 5 |   |   | X | X |   | ☐ |

shown by the Table 11, in which $\langle 1,c \rangle, \langle 1,d \rangle, \langle 2,a \rangle, \langle 2,d \rangle$ are covered. This disturbance's inactive objects are 3,4,5 and inactive attributes are $a,b,e,f$.

## Theorem 4.3

Assume that $\mathbb{K} = (U, M, I)$ is a context, $J$ is a response of the disturbance $J_0$, $V$ is the set of all inactive objects, $N$ is the set of all inactive attributes. Then the tolerance relation defined by response $J$ is a congruence relation with characteristic value $(V, N)$.

By Theorem 4.3, by using the disturbance and response mechanism to find out all tolerance relations, there if only exists some inactive objects or some inactive attributes, then tolerance relations generated are still congruence relations, granular spaces generated are also congruence granular spaces. In order to find out "real" tolerance relation (tolerance relation but not congruence relation) it must operate on the disturbance in which all $\swarrow$, $\nearrow$ and $\swarrow\nearrow$ are covered by "×".

## Example 4.7

Finding out all real tolerance relations and their granular spaces on the context shown by Table 7. By Theorem 4.3, we should begin to find one by one from the disturbance shown as Table 12 in which all $\swarrow$, $\nearrow$ and $\swarrow\nearrow$ are just covered by "×". By the definition of $\nearrow$, $\swarrow$ and $\swarrow\nearrow$, every row and every column in

*Figure 25. Real tolerance granular space*

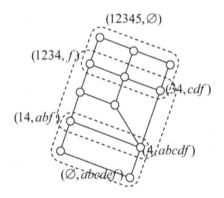

*Table 12. Just all covered arrows' occasion*

|   | a | b | c | d | e | f |
|---|---|---|---|---|---|---|
| 1 | × | × | × |   | × | × |
| 2 | × | × | × | × |   | × |
| 3 | × | × | × | × |   | × |
| 4 | × | × | × | × | × | × |
| 5 |   |   | × | × |   | × |

*Table 13. Further disturbance space*

|   | a | b | c | d | e | f |
|---|---|---|---|---|---|---|
| 1 | X | X | X | X | X | X |
| 2 | X | X | X | X | ① | X |
| 3 | X | X | X | X | ② | X |
| 4 | X | X | X | X | X | X |
| 5 | ⑤ | ④ | X | X | ③ | X |

*Figure 26. Six different responses*

|   | a | b | c | d | e | f |
|---|---|---|---|---|---|---|
| 1 | × | × | × | × | × | × |
| 2 | × | × | × | × | × | × |
| 3 | × | × | × | × |   | × |
| 4 | × | × | × | × | × | × |
| 5 |   | × | × |   |   | × |

(a)

|   | a | b | c | d | e | f |
|---|---|---|---|---|---|---|
| 1 | × | × | × | × | × | × |
| 2 | × | × | × | × | × | × |
| 3 | × | × | × | × | × | × |
| 4 | × | × | × | × | × | × |
| 5 |   | × | × |   |   | × |

(b)

|   | a | b | c | d | e | f |
|---|---|---|---|---|---|---|
| 1 | × | × | × | × | × | × |
| 2 | × | × | × | × | × | × |
| 3 | × | × | × | × | × | × |
| 4 | × | × | × | × | × | × |
| 5 | × | × | × | × | × | × |

(c)

|   | a | b | c | d | e | f |
|---|---|---|---|---|---|---|
| 1 | × | × | × | × | × | × |
| 2 | × | × | × | × |   | × |
| 3 | × | × | × | × |   | × |
| 4 | × | × | × | × | × | × |
| 5 | × | × | × | × |   |   |

(d)

|   | a | b | c | d | e | f |
|---|---|---|---|---|---|---|
| 1 | × | × | × | × | × | × |
| 2 | × | × | × | × | × | × |
| 3 | × | × | × | × |   | × |
| 4 | × | × | × | × | × | × |
| 5 | × | × | × | × |   | × |

(e)

|   | a | b | c | d | e | f |
|---|---|---|---|---|---|---|
| 1 | × | × | × | × | × | × |
| 2 | × | × | × | × | × | × |
| 3 | × | × | × | × | × | × |
| 4 | × | × | × | × | × | × |
| 5 | × | × | × | × |   | × |

(f)

Table10 is just an intent and an extent of original context, respectively. So the response of this disturbance is itself. The tolerance granules of tolerance relations $\theta$ generated by the response in Example 4.5 are the intervals: $[(34, cdf), (12345, \varnothing)]$, $[(4, abcdf), (1234, f)]$ and $[(\varnothing, abcdef), (14, abf)]$ shown by Figure 25.

Next step is to add "×" again at others blank position to make further disturbance. The position can be added "×" are ①②③④ and ⑤ in Table 13, so it has $32\ (= 2^5)$ disturbances. But many disturbances have the same response. There exists only 6 responses really. They are shown by Figure 26 (a) (b)(c)(d)(e)(f), the tolerance granular spaces generated by them are shown in Figure 27(a)(b)(c)(d)(e) (f).

In this section we studied various properties of the granular spaces which are generated by the tolerance relations and showed the method to get all tolerance granular spaces in a concept lattice through the disturbance and response of context.

*Figure 27. Granular spaces of responses*

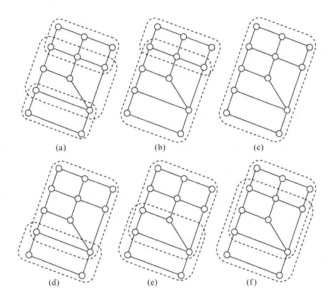

(a)          (b)          (c)

(d)          (e)          (f)

## 5. PROSPECT

The research about granular computing in formal concept is just at the very beginning. There are many topics being studied and paid increasingly attention on them. For example, Concept Algebra had been put forward by Wille in 2000. Let $\mathbb{K} = (U, M, I)$ be a context, $\Delta$ and $\nabla$ are two operations defined on the concept lattice $\underline{\mathfrak{B}}(U, M, I)$. For two arbitrary concepts $(A, B), (C, D) \hat{\mathbb{1}} \underline{\mathfrak{B}}(U, M, I)$, it follows that:

(1) $(A, B)^{\Delta\Delta} \leq (A, B)$ (1') $(A, B)^{\nabla\nabla} \geq (A, B)$

(2) $(A, B) \leq (C, D) \Rightarrow (A, B)^{\Delta} \geq (C, D)^{\Delta}$

(2') $(A, B) \leq (C, D) \Rightarrow (A, B)^{\nabla} \geq (C, D)^{\nabla}$

(3) $\left( (A, B) \wedge (C, D) \right) \vee \left( (A, B) \wedge (C, D)^{\Delta} \right) = (A, B)$

(3') $\left( (A, B) \vee (C, D) \right) \wedge \left( (A, B) \vee (C, D)^{\nabla} \right) = (A, B)$

Then, $\left( \underline{\mathfrak{B}}(U, M, I), \Delta, \nabla \right)$ is called a **Concept Algebra**. The method of ↙,↗,↙↗ was extended to the field of Concept Algebra. Canter suggested add two new symbols $\diagdown$ and $\diagup$ to {↙,↗,↙↗ } in 2004. And let $S_1 = \{ ↙, \diagdown \}, S_2 = \{ ↗, \diagup \}$. Define a relation denoted by $trans(S_1, S_2)$ is similar to the relation ↙↙:

$(u,m) \in trans(S_1, S_2)$

$$\Leftrightarrow \begin{cases} u = u_1, u_2, \cdots, u_k \in U \quad m_1, m_2, \cdots, m_k = m \in M \\ u_i d m_i \ (d \in S_1) i = 1, 2, \cdots, k \quad u_i c m_{i-1} \ (c \in S_2) i = 2, \cdots, k \end{cases}$$

By $\neg trans(S_1, S_2) = U \times M - trans(S_1, S_2)$, we would find out the concepts of the context. $(U, M, \neg trans(S_1, S_2))$. For each concept $(A, B)$ of, $(U, M, \neg trans(S_1, S_2))$ let $V = U - A$, $N = B$, then $(V, N, I \cap V \times N)$ is called $(S_1, S_2)$ **compatible**. If $\varphi$ is a homomorphous map from $\mathfrak{B}(U, M, I)$ to $\mathfrak{B}(U, M, I \cap V \times N)$, the homomorphism kernel $Ker\varphi$ of $\varphi$ can be regard as a new kind of granular space which is similar to the congruence granular space. The researches on this kind of granular space have obtained many achievements. And people will keep focus on it.

In addition, it is still similar to congruence granule, for an arbitrary $X \in U$ (or $X \in M$), we can more generally define the follows as:

$$R_X = \{((A,B),(C,D)) \in \mathfrak{B}(\mathbb{K}) \times \mathfrak{B}(\mathbb{K}) \mid A \cap X = C \cap X\}$$

or $R_X = \{((A,B),(C,D)) \in \mathfrak{B}(\mathbb{K}) \times \mathfrak{B}(\mathbb{K}) \mid B \cap X = D \cap X\}$

Then $R_X$ is equivalence relation. It is proved easily that their equivalence classes are infimum-semisublattices (or supremum-semisublattices), then, they are infimum granules (or the supremum granules). We say that the set $\mathscr{V} / R_X$ of all equivalence class of $R_X$ is an **object projection granular space** (or **attribute projection granular space**). For example, Figure 28(a) is the concept lattice of the context shown by Table 3. The object projection granular space of $X_1 = 25$, and the attribute projection granular space of $X_2 = bdef$ are shown by Figure 28 (b), (c) respectively.

Let $\mathscr{V} / R_X, \mathscr{V} / R_Y, \mathscr{V} / R_Z, \cdots, \mathscr{V} / R_W$ be the family of object (or attribute) projection granular spaces on concept lattice $\mathscr{V} = \mathfrak{B}(U, M, I)$ Each two of the granules from the different projection granu-

*Figure 28. Infinum-granular-space and supremum-granular-space*

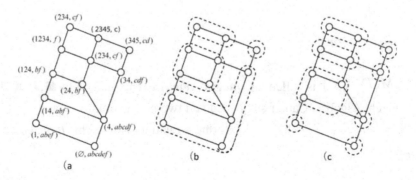

lar spaces in the family of granular spaces always have only one common element at most, then, a **granular coordinate** system can generated from them. For example, in Table 3, let $X = ac$, $Y = bf$, $Z = de$, the attribute projection granular spaces $\mathscr{V} / R_X, \mathscr{V} / R_Y, \mathscr{V} / R_Z$ determined by $X, Y, Z$ are Figure 29 (a), (b), (c), respectively.

It can be observed from Figure 30 that if get one granule at random in each of attribute projection granular spaces, these granules have only one common element at most, thus a coordinate can begenerated. A coordinate of a concept, which is the common element of granules and which is respectively in $\mathscr{V} / R_{ac}, \mathscr{V} / R_{bf}, \mathscr{V} / R_{de}$ (coded numbers of the granules are shown by Figure 29, $\langle x, y, z \rangle$ can be generated as Figure 31 (Figures 29 and 30 for reference).

This kind of coordinate lead people associate it with the design of orthogonal Latin square and Hadamard matrix immediately. There are many questions need to be solved in these domains. For example, in 1782 Euler suspected that the orthogonal Latin squares whose order is $4n + 2$ do not exist. In 1900

*Figure 29. Attribute-projection-granular-space-race and granular code in various spaces*

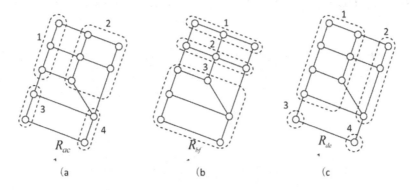

*Figure 30. Meet of attribute projection granular space race*

*Figure 31. Coordinates of concept lattice*

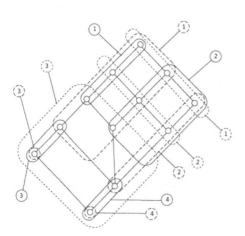

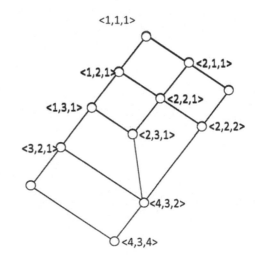

G. Tarry proved that the orthogonal Latin square of order 6 did not exist $(n = 1)$. This strengthens people's confidence to the correctness of Euler's conjecture. However, in 1959 E. T. Parker got the orthogonal Latin square of 10 orders $(n = 2)$. The correctness of Euler's conjecture was vacillated. In 1960 R. C. Rose and some others had proved that orthogonal Latin squares of all orders are exists besides of the 2 order one and the 6 order one. Euler's conjecture was overthrown. It is very difficult to construct these orthogonal Latin squares of $(4n + 2)$ order. To look for a practical method, obviously, is a very necessary and meaningful research topic. It is very interesting whether we can finish the design of such orthogonal Latin square using the family of projection granular space of different concept lattices.

On the other hand, many years ago people had proved that the orders of the Hadamard matrix must be multiple of 4. But nobody knows whether all Hadamard matrixs of multiple of 4 orders exist until now, since many Hadamard matrixs of multiple of 4 order have not been worked out by any one. Hence, it is also a very meaningful research topic to complete the design of Hadamard matrix by these different families of concept lattice. We deeply believed that the research about these questions will apply the research of granular computing in formal concept to more domains.

There are also some questions need to be studied in these projection granular space. For example, the number of subsets of $U$ that is the object set of the context shown in Table 3 is $2^5 = 32$. In the

*Figure 32. The infimum granular spaces generated by 12 subsets*

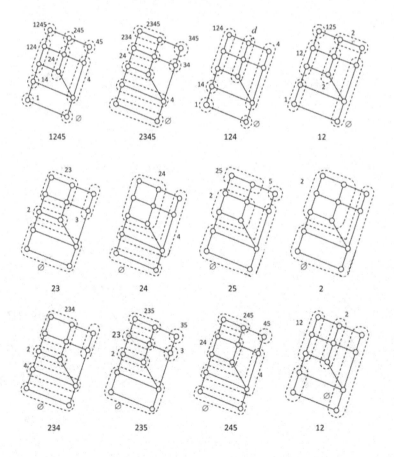

power set of object set, among the object projection granular spaces, the congruence granular spaces (see Example 3.4) are generated by 20 subsets:

$$\varnothing, 5, 4, 1, 3, 145, 45, 15, 35, 135, 14, 345, 34,$$
$$13, 134, 123, 1235, 1234, 1345, 12345 \qquad .$$

The remainder 12 subsets are

$$1245, 2345, 124, 125, 23,$$
$$24, 25, 2, 234, 235, 245, 12$$

The infimum granular spaces generated by these 12 subsets are as shown in Figure 32, the text under each granular space is the object subset $X$ which generated this space, the text next to each granule is the common value of each extent in this granule and $X$. Among these 12 infimumgranular spaces, many are not only infimum granular spaces but also regular granular spaces (see the granular spaces generated by $1245, 2345, 124, 125, 23, 234, 235$ in Figure 32). Containing the tolerance granular spaces, we may obtain the subordinate relations of granular space shown by Figure 33. It is difficult to use the form of a general formula to present the boundary of the **regular projection granular space**s in projection granular spaces. At the present time, we can only judge them one by one concretely, the one belongs to the regular at here and the other one belongs to the supremum granules at there. Obviously, it is also a very meaningful research topic to discover this general abstract formula.

Above, we only gave some questions that can be seen from the former content of this chapter directly and need to be studied further. In fact, there are also many other questions being worth to discuss here. For example, the granular spaces in Horn context and the granular spaces in Q- Horn context cannot be discussed in this chapter. They gave rise to some burning question.

In this section we gave 4 further research directions about granular computing in formal concepts and showed the prospect of these studies.

## DEVELOPING TRENDS IN THE FUTURE

The research of granular computing in formal concept is significant and arduous. Firstly,granular computing is a multidisciplinary research, and we have to study, analyze, understand and apply it in

*Figure 33. Subset subordination relations among various granular spaces*

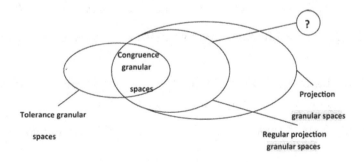

the practical world. Secondly, formal concept analysis also has a widespread application. Then, it also associates with corresponding knowledge in many fields. Hence, there are many multidisciplinary and the cross domain various findings production in future. The most essential fundamental viewpoint that we proposed in this paper is to unify the most basic and diverse set, such as supremum semisublattice, infimum semisublattice and sublattice, in formal concept analysis to granule which can be studied at an abstract mathematics level. It provides a good foundation and the platform for exploring the idea of other granular computing in future research of formal concept analysis. Obviously on the fundamental platform, it will unfold entirely for the research of granular space level (Limited by the length of this paper, we abridged the depiction on hierarchy of these granular spaces) and granular computing application in formal concept analysis. To many other fields, such as orthogonal Latin square and the Hadamard matrix, it will be discussed intensely because powerful new tools supported, moreover it may have more breakthroughs. In summary, future prospects and advancements of granular computing will be very expansive and profound in the formal concept analysis, no matter which direction we have discussed.

## CONCLUSION

In this chapter, we study mainly the consanguineous relations between formal concept and granular computing, and propose three methods generating ideal-filter granular spaces, congruence granular spaces and tolerance granular spaces in concept lattice. It deeply explains that the properties, relations and essences of various sublattices. We not only connected the idea of granular computing and formal concept, but also promoted the application of granular computing into a further field. In brief, the research about granular computing in formal concept had begun. However, there are still many important topics expected people's further studying. We would like to draw forth the research and offer the strength for the researcher by the content of this section.

## ACKNOWLEDGMENT

The graduate students of Professor Ma Yuan, Li-Guodong, Zhang-Wei, Chen-Yongli, Mo-Yuhong, Su-Chaozong, Li-Meixue, took part in the typing work and interpreting word of this chapter.

## REFERENCES

Bose, R. C., Shrikhande, S. S., & Parker, E. T. (1960). Further results on the construction of mutually orthogonal Latin squares and the falsity of Euler's conjecture. *Canadian J. Math.*, *12*, 189–203.

Canter, B. (2004). Congruences of finite distributive concept algebras. In. *Proceedings of ICFCA*, *04*, 128–141.

Du, W. L., Miao, D. Q., Li, D. G., & Zhang, N. Q. (2005). *Analysis on relationship between concept lattice and granule partition lattice*. Beijing, China: Computer Science.

Ganter, B., & Wille, R. (1999). *Formal concept analysis: Mathematical Foundations*. Berlin, Germany: Springer.

Lin, T. Y. (2003). Granular computing, (LNCS 2639, pp. 16-24). Springer, Berlin.

Parker, E. T. (1959). Orthogonal latin squares. *Proceedings of the National Academy of Sciences of the United States of America, 45,* 859–862. doi:10.1073/pnas.45.6.859

Pedrycz, W. (2006). *Granular Computing: An Overview, Applied Soft Computing Technologies: The Challenge of Complexity.* Berlin, Germany: Springer.

Peters, J. F., Pawlak, Z., & Skowron, A. (2002). A rough set approach to measuring information granules. In. *Proceedings of COMPSAC, 2002,* 1135–1139.

Wille, R. (1982). Restructuring lattice theory: An approach based on hierarchies of concepts. In Proceedings of Rival I, ed. Ordered Sets (pp. 445-470). Boston: Reidel.

Wille, R. (2000). Boolean concept logic, In B. Canter and G. W. Mineau (Eds.), *Conceptual Structures: Logical, Linguistic, and Computational Issues* (LNAI 1867). Berlin, Germany: Springer

Yao, Y. Y. (2001). Information granulation and rough set approximation. *International Journal of Intelligent Systems,* 87–104. doi:10.1002/1098-111X(200101)16:1<87::AID-INT7>3.0.CO;2-S

Yao, Y. Y. (2001). Modeling data mining with granular computing. In. *Proceedings of COMPSAC, 2001,* 638–643.

Yao, Y. Y., & Liau, C.-J. (2002). A generalized decision logic language for granular computing. In. *Proceedings of FUZZ-IEEE, 02,* 1092–1097.

Yao, Y. Y., Liau, C.-J., & Zhong, N. (2003). Granular computing based on rough sets, quotient space theory, and belief functions. In. *Proceedings of ISMIS, 03,* 152–159.

Yao, Y. Y., & Yao, J. T. (2002). *Granular computing as a basis for consistent classification problems.* Taiwan, China: Institute of Information and Computing Machinery.

Yao, Y. Y., & Zhong, N. (2002). Granular computing using information tables. In Lin, T. Y., Yao, Y. Y., & Zadeh, L. A. (Eds.), *Data Mining, Rough Sets and Granular Computing* (pp. 102–124). Berlin, Germany: Springer.

Yixian, Y. (2006). *Theory and applications of higher-dimensional Hadamard Matrices.* Beijin, China: Science Press.

Zadeh, L. A. (1998). Some reflections on soft computing, granular computing and their roles in the conception, design and utilization of information/ intelligent systems. *Soft Computing, 2,* 23–25. doi:10.1007/s005000050030

Zheng, Z., Hu, H., & Shi, Z. (2005). *Tolerance granular space and its applications.* Washington, DC: IEEE Press.

# Chapter 17
# Granular Synthesis of Rule–Based Models and Function Approximation Using Rough Sets

**Carlos Pinheiro**
*Federal University of Itajubá, Brazil*

**Fernando Gomide**
*State University of Campinas, Brazil*

**Otávio Carpinteiro**
*Federal University of Itajubá, Brazil*

**Isaías Lima**
*Federal University of Itajubá, Brazil*

## ABSTRACT

*This chapter suggests a new method to develop rule-based models using concepts about rough sets. The rules encapsulate relations among variables and give a mechanism to link granular descriptions of the models with their computational procedures. An estimation procedure is suggested to compute values from granular representations encoded by rule sets. The method is useful to develop granular models of static and dynamic nonlinear systems and processes. Numerical examples illustrate the main features and the usefulness of the method.*

## 1. INTRODUCTION

Information granules are key components of knowledge representation and processing. Granular computing forms a unified conceptual and computing platform that benefits from existing and known concepts of information granules in the realm of set theory, fuzzy sets and rough sets. The comput-

DOI: 10.4018/978-1-60566-324-1.ch017

ing framework that includes these concepts comprises the emerging paradigm of granular computing. Granular computing identifies essential commonalities between diversified problems and technologies, gives a better grasp to the role of interaction between various formalisms, and brings together the existing formalisms of interval analysis, fuzzy sets and rough sets under the same roof. Moreover, it helps to build heterogeneous and multifaceted models, acknowledges the notion of variable granularity covering from numerical entities to abstract information granules, and is a fundamental paradigm of abstraction (Pedrycz and Gomide, 2007).

The description of information granules usually is imprecise. One mechanism to approach imprecision is to look at the descriptions as an approximation and use lower and upper bounds. Intervals are examples of such a mechanism. However, often imprecision is caused by the conceptual incompatibilities between the description of a notion with respect to a collection of simpler notions. The notion may either fully cover or have limited overlaps with simpler notions. In this case, the notion, when characterized in terms of the simpler notions, does not lend itself to a unique description and the best we can do is to give an approximation in the form of some boundaries. Rough Set Theory (Pawlak, 1982) offers the appropriate formal and computational framework to approximation.

Rule-based models (Hofestädt and Meinecke, 1995) play a fundamental role in system modeling. In general, rules encapsulate relations among variables and give a mechanism to link granular descriptions of systems with their computational procedures. For instance, many rule-based models can uniformly approximate continuous functions to any degree of accuracy on closed and bounded sets. Another important issue concerns rule-based interpolation. Methods of interpolative reasoning are particularly useful to reduce complexity of rule-based models (Pedrycz and Gomide, 2007).

Due to its own nature, rule-based systems rely on the computation with information granules. Information granules are in the center of the development of the individual rules. There are two main schemes to construct rule-based models, expert knowledge-based and data-driven, respectively. There are several hybrid schemes that could be somewhere in between. Knowledge-based development assumes that an expert can provide domain knowledge. Experts are individuals who can quantify knowledge about the basic concepts and variables to solve a problem and link them in the form of a set of rules. Knowledge-based approach has some advantages: knowledge becomes available and information granules help to the quantification process. However, in many applications the information required to develop the rules may not be easily available and humans may be unable to extract all relevant knowledge from large amount of data. In these circumstances, data-driven computational procedures must be used to extract knowledge and to encode it in the form of rules. Data-driven development is guided by the use of data. The resulting design captures the structure existing in the data themselves. Rules derived from data should provide a model to describe the underlying behavior mirrored by the data.

This chapter suggests a new data-driven method to develop rule-based models based on rough set theory. The method is useful to develop granular models of static and dynamic nonlinear systems and processes. We assume that the rule-based model is a granular representation of a function. More importantly, we shown that the behavior captured by the rules provides information to estimate the values of the function embedded in the set of rules. An estimation procedure is suggested to compute function values from its granular representation encoded by the set of rules. Therefore, differently from most classic and alternative modeling schemes such as interpolation and approximation using, for example, neural networks and fuzzy systems, the method developed in this chapter simultaneously offers a granular model of a system and a mechanism to compute system output estimates.

The purpose of the title of this chapter is related with the fact that information granules and granular computing are key components in the computation of the rough sets. Considering that rule-based models will be obtained via concepts of rough sets, the title of this chapter seems to be adequate.

This chapter is organized as follows. Section 2 gives background material and reviews related works that have been addressed in the literature. Section 3 shows the procedure to construct the granular model from data and details the method to estimate values of the underlying function encoded in the rule base. Computational results illustrate the main features and the usefulness of the method in Section 4. Finally, Section 5 concludes the chapter summarizing its main contribution and suggesting issues to be addressed in the future.

## 2. BACKGROUND

Rough Set Theory (Pawlak, 1991) has been successfully used in several areas such as data mining (Ilczuk and Wakulicz-Deja, 2007$_a$), decision analysis (Ilczuk and Wakulicz-Deja, 2007$_b$), expert systems (Jeon, Kim, and Jeong, 2006), security information (Yao et al., 2005), and in other domains.

Rough set theory (RST) was developed aiming at the manipulation of uncertainties and inaccuracy in data sets, a context inherent in many practical problems. One of the main advantages of RST is that it does not need detailed and high quality information about the data to be manipulated, such as probability distributions, belief intervals, and possibilities values.

The main concept involved in RST is the indiscernibility relation (Pawlak and Skowron, 2007$_a$). Through indiscernibility relations it is simple to define redundant or superfluous attributes in databases, decision rules, and systems, allowing reduction of data into more consistent sets (Sakai and Nakata, 2006). RST also provides an effective way to analyze and summarize data sets in the form of information granules, and therefore, a way to compress information of precise concepts in practical applications (Sankar and Mitra, 2002).

Information granules as subsets, objects, elements and classes of a universe are the basic ingredients of granular computing (Yao, 2005). For instance, decision rules encoded in attribute-value tables are examples of granules (Yao and Yao, 2002; Pawlak and Skowron, 2007$_b$). Granular computing covers theory, methodology, techniques, and tools that use information granules to solve complex problems (Yao, 2007).

Currently, there are computational tools especially tailored to process information using RST, most of which are easily accessible. Among well known tools one can mention RSL (Rough Sets Library); Rough Enough; CI (Column Importance facility); and Rosetta (Øhrn and Komorowski, 1997).

Several papers have shown the potential of RST in different application areas including control and system modeling using discrete variables (Yun and Yuanbin, 2004) and symbolic information (Ziarko and Katzberg, 1993). However, few studies have addressed rule-based modeling of static and dynamic systems using real-valued data sets instead of binary or symbolic variables of the type 1/0, true/false, on/off, hot/cold. Pawlak and Munakata (1996) have suggested system modeling as promising area for future development of RST, both theoretical and practical. As far as the knowledge of the authors is concerned, applications of RST in systems and processes modeling still are to be developed. Before to proceed, let us recall some basic notions of RST.

An *approximation space* is understood as a pair $S = (U,A)$, where $U$ is a finite set of objects called universe and $A$ is a set of attributes. Let $S$ be an *information system* (IS) in the form of a decision system viewed as an attribute-value table where the attributes $a \in A$ and the corresponding values $V_a$ determine a classification function $F:U \times A \to V_a$. Let $R$ be an equivalence relation on $U$ denominated *indiscernibility relation*. Every subset of attributes determines an indiscernibility relation. An equivalence relation $R$ is a relation which is reflexive (*i.e.*, $xRx$), symmetrical (if $xRz$ then $zRx$) and transitive (if $xRz$ and $zRx$, then $xRq$). The equivalence class of an element $x \in X$ consists of all the objects $z \in X$ for which $xRz$. Objects that belong to the same equivalence class of $R$ are indiscernible. In fact, if $xRz$, then $x$ and $z$ are indiscernible because equivalence class generalizes the notion of equality. The equivalence classes of $R$, denoted by $U/R$, are called elementary sets. Objects of $U$ belonging to the same elementary set are indiscernible. Let $I(x)$ be a set of all $z$ such that $xIz$ is an equivalence class of the relation $I$ containing $x$. Given $X \subseteq U$, it is important to know how many of the elements of $X$ can be defined by the elementary sets of $S$. To know how many elements, we define the *lower* ($I_*$) and *upper* ($I^*$) approximations as in (1). If $I_*(X) = I^*(X)$ the set $X$ is $I$-exact, otherwise the set is $I$-rough.

$$I_*(X) = \{x \in U : I(x) \subseteq X\};$$

$$I^*(X) = \{x \in U : I(x) \cap X \neq \varphi\}. \tag{1}$$

Let $P$ and $Q$ be sets of attributes. The *P-positive* region of $Q$ is the set of all objects of the universe $U$ which can be properly classified to classes of $U/Q$ employing knowledge expressed by the classification $U/P$.

$$POS_P(Q) = \bigcup_{X \in U/Q} P_*(X) \tag{2}$$

Let the *degree of dependence* $\gamma(P,Q)$ of a set of attributes $P$ with respect to a set of attributes $Q$ be

$$\gamma(P,Q) = \frac{|POS_P(Q)|}{|U|}. \tag{3}$$

The degree of dependency provides a measure of how important $P$ is mapping the dataset examples in $Q$. If $\gamma(P,Q) = 0$, then $Q$ is not associated with $P$. If $\gamma(P,Q) = 1$, then $Q$ is fully associated with $P$.

Given $K$ and $L$, a *reduct* is a minimal set of attributes for which $\gamma(K,L) = \gamma(M,L)$, $M \subseteq K$. Decision rules are generated by computing reducts, a key concept of rough set theory in data analysis (Pawlak and Skowron, 2007a). For $P$, $Q$ and an object $x \in P$, an attribute $x$ is dispensable if $\gamma(P,Q) = \gamma(P-\{x\},Q)$.

The computation of all reducts in large information systems (with high dimensionality) is a NP-hard computational problem (Skowron and Rauszer, 1992). Some approaches are applied to solve this problem like ant colony algorithm (Quan and Biao, 2008), similarity relation (Huang et al., 2007), supervised learning (Shen and Chouchoulas, 2001), and genetic algorithms (Wróblewski, 1995).

The relation among the equivalence relations associated with the sets of attributes is used to generate decision rules in form

*Figure 1. Procedures for rule base generation*

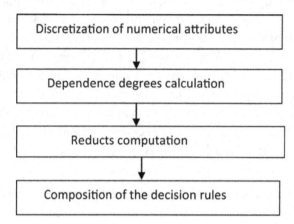

IF $F(x,a_1) = a_1$ AND..AND $F(x,a_v) = a_v$ THEN $\quad F(x,b_1) = b_1$ OR..OR $F(x,b_m) = b_m$. $\hspace{2em}$ (4)

Where $F$ is a classification function of the information system, $a_1$, $a_2$, and $a_v$ are condition attributes, and $b_1$, $b_2$, and $b_m$ decision attributes. Figure 1 summarizes the main steps of the procedures to obtain a set of rules. Computational tools (Rosetta, RSL, CI, etc.) especially tailored to compute information via RST use these procedures.

The concept of *rough function* (Pawlak, 1997) was introduced to overcome the limitations when using real variables in applications of RST. Suppose a real function $f: X{\rightarrow}Y$, where $X$ and $Y$ are sets of real numbers, and let $D = (X,B)$ and $E = (Y,C)$ be two approximation spaces. Functions $f_*{:}X{\rightarrow}Y$ and $f^*{:}X{\rightarrow}Y$ are defined from the definition of $(B,C)$-lower approximation and $(B,C)$-upper approximation of $f$, such that

$$f_*(x) = C_*(f(x)),$$
$$f^*(x) = C^*(f(x)), \quad \forall x \in X. \hspace{2em} (5)$$

Function $f$ is exact in $x$ if and only if $f_*(x) = f^*(x)$, otherwise $f$ is inexact (rough) in $x$. Intermediary values of $f$, namely, those values between the upper and lower approximations, can be estimated using interpolation functions (6) that employ the definition of *rough membership function* (7) (Pawlak, 1997).

$$f_I(x) = \psi(\mu(x), f_*(x), f^*(x)) \hspace{2em} (6)$$

$$\mu(x) = \frac{card(X \cap I(x))}{card(I(x))} \hspace{2em} (7)$$

Next section presents a procedure to develop a granular model from a data set in the form of rules viewed as rough functions, and suggests a mechanism to estimate output values of the model for given inputs. The distinctive advantage of the procedure is that it does not depend on the rough membership function computations. We show that estimation of output/input behavior model in the form of rules can be done straightforwardly using classic function approximation formulas. This is particularly attractive when handling complex systems and processes, because it improves computational performance, model accuracy, and transparency.

## 3. RULE-BASED MODEL DEVELOPMENT AND FUNCTION APPROXIMATION

This section summarizes the basic procedure to develop a rule-based model from data provided by an IS. A set of rules may supply a granular representation of an underlying function $f(x_n)$. To estimate the value of $f(x_n)$, given $x_n^{(k)} \leq x_n \leq x_n^{(m)}$ and a lower and upper approximation $y^{(k)} \leq y \leq y^{(m)}$, we may employ a general function approximation procedure. In particular, if we assume that $f$ is an arbitrary continuous real valued function, then it can be uniformly approximated in $x_n^{(k)} \leq x_n \leq x_n^{(m)}$ using an algebra of continuous real valued functions (Stone-Weierstrass theorem; see Davis, 1975 for details). For instance, if we assume that $f$ is real and continuous, then it can be approximated by polynomials in $x_1, x_2, \ldots, x_N$ as

$$f(x_1, \ x_2, \ \ldots, x_N) = y^{(k)} + \frac{(y^{(m)} - y^{(k)})}{\sum\limits_{n=1}^{N} d_n} \sum_{n=1}^{N} c_n (x_n - x_n^{(k)})$$

where $x_1, x_2, \ldots, x_N$ are the values of the variables, the indices $k$ and $m$ represent the lower and upper bound values, $N$ is the number of variables, $c_n = (x_n^{(m)} - x_n^{(k)})$ and $d_n = (x_n^{(m)} - x_n^{(k)})^2$ are coefficients calculated with the bound parameters of the variables. Equation (8) is an equivalent formula that supplies the same numeric values.

$$f(x_1, \ x_2, \ \ldots, \ x_N) = y(x_n, x_n^{(i)}, y^{(i)})_{\substack{i=k,m \\ n=1,N}}$$

$$= y^{(k)} + \frac{(y^{(m)} - y^{(k)})}{N} \sum_{n=1}^{N} \frac{(x_n - x_n^{(k)})}{c_n} \tag{8}$$

Therefore, since any system has a specific function governing its behavior, from the set of rules obtained using attribute-value tables, filled with input and output data, we can estimate system outputs using interpolation functions.

To clarify the main idea and to grasp the procedure behind granular rule-based model development and system modeling using function approximation suggested here, let us consider the information systems table illustrated in Table 1.

Clearly, the following set of rules can be straightforwardly derived from the IS table:

- $s_1$: IF $x_1 = x_1^{(a)}$ AND $x_2 = x_2^{(a)}$ AND ... AND $x_N = x_N^{(a)}$ THEN $y = y^{(a)}$
- $s_2$: IF $x_1 = x_1^{(b)}$ AND $x_2 = x_2^{(b)}$ AND ... AND $x_N = x_N^{(b)}$ THEN $y = y^{(b)}$
- ... ... ...
- $s_k$: IF $x_1 = x_1^{(k)}$ AND $x_2 = x_2^{(k)}$ AND ... AND $x_N = x_N^{(k)}$ THEN $y = y^{(k)}$
- ... ... ...

*Table 1. Information system*

| $x_1$ | $x_2$ | $x_3$ | ... | $x_N$ | $Y$ |
|---|---|---|---|---|---|
| $x_1^{(a)}$ | $x_2^{(a)}$ | $x_3^{(a)}$ | ... | $x_N^{(a)}$ | $y^{(a)}$ |
| $x_1^{(b)}$ | $x_2^{(b)}$ | $x_3^{(b)}$ | ... | $x_N^{(b)}$ | $y^{(b)}$ |
| ... | ... | ... | ... | ... | ... |
| $x_1^{(k)}$ | $x_2^{(k)}$ | $x_3^{(k)}$ | ... | $x_N^{(k)}$ | $y^{(k)}$ |
| ... | ... | ... | ... | ... | ... |
| $x_1^{(m)}$ | $x_2^{(m)}$ | $x_3^{(m)}$ | ... | $x_N^{(m)}$ | $y^{(m)}$ |
| ... | ... | ... | ... | ... | ... |
| $x_1^{(v)}$ | $x_2^{(v)}$ | $x_3^{(v)}$ | ... | $x_N^{(v)}$ | $y^{(v)}$ |

- $s_m$: IF $x_1 = x_1^{(m)}$ AND $x_2 = x_2^{(m)}$ AND ... AND $x_N = x_N^{(m)}$ THEN $y = y^{(m)}$

- ... ... ...

- $s_v$: IF $x_1 = x_1^{(v)}$ AND $x_2 = x_1^{(v)}$ AND ... AND $x_N = x_N^{(v)}$ THEN $y = y^{(v)}$.(9)

For example, if $x_1 = x_1^{(k)}$, $x_2 = x_2^{(k)}$, $x_3 = x_3^{(k)}$, and $x_N = x_N^{(k)}$ then we have $y = y^{(k)}$ expressed as $s_k$, and if $x_1 = x_1^{(m)}$, $x_2 = x_2^{(m)}$, $x_3 = x_3^{(m)}$, and $x_N = x_N^{(m)}$ then $y = y^{(m)}$ expressed as $s_m$. Values between $x_1^{(k)} \leq x_1 \leq x_1^{(m)}$, $x_2^{(k)} \leq x_2 \leq x_2^{(m)}$, $x_3^{(k)} \leq x_3 \leq x_3^{(m)}$, and $x_N^{(k)} \leq x_N \leq x_N^{(m)}$ can be obtained combining $s_k$ and $s_m$ to get a general rule of the form

- $r_g$: IF $x_1^{(k)} \leq x_1 \leq x_1^{(m)}$ AND $x_2^{(k)} \leq x_2 \leq x_2^{(m)}$ AND ... AND $x_N^{(k)} \leq x_N \leq x_N^{(m)}$
- THEN $\min\{y^{(k)},...,y^{(m)}\} \leq y \leq \max\{y^{(k)},...,y^{(m)}\}$. (10)

Next, if we adopt the simplest approximation case, namely, linear approximation, then we can use expression (8) to estimate the value of the underlying function of the model for any $x_n$. If two or more rules produce approximation results for the same attribute values, the respective estimated function values can be averaged to give a single value. For multi output models we can to compile distinct rules for each input variable. The procedure to develop a rule-based model and to estimate model outputs using function approximation is as follows:

- Step 1: Select system input/output data;
- Step 2: Translate the I/O data into an attribute-value table;
- Step 3: Develop the rules from the attribute-value table;
- Step 4: Select the intervals of the values for each attribute of the rules;
- Step 5: Select the upper and lower limits of the decision values;
- Step 6: Put the rules in the form of (10);
- Step 7: Given an input, compute system output by using (8).

Step 3 is accomplished with the use of computational tools like Rosetta, RSL, CI, etc.

One of the advantages of the structure for rule-based models suggested in this work (Step 6 and Step 7), compared to fuzzy models, is that the use of specific procedures like fuzzification or defuzzification are unnecessary in the computation of the models.

An additional advantage of the proposed methodology is also to enable development of fuzzy models as to the generation of rules and in the estimation of membership functions.

Some examples will illustrate these concepts.

For instance, assume that the underlying function of a IS given in Table 2 is $g(x_1,x_2) = x_1 + x_2$, where $x_1, x_2 \in [0, 2]$.

Using the structure of the general rule (10) and data of Table 2 we get the set of rules (11), which gives a granular model of the linear function $g(.)$.

- $r_1$: IF $0 \leq x_1 \leq 1$ AND $0 \leq x_2 \leq 1$ THEN $0 \leq y \leq 2$
- $r_2$: IF $0 \leq x_1 \leq 1$ AND $1 \leq x_2 \leq 2$ THEN $1 \leq y \leq 3$
- $r_3$: IF $1 \leq x_1 \leq 2$ AND $0 \leq x_2 \leq 1$ THEN $1 \leq y \leq 3$
- $r_4$: IF $1 \leq x_1 \leq 2$ AND $1 \leq x_2 \leq 2$ THEN $2 \leq y \leq 4$ (11)

If we set the inputs as $x_1 = 0.8$ and $x_2 = 1.3$, then the value of $g(x_1, x_2)$ can be estimated using rule $r_2$ and (8) in which $x_1^{(k)} = 0$, $x_1^{(m)} = 1$, $x_2^{(k)} = 1$, $x_2^{(m)} = 2$, $y^{(k)} = 1$, and $y^{(m)} = 3$, that is,

$$f(1.3, \ 0.8) = y(x_1, x_2, x_1^{(i)}, x_2^{(i)}, y^{(i)})_{\substack{i=k,m \\ n=1,2}}$$
$$= 1 + \frac{(3-1)}{2}\left(\frac{(0.8-0)}{(1-0)} + \frac{(1.3-1)}{(2-1)}\right) = 2.1$$

In this simple case, the estimated value corresponds to the value of the original function $g(x_1, x_2) = x_1 + x_2$, exactly, as it would be expected.

## 4. COMPUTATIONAL RESULTS

In this section we present selected examples to illustrate the modeling method to develop rule-based models and functions approximation. We address static and dynamic models. Performances of the models are evaluated against fuzzy models using squared error criterion.

*Table 2. IS of g(x₁,x₂)*

| $x_1$ | $x_2$ | $y$ |
|---|---|---|
| 0 | 0 | 0 |
| 0 | 1 | 1 |
| 0 | 2 | 2 |
| 1 | 0 | 1 |
| 1 | 1 | 2 |
| 1 | 2 | 3 |
| 2 | 0 | 2 |
| 2 | 1 | 3 |
| 2 | 2 | 4 |

*Table 3. Process input and output values*

| $x$ | $y = h(x)$ |
|---|---|
| 0.00 | 2.0000 |
| ... | ... |
| 3.00 | 3.7345 |
| ... | ... |
| 5.25 | 6.9608 |
| ... | ... |
| 8.50 | 10.8862 |
| ... | ... |
| 10.0 | 11.0000 |

## 4.1 Static System Modeling

Assume data (measurements) of a process as shown in Figure 2. Suppose that the information granules are the subsets of points in the regions A-B, B-C, and C-D. In this case, we notice that implicitly they suggest a piecewise linear function we denote by $h(x)$. Function $h(x)$ is assumed to be the underlying function. Table 3 gives samples of the data that assemble the information system of the process. Next we show how the set of rules is associated with the function $h(x)$.

The rules can be obtained using Rosetta (http://www.idi.ntnu.no/~aleks/rosetta/). Data of Figure 2 were input to Rosetta and the following processing steps were performed: *Discretization → Equal frequency binning → Intervals = 3; Reduction → Exhaustive calculation (RSES) → Full; Rule generator (RSES)*. Rosetta output the three rules shown below (12).

- $x([*, 3.3750]) \Rightarrow y(2.0000)$ OR $y(2.2197)$ OR $y(2.3811)$ OR $y(2.5136)$ OR $y(2.7310)$ OR $y(2.7827)$ OR $y(2.8327)$ OR $y(3.0351)$ OR $y(2.9551)$ OR $y(3.3973)$ OR $y(3.5117)$ OR $y(3.5909)$ OR $y(3.7345)$ OR $y(3.8419)$
- $x([3.3750, 6.8750]) \Rightarrow y(4.0952)$ OR $y(4.2879)$ OR $y(4.4000)$ OR $y(4.8764)$ OR $y(5.2843)$ OR $y(5.9241)$ OR $y(6.3302)$ OR $y(6.9608)$ OR $y(7.3044)$ OR $y(7.6791)$ OR $y(8.2819)$ OR $y(9.0139)$ OR $y(9.3387)$ OR $y(10.0420)$
- $x([6.8750,*]) \Rightarrow y(10.4000)$ OR $y(10.6437)$ OR $y(10.4786)$ OR $y(10.4928)$ OR $y(10.7082)$ OR $y(10.6233)$ OR $y(10.8862)$ OR $y(10.6830)$ OR $y(10.8393)$ OR $y(10.9186)$ OR $y(10.8814)$ OR $y(10.9779)$ OR $y(11.0000)$ (12)

The usage of the rules given in (12) is direct. The values in the rules antecedents are the lower and upper bound values of the attribute ($x^{(k)}$, $x^{(m)}$, etc.). Symbol "*" represents the limit values of the variables (lower bound = 0 and upper bound = 10). For the rules consequents, the minimum and the maximum values of the consequents of each rule are selected to give the values of $y^{(k)}$ and $y^{(m)}$ (the lower approximation and the upper approximation, respectively). After performing these steps we get the set of rules given in (13) with $x^{(a)} = 0$, $x^{(b)} = 3.375$, $x^{(c)} = 6.875$, $x^{(d)} = 10$, $y^{(a)} = 2$, $y^{(b)} = 3.8419$, $y^{(c)} = 4.0952$, $y^{(d)} =$

*Figure 2. Information granules and the underlying function h(x)*

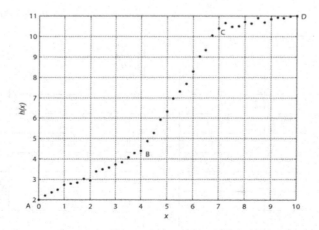

10.042, $y^{(e)} = 10.4$, and $y^{(f)} = 11$. The set of rules constitutes a granular model of the underlying function. In this particular example we see that rules $r_1$, $r_2$, and $r_3$ are granular models of the line segments L1, L2, and L3, as depicted in Figure 3.

- $r_1$: IF $x^{(a)} \leq x \leq x^{(b)}$ THEN $y^{(a)} \leq y \leq y^{(b)}$
- $r_2$: IF $x^{(b)} \leq x \leq x^{(c)}$ THEN $y^{(c)} \leq y \leq y^{(d)}$
- $r_3$: IF $x^{(c)} \leq x \leq x^{(d)}$ THEN $y^{(e)} \leq y \leq y^{(f)}$ (13)

Given a value of an input $x$, we compute the corresponding output using (8). For instance, if $x = 3$, then $f(x) = 2 + (3.8419 - 2)(3 - 0) / (3.375 - 0) = 3.6372$. If $x = 5.25$ then $f(x) = 4.0952 + (10.042 - 4.0952)(5.25 - 3.375) / (6.875 - 3.375) = 7.281$. If $x = 8.5$, then $f(x) = 10.4 + (11 - 10.4)(8.5 - 6.875) / (10 - 6.875) = 10.712$.

To evaluate the performance of the rule-based model development and function approximation method, Table 4 shows the squared error, the quadratic sum of the differences between values of the Table 3 and the results estimated by the rough model. They are compared against models developed for the same data using linguistic and functional fuzzy rule-based models, and a feedforward neural network. We notice that error values indicate similar performance from the approximation error point of view.

The fuzzy model I is linguistic model (Mamdani type) whose rules are

- $r_1$: IF $x = A^{(1)}$ THEN $y = E^{(1)}$
- $r_2$: IF $x = A^{(2)}$ THEN $y = E^{(2)}$
- $r_3$: IF $x = A^{(3)}$ THEN $y = E^{(3)}$
- $r_4$: IF $x = A^{(4)}$ THEN $y = E^{(4)}$ (14)

*Table 4. Performance of the models (squared errors)*

| Rough | Linguistic fuzzy | Functional fuzzy | Neural network |
|-------|------------------|------------------|----------------|
| 1.61  | 1.63             | 1.60             | 1.44           |

*Figure 3. Granular model and the underlying function*

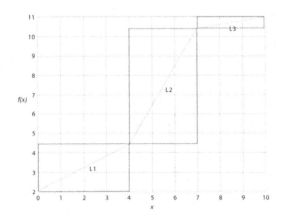

The membership functions of the fuzzy sets of (14) are shown in Figure 4. The parameters of the fuzzy model are the same as of the rough model, that is, $x^{(1)} = x^{(a)}$, $x^{(2)} = x^{(b)}$, $x^{(3)} = x^{(c)}$, and $x^{(4)} = x^{(d)}$. The values of $y^{(1)} = 2$, $y^{(2)} = 3.9686$, $y^{(3)} = 10.221$, and $y^{(4)} = 11$ were obtained using data of the rough model (13) with the interpolation (8).

Fuzzy model II is a functional fuzzy model (Takagi-Sugeno type) whose rules are

- $r_1$: IF $x = C^{(1)}$ THEN $y_1 = 0.5457x + 2$
- $r_2$: IF $x = C^{(2)}$ THEN $y_2 = 1.6991x - 1.6392$
- $r_3$: IF $x = C^{(3)}$ THEN $y_3 = 0.1920x + 9.08$ (15)

The fuzzy sets of the antecedents have the membership functions depicted in Figure 5, where $x^{(1)} = x^{(a)}$, $x^{(2)} = x^{(b)}$, $x^{(3)} = x^{(c)}$, $x^{(4)} = x^{(d)}$. The parameters of $y_1$, $y_2$, and $y_3$ were obtained using the data of the rule-based model (13) and (8).

The neural network has one input and one output, twenty neurons in the hidden layer whose activation function is the sigmoid function. Training was done using the back-propagation and half of the data of the Table 3 for training and the remaining part for validation. The learning rate was 0.005 and the stop criterion is the squared error smaller 0.01.

## 4.2 Dynamic Systems Modeling

Figure 6 shows a general structure of rule-based models of dynamic systems, where the variable $u$ is the system input, $c$ is the output of the process, and $z^j$, $z^p$ denote the $j$-th and $p$-th delay operators.

*Figure 4. Fuzzy sets of the linguistic model*

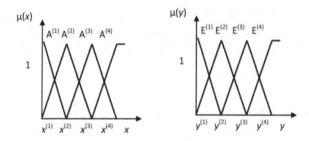

*Figure 5. Fuzzy sets of the functional model*

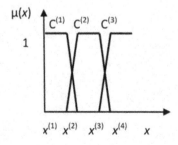

The aim of this section is to develop a rule-based model of a dynamic system. For instance, equation (16) is typical in modeling of dynamic systems such as electric, mechanical, thermal, and chemical processes.

$$c(t) = b_1 u(t-1) + a_1 c(t-1) \qquad (16)$$

System outputs were computed for randomly chosen inputs in the unit interval [0,1] at each time step. Three hundred pairs of input and output values were generated. Table 5 gives examples of these values. The original model parameters are $a_1 = 0.3679$ and $b_1 = 0.6321$.

The procedure to obtain the rule-based model of dynamic systems is basically the same as the one for static systems: we just define $x_1 = u(t-1)$; $x_2 = c(t-1)$; $y = c(t)$ and proceed similarly. Given the IS system shown in Table 5 Rosetta outputs the following rules

- $x_1([*, 0.3410])$ AND $x_2([*, 0.4096]) \Rightarrow y(0.0000)$ OR $y(0.3163)$ OR... OR $y(0.3247)$ OR ... OR $y(0.3257)$ OR ... OR $y(0.0996)$
- $x_1([0.3410, 0.6637])$ AND $x_2([*, 0.4096]) \Rightarrow y(0.2278)$ OR $y(0.4305)$ OR ... OR y$(0.4323)$ OR ... OR $y(0.5122)$ OR ... OR $y(0.4240)$
- ... ... ...
- $x_1([0.6637, *])$ AND $x_2([*, 0.4096]) \Rightarrow y(0.7159)$ OR $y(0.6744)$ OR ... OR $y(0.4812)$ OR ... OR $y(0.7318)$ OR ... OR $y(0.7236)$ (17)

In (17) we give the first, second, and the ninth rules of the model, for short. The method of section 3 builds the rules (18), where $x_1^{(a)} = 0$, $x_1^{(b)} = 0.341$, $x_1^{(c)} = 0.6637$, $x_1^{(d)} = 1$, $x_2^{(a)} = 0$, $x_2^{(b)} = 0.4096$, $x_2^{(c)} = 0.609$, and $x_2^{(d)} = 0.9$. A simulation was conducted to compare the results of the model given by the

*Figure 6. General structure of dynamic rule-based models*

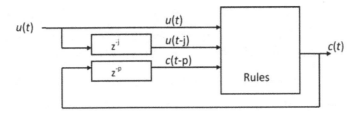

*Table 5. IS of the dynamic system*

| $t$ | $u(t-1)$ | $c(t-1)$ | $c(t)$ |
|---|---|---|---|
| 1 | 0.0000 | 0.0000 | 0.0000 |
| 2 | 0.3603 | 0.0000 | 0.2278 |
| 3 | 0.5485 | 0.2278 | 0.4305 |
| ... | ... | ... | ... |
| 299 | 0.9339 | 0.3625 | 0.7236 |
| 300 | 0.1372 | 0.7236 | 0.3529 |

rule-based model against the original model expressed by (16). Figure 7 depicts the result.

- $r_1$: IF $x_1^{(a)} \le x_1 \le x_1^{(b)}$ AND $x_2^{(a)} \le x_2 \le x_2^{(b)}$ THEN $0.0000 \le y \le 0.3257$
- $r_2$: IF $x_1^{(b)} \le x_1 \le x_1^{(c)}$ AND $x_2^{(a)} \le x_2 \le x_2^{(b)}$ THEN $0.2278 \le y \le 0.5122$
- $r_3$: IF $x_1^{(a)} \le x_1 \le x_1^{(b)}$ AND $x_2^{(b)} \le x_2 \le x_2^{(c)}$ THEN $0.1670 \le y \le 0.4263$
- $r_4$: IF $x_1^{(c)} \le x_1 \le x_1^{(d)}$ AND $x_2^{(b)} \le x_2 \le x_2^{(c)}$ THEN $0.5993 \le y \le 0.8507$
- $r_5$: IF $x_1^{(c)} \le x_1 \le x_1^{(d)}$ AND $x_2^{(c)} \le x_2 \le x_2^{(d)}$ THEN $0.6635 \le y \le 0.8846$
- $r_6$: IF $x_1^{(b)} \le x_1 \le x_1^{(c)}$ AND $x_2^{(c)} \le x_2 \le x_2^{(d)}$ THEN $0.4867 \le y \le 0.7065$
- $r_7$: IF $x_1^{(b)} \le x_1 \le x_1^{(c)}$ AND $x_2^{(b)} \le x_2 \le x_2^{(c)}$ THEN $0.3761 \le y \le 0.6277$
- $r_8$: IF $x_1^{(a)} \le x_1 \le x_1^{(b)}$ AND $x_2^{(c)} \le x_2 \le x_2^{(d)}$ THEN $0.2600 \le y \le 0.4700$
- $r_9$: IF $x_1^{(c)} \le x_1 \le x_1^{(d)}$ AND $x_2^{(a)} \le x_2 \le x_2^{(b)}$ THEN $0.4812 \le y \le 0.7318$ (18)

The top of Figure 7 shows the input (each input value was generated randomly at intervals of one step), and the bottom the corresponding outputs of the original model (solid line) and the output of the rule-based model (dotted line). Clearly, the values of the original and rule-based models are very close. The resulting approximation error, in the squared error sense, is 0.04. Figure 8 shows the result when the input is computed using the expression $u(t) = 0.4[1 + \sin(t)]$. Notice that the rule-based model with estimation adequately captures the actual behavior, introducing practically the same level of attenuation and of phase difference as in the original model.

The Takagi-Sugeno model with a rule base given in (19) achieved the same degree of accuracy. The antecedent membership functions are shown in Figure 9. The parameters of the fuzzy model were obtained using the data of the rough model.

- $r_1$: IF $x_1 = C^{(1)}$ AND $x_2 = D^{(1)}$ THEN $y_1 = 0.4776x_1 + 0.3976x_2$
- $r_2$: IF $x_1 = C^{(2)}$ AND $x_2 = D^{(1)}$ THEN $y_2 = 0.4362x_1 + 0.3472x_2 + 0.0791$
- $r_3$: IF $x_1 = C^{(1)}$ AND $x_2 = D^{(2)}$ THEN $y_3 = 0.3802x_1 + 0.6502x_2 - 0.0993$
- $r_4$: IF $x_1 = C^{(3)}$ AND $x_2 = D^{(2)}$ THEN $y_4 = 0.3940x_1 + 0.6304x_2 + 0.0783$

*Figure 7. Original model versus the rule-based model*

*Figure 8. Original versus rule based model using $u(t) = 0.4[1+\sin(t)]$*

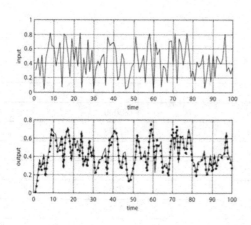

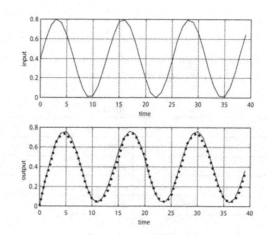

- $r_5$: IF $x_1 = C^{(3)}$ AND $x_2 = D^{(3)}$ THEN $y_5 = 0.3466x_1 + 0.3799x_2 + 0.201$
- $r_6$: IF $x_1 = C^{(2)}$ AND $x_2 = D^{(3)}$ THEN $y_6 = 0.3371x_1 + 0.3777x_2 + 0.1417$
- $r_7$: IF $x_1 = C^{(2)}$ AND $x_2 = D^{(2)}$ THEN $y_7 = 0.3859x_1 + 0.6309x_2 - 0.0139$
- $r_8$: IF $x_1 = C^{(3)}$ AND $x_2 = D^{(3)}$ THEN $y_8 = 0.3079x_1 + 0.3608x_2 + 0.0403$
- $r_9$: IF $x_1 = C^{(3)}$ AND $x_2 = D^{(1)}$ THEN $y_9 = 0.3928x_1 + 0.3059x_2 + 0.2192$ (19)

A linguistic fuzzy model (Mamdani) whose rules are given in (20) and membership functions of the fuzzy sets of Figure 10 was also developed. The linguistic fuzzy model uses the same parameters as those of the rough model: modal values $E^{(1)}$ up to $E^{(16)}$ are 0, 0.1649, 0.1953, 0.3421, 0.4256, 0.5418, 0.2783, 0.4318, 0.6269, 0.7403, 0.7284, 0.8124, 0.8846, 0.5333, 0.365, and 0.6065, respectively. The linguistic model outputs are computed using the max-min composition center of gravity defuzzification ((Pedrycz and Gomide, 2007).

- $r_1$: IF $x_1 = A^{(1)}$ AND $x_2 = B^{(1)}$ THEN $y = E^{(1)}$
- $r_2$: IF $x_1 = A^{(1)}$ AND $x_2 = B^{(2)}$ THEN $y = E^{(2)}$
- $r_3$: IF $x_1 = A^{(2)}$ AND $x_2 = B^{(1)}$ THEN $y = E^{(3)}$
- $r_4$: IF $x_1 = A^{(2)}$ AND $x_2 = B^{(2)}$ THEN $y = E^{(4)}$
- $r_5$: IF $x_1 = A^{(3)}$ AND $x_2 = B^{(1)}$ THEN $y = E^{(5)}$
- $r_6$: IF $x_1 = A^{(3)}$ AND $x_2 = B^{(2)}$ THEN $y = E^{(6)}$
- $r_7$: IF $x_1 = A^{(1)}$ AND $x_2 = B^{(3)}$ THEN $y = E^{(7)}$
- $r_8$: IF $x_1 = A^{(2)}$ AND $x_2 = B^{(3)}$ THEN $y = E^{(8)}$

*Figure 9. Fuzzy sets of Takagi-Sugeno model*

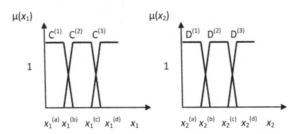

*Figure 10. Fuzzy sets of the fuzzy linguistic model*

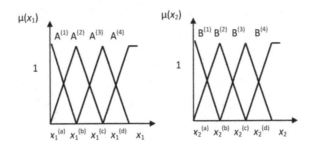

- $r_9$: IF $x_1 = A^{(3)}$ AND $x_2 = B^{(3)}$ THEN $y = E^{(9)}$
- $r_{10}$: IF $x_1 = A^{(3)}$ AND $x_2 = B^{(4)}$ THEN $y = E^{(10)}$
- $r_{11}$: IF $x_1 = A^{(4)}$ AND $x_2 = B^{(2)}$ THEN $y = E^{(11)}$
- $r_{12}$: IF $x_1 = A^{(4)}$ AND $x_2 = B^{(3)}$ THEN $y = E^{(12)}$
- $r_{13}$: IF $x_1 = A^{(4)}$ AND $x_2 = B^{(4)}$ THEN $y = E^{(13)}$
- $r_{14}$: IF $x_1 = A^{(2)}$ AND $x_2 = B^{(4)}$ THEN $y = E^{(14)}$
- $r_{15}$: IF $x_1 = A^{(1)}$ AND $x_2 = B^{(4)}$ THEN $y = E^{(15)}$
- $r_{16}$: IF $x_1 = A^{(4)}$ AND $x_2 = B^{(1)}$ THEN $y = E^{(16)}$ (20)

## 4.3 Non-Linear System Modeling

Consider the non-linear model (21) and inputs randomly chosen in [0, 1] at each time step as shown in Figure 11.

$$c(t) = 0.4c(t-1) + 0.6u^2(t-1) \qquad (21)$$

An IS system table was constructed with the values of the inputs $u(t)$ and the outputs $c(t)$ of the model. In the table we set $x_1 = u(t\text{-}1)$; $x_2 = c(t\text{-}1)$; $y = c(t)$. The resulting IS table constitutes a representation of the process. Similarly to the examples of previous sections, we use *Rosetta* with the option: *Discretization → Equal frequency binning → Intervals* = 4) to generate the following rules

- $r_1$: IF $x_1^{(a)} \leq x_1 \leq x_1^{(b)}$ AND $x_2^{(a)} \leq x_2 \leq x_2^{(b)}$ THEN $0.0000 \leq y \leq 0.0841$
- $r_2$: IF $x_1^{(b)} \leq x_1 \leq x_1^{(c)}$ AND $x_2^{(a)} \leq x_2 \leq x_2^{(b)}$ THEN $0.0630 \leq y \leq 0.1977$
- $r_3$: IF $x_1^{(d)} \leq x_1 \leq x_1^{(e)}$ AND $x_2^{(a)} \leq x_2 \leq x_2^{(b)}$ THEN $0.3750 \leq y \leq 0.6151$
- $r_4$: IF $x_1^{(b)} \leq x_1 \leq x_1^{(c)}$ AND $x_2^{(c)} \leq x_2 \leq x_2^{(d)}$ THEN $0.1832 \leq y \leq 0.2793$
- $r_5$: IF $x_1^{(a)} \leq x_1 \leq x_1^{(b)}$ AND $x_2^{(b)} \leq x_2 \leq x_2^{(c)}$ THEN $0.0790 \leq y \leq 0.1322$
- $r_6$: IF $x_1^{(c)} \leq x_1 \leq x_1^{(d)}$ AND $x_2^{(a)} \leq x_2 \leq x_2^{(b)}$ THEN $0.1614 \leq y \leq 0.4102$

*Figure 11. Input and output data of the nonlinear system*

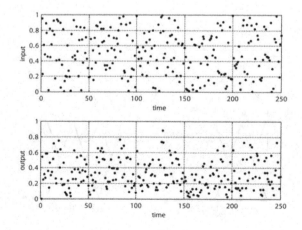

- $r_7$: IF $x_1^{(b)} \le x_1 \le x_1^{(c)}$ AND $x_2^{(b)} \le x_2 \le x_2^{(c)}$ THEN $0.1255 \le y \le 0.2328$
- $r_8$: IF $x_1^{(d)} \le x_1 \le x_1^{(e)}$ AND $x_2^{(c)} \le x_2 \le x_2^{(d)}$ THEN $0.4965 \le y \le 0.7379$
- $r_9$: IF $x_1^{(b)} \le x_1 \le x_1^{(c)}$ AND $x_2^{(d)} \le x_2 \le x_2^{(e)}$ THEN $0.2886 \le y \le 0.4100$
- $r_{10}$: IF $x_1^{(d)} \le x_1 \le x_1^{(e)}$ AND $x_2^{(b)} \le x_2 \le x_2^{(c)}$ THEN $0.4719 \le y \le 0.6728$
- $r_{11}$: IF $x_1^{(c)} \le x_1 \le x_1^{(d)}$ AND $x_2^{(c)} \le x_2 \le x_2^{(d)}$ THEN $0.2918 \le y \le 0.4870$
- $r_{12}$: IF $x_1^{(a)} \le x_1 \le x_1^{(b)}$ AND $x_2^{(c)} \le x_2 \le x_2^{(d)}$ THEN $0.1334 \le y \le 0.2161$
- $r_{13}$: IF $x_1^{(c)} \le x_1 \le x_1^{(d)}$ AND $x_2^{(b)} \le x_2 \le x_2^{(c)}$ THEN $0.2288 \le y \le 0.4578$
- $r_{14}$: IF $x_1^{(a)} \le x_1 \le x_1^{(b)}$ AND $x_2^{(d)} \le x_2 \le x_2^{(e)}$ THEN $0.2093 \le y \le 0.3463$
- $r_{15}$: IF $x_1^{(c)} \le x_1 \le x_1^{(d)}$ AND $x_2^{(d)} \le x_2 \le x_2^{(e)}$ THEN $0.3639 \le y \le 0.5994$
- $r_{16}$: IF $x_1^{(d)} \le x_1 \le x_1^{(e)}$ AND $x_2^{(d)} \le x_2 \le x_2^{(e)}$ THEN $0.5921 \le y \le 0.8405$ (22)

where $x_1^{(a)} = 0$; $x_1^{(b)} = 0.2521$; $x_1^{(c)} = 0.4893$; $x_1^{(d)} = 0.7787$; $x_1^{(e)} = 1$; $x_2^{(a)} = 0$; $x_2^{(b)} = 0.1703$; $x_2^{(c)} = 0.2951$; $x_2^{(d)} = 0.4913$; $x_2^{(e)} = 0.8405$.

Figure 12 shows the input and the output of the non-linear model in solid line and the output of the rule-based model in dotted line. The squared error approximation is 0.07. The generalization capability of the rule-based model is illustrated in Figure 13 where steps were used as inputs for the model given in (22). The rule-based model (dotted line) is able to reproduce the behavior of the original model (solid line) with a squared error approximation of 0.06.

The results of this section indicate that the modeling method suggested in this chapter can model linear and non-linear systems adequately, constituting a powerful option to develop models of complex systems.

## 5. CONCLUSION

This chapter has shown how concepts of rough sets can be used to model static and dynamic nonlinear systems. The granular modeling methodology introduced here gives rule-based models associated with a functional representation that can uniformly approximate continuous function with a certain degree of

*Figure 12. Original non-linear model versus rule-based model, random inputs*

*Figure 13. Original non-linear model versus rule-based model, step inputs*

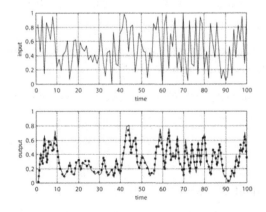

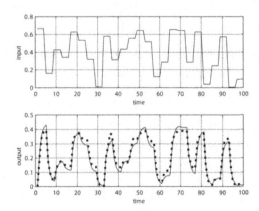

accuracy. Therefore, it gives an alternative form to construct universal approximators similar to neural and rule-based fuzzy models.

Experiments and examples testify that granular models with function approximation and estimation capabilities can model continuous linear and nonlinear systems. The main advantage of the method relies on its computational simplicity and efficiency. In addition it gives models that are transparent and, at the same time, precise because estimation of system outputs can be found through an approximation scheme whose parameters are easily obtained from the set of rules.

Future work shall consider the use of the methodology developed in this chapter to construct evolving models and adaptive rule-based controllers for nonlinear systems.

## ACKNOWLEDGMENT

The second, the third and the fourth author are grateful to CNPq, the Brazilian National Research Council, for grant 304857/2006-8, 305863/2006-1 and 35942/2006-9, respectively.

## REFERENCES

Davis, P. J. (1975). *Interpolation & Approximation*. New York: Dover Publications Inc.

Hofestädt, R., & Meinecke, F. (1995). Interactive Modelling and Simulation of Biochemical Networks. *Computers in Biology and Medicine, 25*, 321–334. doi:10.1016/0010-4825(95)00019-Z

Huang, B., Guo, L., & Zhou, X. (2007). Approximation Reduction Based on Similarity Relation. In *Proceedings of theIEEE Fourth International Conference on Fuzzy Systems and Knowledge Discovery* (pp. 124-128).

Ilczuk, G., & Wakulicz-Deja, A. (2007). $_a$). Data preparation for data mining in medical data sets. *LNCS Transactions on Rough Sets, 6*, 83–93. doi:10.1007/978-3-540-71200-8_6

Ilczuk, G., & Wakulicz-Deja, A. (2007). $_b$). Selection of important attributes for medical diagnosis systems. *LNCS Transactions on Rough Sets, 7*, 70–84.

Jeon, G., Kim, D., & Jeong, J. (2006). Rough sets attributes reduction based expert system in interlaced video sequences. *IEEE Transactions on Consumer Electronics, 52*, 1348–1355. doi:10.1109/TCE.2006.273155

Øhrn, A., & Komorowski, J. (1997). ROSETTA: A rough set toolkit for analysis of data. In *Proceeding of the Third International Joint Conference on Information Sciences* (pp. 403-407).

Pawlak, Z. (1982). Rough sets. *International Journal of Computer and Information Sciences*, 341-356.

Pawlak, Z. (1991). *Rough Sets: Theoretical Aspects of Reasoning about Data*. Dordrecht, The Netherlands: Kluwer Academic Publishers.

Pawlak, Z. (1997). *Rough real functions and rough controllers. Rough sets and data mining: Analysis of imprecise data* (pp. 139–147). Boston: Kluwer Academic Publishers.

Pawlak, Z., & Munakata, T. (1996). Rough control: Application of Rough Set Theory to control. In *Proceeding of the Fourth European Congress on Intelligent Techniques and Soft Computing (EUFIT'96)*, (pp. 209-218).

Pawlak, Z., & Skowron, A. (2007). ₐ). Rudiments of rough sets. *Information Sciences, 177*, 3–27. doi:10.1016/j.ins.2006.06.003

Pawlak, Z., & Skowron, A. (2007). ᵦ). Rough sets: Some extensions. *Information Sciences, 177*, 28–40. doi:10.1016/j.ins.2006.06.006

Pedrycz, W., & Gomide, F. (2007). *Fuzzy Systems Engineering: Toward Human-Centric Computing*. New York: Wiley Interscience.

Quan, X., & Biao, M. (2008). Self-Adaptive Ant Colony Algorithm for Attributes Reduction. In Proceedings of the *IEEE International Conference on Granular Computing* (pp. 686-689).

Sakai, H., & Nakata, M. (2006). On Rough sets based rule generation from tables. *International Journal of Innovative Computing. Information and Control, 2*, 3–31.

Sankar, K. P., & Mitra, P. (2002). Multispectral image segmentation using the rough-set-initialized EM algorithm. *IEEE Transactions on Geoscience and Remote Sensing, 40*, 2495–2501. doi:10.1109/TGRS.2002.803716

Shen, Q., & Chouchoulas, A. (2001). Rough set-based dimensionality reduction for supervised and unsupervised learning. *Int. J. Appl. Comput. Sci., 11*, 583–601.

Skowron, A., & Rauszer, C. (1992). The Discernibility Matrices and Functions in Information Systems. In Slowinski, R. (Ed.), *Intelligent Decision Support: Handbook of Application and Advances of Rough Sets Theory*. Dordrecht, The Netherlands: Kluwer Academic Publishers.

Wróblewski, J. (1995). Finding minimal reducts using genetic algorithms. In *Proceedings of Second International Joint Conference on Information Science* (pp. 186-189).

Yao, J. T. (2005). Information granulation and granular relationships. In *Proceedings of the IEEE - Conference on Granular Computing*, (pp.326-329).

Yao, J. T. (2007). A ten-year review of granular computing. In *Proceedings of the IEEE - Conference on Granular Computing* (pp. 734-739).

Yao, J. T., & Yao, Y. Y. (2002). Induction of classification rules by granular computing. In Alpigini, J.J., Peters, J.F., Skowron, A., & Zhong, N. (Eds.), *Proceedings of the Third International Conference on Rough Sets and Current Trends in Computing, Lecture Notes in Artificial Intelligence* (pp. 331-338).

Yao, Y. Y., Wang, F. Y., Wang, J., & Zeng, D. (2005). Rule + exception strategies for security information analysis. *IEEE Transactions on Intelligent Systems, 20*, 52–57. doi:10.1109/MIS.2005.93

Yun, G., & Yuanbin, H. (2004). Application of Rough Set Theory on system modeling. In *Proceedings of the IEEE - 5ᵗʰ World Congress on Intelligent Control and Automation* (pp. 2352-2354).

Ziarko, W., & Katzberg, J. D. (1993). Rough sets approach to system modeling and control algorithm acquisition. In *Proceedings of the IEEE - Communications, Computers and Power in the Modern Environment* (pp. 154-164).

# Chapter 18
# A Genetic Fuzzy Semantic Web Search Agent Using Granular Semantic Trees for Ambiguous Queries

**Yan Chen**
*Georgia State University, USA*

**Yan-Qing Zhang**
*Georgia State University, USA*

## ABSTRACT

*For most Web searching applications, queries are commonly ambiguous because words or phrases have different linguistic meanings for different Web users. The conventional keyword-based search engines cannot disambiguate queries to provide relevant results matching Web users' intents. Traditional Word Sense Disambiguation (WSD) methods use statistic models or ontology-based knowledge systems to measure associations among words. The contexts of queries are used for disambiguation in these methods. However, due to the fact that numerous combinations of words may appear in queries and documents, it is difficult to extract concepts' relations for all possible combinations. Moreover, queries are usually short, so contexts in queries do not always provide enough information to disambiguate queries. Therefore, the traditional WSD methods are not sufficient to provide accurate search results for ambiguous queries. In this chapter, a new model, Granular Semantic Tree (GST), is introduced for more conveniently representing associations among concepts than the traditional WSD methods. Additionally, users' preferences are used to provide personalized search results that better adapt to users' unique intents. Fuzzy logic is used to determine the most appropriate concepts related to queries based on contexts and users' preferences. Finally, Web pages are analyzed by the GST model. The concepts of pages for the queries are evaluated, and the pages are re-ranked according to similarities of concepts between pages and queries.*

DOI: 10.4018/978-1-60566-324-1.ch018

## 1. INTRODUCTION

Nowadays, Web search engines play a key role in retrieving information from the Internet to provide useful Web documents in response to users' queries. The keywords-based search engines, like GOOGLE, YAHOO Search and MSN Live Search, explore documents by matching keywords in queries with words in documents. However, some keywords have more than one meaning, and such words may be related to different concepts in different contexts, so they are potentially ambiguous. Since current search engines simply search keywords separately and do not consider the contexts of queries, word sense ambiguity may result in searching errors for Web search applications. For example, if a user searches "drawing tables in a document" by MSN Live Search, five useless results related to the furniture table will be shown in the first result page. Therefore, an exact concept of a query may be determined by the contexts. Moreover, queries are usually short and contexts in queries do not always provide enough information for disambiguating queries. Under these circumstances, users' preferences may be helpful for determining an appropriate concept for an ambiguous word. For an example, if a biologist searches "mouse", we can speculate that the biologist is interested in Web pages related to a rodent "mouse" instead of a computer device "mouse." Thus, both contexts of queries and users' preferences are useful for disambiguating queries in Web search applications.

In fact, Query Disambiguation (QD) is a special application of Word Sense Disambiguation (WSD) problems. For most WSD problems, usually a set of possible meanings for a word is known ahead of time, and stored in a lexical database. Then, the meaning for the word is assigned depending on its contexts.

In this chapter, we propose a new model called Granular Semantic Tree to represent semantic relations between concepts. Each concept is represented as one granule in the tree structure. If concept A contains concept B, then granule B is represented as a child of granule A. Thus, a granular semantic tree that contains hierarchical structures can be constructed. Then, any concepts' relations in the granular semantic tree can be evaluated based on the hops between them. The exact concept for an ambiguous word is assigned depending on the concepts of its nearby words.

This chapter firstly discusses conventional effective methods for solving QD problems. Different from those methods, the GST model for easily expressing relations among words in contexts is proposed. Then, fuzzy logic is used for determine the most appropriate concepts related to queries based on contexts and users' interests. Experiments and evaluations are given. Finally conclusions are described.

## 2. RELATED WORKS

Based on the theory of granular computing, the granules, such as subsets, classes, objects, and elements of a universe, are basic ingredients of granular computing (Yao, 2007). The general granules are constructed by grouping finer granules based on available information and knowledge, such as similarity or functionality. The term-space granulation is used in the information retrieval and WSD areas (Yao, 2003). Terms are basic granules and term hierarchy is constructed by clustering terms. Then, new terms may be assigned to clusters as labels. Usually, those labels are more general than the terms in the cluster. The notion of term-space granulation serves as an effective tool for the QD applications. Many researchers have used term clustering with its application in disambiguating queries.

One of the frequently used techniques for term clustering is Statistical Association method (Brena and Ramirez, 2006). Through measuring the co-occurrences of words in the large quantities of Web pages on the Internet, collections of word clusters can be made. For example, through statistical analysis, the words "beach", "resort", "Florida" and "hotel" usually appear in the same Web pages, so they can be in the same cluster. Keyword palm has three meanings: beach, tree, and electrical device. If palm and resort co-occur in one Web page, then Palm should be interpreted as a beach, neither a tree nor an electrical device in that page. This algorithm uses a statistical approach, instead of a knowledge-based approach, to express words relations. Therefore, human knowledge or intervene is not needed in this algorithm. However, since billions of Web pages exist on the Internet, it is very difficult to select samples for measuring the co-occurrence degrees of words.

Another frequently used technique for matching contexts-dependent keywords and concepts is Concept Fuzzy Sets (CFS) model (Takagi and Tajima, 2001). The fuzzy ontology can be constructed by CFS for resolving the ambiguity of queries. In the CFS approach, each concept is connected by a series of keywords with different weights depending on the semantic similarities between the concept and keywords. Also, each keyword is connected by concepts with different weights. By constructing the ontology and fine-tuning the strength of links, a fuzzy set can be constructed for defining the ambiguous keywords. From the previous example, keyword palm has three meanings: beach, tree, and electrical device. If palm and computer co-occur in context, then concept electrical device is activated, and weight between the concept and the context is calculated. In the CFS model, relations between words and concepts are well pre-defined. However, due to the fact that numerous combinations of words may appear in queries and documents, it is difficult to create a complete fuzzy ontology for representing the relations between any two concepts in all possible combinations.

Different from the CFS model, our search agent applies the GST model to represent the concepts and their relations with other concepts. In the GST model, one concept only has the direct relation to its parent granule (super concept) and children granules (sub concepts), and the relation between any two concepts can be explored along with the edges of the tree. Therefore, for one concept, once the parent granule and children granules are identified, the semantic relations between this concept and any other concepts can be simply found in the tree.

## 3. GRANULAR SEMANTIC TREES FOR QUERIES DISAMBIGUATION

Granular Semantic Trees (GSTs) are tree models that represent relations between concepts. Each unique concept is represented as one granule in one GST. Sub concepts are represented as children nodes of super concepts. For example, in Figure 1, "Fruit" is a child node of "Food."

*Figure 1. A granular semantic tree model*

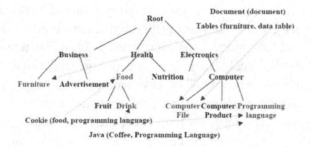

In the query "java and cookies," "java" is related to two concepts: coffee and programming language. "Cookie" is related to two concepts: food and programming language. By calculating the distances between the concepts associated with "java" and the concepts associated with "cookie" in the GST model, the most appropriate concepts for "java" and "cookie" can be determined. In our GST model, distances between concepts relative to "java" and "cookie" are shown in Table 1.

After the distances are obtained between concepts, fuzzy logic is then used to calculate the semantic similarities between concepts and words. Fuzzy logic is derived from the development of theory of fuzzy sets (Zadeh, 1965). Fuzzy logic deals with approximate reasoning with uncertain, ambiguous, incomplete or partially true knowledge and information.

The basic structure of a fuzzy system consists of four components: (1) a fuzzifier that converts crisp inputs into fuzzy values, (2) a fuzzy rule base that contains a collection of fuzzy IF-THEN rules for approximate reasoning, (3) an inference engine that performs fuzzy reasoning, and (4) a defuzzifier that generates crisp outputs. The structure of a fuzzy system is shown in Figure 2.

The distances between concepts are crisp inputs and semantic similarities between keywords and concepts are crisp outputs. The membership functions of the distance variable and the semantic similarity variable are shown in Figure 3. For simplicity, the universe for the distance variable is defined from 0 to 10. The universe for the semantic similarity variable is from 0 to 1. The fuzzy rule base for determining semantic similarities is given in Table 2.

## Step 1: Fuzzification

The first step is to convert crisp values of distance variables into fuzzy values. The linguist values of the distance variable are short, medium and long. Each one is represented by a triangle membership function.

*Table 1. Concept distances between Java and Cookie*

|  | Java (drink) | Java (programming language) |
|---|---|---|
| Cookie (food) | 1 | 7 |
| Cookie (programming language) | 8 | 0 |

*Table 2. The fuzzy rule base for the distance and semantic similarity variables*

| Rule Num. | Distance | Semantic Similarity |
|---|---|---|
| 1 | short | high |
| 2 | medium | medium |
| 3 | long | low |

*Figure 2. The structure of a type-1 fuzzy system*

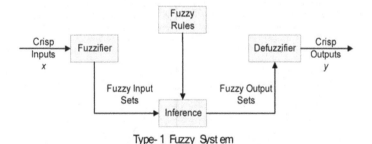

*Figure 3. Membership functions for the distance and semantic similarity variables*

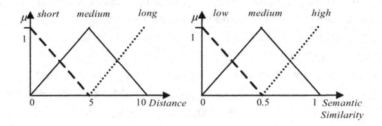

The corresponding linguist values for the distances of concept pairs are shown in Table 3.

## Step 2: Fuzzy Inference

The second step is to perform fuzzy reasoning based on the fuzzy rule base shown in Table 2. The linguist values of semantic similarities can be obtained by fuzzy reasoning.

- Drink-Food
    - Rule 1: If *distance* is 0.8 *short*, then *semantic similarity* is 0.8 *high*.
    - Rule 2: If *distance* is 0.2 *medium*, then *semantic similarity* is 0.2 *medium*.

*Table 3. Crisp and linguist inputs for the distance variable*

| Distance | Crisp Input | Linguist Input |
|---|---|---|
| Drink-Food | 1 | 0.8 short, 0.2 medium |
| P. L. - Food | 7 | 0.6 medium, 0.4 long |
| Drink-P. L. | 8 | 0.4 medium, 0.6 long |
| P. L. – P. L. | 0 | 1 short |

*Figure 4. Fuzzification*

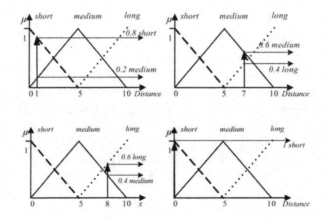

- P. L. - Food
    - Rule 2: If *distance* is 0.6 *medium*, then *semantic similarity* is 0.6 *medium*.
    - Rule 3: If *distance* is 0.4 *long*, then *semantic similarity* is 0.2 *low*.
- Drink - P.L.
    - Rule 2: If *distance* is 0.4 *medium*, then *semantic similarity* is 0.4 *medium*.
    - Rule 3: If *distance* is 0.6 *long*, then *semantic similarity* is 0.6 *low*.
- P.L. – P.L.
    - Rule 1: If *distance* is 1 short, then *semantic similarity* is 1 high.

## Step 3: Defuzzification

The final crisp value of the output score is calculated by using the Average Of Gravities (AOG) method:

$$
Y = \frac{\sum_{i=1}^{n} G_i \mu^i(x)}{\sum_{i=1}^{n} \mu^i(x)}, \tag{1}
$$

where $G_i$ is the value of the center of gravity of the membership function, Y (semantic similarities) is the output, and $x$ (the distance between node m and n) is the input, $\mu^i(x)$ represents the membership functions of $x$, and $n$ is the number of fired rules. The normalized crisp semantic similarities, whose sum is 1, are shown in Table 4.

Based on Table 4, for the query "java and cookie", we can conclude that java means "drink" while cookie means "food", or java means "programming language" while cookie also means "programming language." Therefore, we cannot determine which concept, coffee or programming language, should be associated with "java." Also, we cannot determine which concept, computer file or food, should be associated with the "cookie." If we consider users' preferences in QD, then we can use both semantic similarities and users' preferences to determine the most appropriate concepts associated with queries.

*Table 4. Crisp outputs for the semantic similarity variable*

| Distance | Crisp Output |
|---|---|
| Drink-Food | 0.37 |
| P. L. - Food | 0.15 |
| Drink-P. L. | 0.08 |
| P. L. – P. L. | 0.40 |

*Table 5. Personal preferences for Bob and Tom*

| | Bob | Tom |
|---|---|---|
| Computer | very interested | little interested |
| Food | little interested | very interested |

*Figure 5. The interface of users' preferences*

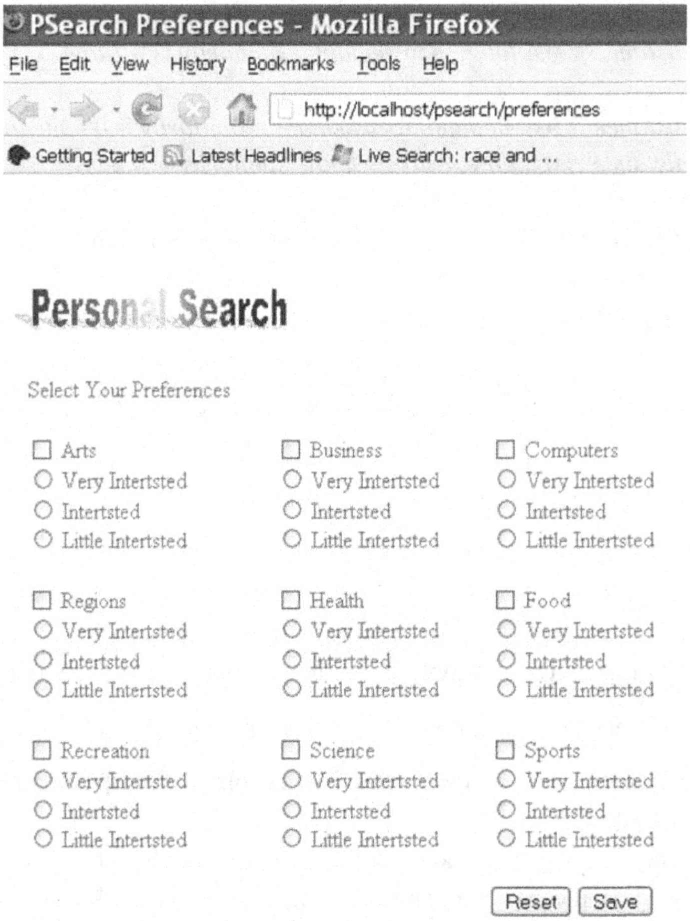

## 4. USING USERS' PREFERENCES TO PERFORM PERSONALIZED QUERIES DISAMBIGUATION

Assume that two users, Bob and Tom, specify their interests through the interface of users' preferences. Then, we can use both semantic similarities and users' preferences to determine the personalized semantic similarities by fuzzy logic. In this step, semantic similarities and user preferences are inputs, while personalized semantic similarities are outputs. The membership functions for personalized semantic similarities are shown in Figure 6. The fuzzy rule base for determining personalized semantic similarities is given in Table 6.

The final crisp value of the output score is calculated by using the AOG method. Based on the calculation of the fuzzy system, for Bob, the relations between "java" and concepts programming language and coffee are 0.71 and 0.29 respectively, while the relation between "cookie" and concepts computer file and food are 0.71 and 0.29. However, for Tom, the relations between "java" and concepts programming language and coffee are 0.33, 0.64 respectively, while the relation between "cookie" and concepts com-

*Figure 6. Membership functions for the personalized semantic similarity variable*

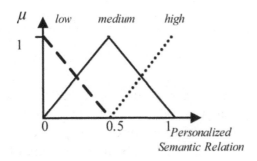

*Table 6. The fuzzy rule base for the personalized semantic similarity variable*

| Rule Num. | S.R. | Preference | P.S.R. |
|-----------|--------|------------------|--------|
| 1 | low | little interested | low |
| 2 | low | interested | low |
| 3 | low | very interested | medium |
| 4 | medium | little interested | low |
| 5 | medium | interested | medium |
| 6 | medium | very interested | high |
| 7 | high | little interested | medium |
| 8 | high | interested | high |
| 9 | high | very interested | high |

puter file and food are 0.33 and 0.64. Therefore, for Bob, "java" should be interpreted as a programming language and "cookie" should be interpreted as a computer file. For Tom, "java" should be interpreted as coffee and "cookie" should be interpreted as food.

## 5. SEMANTIC SEARCH AGENT OPTIMIZED BY GENETIC ALGORITHMS

Some users may consider semantic similarities as a dominant factor for determining an ambiguous word's concept, while others may consider users' preferences as a dominant factor. Thus, these two factors should be leveraged based on users' real intents. A set of semantic similarities, $S$, is defined in (2), and a set of users' preferences, $P$, is defined in (3).

$$S = \left\{ s_1, s_2, ..., s_m \right\} \tag{2}$$

$$P = \left\{ p_1, p_2, ..., p_n \right\} \tag{3}$$

In (2), $s_m$ denotes the semantic similarity between concept $m$ and the keyword. In (3), $p_n$ denotes the personal preferences for category $n$. For leveraging factors, factors' weights are added. The ranges for the weight of semantic similarities, $S\_Weight$, and the weight of users' preferences, $P\_Weight$, are defined in (4).

$$\begin{aligned} S\_Weight + P\_Weight &= 1 \\ S\_Weight \geq 0, P\_Weight &\geq 0 \end{aligned} \tag{4}$$

The initial values of $S\_Weight$ and $P\_Weight$ are both 0.5. Based on the values of $S\_Weight$ and $P\_Weight$, $S$ and $P$ should be updated by (5) and (6).

$$s'_i = Max\left(\frac{\sum_{k=1}^{m} s_k}{m} + \left(s_i - \frac{\sum_{k=1}^{m} s_k}{m}\right) \times \frac{S\_Weight}{0.5}, 0\right), \ i \in (1, 2, ..., m) \tag{5}$$

$$p'_j = Max\left(\frac{\sum_{k=1}^{n} p_k}{n} + \left(p_j - \frac{\sum_{k=1}^{n} p_k}{n}\right) \times \frac{p\_Weight}{0.5}, 0\right), \ j \in (1, 2, ..., n) \tag{6}$$

In (5), $s_i$ denotes the original semantic similarity between the concept $i$ and the keyword; $s'_i$ denotes the updated semantic similarity between the concept $i$ and the keyword; $m$ denotes m concepts are relative to the keyword. In (6), $p_j$ denotes the original personal preference for category $j$; $p'_j$ denotes the updated personal preference for category $j$. (5) and (6) are used to reduce or enlarge differences of semantic similarities and personal preferences. If *S_Weight* is smaller than 0.5, the differences of semantic similarities between concepts and the keyword become smaller. If *S_Weight* is larger than 0.5, the differences become larger.

Through analysis of users' search history, Genetic Algorithms (GAs) are applied to adjust *S_Weight* and *P_Weight* for adapting to users' actual selections. Predicted concepts and actual selecting concepts are both represented by value vectors in the training data set. In this case, the Fitness value is a sum of these two similarity measures. By adjusting the *S_Weight* and *P_Weight*, GAs maximize the similarity of vectors.

## 6. ANALYZING WEB PAGES USING GRANULAR SEMANTIC TREES

Using GST, the concepts related to the keywords in a page can be extracted. In Figure 8, for the query "java and cookie", the first result page gathered by keyword-based search engines is "HTTP Cookie Parser in Java." By analyzing the title and the abstract of this page, two words, "HTTP" and "URL", are related to the concept computer. Thus, keywords "java" and "cookie" in this page are associated with concepts programming language and computer file respectively.

In the second result page "Our Favorite Deals for Food and Wine–CouponCabin", three words "Food", "Wine" and "Chocolate" are related to the concept Food. Thus, keywords "java" and "cookie" in this page are associated with coffee and food respectively.

*Figure 7. The structure of genetic algorithms-based optimizer*

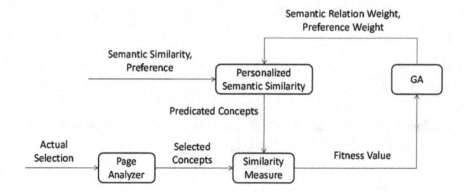

## 7. SIMULATIONS

We implemented the personalized semantic search agent in Java, and deployed it on a TOMCAT Web server. Once a user submits one query to our search engine, the query is transmitted simultaneously to GOOGLE, YAHOO, and MSN Live Search. The first ten results are downloaded and stored in one XML file, in which the titles, abstracts and links of pages are enclosed by meaningful tags.

In our agent, WordNet is referred for creating the conceptual dictionary (Miller, 1985). WordNet is a large lexical database of English, in which synonymous words are grouped together into synonym sets. Each synonym set represents a single distinct sense or concept. In WordNet 3.0, there are 155,287 words organized in 117,659 synonym set, approximate 18% of the words in WordNet are polysemous. Each WordNet sense is associated with a tree structure in the WordNet Is-A hierarchy. The nodes in these tree structures are WordNet hyponyms, and each hyponym has a unique identifier in WordNet. Therefore, each sense can be related to the unique hyponyms above the sense in the tree structure. Open Directory Project (ODP) is referred to establishing the Semantic Tree (Skrenta and Truel, 1998). The ODP is a manually edited directory of 4.6 million URLs that have been categorized into 787,774 categories by 68,983 human editors.

Four users, Joe, Bob, Tom and Susan, use this personalized semantic search agent. Their preferences are shown in Table 7.

148 queries are submitted by those four users and 3779 Web pages are returned by the keyword-based search engines. Table 8. shows the part results of semantic similarities between the words and the concepts in different queries for different users.

After Web pages are gathered by keyword-based search engines, the page analyzer analyzes Web pages, and only returns the associated results to the users. Figure 9. shows the precisions, recalls and $F_1$ measures of the GST model and the TF-IDF method.

In order to evaluate the optimized semantic search agent, Joe submits 10 group queries, 50 queries each group, to our search agent. For every group, GAs update the weights of semantic similarities and

*Figure 8. An example of web page analysis*

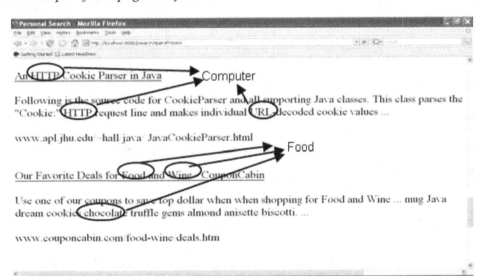

*Table 7. Preferences of Joe, Bob, Tom, and Susan*

|  | Computer | Food | Science | Region | Business |
|---|---|---|---|---|---|
| Joe | 0.3 | 0.1 | 0.1 | 0.3 | 0.2 |
| Bob | 0.7 | 0.3 | 0 | 0 | 0 |
| Tom | 0.3 | 0.7 | 0 | 0 | 0 |
| Susan | 0.6 | 0 | 0.4 | 0 | 0 |

*Table 8. Semantic similarities between words and concepts*

| Words | Query | Related Concepts | | | |
|---|---|---|---|---|---|
|  |  | Joe | Bob | Tom | Susan |
| shell | animal shell | animal organ 0.82 | animal organ 0.71 | animal organ 0.71 | animal organ 0.85 |
|  |  | oil 0.12 | oil 0.19 | oil 0.19 | oil 0.15 |
|  | shell oil | oil 0.79 | oil 0.71 | oil 0.71 | oil 0.76 |
|  |  | animal organ 0.21 | animal organ 0.29 | animal organ 0.29 | animal organ 0.14 |
| office | Microsoft office | software 0.75 | software 0.79 | software 0.75 | software 0.77 |
|  |  | building 0.25 | building 0.21 | building 0.25 | building 0.23 |
|  | office furniture | building 0.81 | building 0.76 | building 0.81 | building 0.79 |
|  |  | software 0.19 | software 0.24 | software 0.19 | software 0.21 |
| palm | coconut palm | fruit 0.74 | fruit 0.77 | fruit 0.8 | fruit 0.71 |
|  |  | telephone 0.26 | telephone 0.23 | telephone 0.2 | telephone 0.29 |
|  | palm phone | telephone 0.70 | telephone 0.71 | telephone 0.54 | telephone 0.74 |
|  |  | fruit 0.30 | fruit 0.29 | fruit 0.46 | fruit 0.26 |
| table | drawing tables in a document | computer file 0.78 | computer file 0.71 | computer file 0.78 | computer file 0.76 |
|  |  | furniture 0.22 | furniture 0.29 | furniture 0.22 | furniture 0.24 |
| mouse | mouse research | rodent 0.53 | rodent 0.36 | rodent 0.48 | rodent 0.52 |
|  |  | computer product 0.47 | computer product 0.64 | computer product 0.52 | computer product 0.48 |
| java | java history | region 0.54 | programming language 0.45 | coffee 0.45 | programming language 0.47 |
|  |  | programming language 0.25 | region 0.33 | region 0.33 | region 0.36 |
|  |  | Coffee 0.21 | coffee 0.22 | programming language 0.22 | coffee 0.17 |

users' preferences according to users' selection. Figure 10. shows that the precisions of prediction become higher after several iterations.

## 8. CONCLUSION

This chapter presents a new personalized semantic search agent. Compared with the CFS, the GST model does not define the relations between all words. In addition, this system personalizes searches by

*Figure 9. Precisions, recalls, F1 measures and fall-out of GST and TF-IDF*

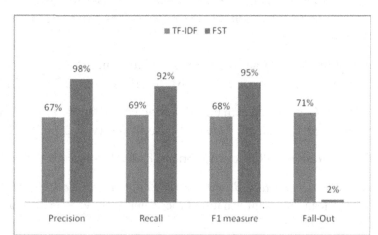

*Figure 10. Optimized precisions of prediction*

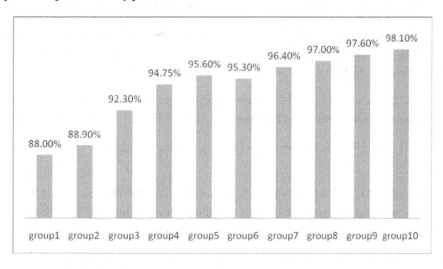

considering users' preferences. GAs are applied to leverage weights of semantic similarities and users' preferences. The simulation results show that this model is a good option for personalizing semantic Web search.

## REFERENCES

Brena, R. F., & Ramirez, E. Z. (2006). A Soft Semantic Web. In *Proceedings of the 2006 1st IEEE Workshop on Hot Topics in Web Systems and Technologies*, (pp. 1-8).

Cheng, Y., & Xu, D. (2002). Content-based semantic associative video model. *2002 6th International Conference on Signal Processing*, (vol. 1, pp. 727-730).

Ding, Y., & Embley, D. W. (2006). Using Data-Extraction Ontologies to Foster Automating Semantic Annotation. In *Proceedings and 22nd International Conference on Data Engineering Workshops*, (pp. 138-146).

Kraft, D., & Bautista, M. (2003). Rules and fuzzy rules in text: Concept, extraction and usage. *International Journal of Approximate Reasoning, 34*, 145–161. doi:10.1016/j.ijar.2003.07.005

Liu, C., & Zhou, Q. (2003). Class-based semantic cohesion computation. In *Proceedings of the 2003 IEEE International Conference on Systems, Man and Cybernetics,* (vol. *2*, pp. 1673- 1678).

Miller, G. (1985). *WordNet Research*. Retrieved February 8, 2008, from http://wordnet.princeton.edu/

Nikravesh, M. (2002). *Fuzzy Conceptual-Based Search Engine using Conceptual Semantic Indexing* (pp. 146–151). North American Fuzzy Information Processing Society - The Special Interest Group on Fuzzy Logic and the Internet.

Ohgaya, R., Fukano, K., Taniguchi, K., Takagi, T., Aizawa, A., & Nikravesh, M. (2002). *Conceptual Fuzzy Sets-Based Menu Navigation System for Yahoo* (pp. 274–279). North American Fuzzy Information Processing Society - The Special Interest Group on Fuzzy Logic and the Internet.

Paliwal, A. V., Adam, N. R., Xiong, H., & Bornhovd, C. (2006). Web Service Discovery via Semantic Association Ranking and Hyperclique Pattern Discovery. In *Proceedings of the 2006 IEEE/WIC/ACM International Conference on Web Intelligence,* (vol. 18, pp. 649-652).

Patil, L., Dutta, D., & Sriram, R. (2005). Ontology-based exchange of product data semantics. *IEEE Transactions on Automation Science and Engineering, 2*(3), 213–225. doi:10.1109/TASE.2005.849087

Skrenta, R., & Truel, B. (1998). *Open Directory Project*. Retrieved February 10, 2008, from http://www.dmoz.org/

Sudha, R., Rajagopalan, M. R., Selvanayaki, M., & Selvi, S. T. (2007). Ubiquitous Semantic Space: A context-aware and coordination middleware for Ubiquitous Computing. In *Proceedings of COMSWARE 2007 and 2nd International Conference on Communication Systems Software and Middleware.* (pp. 1-7).

Sugiyama, K., Hatano, K., & Yoshikawa, M. (2004). Adaptive Web Search Based on User Profile Constructed Without any Effort from Users. In Feldman, S., Uretsky, M., Najork, M. & Wills, C. (Ed.), *Proceedings of the 13th International Conference on World Wide Web,* (pp. 675-684). ACM Press.

Yao, J. T. (2007). A Ten-year Review of Granular Computing. In *Proceedings of the IEEE International Conference on Granular Computing*, (pp. 734-739).

Yao, Y. Y. (2003). Granular computing for the design of information retrieval support systems. In Wu, W., Xiong, H., & Shekhar, S. (Eds.), *Information Retrieval and Clustering* (pp. 299–329). Boston: Kluwer Academic Publishers.

# Chapter 19
# Dominance–Based Rough Set Approach to Granular Computing

**Salvatore Greco**
*University of Catania, Italy*

**Benedetto Matarazzo**
*University of Catania, Italy*

**Roman Słowiński**
*Poznań University of Technology, Poland*

## ABSTRACT

*Dominance-based Rough Set Approach (DRSA) was introduced as a generalization of the rough set approach for reasoning about preferences. While data describing preferences are ordinal by the nature of decision problems they concern, the ordering of data is also important in many other problems of data analysis. Even when the ordering seems irrelevant, the presence or the absence of a property (possibly graded or fuzzy) has an ordinal interpretation. Since any granulation of information is based on analysis of properties, DRSA can be seen as a general framework for granular computing. After recalling basic concepts of DRSA, the article presents their extensions in the fuzzy context and in the probabilistic setting. This permits to define the rough approximation of a fuzzy set, which is the core of the subject. The article continues with presentation of DRSA for case-based reasoning, where granular computing based on DRSA has been successfully applied. Moreover, some basic formal properties of the whole approach are presented in terms of several algebras modeling the logic of DRSA. Finally, it is shown how the bipolar generalized approximation space, being an abstraction of the standard way to deal with roughness within DRSA, can be induced from one of the algebras modeling the logic of DRSA, the bipolar Brower-Zadeh lattice.*

DOI: 10.4018/978-1-60566-324-1.ch019

## INTRODUCTION

This article describes Dominance-based Rough Set Approach (DRSA) to granular computing and data mining. DRSA was first introduced as a generalization of the rough set approach for dealing with multiple criteria decision analysis, where preference order has to be taken into account. The ordering is also important, however, in many other problems of data analysis. Even when the ordering seems irrelevant, the presence or the absence of a property has an ordinal interpretation, because if two properties are related, the presence, rather than the absence, of one property should make more (or less) probable the presence of the other property. This is even more apparent when the presence or the absence of a property is graded or fuzzy, because in this case, the more credible the presence of a property, the more (or less) probable the presence of the other property. Since the presence of properties, possibly fuzzy, is the basis of any granulation, DRSA can be seen as a general framework for granular computing.

The article is organized as follows. First, we introduce DRSA in the context of decision making. After presenting the main ideas sketching a philosophical basis of DRSA and its importance for granular computing, the article introduces basic concepts of DRSA, followed by their extensions in the fuzzy context and in the probabilistic setting. This prepares the ground for defining the rough approximation of a fuzzy set, which is the core of the subject. It is also explained why the classical rough set approach is a specific case of DRSA. The article continues with presentation of DRSA for case-based reasoning, where granular computing based on DRSA has been successfully applied. Finally, some basic formal properties of the whole approach are presented in terms of several algebras modeling the logic of DRSA. Moreover, we show how the bipolar generalized approximation space, being an abstraction of the standard way to deal with roughness within DRSA, can be induced from one of the algebras modeling the logic of DRSA, the bipolar Brower-Zadeh lattice.

## DOMINANCE-BASED ROUGH SET APPROACH

This section presents the main concepts of the Dominance-based Rough Set Approach (DRSA) (for a more complete presentation see, for example, Greco et al. (1999, 2001a, 2004b,c, 2005a); Słowiński et al. (2005)).

Information about objects is represented in the form of an information table. The rows of the table are labeled by objects, whereas columns are labeled by attributes and entries of the table are attribute-values. Formally, an information table (system) is the 4-tuple $S = \langle U, Q, V, \varphi \rangle$, where $U$ is a finite set of objects, $Q$ is a finite set of attributes, $V = \bigcup_{q \in Q} V_q$ and $V_q$ is the value set of the attribute $q$, and $\varphi : U \times Q \rightarrow V_q$ is a total function such that $\varphi(x, q) \in V_q$ for every $q \in Q$, $x \in U$, called an information function (Pawlak, 1991). The set $Q$ is, in general, divided into set $C$ of condition attributes and set $D$ of decision attributes.

Condition attributes with value sets ordered according to decreasing or increasing preference of a decision maker are called *criteria*. For criterion $q \in Q$, $\succeq_q$ is a *weak preference* relation on $U$ such that $x \succeq_q y$ means "$x$ is at least as good as $y$ with respect to criterion $q$". It is supposed that $\succeq_q$ is a complete preorder, i.e., a strongly complete and transitive binary relation, defined on $U$ on the basis of evaluations $\varphi(\cdot, q)$. Without loss of generality, the preference is supposed to increase with the value of $\varphi(\cdot, q)$ for every criterion $q \in C$, such that for all $x, y \in U$, $x \succeq_q y$ if and only if $\varphi(x, q) \geq \varphi(y, q)$.

Furthermore, it is supposed that the set of decision attributes $D$ is a singleton $\{d\}$. Values of decision attribute $d$ make a partition of $U$ into a finite number of decision classes, $\boldsymbol{Cl} = \{Cl_t, \ t = 1, \ldots, n\}$, such that each $x \in U$ belongs to one and only one class $Cl_t \in \boldsymbol{Cl}$. It is supposed that the classes are preference-ordered, i.e., for all $r, s \in \{1, \ldots, n\}$, such that $r > s$, the objects from $Cl_r$ are preferred to the objects from $Cl_s$. More formally, if $\succeq$ is a *comprehensive weak preference relation* on $U$, i.e., if for all $x, y \in U$, $x \succeq y$ means "$x$ is comprehensively at least as good as $y$", then it is supposed:

$$[x \in Cl_r, \ y \in Cl_s, \ r > s] \Rightarrow [x \succeq y \quad \text{and} \quad not \ y \succeq x]$$

The above assumptions are typical for consideration of *ordinal classification problems* (also called *multiple criteria sorting problems*).

The sets to be approximated are called *upward union* and *downward union* of classes, respectively:

$$Cl_t^{\geq} = \bigcup_{s \geq t} Cl_s, \quad Cl_t^{\leq} = \bigcup_{s \leq t} Cl_s, \quad t = 1, \ldots, n.$$

The statement $x \in Cl_t^{\geq}$ means "$x$ belongs to at least class $Cl_t$", while $x \in Cl_t^{\leq}$ means "$x$ belongs to at most class $Cl_t$". Let us remark that $Cl_1^{\geq} = Cl_n^{\leq} = U$, $Cl_n^{\geq} = Cl_n$ and $Cl_1^{\leq} = Cl_1$. Furthermore, for $t = 2, \ldots, n$,

$$Cl_{t-1}^{\leq} = U - Cl_t^{\geq} \quad \text{and} \quad Cl_t^{\geq} = U - Cl_{t-1}^{\leq}.$$

The key idea of the rough set approach is representation (approximation) of knowledge generated by decision attributes, using "*granules of knowledge*" generated by condition attributes.

In DRSA, where condition attributes are criteria and decision classes are preference ordered, the knowledge to be represented is a collection of upward and downward unions of classes, and the "granules of knowledge" are sets of objects defined using a dominance relation.

*x dominates y* with respect to $P \subseteq C$ (shortly, *x P -dominates y*), denoted by $x D_P y$, if for every criterion $q \in P$, $\varphi(x, q) \geq \varphi(y, q)$. The relation of $P$-dominance is reflexive and transitive, i.e., it is a partial preorder.

Given a set of criteria $P \subseteq C$ and $x \in U$, the "granules of knowledge" used for approximation in DRSA are:

- a set of objects dominating $x$, called $P$ *-dominating set*, $D_P^+\left(x\right) = \{y \in U : y D_P x\}$

- a set of objects dominated by $x$, called $P$ *-dominated set,* $D_P^-(x) = \{y \in U : xD_py\}$

Remark that the "granules of knowledge" defined above have the form of upward (positive) and downward (negative) *dominance cones* in the evaluation space.

Let us recall that the *dominance principle* (or Pareto principle) requires that an object $x$ dominating object $y$ on all considered criteria (i.e., $x$ having evaluations at least as good as $y$ on all considered criteria) should also dominate $y$ on the decision (i.e., $x$ should be assigned to at least as good decision class as $y$). This principle is the only objective principle that is widely agreed upon in the multiple criteria comparisons of objects.

Given $P \subseteq C$, the inclusion of an object $x \in U$ to the upward union of classes $Cl_t^{\geq}$ ($t = 2, ..., n$) is *inconsistent with the dominance principle* if one of the following conditions holds:

- $x$ belongs to class $Cl_t$ or better, but it is $P$-dominated by an object $y$ belonging to a class worse than $Cl_t$, i.e., $x \in Cl_t^{\geq}$ but $D_P^+(x) \cap Cl_{t-1}^{\leq} \neq \varnothing$,

- $x$ belongs to a worse class than $Cl_t$ but it $P$-dominates an object $y$ belonging to class $Cl_t$ or better, i.e., $x \notin Cl_t^{\geq}$ but $D_P^-(x) \cap Cl_t^{\geq} \neq \varnothing$.

If, given a set of criteria $P \subseteq C$, the inclusion of $x \in U$ to $Cl_t^{\geq}$, where $t = 2, ..., n$, is inconsistent with the dominance principle, then $x$ belongs to $Cl_t^{\geq}$ *with some ambiguity*. Thus, $x$ belongs to $Cl_t^{\geq}$ *without any ambiguity* with respect to $P \subseteq C$, if $x \in Cl_t^{\geq}$ and there is no inconsistency with the dominance principle. This means that all objects $P$-dominating $x$ belong to $Cl_t^{\geq}$, i.e., $D_P^+(x) \subseteq Cl_t^{\geq}$.

Furthermore, $x$ *possibly belongs to* $Cl_t^{\geq}$ with respect to $P \subseteq C$ if one of the following conditions holds:

- according to decision attribute $d$, object $x$ belongs to $Cl_t^{\geq}$,

- according to decision attribute $d$, object $x$ does not belong to $Cl_t^{\geq}$, but it is inconsistent in the sense of the dominance principle with an object $y$ belonging to $Cl_t^{\geq}$.

In terms of ambiguity, $x$ possibly belongs to $Cl_t^{\geq}$ with respect to $P \subseteq C$, if $x$ belongs to $Cl_t^{\geq}$ with or without any ambiguity. Due to the reflexivity of the dominance relation $D_P$, the above conditions can be summarized as follows: $x$ *possibly belongs* to class $Cl_t$ or better, with respect to $P \subseteq C$, if among the objects $P$-dominated by $x$ there is an object $y$ belonging to class $Cl_t$ or better, i.e., $D_P^-(x) \cap Cl_t^{\geq} \neq \varnothing$.

The $P$ *-lower approximation* of $Cl_t^{\geq}$, denoted by $\underline{P}(Cl_t^{\geq})$, and the $P$ *-upper approximation* of $Cl_t^{\geq}$, denoted by $\overline{P}(Cl_t^{\geq})$, are defined as follows ($t = 1, ..., n$):

$$\underline{P}(Cl_t^{\geq}) = \{x \in U : D_P^+(x) \subseteq Cl_t^{\geq}\},$$

$$\overline{P}(Cl_t^{\geq}) = \{x \in U : D_P^-(x) \cap Cl_t^{\geq} \neq \varnothing\}.$$

Analogously, one can define the $P$ -*lower approximation* and the $P$ -*upper approximation* of $Cl_t^{\leq}$ as follows ( $t = 1, ..., n$ ):

$$\underline{P}(Cl_t^{\leq}) = \{x \in U : D_P^-(x) \subseteq Cl_t^{\leq}\},$$

$$\overline{P}(Cl_t^{\leq}) = \{x \in U : D_P^+(x) \cap Cl_t^{\leq} \neq \varnothing\}.$$

The $P$ -lower and $P$ -upper approximations so defined satisfy the following *inclusion property* for each $t \in \{1, ..., n\}$ and for all $P \subseteq C$ :

$$\underline{P}(Cl_t^{\geq}) \subseteq Cl_t^{\geq} \subseteq \overline{P}(Cl_t^{\geq}), \quad \underline{P}(Cl_t^{\leq}) \subseteq Cl_t^{\leq} \subseteq \overline{P}(Cl_t^{\leq}).$$

The $P$ -lower and $P$ -upper approximations of $Cl_t^{\geq}$ and $Cl_t^{\leq}$ have an important *complementarity property*, according to which,

$$\underline{P}(Cl_t^{\geq}) = U - \overline{P}(Cl_{t-1}^{\leq}) \text{ and } \overline{P}(Cl_t^{\geq}) = U - \underline{P}(Cl_{t-1}^{\leq}), \, t = 2, ..., n,$$

$$\underline{P}(Cl_t^{\leq}) = U - \overline{P}(Cl_{t+1}^{\geq}) \text{ and } \quad \overline{P}(Cl_t^{\leq}) = U - \underline{P}(Cl_{t+1}^{\geq}), \, t = 1, ..., n - 1.$$

The $P$ -*boundaries* of $Cl_t^{\geq}$ and $Cl_t^{\leq}$, denoted by $Bn_P(Cl_t^{\geq})$ and $Bn_P(Cl_t^{\leq})$ respectively, are defined as follows ( $t = 1, ..., n$ ):

$$Bn_P(Cl_t^{\geq}) = \overline{P}(Cl_t^{\geq}) - \underline{P}(Cl_t^{\geq}), \, Bn_P(Cl_t^{\leq}) = \overline{P}(Cl_t^{\leq}) - \underline{P}(Cl_t^{\leq}).$$

Due to complementarity property, $Bn_P(Cl_t^{\geq}) = Bn_P(Cl_{t-1}^{\leq})$, for $t = 2, ..., n$.

For every $P \subseteq C$ , the *quality of approximation* of the ordinal classification *Cl* by a set of criteria $P$ is defined as the ratio of the number of objects $P$ -consistent with the dominance principle and the number of all the objects in $U$. Since the $P$ -consistent objects are those which do not belong to any $P$-boundary $Bn_P(Cl_t^{\geq})$, $t = 2, ..., n$, or $Bn_P(Cl_t^{\leq})$, $t = 1, ..., n - 1$, the quality of approximation of the ordinal classification *Cl* by a set of criteria $P$ , can be written as

$$\gamma_P\left(\mathbf{Cl}\right) = \frac{\left| U - \left( \bigcup_{t=2,\dots,n} Bn_P\left(Cl_t^{\geq}\right) \right) \right|}{|U|} = \frac{\left| U - \left( \bigcup_{t=1,\dots,n-1} Bn_P\left(Cl_t^{\leq}\right) \right) \right|}{|U|}$$

$\gamma_P(\mathbf{Cl})$ can be seen as a degree of consistency of the objects from $U$, where $P$ is the set of criteria and $\mathbf{Cl}$ is the considered ordinal classification.

Each minimal (with respect to inclusion) subset $P \subseteq C$, such that $\gamma_P(\mathbf{Cl}) = \gamma_C(\mathbf{Cl})$, is called a *reduct* of $\mathbf{Cl}$, and is denoted by $RED_{Cl}$. Let us remark that for a given set $U$ one can have more than one reduct. The intersection of all reducts is called the *core*, and is denoted by $CORE_{Cl}$. Criteria in $CORE_{Cl}$ cannot be removed from consideration without deteriorating the quality of approximation. This means that, in set $C$, there are three categories of criteria:

* *indispensable* criteria included in the core,
* *exchangeable* criteria included in some reducts, but not in the core,
* *redundant* criteria, neither indispensable nor exchangeable, and thus not included in any reduct.

The dominance-based rough approximations of upward and downward unions of classes can serve to induce "*if..., then...*" decision rules. It is meaningful to consider the following five types of decision rules:

1) Certain $D_\geq$-decision rules: *if* $x_{q_1} \succeq_{q_1} r_{q_1}$ *and* $x_{q_2} \succeq_{q_2} r_{q_2}$ *and...* $x_{q_p} \succeq_{q_p} r_{q_p}$, *then* $x$ *certainly belongs to* $Cl_t^{\geq}$, where, for each $w_q, z_q \in X_q$, "$w_q \succeq_q z_q$" means "$w_q$ *is at least as good as* $z_q$", and

$$P = \{q_1,\dots,q_p\} \subseteq C, \ (r_{q_1},\dots,r_{q_p}) \in V_{q_1} \times \dots \times V_{q_p}, \ t \in \{2,\dots,n\}$$

2) Possible $D_\geq$-decision rules: *if* $x_{q_1} \succeq_{q_1} r_{q_1}$ *and* $x_{q_2} \succeq_{q_2} r_{q_2}$ *and...* $x_{q_p} \succeq_{q_p} r_{q_p}$, *then* $x$ *possibly belongs to* $Cl_t^{\geq}$, where

$$P = \{q_1,\dots,q_p\} \subseteq C, \ (r_{q_1},\dots,r_{q_p}) \in V_{q_1} \times \dots \times V_{q_p}, \ t \in \{2,\dots,n\}$$

3) Certain $D_\leq$-decision rules: *if* $x_{q_1} \preceq_{q_1} r_{q_1}$ *and* $x_{q_2} \preceq_{q_2} r_{q_2}$ *and...* $x_{q_p} \preceq_{q_p} r_{q_p}$, *then* $x$ *certainly belongs to* $Cl_t^{\leq}$, where, for each $w_q, z_q \in X_q$, "$w_q \preceq_q z_q$" means "$w_q$ *is at most as good as* $z_q$", and

$$P = \{q_1,\dots,q_p\} \subseteq C, \ (r_{q_1},\dots,r_{q_p}) \in V_{q_1} \times \dots \times V_{q_p}, \ t \in \{1,\dots,n-1\}$$

4) Possible $D_\leq$-decision rules: *if* $x_{q_1} \prec_{q_1} r_{q_1}$ *and* $x_{q_2} \prec_{q_2} r_{q_2}$ *and...* $x_{q_p} \prec_{q_p} r_{q_p}$, *then* $x$ *possibly belongs to* $Cl_t^{\leq}$, where

$$P = \{q_1, \ldots, q_p\} \subseteq C, \ (r_{q_1}, \ldots, r_{q_p}) \in V_{q_1} \times \ldots \times V_{q_p}, \ t \in \{1, \ldots, n-1\}$$

5) Approximate $D_{\leq\leq}$-decision rules: *if* $x_{q_1} \succeq_{q_1} r_{q_1}$ *and...* $x_{q_k} \succeq_{q_k} r_{q_k}$ *and* $x_{q_{k+1}} \preceq_{q_{k+1}} r_{q_{k+1}}$ *and...* $x_{q_p} \preceq_{q_p} r_{q_p}$

*then* $x \in Cl_s^{\geq} \cap Cl_t^{\leq}$, where

$$O' = \{q_1, \ldots, q_k\} \subseteq C$$

$$O'' = \{q_{k+1}, \ldots, q_p\} \subseteq C, P = O' \cup O'', O' \text{ and } O'' \text{ not necessarily disjoint,}$$

$(r_{q_1}, \ldots, r_{q_p}) \in V_{q_1} \times \ldots \times V_{q_p}$, and $s, t \in \{1, \ldots, n\}$, such that $s < t$.

The rules of type 1) and 3) represent certain knowledge extracted from the decision table, while the rules of type 2) and 4) represent possible knowledge. Rules of type 5) represent doubtful knowledge.

Since its appearance in the end of 90's, DRSA has inspired many other authors to investigate dominance-based rough set analysis of ordinal data (see, e.g., Fan et al. (2007); Inuiguchi et al. (2009); Liu et al. (2006); Qian et al. (2009); Sai et al. (2001); Yang et al. (2008)).

## Example Illustrating DRSA in the Context of Ordinal Classification

This subsection presents a didactic example which illustrates the main concepts of DRSA. Let us consider the following ordinal classification problem. Students of a college must obtain an overall evaluation on the basis of their achievements in Mathematics, Physics and Literature. The three subjects are clearly criteria (condition attributes) and the comprehensive evaluation is a decision attribute. For simplicity, the value sets of the criteria and of the decision attribute are the same, and they are composed of three values: bad, medium and good. The preference order of these values is obvious. Thus, there are three preference ordered decision classes, so the problem belongs to the category of ordinal classification. In

*Table 1. Exemplary evaluations of students (examples of ordinal classification)*

| Student | Mathematics | Physics | Literature | Overall Evaluation |
|---------|-------------|---------|------------|--------------------|
| $S1$ | good | medium | bad | bad |
| $S2$ | medium | medium | bad | medium |
| $S3$ | medium | medium | medium | medium |
| $S4$ | good | good | medium | good |
| $S5$ | good | medium | good | good |
| $S6$ | good | good | good | good |
| $S7$ | bad | bad | bad | bad |
| $S8$ | bad | bad | medium | bad |

order to build a preference model of the jury, DRSA is used to analyze a set of exemplary evaluations of students provided by the jury. These examples of ordinal classification constitute an input preference information presented as decision table in Table 1.

Note that the dominance principle obviously applies to the examples of ordinal classification, since an improvement of a student's score on one of three criteria, with other scores unchanged, should not worsen the student's overall evaluation, but rather improve it.

Observe that student $S1$ has not worse evaluations than student $S2$ on all the considered criteria, however, the overall evaluation of $S1$ is worse than the overall evaluation of $S2$. This contradicts the dominance principle, so the two examples of ordinal classification, and only those, are inconsistent. One can expect that the quality of approximation of the ordinal classification represented by examples in Table 1 will be equal to 0.75.

One can observe that in result of reducing the set of considered criteria, i.e., the set of considered subjects, some new inconsistencies can occur. For example, removing from Table 1 the evaluation on Literature, one obtains Table 2, where $S1$ is inconsistent not only with $S2$, but also with $S3$ and $S5$. In fact, student $S1$ has not worse evaluations than students $S2$, $S3$ and $S5$ on all the considered criteria (Mathematics and Physics), however, the overall evaluation of $S1$ is worse than the overall evaluation of $S2$, $S3$ and $S5$.

Observe, moreover, that removing from Table 1 the evaluations on Mathematics, one obtains Table 3, where no new inconsistency occurs, comparing to Table 1.

Similarly, after removing from Table 1 the evaluations on Physics, one obtains Table 4, where no new inconsistencies occur, comparing to Table 1.

The fact that no new inconsistency occurs when Mathematics or Physics is removed, means that the subsets of criteria {Physics, Literature} or {Mathematics, Literature} contain sufficient information to

*Table 2. Exemplary evaluations of students excluding Literature*

| Student | Mathematics | Physics | Overall Evaluation |
|---------|-------------|---------|--------------------|
| $S1$ | good | medium | bad |
| $S2$ | medium | medium | medium |
| $S3$ | medium | medium | medium |
| $S4$ | good | good | good |
| $S5$ | good | medium | good |
| $S6$ | good | good | good |
| $S7$ | bad | bad | bad |
| $S8$ | bad | bad | bad |

*Table 3. Exemplary evaluations of students excluding Mathematics*

| Student | Physics | Literature | Overall Evaluation |
|---------|---------|------------|--------------------|
| $S1$ | medium | bad | bad |
| $S2$ | medium | bad | medium |
| $S3$ | medium | medium | medium |
| $S4$ | good | medium | good |
| $S5$ | medium | good | good |
| $S6$ | good | good | good |
| $S7$ | bad | bad | bad |
| $S8$ | bad | medium | bad |

*Table 4. Exemplary evaluations of students excluding Physics*

| Student | Mathematics | Literature | Overall Evaluation |
|---------|-------------|------------|--------------------|
| $S1$ | good | bad | bad |
| $S2$ | medium | bad | medium |
| $S3$ | medium | medium | medium |
| $S4$ | good | medium | good |
| $S5$ | good | good | good |
| $S6$ | good | good | good |
| $S7$ | bad | bad | bad |
| $S8$ | bad | medium | bad |

represent the overall evaluation of students with the same quality of approximation as using the complete set of three criteria. This is not the case, however, for the subset {Mathematics, Physics}. Observe, moreover, that subsets {Physics, Literature} and {Mathematics, Literature} are minimal, because no other criterion can be removed without new inconsistencies occur. Thus, {Physics, Literature} and {Mathematics, Literature} are the reducts of the complete set of criteria {Mathematics, Physics, Literature}. Since Literature is the only criterion which cannot be removed from any reduct without introducing new inconsistencies, it constitutes the core, i.e., the set of indispensable criteria. The core is, of course, the intersection of all reducts, i.e., in our example:

{Literature} = {Physics, Literature} ∩ {Mathematics, Literature}.

In order to illustrate in a simple way the concept of rough approximation, let us limit our analysis to the reduct {Mathematics, Literature}. Let us consider student $S4$. His positive dominance cone $D^+_{\{Mathematics, Literature\}}(S4)$ is composed of all the students having evaluations not worse than him on Mathematics and Literature, i.e., of all the students dominating him with respect to Mathematics and Literature. Thus,

$$D^+_{\{Mathematics, Literature\}}(S4) = \{S4, S5, S6\}.$$

On the other hand, the negative dominance cone of student $S4$, $D^-_{\{Mathematics, Literature\}}(S4)$, is composed of all the students having evaluations not better than him on Mathematics and Literature, i.e., of all the students dominated by him with respect to Mathematics and Literature. Thus,

$D^-_{\{Mathematics,Literature\}}(S4) = \{S1, S2, S3, S4, S7, S8\}.$

Similar dominance cones can be obtained for all the students from Table 6. For example, for $S2$, the dominance cones are

$D^+_{\{Mathematics,Literature\}}(S2) = \{S1, S2, S3, S4, S5, S6\}$

and

$D^-_{\{Mathematics,Literature\}}(S2) = \{S2, S7\}.$

The rough approximations can be calculated using dominance cones. Let us consider, for example, the lower approximation of the set of students having a "good" overall evaluation $\underline{P}(Cl^{\geq}_{good})$, with $P=\{Mathematics, Literature\}$. Notice that $\underline{P}(Cl^{\geq}_{good}) = \{S4, S5, S6\}$, because positive dominance cones of students $S4$, $S5$ and $S6$ are all included in the set of students with an overall evaluation "good". In other words, this means that there is no student dominating $S4$ or $S5$ or $S6$ while having an overall evaluation worse than "good". From the viewpoint of decision making, this means that, taking into account the available information about evaluation of students on Mathematics and Literature, the fact that student $y$ dominates $S4$ or $S5$ or $S6$ is a *sufficient* condition to conclude that $y$ is a "good" student.

The upper approximation of the set of students with a "good" overall evaluation is $\overline{P}(Cl^{\geq}_{good}) = \{S4, S5, S6\}$, because negative dominance cones of students $S4$, $S5$ and $S6$ have a nonempty intersection with the set of students having a "good" overall evaluation. In other words, this means that for each one of the students $S4$, $S5$ and $S6$, there is at least one student dominated by him with an overall evaluation "good". From the point of view of decision making, this means that, taking into account the available information about evaluation of students on Mathematics and Literature, the fact that student $y$ dominates $S4$ or $S5$ or $S6$ is a *possible* condition to conclude that $y$ is a "good" student.

Let us observe that for the set of criteria $P=\{Mathematics, Literature\}$, the lower and upper approximations of the set of "good" students are the same. This means that examples of ordinal classification concerning this decision class are all consistent. This is not the case, however, for the examples concerning the union of decision classes "at least medium". For this upward union the rough approximations are $\underline{P}(Cl^{\geq}_{medium}) = \{S3, S4, S5, S6\}$ and

$\overline{P}(Cl^{\geq}_{medium}) = \{S1, S2, S3, S4, S5, S6\}.$

The difference between $\overline{P}(Cl^{\geq}_{medium})$ and $\underline{P}(Cl^{\geq}_{medium})$, i.e., the boundary $Bn_P(Cl^{\geq}_{medium}) = \{S1, S2\}$, is composed of students with inconsistent overall evaluations, which has already been noticed above. From the viewpoint of decision making, this means that, taking into account the available information about evaluation of students on Mathematics and Literature, the fact that student $y$ is dominated by $S1$

and dominates $S2$ is a condition to conclude that $y$ can obtain an overall evaluation "at least medium" with some doubts.

Until now, rough approximations of only upward unions of decision classes have been considered. It is interesting, however, to calculate also rough approximations of downward unions of decision classes. Let us consider first the lower approximation of the set of students having "at most medium" overall evaluation $\underline{P}(Cl_{medium}^{\leq})$

Observe that

$$\underline{P}(Cl_{medium}^{\leq}) = \{S1, S2, S3, S7, S8\},$$

because the negative dominance cones of students $S1, S2, S3, S7,$ and $S8$ are all included in the set of students with overall evaluation "at most medium". In other words, this means that there is no student dominated by $S1$ or $S2$ or $S3$ or $S7$ or $S8$ while having an overall evaluation better than "medium". From the viewpoint of decision making, this means that, taking into account the available information about evaluation of students on Mathematics and Literature, the fact that student $y$ is dominated by $S1$ or $S2$ or $S3$ or $S7$ or $S8$ is a *sufficient* condition to conclude that $y$ is an "at most medium" student.

The upper approximation of the set of students with an "at most medium" overall evaluation is $\overline{P}(Cl_{medium}^{\leq}) = \{S1, S2, S3, S7, S8\}$, because the positive dominance cones of students $S1, S2, S3, S7,$ and $S8$ have a nonempty intersection with the set of students having an "at most medium" overall evaluation. In other words, this means that for each one of the students $S1, S2, S3, S7,$ and $S8$, there is at least one student dominating him with an overall evaluation "at most medium". From the viewpoint of decision making, this means that, taking into account the available information about evaluation of students on Mathematics and Literature, the fact that student $y$ is dominated by $S1$ or $S2$ or $S3$ or $S7$ or $S8$ is a *possible* condition to conclude that $y$ is an "at most medium" student.

Finally, the lower and upper approximations of the set of students having a "bad" overall evaluation are $\underline{P}(Cl_{bad}^{\leq}) = \{S7, S8\}$ and $\overline{P}(Cl_{bad}^{\leq}) = \{S1, S2, S7, S8\}$. The difference between $\overline{P}(Cl_{bad}^{\leq})$ and $\underline{P}(Cl_{bad}^{\leq})$, i.e., the boundary $Bn_P(Cl_{bad}^{\leq}) = \{S1, S2\}$ is composed of students with inconsistent overall evaluations, which has already been noticed above. From the viewpoint of decision making, this means that, taking into account the available information about evaluation of students on Mathematics and Literature, the fact that student $y$ is dominated by $S1$ and dominates $S2$ is a condition to conclude that $y$ can obtain an overall evaluation "bad" with some doubts. Observe, moreover, that

$$Bn_P(Cl_{medium}^{\geq}) = Bn_P(Cl_{bad}^{\leq}) = \{S1, S2\}.$$

Given the above rough approximations with respect to the set of criteria $P =$ {Mathematics, Literature}, one can induce a set of decision rules representing the preferences of the jury. The idea is that evaluation profiles of students belonging to the lower approximations can serve as a base for some certain rules, while evaluation profiles of students belonging to the boundaries can serve as a base for some approximate rules. The following decision rules have been induced (between parentheses there are id's of students supporting the corresponding rule; the student being a rule base is underlined):

- rule 1) *if* the evaluation on Mathematics is (at least) good, and the evaluation on Literature is at least medium, *then* the overall evaluation is (at least) go
  { $\underline{S4}, S5, S6$ },

- rule 2) *if* the evaluation on Mathematics is at least medium, and the evaluation on Literature is at least medium, *then* the overall evaluation is at least medium,
  { $\underline{S3}, S4, S5, S6$ },

- rule 3) *if* the evaluation on Mathematics is at least medium, and the evaluation on Literature is (at most) bad, *then* the overall evaluation is bad or medium, { $\underline{S1}, \underline{S2}$ },

- rule 4) *if* the evaluation on Mathematics is at most medium, *then* the overall evaluation is at most medium, { $\underline{S2}, \underline{S3}, S7, S8$ },

- rule 5) *if* the evaluation on Literature is (at most) bad, *then* the overall evaluation is at most medium, { $\underline{S1}, \underline{S2}, \underline{S7}$ },

- rule 6) *if* the evaluation on Mathematics is (at most) bad, *then* the overall evaluation is (at most) bad, { $\underline{S7}, \underline{S8}$ }.

Notice that rules 1)-2), 4)-6) are certain, while rule 3) is an approximate one. These rules represent knowledge discovered from the available information. In the current context, the knowledge is interpreted as a preference model of the jury. A characteristic feature of the syntax of decision rules representing preferences is the use of expressions "at least" or "at most" a value; in case of extreme values ("good" and "bad"), these expressions are put in parentheses because there is no value above "good" and below "bad".

Even if one can represent all the knowledge using only one reduct of the set of criteria (as it is the case using $P$ ={Mathematics, Literature}), when considering a larger set of criteria than a reduct, one can obtain a more synthetic representation of knowledge, i.e., the number of decision rules or the number of elementary conditions, or both of them, can get smaller. For example, considering the set of all three criteria, {Mathematics, Physics, Literature}, one can induce a set of decision rules composed of the above rules 1), 2), 3) and 6), plus the following:

- rule 7) *if* the evaluation on Physics is at most medium, and the evaluation on Literature is at most medium, *then* the overall evaluation is at most medium, { $S1, S2, \underline{S3}, S7, S8$ }.

Thus, a complete set of decision rules induced from Table 1 is composed of 5 instead of 6 rules.

Once accepted by the jury, these rules represent its preference model. Assuming that rules 1)-7) in our example represent the preference model of the jury, it can be used to evaluate new students. For example, student $S9$ who is "medium" in Mathematics and Physics and "good" in Literature, would be evaluated as "medium" because his profile matches the premise of rule 2), having as consequence an overall evaluation at least "medium". The overall evaluation of $S9$ cannot be "good", because his profile does not match any rule having as consequence an overall evaluation "good" (in the considered example, the only rule of this type is rule 1), whose premise is not matched by the profile of $S9$ ).

## PHILOSOPHICAL BASIS OF DRSA GRANULAR COMPUTING

It is interesting to analyze the relationships between DRSA and granular computing from the point of view of the philosophical basis of rough set theory proposed by Pawlak. Since according to Pawlak (2001), rough set theory refers to some ideas of Gottlob Frege (vague concepts), Gottfried Leibniz (indiscernibility), George Boole (reasoning methods), Jan Łukasiewicz (multi-valued logic), and Thomas Bayes (inductive reasoning), it is meaningful to give an account for DRSA generalization of rough sets, justifying it in reference to some of these main ideas recalled by Pawlak.

The *identity of indiscernibles* is a principle of analytic ontology first explicitly formulated by Gottfried Leibniz in his Discourse on Metaphysics, section 9 (Loemker & Leibniz, 1969). Two objects $x$ and $y$ are defined indiscernible if $x$ and $y$ have the same properties. The principle of identity of indiscernibles states that

*if $x$ and $y$ are indiscernible, then $x=y$*. (II1)

This can be expressed also as *if $x \neq y$, then $x$ and $y$ are discernible*, i.e., there is at least one property that $x$ has and $y$ does not, or vice versa. The converse of the principle of identity of indiscernibles is called *indiscernibility of identicals* and states that *if $x = y$, then $x$ and $y$ are indiscernible*, i.e., they have the same properties. This is equivalent to say that if there is at least one property that $x$ has and $y$ does not, or vice versa, then $x \neq y$. The conjunction of both principles is often referred to as "Leibniz's law".

Rough set theory is based on a weaker interpretation of Leibniz's law, having as objective the ability to classify objects falling under the same concept. This reinterpretation of the Leibniz's law is based on a reformulation of the principle of identity of indiscernibles as follows:

*if $x$ and $y$ are indiscernible, then $x$ and $y$ belong to the same class*. (II2)

Let us observe that the word "class" in the previous sentence can be considered as synonymous of "granule". Thus, from the point of view of granular computing, II2 can be rewritten as

*if $x$ and $y$ are indiscernible, then $x$ and $y$ belong to the same granule of classification*. (II2')

Notice also that the principle of indiscernibility of identicals cannot be reformulated in analogous terms. In fact, such an analogous reformulation would amount to state that *if $x$ and $y$ belong to the same class, then $x$ and $y$ are indiscernible*. This principle is too strict, however, because there can be two discernible objects $x$ and $y$ belonging to the same class. Thus, within rough set theory, the principle of indiscernibility of identicals should continue to hold in its original formulation (i.e., *if $x = y$, then $x$ and $y$ are indiscernible*). It is worthwhile to observe that the relaxation in the consequence of the implication from II1 to II2, implies an implicit relaxation also in the antecedent. In fact, one could say that two objects are identical if they have the same properties, if one would be able to take into account all conceivable properties. For human limitations this is not the case, therefore, one can imagine that II2' can be properly reformulated as

*if $x$ and $y$ are indiscernible taking into account a given set of properties, then $x$ and $y$ belong to the same class*. (II2")

This weakening in the antecedent of the implication means also that the objects indiscernible with respect to a given set of properties can be seen as a granule, such that, finally, the II2 could be rewritten in terms of granulation as *if x and y belong to the same granule with respect to a given set of properties, then x and y belong to the same classification granule.* (II2''')

For this reason, rough set theory needs a still weaker form of the principle of identity of indiscernibles. Such a principle can be formulated using the idea of vagueness due to Gottlob Frege. According to Frege "the concept must have a sharp boundary – to the concept without a sharp boundary there would correspond an area that had not a sharp boundary-line all around". Therefore, following this intuition, the principle of identity of indiscernibles can be further reformulated as

*if x and y are indiscernible, then x and y should belong to the same class.* (II3)

In terms of granular computing, II3 can be rewritten as

*if x and y belong to the same granule with respect to a given set of properties, then x and y should belong to the same classification granule.* (II3')

This reformulation of the principle of identity of indiscernibles implies that there could be an inconsistency in the statement that x and y are indiscernible, and x and y belong to different classes. Thus, the Leibniz's principle of identity of indiscernibles and the Frege's intuition about vagueness found the basic idea of the rough set concept proposed by Pawlak.

The above reconstruction of the basic idea of the Pawlak's rough set should be completed, however, by referring to another basic idea. This is the idea of George Boole that concerns a property which is satisfied or not satisfied. It is quite natural to weaken this principle admitting that a property can be satisfied to some degree. This idea of graduality can be attributed to Jan Łukasiewicz and his proposal of many-valued logic where, in addition to well-known truth values "true" and "false", other truth values representing partial degrees of truth were present. The Łukasiewicz's idea of graduality has been reconsidered, generalized and fully exploited by Zadeh (1965, 1979, 1997) within fuzzy set theory, where graduality concerns membership to a set.

In this sense, any proposal of putting rough sets and fuzzy sets together can be seen as a reconstruction of the rough set concept, where the Boole's idea of binary logic is abandoned in favor of the Łukasiewicz's idea of many-valued logic, such that the Leibniz's principle of identity of indiscernibles and the Frege's intuition about vagueness are combined with the idea that a property is satisfied to some degree.

Putting aside, for the moment, the Frege's intuition about vagueness, but taking into account the concept of graduality, the principle of identity of indiscernibles can be reformulated as follows:

*if the grade of each property for x is greater than or equal to the grade for y, then x belongs to the considered class in a grade at least as high as y.* (II4)

Taking into account the paradigm of granular computing, II4 can be rewritten as

*if x belongs to the granules defined by considered properties more than y, because the grade of each property for x is greater than or equal to the grade for y, then x belongs to the considered classification granule in a grade at least as high as y.* (II4')

Considering the concept of graduality together with the Frege's intuition about vagueness, one can reformulate the principle of identity of indiscernibles as follows:

*if the grade of each property for x is greater than or equal to the grade for y, then x should belong to the considered class in a grade at least as high as y.* (II5)

In terms of granular computing, II5 can be rewritten as

*if x belongs to the granules defined by considered properties more than y, because the grade of each property for x is greater than or equal to the grade for y, then x should belong to the considered classification granule in a grade at least as high as y.* (II5')

The formulation II5' of the principle of identity of indiscernibles is perfectly concordant with the rough set concept defined within the Dominance-based Rough Set Approach (DRSA) (Greco et al., 2001a).

DRSA has been proposed by the authors to deal with ordinal properties of data related to preferences in decision problems (Greco et al., 2005a; Słowiński et al., 2005). The fundamental feature of DRSA is that it handles monotonicity of comprehensive evaluation of objects with respect to preferences relative to evaluation of these objects on particular attributes. For example, the more preferred is a car with respect to such attributes as maximum speed, acceleration, fuel consumption, and price, the better is its comprehensive evaluation. The type of monotonic relationships within DRSA is also meaningful for problems where relationships between different aspects of a phenomenon described by data are to be taken into account, even if preferences are not considered. Indeed, monotonicity concerns, in general, mutual trends existing between different variables, like distance and gravity in physics, or inflation rate and interest rate in economics. Whenever a relationship between different aspects of a phenomenon is discovered, this relationship can be represented by a monotonicity with respect to some specific measures or perception of the considered aspects. Formulation II5 of the principle of identity of indiscernibles refers to this type of monotonic relationships. So, in general, the monotonicity permits to translate into a formal language a primitive intuition of relationships between different concepts of our knowledge corresponding to the principle of identity of indiscernibles formulated as II5'.

Rough set theory has also inspired other philosophical discussions on granular computing. Let us mention, in particular, granular computing on binary relations investigated by Lin (1998a,b), the human-centered information processing discussed by Bargiela & Pedrycz (2008), rough-granular computing considered and reviewed by Yao (2007, 2008a, 2001) and triarchic theory of granular computing studied by Yao (2008b).

## FUZZY SET EXTENSIONS OF THE DOMINANCE-BASED ROUGH SET APPROACH

The concept of dominance can be refined by introducing gradedness through the use of fuzzy sets. Here are basic definitions of fuzzy connectives (Fodor & Roubens, 1994; Klement et al., 2000). For each proposition $p$, one can consider its truth value $v(p)$ ranging from $v(p) = 0$ ($p$ is definitely false) to $v(p) = 1$ ($p$ is definitely true); and for all intermediate values, the greater $v(p)$, the more credible is the truth of $p$. A negation is a non-increasing function $N : [0,1] \to [0,1]$ such that $N(0) = 1$ and $N(1)=0$. Given proposition $p$, $N(v(p))$ states the credibility of the negation of $p$. A t-norm $T$ and a t-conorm $T^*$ are two functions $T : [0,1] \times [0,1] \to [0,1]$ and $T^* : [0,1] \times [0,1] \to [0,1]$, such that, given two propositions, $p$ and $q$, $T(v(p), v(q))$ represents the credibility of the conjunction of $p$ and $q$, and $T^*(v(p), v(q))$ represents the credibility of the disjunction of $p$ and $q$. t-norm $T$ and t-conorm $T^*$ must satisfy the following properties:

$$T(\alpha, \beta) = T(\beta, \alpha) \text{ and } T^*(\alpha, \beta) = T^*(\beta, \alpha), \text{ for all } \alpha, \beta \in [0,1],$$

$$T(\alpha, \beta) \le T(\gamma, \delta) \text{ and } T^*(\alpha, \beta) \le T^*(\gamma, \delta), \text{ for all } \alpha, \beta, \gamma, \delta \in [0,1]$$

such that $\alpha \leq \gamma$ and $\beta \leq \delta$,

$$T(\alpha, T(\beta, \gamma)) = T(T(\alpha, \beta), \gamma) \text{ and } T^*(\alpha, T^*(\beta, \gamma)) = T^*(T^*(\alpha, \beta), \gamma),$$

for all $\alpha, \beta, \gamma \in [0,1]$,

$$T(1, \alpha) = \alpha \text{ and } T^*(0, \alpha) = \alpha, \text{ for all } \alpha \in [0,1].$$

A negation is strict iff it is strictly decreasing and continuous. A negation $N$ is involutive iff, for all $\alpha \in [0,1]$, $N(N(\alpha)) = \alpha$. A strong negation is an involutive strict negation. If $N$ is a strong negation, then $(T, T^*, N)$ is a de Morgan triplet iff $N(T^*(\alpha, \beta)) = T(N(\alpha), N(\beta))$. A fuzzy implication is a function $I : [0,1] \times [0,1] \to [0,1]$ such that, given two propositions $p$ and $q$, $I(v(p), v(q))$ represents the credibility of the implication of $q$ by $p$. A fuzzy implication must satisfy the following properties (see Fodor & Roubens (1994)):

$I(\alpha, \beta) \geq I(\gamma, \beta)$ for all $\alpha, \beta, \gamma \in [0,1]$, such that $\alpha \leq \gamma$,

$I(\alpha, \beta) \geq I(\alpha, \gamma)$ for all $\alpha, \beta, \gamma \in [0,1]$, such that $\beta \geq \gamma$,

$I(0, \alpha) = 1, I(\alpha, 1) = 1$ for all $\alpha \in [0,1]$,

$I(1, 0) = 0$.

An implication $I_{N,T^*}^{\to}$ is a $T^*$-implication if there is a t-conorm $T^*$ and a strong negation $N$ such that $I_{N,T^*}^{\to}(\alpha, \beta) = T^*(N(\alpha), \beta)$. A fuzzy similarity relation on the universe $U$ is a fuzzy binary relation (i.e., function $R : U \times U \to [0,1]$ reflexive ($R(x, x) = 1$ for all $x \in U$), symmetric ($R(x, y) = R(y, x)$ for all $x, y \in U$) and transitive (given t-norm $T$, $T(R(x, y), R(y, z)) \leq R(x, z)$ for all $x, y, z \in U$

Let $\succeq_q$ be a fuzzy weak preference relation on $U$ with respect to criterion $q \in C$, i.e., $\succeq_q : U \times U \to [0,1]$, such that, for all $x, y \in U$, $\succeq_q(x, y)$ represents the credibility of the proposition "$x$ is at least as good as $y$ with respect to criterion $q$". Suppose that $\succeq_q$ is a fuzzy partial $T$-preorder, i.e., that it is reflexive ($\succeq_q(x, x) = 1$ for each $x \in U$) and $T$-transitive $T(\succeq_q(x, y), \succeq_q(y, z)) \leq \succeq_q(x, z)$, for each $x, y, z \in U$ (see Fodor & Roubens (1994)). Using the fuzzy weak preference relations $\succeq_q$, $q \in C$, a fuzzy dominance relation on $U$ (denotation $D_p(x, y)$) can be defined, for all $P \subseteq C$, as follows:

$$D_P(x,y) = T_{q \in P}\left(\succeq_q (x,y)\right).$$

Given $(x,y) \in U \times U$, $D_P(x,y)$ represents the credibility of the proposition "$x$ is at least as good as $y$ with respect to each criterion $q$ from $P$". Since the fuzzy weak preference relations $\succeq_q$ are supposed to be partial $T$-preorders, then also the fuzzy dominance relation $D_P$ is a partial $T$-preorder. Furthermore, let $\boldsymbol{Cl} = \{Cl_t, \quad t = 1, \ldots, n\}$ be a set of fuzzy classes in $U$ such that, for each $x \in U$, $Cl_t(x)$ represents the membership function of $x$ to $Cl_t$. It is supposed, as before, that the classes of $\boldsymbol{Cl}$ are increasingly ordered, i.e., that for all $r,s \in \{1, \ldots, n\}$ such that $r > s$, the objects from $Cl_r$ have a better comprehensive evaluation than the objects from $Cl_s$. On the basis of the membership functions of the fuzzy class $Cl_t$, fuzzy membership functions of two other sets can be defined as follows:

1) the upward union fuzzy set $Cl_t^{\geq}$, whose membership function $Cl_t^{\geq}(x)$ represents the credibility of the proposition "$x$ is at least as good as the objects in $Cl_t$":

$$Cl_t^{\geq}(x) = \begin{cases} 1 & \text{if } \exists s \in \{1, \ldots, n\} : Cl_s(x) > 0 \text{ and } s > t, \\ Cl_t(x) & \text{otherwise,} \end{cases}$$

2) the downward union fuzzy set $Cl_t^{\leq}$, whose membership function $Cl_t^{\leq}(x)$ represents the credibility of the proposition "$x$ is at most as good as the objects in $Cl_t$":

$$Cl_t^{\leq}(x) = \begin{cases} 1 & \text{if } \exists s \in \{1, \ldots, n\} : Cl_s(x) > 0 \text{ and } s < t, \\ Cl_t(x) & \text{otherwise.} \end{cases}$$

The $P$-lower and the $P$-upper approximations of $Cl_t^{\geq}$ with respect to $P \subseteq C$ are fuzzy sets in $U$, whose membership functions, denoted by $\underline{P}[Cl_t^{\geq}(x)]$ and $\overline{P}[Cl_t^{\geq}(x)]$ respectively, are defined as:

$$\underline{P}[Cl_t^{\geq}(x)] = T_{y \in U}^*(T^*(N(D_P(y,x)), Cl_t^{\geq}(y))),$$

$$\overline{P}[Cl_t^{\geq}(x)] = T_{y \in U}^*(T(D_P(x,y), Cl_t^{\geq}(y))).$$

$\underline{P}[Cl_t^{\geq}(x)]$ represents the credibility of the proposition "for all $y \in U$, $y$ does not dominate $x$ with respect to criteria from $P$ or $y$ belongs to $Cl_t^{\geq}$", while $\overline{P}[Cl_t^{\geq}(x)]$ represents the credibility of the proposition "there is at least one $y \in U$ dominated by $x$ with respect to criteria from $P$ which belongs to $Cl_t^{\geq}$".

The $P$-lower and $P$-upper approximations of $Cl_t^{\leq}$ with respect to $P \subseteq C$, denoted by $\underline{P}[Cl_t^{\leq}(x)]$ and $\overline{P}[Cl_t^{\leq}(x)]$ respectively, can be defined, analogously, as:

$$\underline{P}[Cl_t^{\leq}(x)] = T_{y \in U}(T^*(N(D_P(x,y)), Cl_t^{\leq}(y))),$$

$$\overline{P}[Cl_t^{\leq}(x)] = T_{y \in U}^*(T(D_P(y,x), Cl_t^{\leq}(y))).$$

$\underline{P}[Cl_t^{\leq}(x)]$ represents the credibility of the proposition "for all $y \in U$, $x$ does not dominate $y$ with respect to criteria from $P$ or $y$ belongs to $Cl_t^{\leq}$", while $\overline{P}[Cl_t^{\leq}(x)]$ represents the credibility of the proposition "there is at least one $y \in U$ dominating $x$ with respect to criteria from $P$ which belongs to $Cl_t^{\leq}$".

Let us remark that, using the definition of the $T^*$-implication, it is possible to rewrite the definitions of $\underline{P}[Cl_t^{\geq}(x)]$, $\overline{P}[Cl_t^{\geq}(x)]$, $\underline{P}[Cl_t^{\leq}(x)]$ and $\overline{P}[Cl_t^{\leq}(x)]$, in the following way:

$$\underline{P}[Cl_t^{\geq}(x)] = T_{y \in U}(I_{T^*,N}^{\rightarrow}(D_P(y,x), Cl_t^{\geq}(y))),$$

$$\overline{P}[Cl_t^{\geq}(x)] = T_{y \in U}^*(N(I_{T^*,N}^{\rightarrow}(D_P(x,y), N(Cl_t^{\geq}(y))))),$$

$$\underline{P}[Cl_t^{\leq}(x)] = T_{y \in U}(I_{T^*,N}^{\rightarrow}(D_P(x,y), Cl_t^{\leq}(y))),$$

$$\overline{P}[Cl_t^{\leq}(x)] = T_{y \in U}^*(N(I_{T^*,N}^{\rightarrow}(D_P(y,x), N(Cl_t^{\leq}(y))))).$$

The following results can be proved:

1)  for each $x \in U$ and for each $t \in \{1, \ldots, n\}$

$$\underline{P}[Cl_t^{\geq}(x)] \leq Cl_t^{\geq}(x) \leq \overline{P}[Cl_t^{\geq}(x)],$$
$$\underline{P}[Cl_t^{\leq}(x)] \leq Cl_t^{\leq}(x) \leq \overline{P}[Cl_t^{\leq}(x)];$$

2)  if $(T, T^*, N)$ constitute a de Morgan triplet and if $N[Cl_t^{\geq}(x)] = Cl_{t-1}^{\leq}(x)$ for each $x \in U$ and $t = 2, \ldots, n$, then

$$\underline{P}[Cl_t^{\geq}(x)] = N(\overline{P}[Cl_{t-1}^{\leq}(x)]), \overline{P}[Cl_t^{\geq}(x)] = N(\underline{P}[Cl_{t-1}^{\leq}(x)]), t = 2, \ldots, n,$$

$$\underline{P}[Cl_t^{\leq}(x)] = N(\overline{P[Cl_{t+1}^{\geq}(x)]}), \overline{P}[Cl_t^{\leq}(x)] = N(\underline{P[Cl_{t+1}^{\geq}(x)]}), t = 1, \ldots, n-1;$$

3)    for all $P \subseteq R \subseteq C$, for all $x \in U$ and for each

$$\underline{P}[Cl_t^{\geq}(x)] \leq \underline{R}[Cl_t^{\geq}(x)], \quad \overline{P}[Cl_t^{\geq}(x)] \geq \overline{R}[Cl_t^{\geq}(x)],$$

$$\underline{P}[Cl_t^{\leq}(x)] \leq \underline{R}[Cl_t^{\leq}(x)], \quad \overline{P}[Cl_t^{\leq}(x)] \geq \overline{R}[Cl_t^{\leq}(x)].$$

Results 1) to 3) can be read as fuzzy counterparts of the following results well-known within the classical rough set approach: 1) (*inclusion property*) says that $Cl_t^{\geq}$ and $Cl_t^{\leq}$ include their $P$-lower approximations and are included in their $P$-upper approximations; 2) (*complementarity property*) says that the $P$-lower ($P$-upper) approximation of $Cl_t^{\geq}$ is the complement of the $P$-upper ($P$-lower) approximation of its complementary set $Cl_t^{\leq}$, (analogous property holds for $Cl_{t-1}^{\leq}$ and $Cl_{t+1}^{\geq}$ ); 3) (*monotonicity with respect to sets of condition attributes*) says that enlarging the set of criteria, the membership to the lower approximation does not decrease and the membership to the upper approximation does not increase.

Greco, Inuiguchi and Słowiński (2002) proposed, moreover, the following fuzzy rough approximations based on dominance, which go in line with the fuzzy rough approximation by Dubois & Prade (1990, 1992), concerning classical rough sets:

$$\underline{P}[Cl_t^{\geq}(x)] = inf_{y \in U}(I(D_P(y, x), Cl_t^{\geq}(y))),$$

$$\overline{P}[Cl_t^{\geq}(x)] = sup_{y \in U}(T(D_P(x, y), Cl_t^{\geq}(y))),$$

$$\underline{P}[Cl_t^{\leq}(x)] = inf_{y \in U}(I(D_P(x, y), Cl_t^{\leq}(y))),$$

$$\underline{P}[Cl_t^{\leq}(x)] = sup_{y \in U}(T(D_P(y, x), Cl_t^{\leq}(y))).$$

Using fuzzy rough approximations based on DRSA, one can induce decision rules having the same syntax as the decision rules obtained from crisp DRSA. In this case, however, each decision rule has a fuzzy credibility.

## VARIABLE-CONSISTENCY DOMINANCE-BASED ROUGH SET APPROACH (VC-DRSA)

The definitions of rough approximations introduced in section 3 are based on a strict application of the dominance principle. However, when defining non-ambiguous objects, it is reasonable to accept a limited proportion of negative examples, particularly for large data tables. Such extended version of DRSA is called Variable-Consistency DRSA model (VC-DRSA) (Greco et al., 2001b; Słowiński et al., 2002). It belongs to the family of probabilistic rough set models considered by Yao et al. (2008).

For any $P \subseteq C$ $x \in U$, belongs to $Cl_t^\geq$ *without any ambiguity* at consistency level $l \in (0,1]$, if $x \in Cl_t^\geq$ and at least $l \times 100\%$ of all objects $y \in U$ dominating $x$ with respect to $P$ also belong to $Cl_t^\geq$, i.e., for $t = 2, \ldots, n$,

$$\frac{\left| D_P^+(x) \cap Cl_t^\geq \right|}{\left| D_P^+(x) \right|} \geq l.$$

The level $l$ is called *consistency level* because it controls the degree of consistency with respect to objects qualified as belonging to $Cl_t^\geq$ without any ambiguity. In other words, if $l < 1$, then at most $(1 - l) \times 100\%$ of all objects $y \in U$ dominating $x$ with respect to $P$ do not belong to $Cl_t^\geq$ and thus contradict the inclusion of $x$ in $Cl_t^\geq$.

Analogously, for any $P \subseteq C$, $x \in U$ belongs to $Cl_t^\leq$ *without any ambiguity* at consistency level $l \in (0,1]$, if $x \in Cl_t^\leq$ and at least $l \times 100\%$ of all the objects $y \in U$ dominated by $x$ with respect to $P$ also belong to $Cl_t^\leq$, i.e., for $t = 1, \ldots, n - 1$,

$$\frac{\left| D_P^-(x) \cap Cl_t^\leq \right|}{\left| D_P^-(x) \right|} \geq l.$$

The concept of non-ambiguous objects at some consistency level $l$ leads naturally to the corresponding definition of $P$-lower approximations of the unions of classes $Cl_t^\leq$ and $Cl_t^\geq$, respectively:

$$\underline{P}^l(Cl_t^\geq) = \left\{ x \in Cl_t^\geq : \frac{\left| D_P^+(x) \cap Cl_t^\geq \right|}{\left| D_P^+(x) \right|} \geq l \right\}, \quad t = 2, \ldots, n,$$

$$\underline{P}^l(Cl_t^\leq) = \left\{ x \in Cl_t^\leq : \frac{\left| D_P^-(x) \cap Cl_t^\leq \right|}{\left| D_P^-(x) \right|} \geq l \right\}, \quad t = 1, \ldots, n - 1.$$

Given $P \subseteq C$ and consistency level $l$, the corresponding $P$ *-upper approximations* of $Cl_t^\leq$ and $Cl_t^\geq$, denoted by $\overline{P}^l(Cl_t^\geq)$ and $\overline{P}^l(Cl_t^\leq)$, respectively, can be defined as a complement of $\underline{P}^l(Cl_{t-1}^\leq)$ and $\underline{P}^l(Cl_{t+1}^\geq)$ with respect to $U$:

$$\overline{P}^l(Cl_t^\geq) = U - \underline{P}^l(Cl_{t-1}^\leq), \quad t = 2, \ldots, n,$$

$$\overline{P}^l(Cl_t^\leq) = U - \underline{P}^l(Cl_{t+1}^\geq), \quad t = 1, \ldots, n - 1.$$

$\overline{P}^{l}(Cl_t^{\geq})$ can be interpreted as a set of all the objects belonging to $Cl_t^{\geq}$, *possibly ambiguous* at consistency level *l*. Analogously, $\overline{P}^{l}(Cl_t^{\leq})$ can be interpreted as a set of all the objects belonging to $Cl_t^{\leq}$, *possibly ambiguous* at consistency level *l*. The *P -boundaries* (*P* -doubtful regions) of $Cl_t^{\leq}$ and $Cl_t^{\geq}$ at consistency level *l* are defined as:

$$Bn_P^l(Cl_t^{\geq}) = \overline{P}^{l}(Cl_t^{\geq}) - \underline{P}^{l}(Cl_t^{\geq}), \quad t = 2,\dots,n$$

$$Bn_P^l(Cl_t^{\leq}) = \overline{P}^{l}(Cl_t^{\leq}) - \underline{P}^{l}(Cl_t^{\leq}), \quad t = 1,\dots,n-1.$$

The *variable consistency* model of the dominance-based rough set approach provides some degree of flexibility in assigning objects to lower and upper approximations of the unions of decision classes. The following properties can be easily proved: for $0 < l' < l \leq 1$,

$$\underline{P}^{l}(Cl_t^{\geq}) \subseteq \underline{P}^{l'}(Cl_t^{\geq}) \text{ and } \overline{P}^{l}(Cl_t^{\geq}) \supseteq \overline{P}^{l'}(Cl_t^{\geq}), \quad t = 2,\dots,n,$$

$$\underline{P}^{l}(Cl_t^{\leq}) \subseteq \underline{P}^{l'}(Cl_t^{\leq}) \text{ and } \overline{P}^{l}(Cl_t^{\leq}) \supseteq \overline{P}^{l'}(Cl_t^{\leq}), \quad t = 1,\dots,n-1.$$

The following two basic types of variable-consistency decision rules can be considered:

1.  $D_{\geq}$ -decision rules with the following syntax: "if $\varphi(x,q_1) \geq r_{q_1}$ and $\varphi(x,q_2) \geq r_{q_2}$ and... $\varphi(x,q_p) \geq r_{q_p}$, then $x \in Cl_t^{\geq}$ " with confidence $\alpha$ (i.e., in fraction $\alpha$ of considered cases), where $P = \{q_1,\dots,q_p\} \subseteq C$ $r_{q_1},\dots,r_{q_p}) \in V_{q_1} \times V_{q_2} \times \dots \times V_{q_p}$ and $t = 2,\dots,n$;

2.  $D_{\leq}$ -decision rules with the following syntax: "if $\varphi(x,q_1) \leq r_{q_1}$ and $\varphi(x,q_2) \leq r_{q_2}$ and... $\varphi(x,q_p) \leq r_{q_p}$, then $x \in Cl_t^{\leq}$ " with confidence $\alpha$, where $P = \{q_1,\dots,q_p\} \subseteq C$, $(r_{q_1},\dots,r_{q_p}) \in V_{q_1} \times V_{q_2} \times \dots \times V_{q_p}$ and $t = 1,\dots,n-1$.

The *variable consistency* model is inspired by the *variable precision* model proposed by Ziarko (1993, 1998) within the classical indiscernibility-based rough set approach.

# ROUGH APPROXIMATIONS OF FUZZY SETS BASED ON THE PROPERTY OF MONOTONICITY

In this section, we show how the DRSA can be used for rough approximation of fuzzy sets (see also Greco et al. (2004a, 2006a)).

A *fuzzy information base* is the 3-tuple $\boldsymbol{B} = \langle U, F, \phi \rangle$, where $U$ is a finite set of *objects* (universe), $F = \{f_1, f_2, \dots, f_m\}$ is a finite set of *properties*, and $\phi : U \times F \to [0,1]$ is a function such that $\phi(x, f_h) \in [0,1]$ expresses the degree in which object $x$ has property $f_h$. Therefore, each object $x$ from $U$ is described by a vector

$$Des_F(x) = [\phi(x, f_1), \dots, \phi(x, f_m)]$$

called *description* of $x$ in terms of the evaluations of the properties from $F$; it represents the available information about $x$. Obviously, $x \in U$ can be described in terms of any non-empty subset $E \subseteq F$ and in this case we have

$$Des_E(x) = [\phi(x, f_h), f_h \in E].$$

Let us remark that the concept of fuzzy information base can be considered as a generalization of the concept of property system (Vakarelov, 1992). Indeed, in a property system an object may either possess a property or not, while in the fuzzy information base an object may possess a property in a given degree between 0 and 1.

With respect to any $E \subseteq F$, we can define the *dominance relation* $D_E$ as follows: for any $x, y \in U$, $x$ dominates $y$ with respect to $E$ (denoted as $xD_Ey$) if, for any $f_h \in E$,

$$\phi(x, f_h) \geq \phi(y, f_h).$$

For any $x \in U$ and for each non-empty $E \subseteq F$ let

$$D_E^+\left(x\right) = \{y \in U : yD_Ex\}, \quad D_E^-\left(x\right) = \{y \in U : xD_Ey\}.$$

Given $E \subseteq F$, for each $X \subseteq U$, we can define its *upward lower approximation* $\underline{E}^{(>)}(X)$ and its *upward upper approximation* $\overline{E}^{(>)}(X)$ as:

$$\underline{E}^{(>)}(X) = \left\{x \in U : D_E^+(x) \subseteq X\right\},$$

$$\overline{E}^{(>)}(X) = \left\{x \in U : D_E^-(x) \cap X \neq \varnothing\right\}.$$

Analogously, given $E \subseteq F$, for each $X \subseteq U$, we can define its *downward lower approximation* $\underline{E}^{(<)}(X)$ and its *downward upper approximation* $\overline{E}^{(<)}(X)$ as:

$$\underline{E}^{(<)}(X) = \left\{x \in U : D_E^-(x) \subseteq X\right\},$$

$$\overline{E}^{(<)}(X) = \left\{ x \in U : D_E^+(x) \cap X \neq \varnothing \right\}.$$

Let us observe that in the above definition of rough approximations $\underline{E}^{(>)}(X)$, $\overline{E}^{(>)}(X)$, $\underline{E}^{(<)}(X)$, $\overline{E}^{(<)}(X)$, the elementary sets, which in the classical rough set theory are equivalence classes of the indiscernibility relation, here are positive and negative dominance cones $D_E^+(x)$ and. According to the following theorem, the rough approximations $\underline{E}^{(>)}(X)$, $\overline{E}^{(>)}(X)$, $\underline{E}^{(<)}(X)$, $\overline{E}^{(<)}(X)$, can be expressed as unions of the elementary sets.

## Theorem 1

For any $X \subseteq U$ and $E \subseteq F$

1. $\underline{E}^{(>)}(X) = \bigcup_{x \in U} \left\{ D_E^+(x) : D_E^+(x) \subseteq X \right\}$

2. $\overline{E}^{(>)}(X) = \bigcup_{x \in U} \left\{ D_E^+(x) : D_E^-(x) \cap X \neq \varnothing \right\}$,

3. $\underline{E}^{(<)}(X) = \bigcup_{x \in U} \left\{ D_E^-(x) : D_E^-(x) \subseteq X \right\}$

4. $\overline{E}^{(<)}(X) = \bigcup_{x \in U} \left\{ D_E^-(x) : D_E^+(x) \cap X \neq \varnothing \right\}$

The rough approximations $\underline{E}^{(>)}(X)$, $\overline{E}^{(>)}(X)$, $\underline{E}^{(<)}(X)$, $\overline{E}^{(<)}(X)$, can be used to analyze data relative to gradual membership of objects to some concepts representing properties of objects and their assignment to decision classes. This analysis takes into account the following monotonicity principle: "the greater the degree to which an object has properties from $E \subseteq F$, the greater its degree of membership to a considered class". This principle can be formalized as follows. Let us consider a fuzzy set $X$ in $U$, characterized by the membership function $\mu_X : U \to [0,1]$. This fuzzy set represents a class of interest, such that function $\mu$ specifies a graded membership of objects from $U$ to considered class $X$. For each cutting level $\alpha \in [0,1]$ we can consider the following sets

- weak upward cut of fuzzy set $X$:

$$X^{\geq \alpha} = \left\{ x \in U : \mu(x) \geq \alpha \right\},$$

- strict upward cut of fuzzy set $X$:

$$X^{> \alpha} = \left\{ x \in U : \mu(x) > \alpha \right\},$$

- weak downward cut of fuzzy set $X$:

$$X^{<\alpha} = \left\{ x \in U : \mu(x) < \alpha \right\}.$$

- strict upward cut of fuzzy set $X$:

$$X^{\le\alpha} = \left\{ x \in U : \mu(x) \le \alpha \right\},$$

Let us remark that, for any fuzzy set $X$ and for any $\alpha \in [0,1]$, we have that

$$U - X^{\ge\alpha} = X^{<\alpha}, \quad U - X^{\le\alpha} = X^{>\alpha},$$

$$U - X^{>\alpha} = X^{\le\alpha}, \quad U - X^{<\alpha} = X^{\ge\alpha}.$$

Given a set of fuzzy sets $\boldsymbol{X} = \left\{ X_1, X_2, \ldots, X_p \right\}$ on $U$, whose respective membership functions are $\mu_1, \mu_2, \ldots, \mu_p$, let $P^>(\boldsymbol{X})$ be the set of all the sets obtained as a union and intersection of weak and strict upward cuts of component fuzzy sets. Analogously, let $P^<(\boldsymbol{X})$ be the set of all the sets obtained as a union and intersection of weak and strict downward cuts of component fuzzy sets.

$P^>(\boldsymbol{X})$ and $P^<(\boldsymbol{X})$ are closed under set union and set intersection operations, i.e., for all $Y_1, Y_2 \in P^>(\boldsymbol{X})$, $Y_1 \cup Y_2$ and $Y_1 \cap Y_2$ belong to $P^>(\boldsymbol{X})$, as well as for all $W_1, W_2 \in P^<(\boldsymbol{X})$ $W_1 \cup W_2$, and $W_1 \cap W_2$ belong to $P^<(\boldsymbol{X})$. Observe, moreover, that the universe $U$ and the empty set $\varnothing$ belong both to $P^>(\boldsymbol{X})$ and to $P^<(\boldsymbol{X})$ because, for any fuzzy set $X_i \in \boldsymbol{X}$,

$$U = X_i^{\ge 0} = X_i^{\le 1}$$

and

$$\varnothing = X_i^{>1} = X_i^{<0}.$$

Let us observe, moreover, that for any $Y \in P^>(\boldsymbol{X})$ we have that $(U - Y) \in P^<(\boldsymbol{X})$ and, vice versa, for any $Y \in P^<(\boldsymbol{X})$ we have that $(U - Y) \in P^>(\boldsymbol{X})$.

Let us remark that we can rewrite the rough approximations $\underline{E}^{(>)}(Y)$ $\overline{E}^{(>)}(Y)$, $\underline{E}^{(<)}(Y)$, and $\overline{E}^{(<)}(Y)$ as follows:

$$\underline{E}^{(>)}(Y) = \{ x \in U : \forall w \in U, wD_E x \Rightarrow w \in Y \}$$

$$\overline{E}^{(>)}(Y) = \{x \in U : \exists w \in U \text{ such that } wD_E x \text{ and } w \in Y\}$$

$$\underline{E}^{(<)}(Y) = \{x \in U : \forall w \in U, xD_E w \Rightarrow w \in Y\}$$

$$\overline{E}^{(<)}(Y) = \{x \in U : \exists w \in U \text{ such that } xD_E w \text{ and } w \in Y\}$$

The following theorem states some important properties of the dominance-based rough approximations.

## Theorem 2

1. For any $Y \in P^>(X)$ and for any $W \in P^<(X)$ and for any $E \subseteq F$ ,

$$\underline{E}^{(>)}(Y) \subseteq Y \subseteq \overline{E}^{(>)}(Y), \quad \underline{E}^{(<)}(W) \subseteq W \subseteq \overline{E}^{(<)}(W).$$

2. For any $E \subseteq F$,

$$\underline{E}^{(>)}(\varnothing) = \overline{E}^{(>)}(\varnothing) = \varnothing, \quad \underline{E}^{(<)}(\varnothing) = \overline{E}^{(<)}(\varnothing) = \varnothing,$$

$$\underline{E}^{(>)}(U) = \overline{E}^{(>)}(U) = U, \quad \underline{E}^{(<)}(U) = \overline{E}^{(<)}(U) = U.$$

3. For any $E \subseteq F$, for any $Y_1, Y_2 \in P^>(X)$ and for any $W_1, W_2 \in P^<(X)$ ,

$$\overline{E}^{(>)}(Y_1 \cup Y_2) = \overline{E}^{(>)}(Y_1) \cup \overline{E}^{(>)}(Y_2),$$

$$\overline{E}^{(<)}(W_1 \cup W_2) = \overline{E}^{(<)}(W_1) \cup \overline{E}^{(<)}(W_2).$$

4. For any $E \subseteq F$, for any $Y_1, Y_2 \in P^>(X)$ and for any $W_1, W_2 \in P^<(X)$ ,

$$\underline{E}^{(>)}(Y_1 \cap Y_2) = \underline{E}^{(>)}(Y_1) \cap \underline{E}^{(>)}(Y_2),$$

$$\underline{E}^{(<)}(W_1 \cap W_2) = \underline{E}^{(<)}(W_1) \cap \underline{E}^{(<)}(W_2).$$

5. For any $E \subseteq F$, for any $Y_1, Y_2 \in P^>(X)$ and for any $W_1, W_2 \in P^<(X)$ ,

$$Y_1 \subseteq Y_2 \Rightarrow \underline{E}^{(>)}(Y_1) \subseteq \underline{E}^{(>)}(Y_2),$$

$$W_1 \subseteq W_2 \Rightarrow \underline{E}^{(<)}(W_1) \subseteq \underline{E}^{(<)}(W_2).$$

6. For any $E \subseteq F$, for any $Y_1, Y_2 \in P^>(X)$ and for any $W_1, W_2 \in P^<(X)$ ,

$$Y_1 \subseteq Y_2 \Rightarrow \overline{E}^{(>)}(Y_1) \subseteq \overline{E}^{(>)}(Y_2),$$

$$W_1 \subseteq W_2 \Rightarrow \overline{E}^{(<)}(W_1) \subseteq \overline{E}^{(<)}(W_2).$$

7.  For any $E \subseteq F$, for any $Y_1, Y_2 \in P^>(X)$ and for any $W_1, W_2 \in P^<(X)$,

$$\underline{E}^{(>)}(Y_1 \cup Y_2) \supseteq \underline{E}^{(>)}(Y_1) \cup \underline{E}^{(>)}(Y_2),$$

$$\underline{E}^{(<)}(W_1 \cup W_2) \supseteq \underline{E}^{(<)}(W_1) \cup \underline{E}^{(<)}(W_2).$$

8.  For any $E \subseteq F$, for any $Y_1, Y_2 \in P^>(X)$ and for any $W_1, W_2 \in P^<(X)$,

$$\overline{E}^{(>)}(Y_1 \cap Y_2) \subseteq \overline{E}^{(>)}(Y_1) \cap \overline{E}^{(>)}(Y_2),$$

$$\overline{E}^{(<)}(W_1 \cap W_2) \subseteq \overline{E}^{(<)}(W_1) \cap \overline{E}^{(<)}(W_2).$$

9.  For any $E \subseteq F$, for any $Y \in P^>(X)$ and for any $W \in P^<(X)$,

$$\underline{E}^{(>)}(U - W) = U - \overline{E}^{(<)}(W),$$

$$\underline{E}^{(<)}(U - Y) = U - \overline{E}^{(>)}(Y).$$

10. For any $E \subseteq F$, for any $Y \in P^>(X)$ and for any $W \in P^<(X)$,

$$\overline{E}^{(>)}(U - W) = U - \underline{E}^{(<)}(W),$$

$$\overline{E}^{(<)}(U - Y) = U - \underline{E}^{(>)}(Y).$$

11. For any $E \subseteq F$, for any $Y \in P^>(X)$ and for any $W \in P^<(X)$,

$$\underline{E}^{(>)}[\underline{E}^{(>)}(Y)] = \overline{E}^{(>)}[\underline{E}^{(>)}(Y)] = \underline{E}^{(>)}(Y),$$

$$\underline{E}^{(<)}[\underline{E}^{(<)}(W)] = \overline{E}^{(<)}[\underline{E}^{(<)}(W)] = \underline{E}^{(<)}(W).$$

12. For any $E \subseteq F$, for any $Y \in P^>(X)$ and for any $W \in P^<(X)$,

$$\overline{E}^{(>)}[\overline{E}^{(>)}(Y)] = \underline{E}^{(>)}[\overline{E}^{(>)}(Y)] = \overline{E}^{(>)}(Y),$$

$$\overline{E}^{(<)}[\overline{E}^{(<)}(W)] = \underline{E}^{(<)}[\overline{E}^{(<)}(W)] = \overline{E}^{(<)}(W)$$

Let us remark that the results given in Theorem 2 correspond to well known properties of classical rough sets (see the original properties numbered in the same way by Pawlak (1991)), however, with the noticeable exception of properties 9 and 10 characterizing the specific nature of complementarity relations within the DRSA.

## CLASSICAL ROUGH SET AS A PARTICULAR CASE OF THE MONOTONIC ROUGH APPROXIMATION OF A FUZZY SET

In this section, we show that the classical rough approximation is a particular case of the rough approximation of a fuzzy set presented in the previous section (see also Greco et al. (2005b, 2007b)).

Let us remember that in classical rough set approach (Pawlak, 1982, 1991), the original information is expressed by means of an *information system*, that is the 4-tuple $S = \langle U, Q, V, \varphi \rangle$, where $U$ is a finite set of *objects* (universe), $Q = \{q_1, q_2, \ldots, q_m\}$ is a finite set of *attributes*, $V_q$ is the set of values of the attribute $q$ $V = \bigcup_{q \in Q} V_q$, and $\varphi : U \times Q \rightarrow V$ is a total function such that $\varphi(x, q) \in V_q$ for each $q \in Q$ $x \in U$, called *information function*.

Therefore, each object $x$ from $U$ is described by a vector

$$Des_Q(x) = [\varphi(x, q_1), \varphi(x, q_2), \ldots, \varphi(x, q_m)]$$

called *description* of $x$ in terms of the evaluations of the attributes from $Q$; it represents the available information about $x$. Obviously, $x \in U$ can be described in terms of any non-empty subset $P \subseteq Q$.

With every (non-empty) subset of attributes $P$ there is associated an *indiscernibility relation* on $U$, denoted by $I_P$:

$$I_P = \{(x, y) \in U \times U : \varphi(x, q) = \varphi(y, q), \forall q \in P\}$$

If $(x, y) \in I_P$, it is said that the objects $x$ and $y$ are $P$-indiscernible. Clearly, the indiscernibility relation thus defined is an equivalence relation (reflexive, symmetric and transitive). The family of all the equivalence classes of the relation $I_P$ is denoted by $U \mid I_P$, and the equivalence class containing an element $x \in U$ by $I_P(x)$, i.e.,

$$I_P(x) = \{y \in U : \varphi(y, q) = \varphi(x, q), \forall q \in P\}.$$

The equivalence classes of the relation $I_P$ are called $P$-*elementary sets*.

Let $S$ be an information system, $X$ a non-empty subset of $U$ and $\varnothing \neq P \subseteq Q$. The $P$-*lower approximation* and the $P$-*upper approximation* of $X$ in $S$ are defined, respectively, as:

$$\underline{P}(X) = \{x \in U : I_P(x) \subseteq X\},$$

$$\overline{P}(X) = \{x \in U : I_P(x) \cap X \neq \varnothing\}.$$

The elements of $\underline{P}(X)$ are all and only those objects $x \in U$ which belong to the equivalence classes generated by the indiscernibility relation $I_P$ , *contained* in $X$; the elements of $\overline{P}(X)$ are all and only those objects $x \in U$ which belong to the equivalence classes generated by the indiscernibility relation $I_P$ , *containing at least one* object $x$ belonging to $X$ . In other words, $\underline{P}(X)$ is the largest union of the $P$ -elementary sets included in $X$ , while $\overline{P}(X)$ is the smallest union of the $P$ -elementary sets containing $X$.

Now, we prove that any information system can be expressed in terms of a specific type of an information base (see section 6). An *information base* is called *Boolean* if $\phi : U \times F \to \{0,1\}$. A partition $\boldsymbol{F} = \{F_1,...,F_r\}$ of the set of properties $F$ ,with $card(F_k) \geq 2$ for all $k = 1,...,r$ , is called *canonical* if, for each $x \in U$ and for each $F_k \subseteq \boldsymbol{F}$ , $k = 1,...,r$ , there exists only one $f_j \in F_k$ for which $\phi(x,f_j) = 1$ (and, therefore, for all $f_i \in F_k - \{f_j\}$ , $\phi(x,f_i) = 0$. The condition $card(F_k) \geq 2$ for all $k = 1,...,r$ , is necessary because, otherwise, we would have at least one element of the partition $F_k = \{f'\}$ such that $\phi(x,f') = 1$ for all $x \in U$ , and this would mean that property $f'$ gives no information and can be removed. We can observe now that any *information system* $\boldsymbol{S} = \langle U,Q,V,\varphi \rangle$ can be transformed to a Boolean information base $\boldsymbol{B} = \langle U,F,\phi \rangle$ assigning to each $v \in V_q$ , $q \in Q$ , one property $f_{qv} \in F$ such that $\phi(x,f_{qv}) = 1$ if $\varphi(x,q) = v$ , and $\phi(x,f_{qv}) = 0$ , otherwise. Let us remark that $\boldsymbol{F} = \{F_1,...,F_r\}$ ,with $F_q = \{f_{qv}, v \in V_q\}$ , $q \in Q$ is a canonical partition of $F$ . The opposite transformation, from a Boolean information base to an information system, is not always possible, i.e., there may exist Boolean information bases which cannot be transformed into information systems because their sets of properties do not admit any canonical partition, as shown by the following example.

## Example

Let us consider a Boolean information base, such that $U = \{x_1,x_2,x_3\}$ , $F = \{f_1,f_2\}$ and function $\phi$ is defined by Table 5. One can see that $\boldsymbol{F} = \{\{f_1,f_2\}\}$ is not a canonical partition because $\phi(x_3,f_1) = \phi(x_3,f_2) = 1$ ,while definition of canonical partition $\boldsymbol{F}$ does not allow that for an object $x \in U$ , $\phi(x,f_1) = \phi(x,f_2) = 1$ . Therefore, this Boolean information base has no equivalent information system. Let us remark that also the Boolean information base presented in Table 6, where $U = \{x_1,x_2,x_4\}$ and $F = \{f_1,f_2\}$ , cannot be transformed to an information system, because partition $\boldsymbol{F} = \{\{f_1,f_2\}\}$ is not canonical. Indeed, $\phi(x_4,f_1) = \phi(x_4,f_2) = 0$ , while definition of canonical partition $\boldsymbol{F}$ does not allow that for an object $x \in U$ , $\phi(x,f_1) = \phi(x,f_2) = 0$ .

*Table 5. Information base* **B**

|         | $f_1$ | $f_2$ |
|---------|-------|-------|
| $x_1$   | 0     | 1     |
| $x_2$   | 1     | 0     |
| $x_3$   | 1     | 1     |

*Table 6. Information base* **B'**

|         | $f_1$ | $f_2$ |
|---------|-------|-------|
| $x_1$   | 0     | 1     |
| $x_2$   | 1     | 0     |
| $x_4$   | 0     | 0     |

The above says that consideration of rough approximation in the context of a Boolean information base is more general than the same consideration in the context of an information system. This means, of course, that the rough approximation considered in the context of a fuzzy information base is yet more general.

It is worth stressing that the Boolean information bases **B** and **B'** are not Boolean information systems. In fact, on one hand, a Boolean information base provides information about absence $\big(\phi(x,f)=0\big)$ or presence $\big(\phi(x,f)=1\big)$ of properties $f \in F$ in objects $x \in U$. On the other hand, a Boolean information system provides information about values assigned by attributes $q \in Q$, whose sets of values are $V_q = \{0,1\}$, to objects $x \in U$, such that $\varphi(x,q)=1$

**Index** 1 or $\varphi(x,q)=0$ for all $x \in U$ and $q \in Q$. Observe, therefore, that to transform a Boolean information system **S** into a Boolean information base **B**, each attribute $q$ of **S** corresponds to two properties $f_{q0}$ and $f_{q1}$ of **B**, such that for all $x \in U$

- $\phi(x, f_{q0}) = 1$ and $\phi(x, f_{q1}) = 0$ if $\varphi(x,q) = 0$,

- $\phi(x, f_{q0}) = 0$ and $\phi(x, f_{q1}) = 1$ if $\varphi(x,q) = 1$.

Thus, the Boolean information base **B** in Table 5 and the Boolean information system **S** in Table 7 are different, despite they could seem identical. In fact, the Boolean information system **S** in Table 7 can be transformed into the Boolean information base **B''** in Table 8, which is clearly different from **B**.

What are the relationships between the rough approximation considered in the context of a fuzzy information base and the classical definition of rough approximation in the context of an information system? The following theorem is useful for answering this question.

## Theorem 3

Let us consider an information system and the corresponding Boolean information base. For each $P \subseteq Q$, let $E^P$ be the set of all the properties $f_{qv}$ corresponding to values $v \in V_q$ of each particular

*Table 7. Information system **S***

| | $q_1$ | $q_2$ |
|---|---|---|
| $x_1$ | 0 | 1 |
| $x_2$ | 1 | 0 |
| $x_3$ | 1 | 1 |

*Table 8. Information base **B**"*

| | $f_{q_1 0}$ | $f_{q_1 1}$ | $f_{q_2 0}$ | $f_{q_2 1}$ |
|---|---|---|---|---|
| $x_1$ | 1 | 0 | 0 | 1 |
| $x_2$ | 0 | 1 | 1 | 0 |
| **B** $x_3$ | 0 | 1 | 0 | 1 |

attribute $q \in P$. For each $X \subseteq U$ we have

$$\underline{E}^{P^{(>)}}(X) = \underline{E}^{P^{(<)}}(X) = \underline{P}(X),$$

$$\overline{E}^{P^{(>)}}(X) = \overline{E}^{P^{(<)}}(X) = \overline{P}(X).$$

The above theorem proves that the rough approximation of a set considered within a Boolean information base admitting a canonical partition is equivalent to the classical rough approximation of the same set considered within the corresponding information system. Therefore, the classical rough approximation of a set is a particular case of the rough approximation of this set considered within a fuzzy information system.

## DOMINANCE-BASED ROUGH SET APPROACH TO CASE-BASED REASONING

This section presents rough approximation of a fuzzy set using a similarity relation in the context of case-based reasoning (Greco et al., 2006b).

Case-based reasoning (for a general introduction to case-based reasoning see, e.g., Kolodner (1993); for a fuzzy set approach to case-based reasoning see Dubois et al. (1998)) is a paradigm in machine learning whose idea is that a new problem can be solved by noticing its similarity to a set of problems previously solved. Case-based reasoning regards the inference of some proper conclusions related to a new situation by the analysis of similar cases from a memory of previous cases. It is based on two principles (Leake, 1996):

a)   similar problems have similar solutions;
b)   types of encountered problems tend to recur.

Gilboa & Schmeidler (2001) observed that the basic idea of case-based reasoning can be found in the following sentence of Hume (1748): "From causes which appear *similar* we expect similar effects. This is the sum of all our experimental conclusions." Rephrasing Hume, one can say that "the more similar are the causes, the more similar one expects the effects." Therefore, measuring similarity is the essential point of all case-based reasoning and, particularly, of fuzzy set approach to case-based reasoning (Dubois et al., 1998). This explains the many problems that measuring similarity generates within case-based reasoning. Problems of modeling similarity are relative to two levels:

- at the level of similarity with respect to single features: how to define a meaningful similarity measure with respect to a single feature?
- at the level of similarity with respect to all features: how to properly aggregate the similarity measures with respect to single features in order to obtain a comprehensive similarity measure?

For the above reasons, Greco et al. (2006b) proposed a DRSA approach to case-based reasoning, which tries to be possibly "neutral" and "objective" with respect to similarity relation. At the level of similarity concerning single features, the DRSA approach to case-based reasoning considers only ordinal properties of similarity, and at the level of aggregation, it does not impose any particular functional aggregation based on some very specific axioms (see, for example, Gilboa & Schmeidler (2001)), but it considers a set of decision rules based on the general monotonicity property of comprehensive similarity with respect to similarity of single features. Therefore, the DRSA approach to case-based reasoning is very little "invasive", comparing to the many other existing approaches.

Let us consider a *fuzzy pairwise information base* being the 3-tuple

$$\boldsymbol{B} = <U, F, \sigma>,$$

where $U$ is a finite set of *objects* (universe), $F = \{f_1, f_2, \ldots, f_m\}$ is a finite set of *features*, and $\sigma : U \times U \times F \to [0,1]$ is a function such that $\sigma(x, y, f_h) \in [0,1]$ expresses the credibility that object $x$ is similar to object $y$ w.r.t. feature $f_h$. The minimal requirement function $\sigma$ must satisfy is that, for all $x \in U$ and for all $f_h \in F$, $\sigma(x, x, f_h) = 1$. Therefore, each pair of objects $(x,y) \in U \times U$ is described by a vector

$$Des_F(x,y) = [\sigma(x, y, f_1), \ldots, \sigma(x, y, f_m)],$$

called *description* of (x,y) in terms of the credibilities of similarity with respect to features from $F$; it represents the available information about similarity between $x$ and $y$. Obviously, similarity between $x$ and $y$, $x, y \in U$, can be described in terms of any non-empty subset $E \subseteq F$ as follows:

$$Des_E(x,y) = [\sigma(x, y, f_h), f_h \in E].$$

With respect to any $E \subseteq F$, the dominance relation $D_E$ can be defined on $U \times U$ as follows: for any $x, y, w, z \in U$, (x,y) dominates (w,z) with respect to $E$ (denotation $(x,y)D_E(w,z)$) if, for any $f_h \in E$,

$$\sigma(x, y, f_h) \geq \sigma(w, z, f_h).$$

Given $E \subseteq F$ and $x, y \in U$, let

$$D_E^+(y, x) = \{w \in U : (w, x)D_E(y, x)\},$$

$$D_E^-(y, x) = \{w \in U : (y, x)D_E(w, x)\}.$$

In the pair $(y, x)$, $x$ is considered to be a *reference object*, while $y$ can be called a *limit object*, because it is conditioning the membership of $w$ in $D_E^+(y, x)$ and in $D_E^-(y, x)$.

For each $x \in U$ and $\alpha \in [0, 1]$ and $* \in \{\geq, >\}$, the lower approximation of $X^{*\alpha}$, $\underline{E}_\sigma(X^{*\alpha})$, and the upper approximation of $X^{*\alpha}$, $\overline{E}_\sigma(X^{*\alpha})$, based on similarity $\sigma$ with respect to $E \subseteq F$ and $x$ can be defined, respectively, as:

$$\underline{E}(x)_\sigma(X^{*\alpha}) = \{y \in U : D_E^+(y, x) \subseteq X^{*\alpha}\},$$

$$\overline{E}(x)_\sigma(X^{*\alpha}) = \{y \in U : D_E^-(y, x) \cap X^{*\alpha} \neq \varnothing\}.$$

For the sake of simplicity, in the following only $\underline{E}(x)_\sigma(X^{\geq\alpha})$ and $\overline{E}(x)_\sigma(X^{\geq\alpha})$ with $x \in X^{\geq\alpha}$ are considered. Of course, analogous considerations hold for $\underline{E}(x)_\sigma(X^{>\alpha})$ and $\overline{E}(x)_\sigma(X^{>\alpha})$. Observe that the lower approximation of $X^{\geq\alpha}$ with respect to $x$ contains all the objects $y \in U$ such that any object $w$, being similar to $x$ at least as much as $y$ is similar to $x$ w.r.t. all the considered features $E \subseteq F$, also belongs to $X^{\geq\alpha}$. Thus, the data from the fuzzy pairwise information base **B** confirm that if $w$ is similar to $x$ not less than $y \in \underline{E}(x)_\sigma(X^{\geq\alpha})$ is similar to $x$ w.r.t. all the considered features $E \subseteq F$, then $w$ belongs to $X^{\geq\alpha}$. In other words, $x$ is a reference object and $y \in \underline{E}(x)_\sigma(X^{\geq\alpha})$ is a limit object which belongs "certainly" to set $X$ with credibility at least $\alpha$; the limit is understood such that all objects $w$ that are similar to $x$ w.r.t. considered features at least as much as $y$ is similar to $x$, also belong to $X$ with credibility at least $\alpha$.

Analogously, the upper approximation of $X^{\geq\alpha}$ with respect to $x$ contains all objects $y \in X$ such that there is at least one object $w$, being similar to $x$ at most as much as $y$ is similar to $x$ w.r.t. all the considered features $E \subseteq F$, which belongs to $X^{\geq\alpha}$. Thus, the data from the fuzzy pairwise information base **B** confirm that if $w$ is similar to $x$ not less than $y \in \overline{E}(x)_\sigma(X^{\geq\alpha})$ is similar to $x$ w.r.t. all the considered features $E \subseteq F$, then it is possible that $w$ belongs to $X^{\geq\alpha}$. In other words, $x$ is a reference object and $y \in \overline{E}(x)_\sigma(X^{\geq\alpha})$ is a limit object which belongs "possibly" to set $X$ with credibility at least $\alpha$; the limit is understood such that all objects $z \in U$ similar to $x$ not less than $y$ w.r.t. considered features, possibly belong to $X^{\geq\alpha}$.

For each $x \in U$ and $\alpha \in [0,1]$ and $\Diamond \in \{\leq,<\}$, the lower approximation of $X^{\Diamond\alpha}$, $\underline{E}(x)_\sigma(X^{\Diamond\alpha})$, and the upper approximation of $X^{\Diamond\alpha}$, $\overline{E}(x)_\sigma(X^{\Diamond\alpha})$, based on similarity $\sigma$ with respect to $E \subseteq F$ and $x$ can be defined, respectively, as:

$$\underline{E}(x)_\sigma(X^{\Diamond\alpha}) = \{y \in U : D_E^-(y,x) \subseteq X^{\Diamond\alpha}\},$$

$$\overline{E}(x)_\sigma(X^{\Diamond\alpha}) = \{y \in U : D_E^+(y,x) \cap X^{\Diamond\alpha} \neq \varnothing\}.$$

For the sake of simplicity, in the following only $\underline{E}(x)_\sigma(X^{\leq\alpha})$ and $\overline{E}(x)_\sigma(X^{\leq\alpha})$ with $x \in X^{\leq\alpha}$ are considered. Of course, analogous considerations hold for $\underline{E}(x)_\sigma(X^{<\alpha})$ and $\overline{E}(x)_\sigma(X^{<\alpha})$. Observe that the lower approximation of $X^{\leq\alpha}$ with respect to $x$ contains all the objects $y\in U$ such that any object $w$, being similar to $x$ at most as much as $y$ is similar to $x$ w.r.t. all the considered features $E \subseteq F$, also belongs to $X^{\leq\alpha}$. Thus, the data from the fuzzy pairwise information base **B** confirm that if $w$ is similar to $x$ not more than $y \in \underline{E}(x)_\sigma(X^{\leq\alpha})$ is similar to $x$ w.r.t. all the considered features $E \subseteq F$, then $w$ belongs to $X^{\leq\alpha}$ In other words, $x$ is a reference object and $y \in \underline{E}(x)_\sigma(X^{\leq\alpha})$ is a limit object which belongs "certainly" to set $X$ with credibility at most $\alpha$; the limit is understood such that all objects $w$ that are similar to $x$ w.r.t. considered features at most as much as $y$ is similar to $x$, also belong to $X$ with credibility at most $\alpha$.

Analogously, the upper approximation of $X^{\leq\alpha}$ with respect to $x$ contains all the objects $y\in X$ such that there is at least one object $w$, being similar to $x$ at least as much as $y$ is similar to $x$ with respect to all the considered features $E \subseteq F$, which belongs to $X^{\leq\alpha}$. Thus, the data from the fuzzy pairwise information base **B** confirm that if $w$ is similar to $x$ not more than $y \in \overline{E}(x)_\sigma(X^{\leq\alpha})$ is similar to $x$ w.r.t. all the considered features $E\subseteq F$, then it is possible that $w$ belongs to $X^{\leq\alpha}$. In other words, $x$ is a reference object and $y \in \overline{E}_\sigma(X^{\leq\alpha})$ is a limit object which belongs "possibly" to set $X$ with credibility at most $\alpha$; the limit is understood such that all objects $z \in U$ similar to $x$ not more than $y$ w.r.t. considered features, possibly belong to $X^{\leq\alpha}$.

Observe that the rough approximations $\underline{E}(x)_\sigma(X^{\geq\alpha})$, $\overline{E}(x)_\sigma(X^{\geq\alpha})$, $\underline{E}(x)_\sigma(X^{\leq\alpha})$ and $\overline{E}(x)_\sigma(X^{\leq\alpha})$ can be rewritten as

$$\underline{E}(x)_\sigma(X^{\geq\alpha}) = \{y \in U : \ \forall w \in U, (w,x)D_E(y,x) \Rightarrow w \in X^{\geq\alpha}\},$$

$$\overline{E}(x)_\sigma(X^{\geq\alpha}) = \{y \in U : \exists w \in U \text{ such that } (y,x)D_E(w,x) \text{ and } w \in X^{\geq\alpha}\},$$

$$\underline{E}(x)_\sigma(X^{\leq\alpha}) = \{y \in U : \ \forall w \in U, (y,x)D_E(w,x) \Rightarrow w \in X^{\leq\alpha}\},$$

$$\overline{E(x)}_\sigma(X^{\leq\alpha}) = \{y \in U : \exists w \in U \text{ such that } (w,x)D_E(y,x) \text{ and } w \in X^{\leq\alpha}\}.$$

This formulation of the rough approximation is concordant with the syntax of the decision rules induced by means of DRSA from a fuzzy pairwise information base. More precisely,

- $\underline{E(x)}_\sigma(X^{\geq\alpha})$ is concordant with decision rules of the type "*if* object $w$ is similar to object $x$ w.r.t. feature $f_{i1}$ to degree at least $h_{i1}$ and w.r.t. feature $f_{i2}$ to degree at least $h_{i2}$ and... and w.r.t. feature $f_{ip}$ to degree at least $h_{ip}$, *then* object $w$ belongs to set $X$ to degree at least $\alpha$",

- $\overline{E(x)}_\sigma(X^{\geq\alpha})$ is concordant with decision rules of the type: "*if* object $w$ is similar to object $x$ w.r.t. feature $f_{i1}$ to degree at least $h_{i1}$ and w.r.t. feature $f_{i2}$ to degree at least $h_{i2}$ and... and w.r.t. feature $f_{ip}$ to degree at least $h_{ip}$, *then* object $w$ could belong to set $X$ to degree at least $\alpha$",

- $\underline{E(x)}_\sigma(X^{\leq\alpha})$ is concordant with decision rules of the type: "*if* object $w$ is similar to object $x$ w.r.t. feature $f_{i1}$ to degree at most $h_{i1}$ and w.r.t. feature $f_{i2}$ to degree at most $h_{i2}$ and... and w.r.t. feature $f_{ip}$ to degree at most $h_{ip}$, *then* object $w$ belongs to set $X$ to degree at most $\alpha$",

- $\overline{E(x)}_\sigma(X^{\leq\alpha})$ is concordant with decision rules of the type: "*if* object $w$ is similar to object $x$ w.r.t. feature $f_{i1}$ to degree at most $h_{i1}$ and w.r.t. feature $f_{i2}$ to degree at most $h_{i2}$ and... and w.r.t. feature $f_{ip}$ to degree at most $h_{ip}$, *then* object $w$ could belong to set $X$ to degree at most $\alpha$",

where $\{i1, ..., ip\} = E$ and $h_{i1}, ..., h_{ip} \in [0,1]$.

The above definitions of rough approximations and the syntax of decision rules are based on ordinal properties of similarity relations only. In fact, no algebraic operation, such as sum or product, involving cardinal properties of function $\sigma$ measuring credibility of similarity relations is considered. This is an important characteristic of our approach in comparison with alternative approaches to case-based reasoning.

Let us remark that, similarly to DRSA approximation in an information base, in the case of DRSA approximation in a fuzzy pairwise information base, even if for two fuzzy sets $X$ and $Y$ it is $X^{\geq\alpha} = Y^{\leq\alpha}$, their approximations may be different due to the different directions of cutting the membership functions of sets $X$ and $Y$.

Given a family of fuzzy sets $\boldsymbol{X} = \{X_1, X_2, ..., X_p\}$ on $U$, whose respective membership functions are $\mu_1, \mu_2, ..., \mu_p$, let $P^>(\boldsymbol{X})$ be the set of all the sets obtained through unions and intersections of weak and strict upward cuts of component fuzzy sets. Analogously, let $P^<(\boldsymbol{X})$ be the set of all the sets obtained through unions and intersections of weak and strict downward cuts of component fuzzy sets.

$P^>(\boldsymbol{X})$ and $P^<(\boldsymbol{X})$ are closed under set union and set intersection operations, i.e., for all $Y_1, Y_2 \in P^>(\boldsymbol{X})$, $Y_1 \cup Y_2$ and $Y_1 \cap Y_2$ belong to $P^>(\boldsymbol{X})$, as well as for all $W_1, W_2 \in P^<(\boldsymbol{X})$, $W_1 \cup W_2$

and $W_1 \cap W_2$ belong to $P^<(X)$. Observe, moreover, that the universe $U$ and the empty set $\varnothing$ belong both to $P^>(X)$ and to $P^<(X)$ because, for any fuzzy set $X_i \in X$,

$$U = X_i^{\geq 0} = X_i^{\leq 1} \text{ and } \varnothing = X_i^{>1} = X_i^{<0}.$$

The following theorem states some important properties of the dominance-based rough approximations for case based reasoning.

## Theorem 4

1.  For any $Y \in P^>(X)$, for any $W \in P^<(X)$ and for any $E \subseteq F$ and for any $x \in U$,

$$\underline{E(x)}_\sigma^{(>)}(Y) \subseteq Y \subseteq \overline{E(x)}_\sigma^{(>)}(Y), \quad \underline{E(x)}_\sigma^{(<)}(W) \subseteq W \subseteq \overline{E(x)}_\sigma^{(<)}(W).$$

2.  For any $E \subseteq F$ and for any $x \in U$,

$$\underline{E(x)}_\sigma^{(>)}(\varnothing) = \overline{E(x)}_\sigma^{(>)}(\varnothing) = \varnothing, \quad \underline{E(x)}_\sigma^{(<)}(\varnothing) = \overline{E(x)}_\sigma^{(<)}(\varnothing) = \varnothing,$$

$$\underline{E(x)}_\sigma^{(>)}(U) = \overline{E(x)}_\sigma^{(>)}(U) = U, \quad \underline{E(x)}_\sigma^{(<)}(U) = \overline{E(x)}_\sigma^{(<)}(U) = U.$$

3.  For any $E \subseteq F$, for any $Y_1, Y_2 \in P^>(X)$, for any $W_1, W_2 \in P^<(X)$, for any $x \in U$

$$\overline{E(x)}_\sigma^{(>)}(Y_1 \cup Y_2) = \overline{E(x)}_\sigma^{(>)}(Y_1) \cup \overline{E(x)}_\sigma^{(>)}(Y_2),$$

$$\overline{E(x)}_\sigma^{(<)}(W_1 \cup W_2) = \overline{E(x)}_\sigma^{(<)}(W_1) \cup \overline{E(x)}_\sigma^{(<)}(W_2).$$

4.  For any $E \subseteq F$, for any $Y_1, Y_2 \in P^>(X)$, for any $W_1, W_2 \in P^<(X)$ and for any $x \in U$

$$\underline{E(x)}_\sigma^{(>)}(Y_1 \cap Y_2) = \underline{E(x)}_\sigma^{(>)}(Y_1) \cap \underline{E(x)}_\sigma^{(>)}(Y_2),$$

$$\underline{E(x)}_\sigma^{(<)}(W_1 \cap W_2) = \underline{E(x)}_\sigma^{(<)}(W_1) \cap \underline{E(x)}_\sigma^{(<)}(W_2).$$

5.  For any $E \subseteq F$, for any $Y_1, Y_2 \in P^>(X)$, for any $W_1, W_2 \in P^<(X)$ and for any $x \in U$

$$Y_1 \subseteq Y_2 \Rightarrow \underline{E(x)}_\sigma^{(>)}(Y_1) \subseteq \underline{E(x)}_\sigma^{(>)}(Y_2),$$

$$W_1 \subseteq W_2 \Rightarrow \underline{E(x)}_\sigma^{(<)}(W_1) \subseteq \underline{E(x)}_\sigma^{(<)}(W_2).$$

6. For any $E \subseteq F$, for any $Y_1, Y_2 \in P^>(\boldsymbol{X})$, for any $W_1, W_2 \in P^<(\boldsymbol{X})$ and for any $x \in U$

$$Y_1 \subseteq Y_2 \Rightarrow \overline{E}(x)_\sigma^{(>)}(Y_1) \subseteq \overline{E}(x)_\sigma^{(>)}(Y_2),$$

$$W_1 \subseteq W_2 \Rightarrow \overline{E}(x)_\sigma^{(<)}(W_1) \subseteq \overline{E}(x)_\sigma^{(<)}(W_2).$$

7. For any $E \subseteq F$, for any $Y_1, Y_2 \in P^>(\boldsymbol{X})$, for any $W_1, W_2 \in P^<(\boldsymbol{X})$ and for any $x \in U$

$$\underline{E}(x)_\sigma^{(>)}(Y_1 \cup Y_2) \supseteq \underline{E}(x)_\sigma^{(>)}(Y_1) \cup \underline{E}(x)_\sigma^{(>)}(Y_2),$$

$$\underline{E}(x)_\sigma^{(<)}(W_1 \cup W_2) \supseteq \underline{E}(x)_\sigma^{(<)}(W_1) \cup \underline{E}(x)_\sigma^{(<)}(W_2).$$

8. For any $E \subseteq F$, for any $Y_1, Y_2 \in P^>(\boldsymbol{X})$, for any $W_1, W_2 \in P^<(\boldsymbol{X})$ and for any $x \in U$

$$\overline{E}(x)_\sigma^{(>)}(Y_1 \cap Y_2) \subseteq \overline{E}(x)_\sigma^{(>)}(Y_1) \cap \overline{E}(x)_\sigma^{(>)}(Y_2),$$

$$\overline{E}(x)_\sigma^{(<)}(W_1 \cap W_2) \subseteq \overline{E}(x)_\sigma^{(<)}(W_1) \cap \overline{E}(x)_\sigma^{(<)}(W_2).$$

9. For any $E \subseteq F$, for any $Y \in P^>(\boldsymbol{X})$, for any $W \in P^<(\boldsymbol{X})$ and for any $x \in U$,

$$\underline{E}(x)_\sigma^{(>)}(U - W) = U - \overline{E}(x)_\sigma^{(<)}(W),$$

$$\underline{E}(x)_\sigma^{(<)}(U - Y) = U - \overline{E}(x)_\sigma^{(>)}(Y).$$

10. For any $E \subseteq F$, for any $Y \in P^>(\boldsymbol{X})$, for any $W \in P^<(\boldsymbol{X})$ and for any $x \in U$,

$$\overline{E}(x)_\sigma^{(>)}(U - W) = U - \underline{E}(x)_\sigma^{(<)}(W),$$

$$\overline{E}(x)_\sigma^{(<)}(U - Y) = U - \underline{E}(x)_\sigma^{(>)}(Y).$$

11. For any $E \subseteq F$, for any $Y \in P^>(\boldsymbol{X})$, for any $W \in P^<(\boldsymbol{X})$ and for any $x \in U$,

$$\underline{E}(x)_\sigma^{(>)}[\underline{E}(x)_\sigma^{(>)}(Y)] = \overline{E}(x)_\sigma^{(>)}[\underline{E}(x)_\sigma^{(>)}(Y)] = \underline{E}(x)_\sigma^{(>)}(Y),$$

$$\underline{E}(x)_\sigma^{(<)}[\underline{E}(x)_\sigma^{(<)}(W)] = \overline{E}(x)_\sigma^{(<)}[\underline{E}(x)_\sigma^{(<)}(W)] = \underline{E}(x)_\sigma^{(<)}(W).$$

12. For any $E \subseteq F$, for any $Y \in P^>(\boldsymbol{X})$, for any $W \in P^<(\boldsymbol{X})$ and for any $x \in U$,

$$\overline{E}(x)_\sigma^{(>)}[\overline{E}(x)_\sigma^{(>)}(Y)] = \underline{E}(x)_\sigma^{(>)}[\overline{E}(x)_\sigma^{(>)}(Y)] = \overline{E}(x)_\sigma^{(>)}(Y),$$

$$\overline{E}(x)_\sigma^{(<)}[\overline{E}(x)_\sigma^{(<)}(W)] = \underline{E}(x)_\sigma^{(<)}[\overline{E}(x)_\sigma^{(<)}(W)] = \overline{E}(x)_\sigma^{(<)}(W).$$

Let us remark that the results given in the above theorem correspond to well known properties of classical rough sets (see the original properties numbered in the same way by Pawlak (1991)), however, with the noticeable exception of properties 9 and 10 characterizing the specific nature of complementarity relations within the DRSA.

## ALGEBRAIC STRUCTURES FOR DOMINANCE-BASED ROUGH SET APPROACH

Many algebraic characterizations of the classical rough set approach have been proposed (for a survey see Polkowski (2002, Chapter 12), and Cattaneo & Ciucci (2004)). In this section we present algebraic representations of DRSA in terms of generalizations of several algebras already used to represent classical rough set approach, namely: bipolar de Morgan Brouwer-Zadeh distributive lattice (Greco et al., 2008a), bipolar Nelson algebra, bipolar Heyting algebra, bipolar double Stone algebra, bipolar three-valued Łukasiewicz algebra, bipolar Wajsberg algebra. We present also an algebraic model for ordinal classification.

In the following, we shall consider a fuzzy information base $\boldsymbol{B}$=<$U$, $F$, $\varphi$>. Given $G \subseteq F$, for each $X \subseteq U$, its *upward lower approximation* $\underline{G}^{(>)}(X)$ and its *upward upper approximation* $\overline{G}^{(>)}(X)$ can be defined as:

$$\underline{G}^{(>)}(X) = \left\{ x \in U : D_G^+(x) \subseteq X \right\},$$

$$\overline{G}^{(>)}(X) = \left\{ x \in U : D_G^-(x) \cap X \neq \varnothing \right\}.$$

Analogously, given $G \subseteq F$, for each $X \subseteq U$, its *downward lower approximation* $\underline{G}^{(<)}(X)$ and its *downward upper approximation* $\overline{G}^{(<)}(X)$ can be defined as:

$$\underline{G}^{(<)}(X) = \left\{ x \in U : D_G^-(x) \subseteq X \right\},$$

$$\overline{G}^{(<)}(X) = \left\{ x \in U : D_G^+(x) \cap X \neq \varnothing \right\}.$$

The algebraic structures that we shall consider for DRSA are based on a representation of DRSA approximations written as

$$\left\langle \underline{G}^{(>)}(X), \ U - \overline{G}^{(>)}(X) \right\rangle$$

and

$$\left\langle \underline{G}^{(<)}(X), \quad U - \overline{G}^{(<)}(X) \right\rangle,$$

which is called *bipolar disjoint representation*. Within bipolar disjoint representation, we consider a set $B^+$ of "positive" concepts, and a set $B^-$ of "negative" concepts. For example, in a problem of evaluation of students, the concept of "good students" is "positive", while the concept of "bad students" is "negative". Within DRSA, each concept is represented by the pair $(I, E)$, where $I$ (the interior) is the lower approximation of set $X \subseteq U$ and $E$ (the exterior) is the complement in $U$ of the upper approximation of $X$. Intuitively, each concept is represented by $I$, which is the set of objects that certainly belong to the concept, and by $E$, which is the set of objects that certainly do not belong to the concept. Therefore, the positive concept "good students" is represented by the pair $(I_G, E_G)$, where $I_G$ represents the set of students "certainly good", and $E_G$ represents the set of students "certainly not good". Analogously, the negative concept "bad students" is represented by the pair $(I_B, E_B)$, where $I_B$ represents the set of students "certainly bad", and $E_B$ represents the set of students "certainly not bad".

In the context of bipolar disjoint representation, it is natural to represent union and intersection of sets by the operation of join $\sqcup$ and meet $\sqcap$ defined as follows below. Let us consider the concepts of "good students in Mathematics", represented by the pair $(I_{G_M}, E_{G_M})$, and "good students in Literature", represented by the pair $(I_{G_L}, E_{G_L})$. In this example, the concept of "good students in Mathematics <u>or</u> Literature" is represented by

$$(I_{G_M}, E_{G_M}) \sqcup (I_{G_L}, E_{G_L}) = (I_{G_M} \cup I_{G_L}, E_{G_M} \cap E_{G_L}).$$

This means that to the concept of "good students in Mathematics or Literature" there certainly belongs the set of students "certainly good in Mathematics" or "certainly good in Literature", i.e., $I_{G_M} \cup I_{G_L}$, while there certainly does not belong the set of students "certainly not good in Mathematics" and "certainly not good in Literature", i.e., $E_{G_M} \cap E_{G_L}$. Analogously, the concept of "good students in Mathematics *and* Literature" is represented by

$$(I_{G_M}, E_{G_M}) \sqcap (I_{G_L}, E_{G_L}) = (I_{G_M} \cap I_{G_L}, E_{G_M} \cup E_{G_L}).$$

This means that to the concept of "good students in Mathematics and Literature" there certainly belongs the set of students "certainly good in Mathematics" and "certainly good in Literature", i.e., $I_{G_M} \cap I_{G_L}$, while there certainly does not belong the set of students "certainly not good in Mathematics" or "certainly not good in Literature", i.e., $E_{G_M} \cup E_{G_L}$.

Moreover, within the context of bipolar disjoint representation, one can imagine different negations. Perhaps, the most interesting of them are two negations that can be called the Kleene negation and the

Brouwer negation. The Kleene bipolar complementation $^{-+}$ of the concept of "good students" $(I_G, E_G)$ is the set $(E_G, I_G)$, that is, to the negation of the concept of "good students" there certainly belongs the set of students "certainly not good" $E_G$, and there certainly does not belong the set of students "certainly good" $I_G$. Considering the Brouwer bipolar complementation $^{\approx+}$, the negation of the concept of "good students" $(I_G, E_G)$ is given by $(E_G, U - E_G)$, that is to the negation of the concept of "good students" there certainly belongs the set of students "certainly not good" $E_G$, as in the case of the Kleene bipolar complementation, and there certainly does not belong the set of all the other students $U - E_G$, differently from the case of the Kleene bipolar complementation. Similar considerations hold for the Kleene bipolar complementation $^{--}$ and for the Brouwer bipolar complementation $^{\approx-}$ of negative concepts. Observe that any negation, either Kleene negation or Brouwer negation, assigns a negative concept belonging to $B^-$ to any positive concept belonging to $B^+$ as well as it assigns a positive concept belonging to $B^+$ to any negative concept belonging to $B^-$

The algebraic models presented below hold under particular conditions which ensure that for any $X, Y \subseteq U$ there exist $Z_1, Z_2, Z_3, Z_4 \subseteq U$, such that

(i) $\left\langle \underline{G}^{(>)}(X), \ U - \overline{G}^{(>)}(X) \right\rangle \sqcup \left\langle \underline{G}^{(>)}(Y), \ U - \overline{G}^{(>)}(Y) \right\rangle = \left\langle \underline{G}^{(>)}(Z_1), \ U - \overline{G}^{(>)}(Z_1) \right\rangle$

(ii) $\left\langle \underline{G}^{(<)}(X), \ U - \overline{G}^{(<)}(X) \right\rangle \sqcup \left\langle \underline{G}^{(<)}(Y), \ U - \overline{G}^{(<)}(Y) \right\rangle = \left\langle \underline{G}^{(<)}(Z_2), \ U - \overline{G}^{(<)}(Z_2) \right\rangle$

(iii) $\left\langle \underline{G}^{(>)}(X), \ U - \overline{G}^{(>)}(X) \right\rangle \sqcap \left\langle \underline{G}^{(>)}(Y), \ U - \overline{G}^{(>)}(Y) \right\rangle = \left\langle \underline{G}^{(>)}(Z_3), \ U - \overline{G}^{(>)}(Z_3) \right\rangle$

(iv) $\left\langle \underline{G}^{(<)}(X), \ U - \overline{G}^{(<)}(X) \right\rangle \sqcap \left\langle \underline{G}^{(<)}(Y), \ U - \overline{G}^{(<)}(Y) \right\rangle = \left\langle \underline{G}^{(<)}(Z_4), \ U - \overline{G}^{(<)}(Z_4) \right\rangle$

This means that join and meet operations on disjoint representations of rough sets give again disjoint representations of rough sets. One of the conditions which permit to satisfy (i)–(iv) is the following: for each object $x \in U$ there exists another object $x' \in U$ which is "indiscernible" with it, i.e., for all $f_h \in F$, $\varphi(x, f_h) = \varphi(x', f_h)$. This condition has an interesting interpretation. Assume that subset $X \subseteq U$ represents the concept of "good students". Then, naturally, one can include or exclude with certainty some students from this concept, but also one can state that the membership of some students to this concept is doubtful. When the above condition holds, this situation can be explained by assigning a pair $(x, x')$ of indiscernible objects to each student. If a student represented by the pair $(x, x')$ belongs with certainty to the set of good students, then both $x$ and $x'$ are included in $X$; if the student represented by $(x, x')$ certainly does not belong to the set of good students, then both $x$ and $x'$ are excluded from $X$; finally, if the membership of the student represented by $(x, x')$ to the set of good students is doubtful, then one object from among $x$ and $x'$ is assigned to the set of good students, and the other is assigned to its complement.

## Bipolar de Morgan Brouwer-Zadeh Distributive Lattices

A *bipolar quasi Brouwer-Zadeh distributive lattice* (Greco et al., 2008a,b), which is a generalization of quasi Brouwer-Zadeh distributive lattice (Cattaneo & Nisticó, 1989), is a system

$$\left\langle \Sigma, \Sigma^+, \Sigma^-, \wedge, \vee, {}'^+, {}'^-, {}^{\sim+}, {}^{\sim-}, 0, 1 \right\rangle$$

in which the following properties (1b)-(4b) hold:

(1b) $\Sigma$ is a distributive lattice with respect to the join and the meet operations $\vee$ and $\wedge$

(1b') $\Sigma^+, \Sigma^- \subseteq \Sigma$ are distributive lattices with respect to the join and the meet operations $\vee$ and $\wedge$. $\Sigma$ is bounded by the least element 0 and the greatest element 1, which implies that also $\Sigma^+$ and $\Sigma^-$ are bounded.

(2b) The unary operations ${}'^+ : \Sigma^+ \to \Sigma^-$ and ${}'^- : \Sigma^- \to \Sigma^+$ are Kleene (also Zadeh or fuzzy) bipolar complementation, that is, for arbitrary $a, b \in \Sigma^+$ and $c, d \in \Sigma^-$.

(K1b) $a^{'+'-} = a$, $c^{'-'+} = c$,

(K2b) $(a \vee b)^{'+} = a^{'+} \wedge b^{'+}$, $(c \vee d)^{'-} = c^{'-} \wedge d^{'-}$

(K3b) $a \wedge a^{'+} \le b \vee b^{'+}$, $c \wedge c^{'-} \le d \vee d^{'-}$.

(3b) The unary operations ${}^{\sim+} : \Sigma^+ \to \Sigma^-$ and ${}^{\sim-} : \Sigma^- \to \Sigma^+$ are Brouwer (or intuitionistic) bipolar complementations, that is, for arbitrary $a, b \in \Sigma^+$ and $c, d \in \Sigma^-$,

(B1b) $a \wedge a^{\sim+\sim-} = a$, $c \wedge c^{\sim-\sim+} = c$,

(B2b) $(a \vee b)^{\sim+} = a^{\sim+} \wedge b^{\sim+}$, $(c \vee d)^{\sim-} = c^{\sim-} \wedge d^{\sim-}$,

(B3b) $a \wedge a^{\sim+} = 0$, $c \wedge c^{\sim-} = 0$.

(4b) Complementation ${}'^+$ and complementation ${}^{\sim+}$ on one hand, and complementation ${}'^-$ and complementation ${}^{\sim-}$ on the other hand, are linked by the interconnection rule, that is, for arbitrary $a \in \Sigma^+$ and arbitrary $b \in \Sigma^-$:

(in-b) $a^{\sim+} \le a^{'+}$, $b^{\sim-} \le b^{'-}$.

A structure $\left\langle \Sigma, \Sigma^+, \Sigma^-, \wedge, \vee, {}'^+, {}'^-, {}^{\sim+}, {}^{\sim-}, 0, 1 \right\rangle$ is a *bipolar Brouwer-Zadeh distributive lattice* if it is a bipolar quasi Brouwer-Zadeh distributive lattice satisfying the stronger interconnection rule, that is, for arbitrary $a \in \Sigma^+$ and arbitrary $b \in \Sigma^-$

(s-in-b) $a^{\sim+'-} = a^{\sim+'-}$, $b^{\sim-\sim+} = b^{\sim-'+}$.

A bipolar Brouwer-Zadeh distributive lattice is a *bipolar de Morgan Brouwer-Zadeh distributive lattice*, if it satisfies also the $\vee$ de Morgan property, that is, for arbitrary $a, b \in \Sigma^+$ and $c, d \in \Sigma^-$:

(B2a-b) $(a \wedge b)^{\sim+} = a^{\sim+} \vee b^{\sim+}$, $(c \wedge d)^{\sim-} = c^{\sim-} \vee d^{\sim-}$

Fixed $G \subseteq F$, for any $X \subseteq U$, let us consider the pairs $\left\langle \underline{G}^{(<)}(X), U - \overline{G}^{(<)}(X) \right\rangle$ and $\left\langle \underline{G}^{(>)}(X), U - \overline{G}^{(>)}(X) \right\rangle$, and the sets

$$B = \left\{ (I, E) : I, E \subseteq U \text{ such that } I \cap E = \varnothing \right\}$$

$$B^- = \left\{ (I, E) : \exists X \subseteq U \text{ for which } I = \underline{G}^{(<)}(X) \text{ and } E = U - \overline{G}^{(<)}(X) \right\}$$

$$B^+ = \left\{ (I, E) : \exists X \subseteq U \text{ for which } I = \underline{G}^{(>)}(X) \text{ and } E = U - \overline{G}^{(>)}(X) \right\}$$

## Theorem 5

(Greco et al., 2008a). The structure $\left\langle B, B^+, B^-, \sqcup, \sqcap, ^{-+}, ^{--}, ^{\approx+}, ^{\approx-}, \langle \varnothing, U \rangle, \langle U, \varnothing \rangle \right\rangle$, where, for any $\left\langle I_1, E_1 \right\rangle, \left\langle I_2, E_2 \right\rangle \in B$, $\left\langle I_3, E_3 \right\rangle \in B^-$, $\left\langle I_4, E_4 \right\rangle \in B^+$,

$$\left\langle I_1, E_2 \right\rangle \sqcap \left\langle I_1, E_2 \right\rangle = \left\langle I_1 \cap I_2, E_1 \cup E_2 \right\rangle,$$

$$\left\langle I_1, E_1 \right\rangle \sqcup \left\langle I_2, E_2 \right\rangle := \left\langle I_1 \cup I_2, E_1 \cap E_2 \right\rangle,$$

$$\left\langle I_3, E_3 \right\rangle^{--} := \left\langle E_3, I_3 \right\rangle, \left\langle I_4, E_4 \right\rangle^{-+} := \left\langle E_4, I_4 \right\rangle,$$

$$\left\langle I_3, E_3 \right\rangle^{\approx-} := \left\langle E_3, U - E_3 \right\rangle, \left\langle I_4, E_4 \right\rangle^{\approx+} := \left\langle E_4, U - E_4 \right\rangle$$

is a bipolar de Morgan Brouwer-Zadeh distributive lattice.

## Bipolar Nelson Algebra

A *bipolar Nelson algebra*, which is a generalization of the Nelson algebra proposed to model the classical rough set approach by Pagliani (1996), is a structure of the form

$$\left\langle \pounds, \pounds^+, \pounds^-, \wedge, \vee, \rightarrow_N^{+-}, \rightarrow_N^{-+}, ^{'+}, ^{'-}, ^{o+}, ^{o-}, 0, 1 \right\rangle,$$

where

- $\rightarrow_N^{+-} : \Sigma^+ \times \Sigma^- \rightarrow \Sigma^-$ $\rightarrow_N^{-+} : \Sigma^- \times \Sigma^+ \rightarrow \Sigma^+$,

- $'^+ : \Sigma^+ \to \Sigma^-$, $'^- : \Sigma^- \to \Sigma^+$,
- $^{o+} : \pounds^+ \to \pounds^-$, $^{o-} : \pounds^- \to \pounds^+$,

satisfy the following properties:

(NLS1.1) $\langle \Sigma, \wedge, \vee, 0, 1 \rangle$ is a distributive bounded lattice,

(NLS1.2) $\langle \Sigma^+, \wedge, \vee, 0, 1 \rangle$ and $\langle \Sigma^-, \wedge, \vee, 0, 1 \rangle$, with $\Sigma^+, \Sigma^- \subseteq \Sigma$, are distributive bounded lattices,

(NLS2.1) for each $a \in \Sigma^+$, $(a'^+)'^- = a$ ,

(NLS2.2) for each $a \in \Sigma^-$, $(a'^-)'^+ = a$ ,

(NLS3.1) for cach $a, b \in \Sigma^+$, $(a \vee b)'^+ = a'^+ \wedge b'^+$

(NLS3.2) for each $a, b \in \Sigma^-$, $(a \vee b)'^- = a'^- \wedge b'^-$

(NLS4.1) for each $a \in \Sigma^+$ and $b \in \Sigma^-$, $a \wedge a'^+ \leq b \vee b'^-$ ,

(NLS4.2) for each $a \in \Sigma^+$ and $b \in \Sigma^-$, $b \wedge b'^- \leq a \vee a'^+$ ,

(NLS5.1) for each $a \in \Sigma^+$ and $b, c \in \Sigma^-$, $a \vee c \leq (a'^+ \wedge b)$ if and only if $c \leq a \to_N^{+-} b$ ,

(NLS5.2) for each $a \in \Sigma^-$ and $b, c \in \Sigma^+$, $a \vee c \leq (a'^- \wedge b)$ if and only if $c \leq a \to_N^{-+} b$ ,

(NLS6.1) for each $a, b \in \Sigma^+$ and $c \in \Sigma^-$, $a \to_N^{+-} (b \to_N^{+-} c) = (a \vee b) \to_N^{+-} c$ ,

(NLS6.2) for each $a, b \in \Sigma^-$ and $c \in \Sigma^+$, $a \to_N^{-+} (b \to_N^{-+} c) = (a \vee b) \to_N^{-+} c$ ,

(NLS7.1) for each $a \in \Sigma^+$, $a^{o+} = a \to_N^{+-} a'^+ = a \to_N^{+-} 0$ ,

(NLS7.2) for each $a \in \Sigma^-$, $a^{o-} = a \to_N^{-+} a'^- = a \to_N^{-+} 0$ .

## Theorem 6

The structure $\langle B, B^+, B^-, \sqcup, \sqcap, \Rightarrow_N^{+-}, \Rightarrow_N^{-+}, {}^{-+}, {}^{--}, {}^{+}, {}^{-}, \langle \varnothing, U \rangle, \langle U, \varnothing \rangle \rangle$, where $\Pi, \amalg, {}^{--}, {}^{-+}, {}^{\approx-}$ and ${}^{\approx+}$ are defined as in above Theorem 5, and for any $\langle I_1, E_1 \rangle \in B^+$ and $\langle I_2, E_2 \rangle \in B^-$,

$$\langle I_1, E_1 \rangle \Rightarrow_N^{+-} \langle I_2, E_2 \rangle := \langle (U - I_1) \cup I_2, I_1 \cap E_2 \rangle$$

$$\langle I_2, E_2 \rangle \Rightarrow_N^{-+} \langle I_1, E_1 \rangle := \langle (U - I_2) \cup I_1, I_2 \cap E_1 \rangle$$

$$\langle I_1, E_1 \rangle^{*+} := \langle (U - I_1), I_1) \rangle, \ \langle I_2, E_2 \rangle^{*-} := \langle (U - I_2) I_2) \rangle$$

is a bipolar Nelson algebra.

## Bipolar Heyting Algebra

A *bipolar Heyting algebra*, which is a generalization of the Heyting algebra proposed to model the classical rough set approach by Pagliani (1998), is a structure of the form

$$\left\langle \Sigma, \Sigma^+, \Sigma^-, \wedge, \vee, \to_G^{+-}, \to_G^{-+}, {}^{\circ+}, {}^{\circ-}, 0, 1 \right\rangle$$

where:

(H1.1) $\left\langle \Sigma, \wedge, \vee, 0, 1 \right\rangle$ is a distributive bounded lattice,

(H1.2) $\left\langle \Sigma^+, \wedge, \vee, 0, 1 \right\rangle$ and $\left\langle \Sigma^-, \wedge, \vee, 0, 1 \right\rangle$, with $\Sigma^+, \Sigma^- \subseteq \Sigma$, are distributive bounded lattices,

(H2.1) $\to_G^{+-} : \Sigma^+ \times \Sigma^- \to_G \Sigma^-$ is a binary operation such that, for all $a \in \Sigma^+$ and $b, c \in \Sigma^-$,

$$a \wedge c \leq b \Leftrightarrow c \leq a \to_G^{+-} b$$

(H2.2) $\to_G^{-+} : \Sigma^- \times \Sigma^+ \to_G \Sigma^+$ is a binary operation such that, for all $a \in \Sigma^-$ and $b, c \in \Sigma^+$,

$$a \wedge c \leq b \Leftrightarrow c \leq a \to_G^{+-} b$$

(H3.1) ${}^{\circ+} : \Sigma^+ \to \Sigma^-$ is a unary operation such that, for all $a \in \Sigma^+$ $a^{\circ+} = a \to_G^{+-} 0$

(H3.2) ${}^{\circ-} : \Sigma^- \to \Sigma^+$ is a unary operation such that, for all $a \in \Sigma^-$ $a^{\circ-} = a \to_G^{-+} 0$

## Theorem 7

The structure

$$\left\langle B, B^+, B^-, \prod, \amalg, \Rightarrow_G^{+-}, \Rightarrow_G^{-+}, {}^{\cdot+}, {}^{\cdot-}, \left\langle \varnothing, U \right\rangle, \left\langle U, \varnothing \right\rangle \right\rangle$$

where $\prod$ and $\amalg$ are defined as in Theorem 5, ${}^{\cdot+}$ and ${}^{\cdot-}$ are defined as in Theorem 6, and for any

$$\Sigma^+ \left\langle \Sigma^-, \wedge, \vee, 0, 1 \right\rangle \Sigma^+, \Sigma^- \subseteq \Sigma^{\sim+}, {}^{\sim-}, {}^{\circ+}, {}^{\circ-},$$
$$a \wedge a^{\sim+} \leq b \vee b^{\circ+} \left\langle \Sigma, \Sigma^+, \Sigma^-, \wedge, \vee, {}^{\prime+}, {}^{\prime-}, {}^{\nabla+}, {}^{\nabla-}, 0, 1 \right\rangle$$
$$\left\langle B, B^+, B^-, \Rightarrow_L, {}^{-+}, {}^{--}, \left\langle \varnothing, U \right\rangle, \left\langle U, \varnothing \right\rangle \right\rangle$$
$$\left\langle I_1, E_1 \right\rangle \Rightarrow_L \left\langle I_2, E_2 \right\rangle := \left\langle (U - I_1) \cap (U - E_2) \cup E_1 \cup I_2, I_1 \cap E_2 \right\rangle$$
$$G \subseteq F, I_1 \cap E_1 = \varnothing, i = 1, \ldots, n-1.$$

and $\left\langle I_2, E_2 \right\rangle \in B^-$,

$$\left\langle I_1, E_1 \right\rangle \Rightarrow_G^{+-} \left\langle I_2, E_2 \right\rangle := \left\langle (U - I_1) \cap (U - E_2) \cup E_1 \cup I_2, (U - E_1) \cap E_2 \right\rangle$$

$$\left\langle I_2, E_2 \right\rangle \Rightarrow_G^{-+} \left\langle I_1, E_1 \right\rangle := \left\langle (U - I_2) \cap (U - E_1) \cup E_2 \cup I_1, (U - E_2) \cap E_1 \right\rangle$$

is a bipolar Heyting algebra.

## Bipolar Double Stone Algebra

A *bipolar double Stone algebra*, which is a generalization of the double Stone algebra proposed to model the classical rough set approach by Pomykała & Pomykała (1988), is a structure of the form

$$\left\langle \Sigma, \Sigma^+, \Sigma^-, \wedge, \vee, ^{\sim+}, ^{\sim-}, ^{\circ+}, ^{\circ-}, 0, 1 \right\rangle$$

where:

(S1.1) $\left\langle \Sigma, \wedge, \vee, 0, 1 \right\rangle$ is a distributive bounded lattice;

(S1.2) $\left\langle \Sigma^+, \wedge, \vee, 0, 1 \right\rangle$ and $\left\langle \Sigma^-, \wedge, \vee, 0, 1 \right\rangle$, with $\Sigma^+, \Sigma^- \subseteq \Sigma$, are distributive bounded lattices;

(S2.1) $^{\sim+}: \Sigma^+ \to \Sigma^-$ is a unary operation such that, for each $a \in \Sigma^+$ and $b \in \Sigma^-$, $a \wedge a^{\sim+} = 0$ and if $a \wedge b = 0$, then $b \le a^{\sim+}$, which means that $a^{\sim+}$ is the greatest among all the elements $b \in \Sigma^-$ with the property that $a \wedge b = 0$; $a^{\sim+}$ is called the pseudo-complement of $a$;

(S2.2) $^{\sim-}: \Sigma^- \to \Sigma^+$ is a unary operation such that, for each $a \in \Sigma^-$ and $b \in \Sigma^+$, $a \wedge a^{\sim-} = 0$ and if $a \wedge b = 0$, then $b \le a^{\sim-}$, which means that $a^{\sim-}$ is the greatest among all the elements $b \in \Sigma^+$ with the property that $a \wedge b = 0$; $a^{\sim-}$ is called the pseudo-complement of $a$;

(S3.1) $^{\circ+}: \Sigma^+ \to \Sigma^-$ is a unary operation such that, for each $a \in \Sigma^+$ and $b \in \Sigma^-$, $a \vee a^{\circ+} = 1$ and if $a \vee b = 1$, then $b \ge a^{\circ+}$, which means that $a^{\circ+}$ is the smallest among all the elements $b \in \Sigma^-$ with the property that $a \vee b = 1$; $a^{\circ+}$ is called the positive dual pseudo-complement of $a$;

(S3.2) $^{\circ-}: \Sigma^+ \to \Sigma^-$ is a unary operation such that, for each $a \in \Sigma^-$ and $b \in \Sigma^+$, $a \vee a^{\circ-} = 1$ and if $a \vee b = 1$, then $b \ge a^{\circ-}$, which means that $a^{\circ-}$ is the smallest among all the elements $b \in \Sigma^+$ with the property that $a \vee b = 1$; $a^{\circ-}$ is called the negative dual pseudo-complement of $a$;

(S4.1) for each $a \in \Sigma^+$, $a^{\sim+} \vee (a^{\sim+})^{\sim-} = 1$ and $a^{\circ+} \wedge (a^{\circ+})^{\circ-} = 0$;

(S4.2) for each $a \in \Sigma^-$, $a^{\sim-} \vee (a^{\sim-})^{\sim+} = 1$ and $a^{\circ-} \wedge (a^{\circ-})^{\circ+} = 0$.

A bipolar double Stone algebra is *regular* if it satisfies the following inequalities:

(S5.1) for each $a, b \in \Sigma^+$, $a \wedge a^{\sim+} \le b \vee b^{\circ+}$;

(S5.2) for each $a, b \in \Sigma^-$, $a \wedge a^{\sim-} \le b \vee b^{\circ-}$.

## Theorem 8

The structure

$$\left\langle B, B^+, B^-, \Pi, \amalg, {}^{\approx+}, {}^{\approx-}, {}^{\cdot+}, {}^{\cdot-}, \langle \varnothing, U \rangle, \langle U, \varnothing \rangle \right\rangle,$$

where $\Pi, \amalg, {}^{\approx-}$ and ${}^{\approx+}$ are defined as in Theorem 5, and ${}^{\cdot+}$ and ${}^{\cdot-}$ are defined as in Theorem 6, is a bipolar regular double Stone algebra.

## Bipolar Three-Valued Łukasiewicz Algebra

A *bipolar* three-*valued Łukasiewicz algebra*, which is a generalization of the Łukasiewicz algebra proposed to model the classical rough set approach by Pagliani (1998), is a structure of the form

$$\left\langle \Sigma, \Sigma^+, \Sigma^-, \wedge, \vee, {}^{\prime+}, {}^{\prime-}, {}^{\nabla+}, {}^{\nabla-}, 0, 1 \right\rangle,$$

where:

(Ł1.1) $\left\langle \Sigma, \wedge, \vee, 0, 1 \right\rangle$ is a distributive bounded lattice;

(Ł1.1) $\left\langle \Sigma^+, \wedge, \vee, 0, 1 \right\rangle$ and $\left\langle \Sigma^-, \wedge, \vee, 0, 1 \right\rangle$, with $\Sigma^+, \Sigma^- \subseteq \Sigma$, are distributive bounded lattices;

(Ł2) ${}^{\prime+}: \Sigma^+ \to \Sigma^-$ and ${}^{\prime-}: \Sigma^- \to \Sigma^+$ are de Morgan complements, that is unary operations that, for each $a, b \in \Sigma^+$ and $c, d \in \Sigma^-$, $(a \vee b)^{\prime+} = a^{\prime+} \wedge b^{\prime+}$, $(c \vee d)^{\prime-} = c^{\prime-} \wedge d^{\prime-}$, $(a^{\prime+})^{\prime-} = a$ and $(c^{\prime+})^{\prime-} = c$;

(Ł3) ${}^{\nabla+}: \Sigma^+ \to \Sigma^-$ and ${}^{\nabla-}: \Sigma^- \to \Sigma^+$ are unary operations that, for all $a, b \in \Sigma^+$ and $c, d \in \Sigma^-$, satisfy the following conditions:

- $a^{\prime+} \vee a^{\nabla+} = 1$, $c^{\prime-} \vee c^{\nabla-} = 1$,
- $a^{\prime+} \wedge a = a^{\prime+} \wedge a^{\nabla+}$, $c^{\prime-} \wedge c = c^{\prime-} \wedge c^{\nabla-}$
- $(a \wedge b)^{\nabla+} = a^{\nabla+} \wedge b^{\nabla+}$ $(c \wedge d)^{\nabla-} = c^{\nabla-} \wedge d^{\nabla-}$.

## Theorem 9

The structure

$$\left\langle B, B^+, B^-, \Pi, \amalg, {}^{-+}, {}^{--}, {}^{\partial+}, {}^{\partial-}, \langle \varnothing, U \rangle, \langle U, \varnothing \rangle \right\rangle,$$

where $\Pi, \amalg, {}^{-+}$ and ${}^{--}$ are defined as in above Theorem 5, and for any and $\left\langle I_2, E_2 \right\rangle \in B^-$,

$$\left\langle I_1, E_1 \right\rangle^{\partial+} := \left\langle (U - E_1), E_1 \right\rangle \left\langle I_2, E_2 \right\rangle^{\partial-} := \left\langle (U - E_2), E_2 \right\rangle$$

is a bipolar three-valued Łukasiewicz algebra.

## Bipolar Wajsberg Algebra

A *bipolar Wajsberg algebra*, which is a generalization of the Wajsberg algebra proposed to model the classical rough set approach by Polkowski (2002), is a structure of the form

$$\left\langle \Sigma, \Sigma^+, \Sigma^-, \rightarrow_L, '+, '-, 0, 1 \right\rangle$$

where, $\Sigma^+, \Sigma^- \subseteq \Sigma \rightarrow_L: \Sigma \times \Sigma \rightarrow \Sigma$, $'+: \Sigma^+ \rightarrow \Sigma^-$ $'-: \Sigma^- \rightarrow \Sigma^+$ satisfy the following axioms: for all, $a, b, c \in \Sigma$ $d \in \Sigma^+, e \in \Sigma^-$

(W1) $1 \rightarrow_L a$,

(W2) $(a \rightarrow_L b) \rightarrow_L ((b \rightarrow_L c) \rightarrow_L (a \rightarrow_L c)) = 1$

(W3) $(a \rightarrow_L b) \rightarrow_L b = (b \rightarrow_L a) \rightarrow_L a$,

(W4.1) $(e^{'-} \rightarrow_L d^{'+}) \rightarrow_L (d \rightarrow_L e) = 1$,

(W4.2) $(d^{'+} \rightarrow_L e^{'-}) \rightarrow_L (e \rightarrow_L d) = 1$.

## Theorem 10

The structure

$$\left\langle B, B^+, B^-, \Rightarrow_L, {}^{-+}, {}^{--}, \left\langle \varnothing, U \right\rangle, \left\langle U, \varnothing \right\rangle \right\rangle$$

where $^{-+}$ and $^{--}$ are defined as in above Theorem 5, and for any $\left\langle I_1, E_1 \right\rangle, \left\langle I_2, E_2 \right\rangle \in B$,

$$\left\langle I_1, E_1 \right\rangle \Rightarrow_L \left\langle I_2, E_2 \right\rangle := \left\langle (U - I_1) \cap (U - E_2) \cup E_1 \cup I_2, I_1 \cap E_2 \right\rangle$$

is a bipolar Wajsberg algebra.

## An Algebra for Ordinal Classification

We consider a universe $U$. $n^u$ is the set of all ordered partitions of $U$ into $n$ classes, i.e.,

$$n^u = \left\{ \left\langle X_1, \dots, X_n \right\rangle : X_1, \dots, X_n \subseteq U, \bigcup_{i=1}^{n} X_i = U, X_i \cap X_j = \varnothing \forall i, j = 1, \dots, n \right\}$$

Observe that $\left\langle X_1, \ldots, X_n \right\rangle$ can be identified with the set of decision classes $\mathbf{Cl} = \left\{ Cl_1, \ldots, Cl_n \right\}$

We consider also the following set $\boldsymbol{B}$, whose elements are $\left\langle I_1, \ldots I_{n-1}, E_1, \ldots, E_{n-1} \right\rangle$, where $I_1, E_1 \subseteq U, I_1 \cap E_1 = \varnothing, i = 1, \ldots, n-1..$

Given $\left\langle X_1, \ldots, X_n \right\rangle \in n^u$, we define upward unions $X^{\geq i}$ and downward unions $X^{\leq i}$, $i = 1, \ldots n$ as follows:

$$X^{\geq i} = \bigcup_{j=1}^{n} X_j, X^{\leq i} = \bigcup_{j=1}^{i} X_j .$$

Fixed $G \subseteq F$, we define sets $B^+$ and $B^-$ as follows:

$$B^+ = \left\{ \left\langle G^{(>)}(X^{\geq i}), i = 2, \ldots, n; U - \bar{G}^{(>)}(X^{\geq i}), i = 2, \ldots, n \right\rangle : \left\langle X_1, \ldots, X_n \right\rangle \in n^u \right\}$$

$$B^- = \left\{ \left\langle G^{(<)}(X^{\leq i}), i = 1, \ldots, n-1; U - \bar{G}^{(<)}(X^{\leq i}), i = 1, \ldots, n-1 \right\rangle : \left\langle X_1, \ldots, X_n \right\rangle \in n^u \right\}$$

## Theorem 11

The structure

$$\left\langle B, B^+, B^-, \Pi, \sqcup, ^{--}, ^{-+}, ^{\approx-}, ^{\approx+}, \left\langle \varnothing, \ldots, \varnothing; U, \ldots, U \right\rangle, \left\langle U, \ldots, U; \varnothing, \ldots, \varnothing \right\rangle \right\rangle$$

where for any $\left\langle I_1^1, \ldots, I_{n-1}^1; E_1^1, \ldots, E_{n-1}^1 \right\rangle, \left\langle I_1^2, \ldots, I_{n-1}^2; E_1^2, \ldots, E_{n-1}^2 \right\rangle \in B$

$\left\langle I_1^3, \ldots, I_{n-1}^3; E_1^3, \ldots, E_{n-1}^3 \right\rangle \in B^-$, $\left\langle I_1^4, \ldots, I_{n-1}^4; E_1^4, \ldots, E_{n-1}^4 \right\rangle \in B^+$,

$$\left\langle I_1^1, \ldots, I_{n-1}^1; E_1^1, \ldots, E_{n-1}^1 \right\rangle \Pi \left\langle I_1^2, \ldots, I_{n-1}^2; E_1^2, \ldots, E_{n-1}^2 \right\rangle :=$$

$$\left\langle I_1^1 \cap I_1^2, \ldots, I_{n-1}^1 \cap I_{n-1}^2; E_1^1 \cup E_1^2, \ldots, E_{n-1}^1 \cup E_{n-1}^2 \right\rangle$$

$$\left\langle I_1^1, \ldots, I_{n-1}^1; E_1^1, \ldots, E_{n-1}^1 \right\rangle \sqcup \left\langle I_1^2, \ldots, I_{n-1}^2; E_1^2, \ldots, E_n^2 \right\rangle :=$$

$$\left\langle I_1^1 \cup I_1^2, \ldots, I_{n-1}^1 \cup I_{n-1}^2; E_1^2 \cap E_1^2, \ldots, E_{n-1}^1 \cap E_{n-1}^2 \right\rangle$$

$$\left\langle I_1^3, \ldots, I_{n-1}^3; E_1^3, \ldots, E_{n-1}^3 \right\rangle^{--} := \left\langle E_1^3, \ldots, E_{n-1}^3; I_1^3, \ldots, I_{n-1}^3 \right\rangle$$

$$\left\langle I_1^4, \ldots, I_{n-1}^4; E_1^4, \ldots, E_{n-1}^4 \right\rangle^{-+} := \left\langle E_1^4, \ldots, E_{n-1}^4; I_1^4, \ldots, I_{n-1}^4 \right\rangle$$

$$\left\langle I_1^3,\ldots,I_{n-1}^3;E_1^3,\ldots,E_{n-1}^3\right\rangle^{\approx-} := \left\langle E_1^3,\ldots,E_{n-1}^3;U-E_1^3\ldots,U-E_{n-1}^3\right\rangle$$

$$\left\langle I_1^4,\ldots,I_{n-1}^4;E_1^4,\ldots,E_{n-1}^4\right\rangle^{\approx+} := \left\langle E_1^4,\ldots,E_{n-1}^4;U-E_1^4\ldots,U-E_{n-1}^4\right\rangle$$

is a bipolar de Morgan Brouwer-Zadeh distributive lattice.

## BIPOLAR APPROXIMATION SPACE INDUCED FROM BIPOLAR QUASI BROUWER-ZADEH LATTICE

The bipolar generalized approximation space is an abstraction of the standard way to deal with roughness within DRSA. Now, we show how a structure of this type can be induced from any bipolar quasi Brouwer-Zadeh lattice (Greco et al., 2008b). Making use of the Kleene complementations $'^+$ and $'^-$, and of the two Brouwer complementations $\sim^+$ and $\sim^-$, it is possible to define the mappings

$$^{\beta+}: a \in \Sigma^+ \mapsto a^{\beta+} := a'^{+\sim-'^+} \in \Sigma^-$$

and

$$^{\beta-}: a \in \Sigma^- \mapsto a^{\beta-} := a'^{-\sim+'^-} \in \Sigma^+,$$

which are anticomplementations, i.e., for any $a,b \in \Sigma^+$ and $c,d \in \Sigma^-$:

$$a^{\beta+\beta-} \le a,\ c^{\beta-\beta+} \le c,$$

$$a \le b \text{ implies } b^{\beta+} \le a^{\beta+},\ c \le d \text{ implies } d^{\beta-} \le c^{\beta-},$$

$$a \vee a^{\beta+} = 1,\ c \vee c^{\beta-} = 1.$$

For any $a \in \Sigma^+$ and any $b \in \Sigma^-$, we have

$$a^{\sim+} \le a'^+ \le a^{\beta+},\ b^{\sim-} \le b'^- \le b^{\beta-}.$$

The following statements are equivalent for a fixed element $a \in \Sigma^+$:

$$a^{\sim+} = a'^+, a = a'^{+\sim-}, a^{\sim+\sim-} = a'^{+\sim-}, a = a^{\sim+'^-}$$

Moreover, the following logical implication holds for a fixed element $a \in \Sigma^+$:

$$a^{\sim+} = a'^{+} \Rightarrow [a = a^{\beta+\beta-} = a^{\sim+\sim-}]$$

Analogously, for a fixed element $b \in \Sigma^{-}$,

$$b^{\sim-} = b'^{-}, b = b'^{-\sim+}, b^{\sim-\sim+} = b'^{-\sim+}, b = b^{\sim-'+},$$

and the following logical implication holds

$$b^{\sim-} = b'^{-} \Rightarrow [b = b^{\beta-\beta+} = b^{\sim-\sim+}].$$

We can introduce the following sets:

- the set of all *upward exact* elements

$$\Sigma_{e}^{+} := \left\{ f \in \Sigma^{+} : f'^{+} = f^{\sim+} \right\},$$

- the set of all *downward exact* elements

$$\Sigma_{e}^{-} := \left\{ f \in \Sigma^{-} : f'^{-} = f^{\sim-} \right\},$$

- the set of all *upward open* elements

$$\Sigma_{o}^{+} := \left\{ f \in \Sigma^{+} : f = f^{\beta+\beta-} \right\},$$

- the set of all *downward open* elements

$$\Sigma_{o}^{-} := \left\{ f \in \Sigma^{-} : f = f^{\beta-\beta+} \right\},$$

- the set of all *upward closed* elements

$$\Sigma_{c}^{+} := \left\{ f \in \Sigma^{+} : f = f^{\sim+\sim-} \right\},$$

- the set of all *downward closed* elements

$$\Sigma_{c}^{-} := \left\{ f \in \Sigma^{-} : f = f^{\sim-\sim+} \right\},$$

- the set of all *upward clopen* elements $\Sigma_{co}^{+} = \Sigma_{c}^{+} \cap \Sigma_{o}^{+}$,

- the set of all *downward clopen* elements $\Sigma_{co}^- = \Sigma_c^- \cap \Sigma_o^+$.

We also have

$$\Sigma_e^+ \subseteq \Sigma_{co}^+, \Sigma_e^- \subseteq \Sigma_{co}^-,$$

$$\Sigma_o^+ = \left\{ f \in \Sigma^+ : f' \in \Sigma_c^- \right\} \Sigma_o^- = \left\{ f \in \Sigma^- : f' \in \Sigma_c^+ \right\},$$

$$\Sigma_c^+ = \left\{ f \in \Sigma^+ : f' \in \Sigma_o^- \right\} \Sigma_c^- = \left\{ f \in \Sigma^- : f' \in \Sigma_o^+ \right\}.$$

Observe that in any bipolar quasi Brouwer-Zadeh lattice we have that, for any $a \in \Sigma^+$ and for any $b \in \Sigma^-$: $a'^{+\sim-}, a^{\sim+\sim-}, \in \Sigma_c^+$, $a^{\beta+\beta-}, a^{\sim+'-}, \in \Sigma_o^+$, $b'^{\sim+}, b^{\sim-\sim+}, \in \Sigma_c^-$, and $b^{\beta-\beta+}, a^{\sim-'+}, \in \Sigma_o^-$. On the basis of these results, eight further unary operators can be introduced:

$$v^+ : a \in \Sigma^+ \mapsto v^+(a) := a'^{+\sim-} \in \Sigma_c^+, \text{ (upward necessity)}$$

$$v^- : a \in \Sigma^- \mapsto v^-(a) := a'^{-\sim+} \in \Sigma_c^-, \text{ (downward necessity)}$$

$$I^+ : a \in \Sigma^+ \mapsto I^+(a) := a^{\beta+\beta-} \in \Sigma_o^+, \text{ (upward interior)}$$

$$I^- : a \in \Sigma^- \mapsto I^-(a) := a^{\beta-\beta+} \in \Sigma_o^-, \text{ (downward interior)}$$

$$C^+ : a \in \Sigma^+ \mapsto C^+(a) := a^{\sim+\sim-} \in \Sigma_c^+, \text{ (upward closure)}$$

$$C^- : a \in \Sigma^- \mapsto C^-(a) := a^{\sim-\sim+} \in \Sigma_o^-, \text{ (downward closure)}$$

$$\mu^+ : a \in \Sigma^+ \mapsto \mu^+(a) := a^{\sim+'-} \in \Sigma_o^+, \text{ (upward possibility)}$$

$$\mu^- : a \in \Sigma^- \mapsto \mu^-(a) := a^{\sim-'+} \in \Sigma_o^-. \text{ (downward possibility)}$$

According to the above definitions, the complementations $^{\sim+}$, $^{\sim-}$, $^{\beta+}$ and $^{\beta-}$ can be interpreted as follows: $a^{\sim+} = \mu^+(a)'^+$ (upward impossibility), $a^{\sim-} = \mu^-(a)'^-$ (downward impossibility), $a^{\beta+} = v^+(a)'^+$ (upward contingency) and $a^{\beta-} = v^-(a)'^-$ (downward contingency).

In any bipolar quasi Brouwer-Zadeh lattice, the mappings

$$I^+ : \Sigma^+ \to \Sigma_o^+, a \mapsto I^+(a) = a^{\beta+\beta-}$$

and

$$I^- : \Sigma^- \to \Sigma_o^-, a \mapsto I^-(a) = a^{\beta - \beta +}$$

are *inner* (normalized, decreasing, idempotent and monotone) operations, i.e., the following holds:

$$1 = I^+(1), 1 = I^-(1)$$

$$\forall a \in \Sigma^+, I^+(a) \le a, \forall b \in \Sigma^-, I^-(b) \le b$$

$$\forall a \in \Sigma^+, I^+(a) = I^+(I^+(a)), \forall b \in \Sigma^-, I^-(b) = I^-(I^-(b))$$

$\forall a, b \in \Sigma^+, a \le b$ implies $I^+(a) \le I^+(b), \forall a, b \in \Sigma^-, a \le b$ implies $I^-(a) \le I^-(b)$ such that for all $a \in \Sigma^+$ and for all $b \in \Sigma^-$:

$$I^+(a) = \vee\left\{ f \in \Sigma_o^+ : f \le a \right\} I^-(b) = \vee\left\{ f \in \Sigma_o^- : f \le b \right\}.$$

In any bipolar quasi Brouwer-Zadeh lattice, the mappings

$$C^+ : \Sigma^+ \to \Sigma_c^+, a \mapsto C^+(a) = a^{\sim + \sim -}$$

and

$$C^- : \Sigma^- \to \Sigma_c^-, a \mapsto C^-(a) = a^{\sim - \sim +}$$

are *outer* (normalized, increasing, idempotent and monotone) operations, i.e., the following holds:

$$0 = C^+(0), 0 = C^-(0),$$

$$\forall a \in \Sigma^+, a \le C^+(a), \forall b \in \Sigma^-, b \le C^-(b),$$

$$\forall a \in \Sigma^+, C^+(a) = C^+(C^+(a)), \forall b \in \Sigma^-, C^-(b) = C^-(C^-(b))$$

$$\forall a, b \in \Sigma^+, a \le b \text{ implies } C^+(a) \le C^+(b), \forall a, b \in \Sigma^-, a \le b \text{ implies } C^-(a) \le C^-(b)$$

such that for all $a \in \Sigma^+$ and for all $b \in \Sigma^-$:

$$C^+(a) = \wedge\left\{ f \in \Sigma_c^+ : f \le a \right\} C^-(b) = \wedge\left\{ f \in \Sigma_c^- : f \le b \right\}$$

Let $\left\langle \Sigma, \Sigma^+, \Sigma^-, \wedge, \vee,^{'+},^{'-},^{\sim +},^{\sim -}, 0, 1 \right\rangle$ be a bipolar complemented quasi Brouwer-Zadeh distributive lattice. Then, the structure

$$\left\langle \left\langle \Sigma, \Sigma^{+}, \Sigma^{-}, \leq, '^{+}, '^{-}, 0 \right\rangle, \Sigma_{o}^{+}, \Sigma_{o}^{-}, \Sigma_{c}^{+}, \Sigma_{c}^{-}, I^{+}, I^{-}, C^{+}, C^{-} \right\rangle$$

is a bipolar approximation space with respect to: the set of upward open definable elements $O(\Sigma^{+})^{+} = \Sigma_{c}^{+}$; the set of downward open definable elements $O(\Sigma^{-})^{-} = \Sigma_{c}^{-}$; the set of upward closed definable elements $C(\Sigma^{+})^{+} = \Sigma_{c}^{+}$; the set of downward closed definable elements $C(\Sigma^{-})^{-} = \Sigma_{c}^{-}$; the upward inner approximation mapping $i^{+}(a) = I^{+}(a) = a^{\beta+\beta-}$; the downward inner approximation mapping $i^{-}(a) = I^{-}(a) = a^{\beta-\beta+}$; the upward outer approximation mapping $o^{+}(a) = C^{+}(a) = a^{\sim+\sim-}$; the downward outer approximation mapping $o^{-}(a) = C^{-}(a) = a^{\sim-\sim+}$. Observe that for all $a \in \Sigma^{+}$, $I^{+}(a) = (C^{-}(a'^{+}))'^{-}$, and for all $b \in \Sigma^{-}$, $I^{-}(b) = (C^{+}(b'^{-}))'^{+}$.

In any bipolar quasi Brouwer-Zadeh lattice, the following chains of inclusions hold for all $a \in \Sigma^{+}$ and $b \in \Sigma^{-}$:

$$v^{+}(a) \leq I^{+}(a) \leq a \leq C^{+}(a) \leq \mu^{+}(a),$$

$$v^{-}(b) \leq I^{-}(b) \leq b \leq C^{-}(b) \leq \mu^{-}(b).$$

## CONCLUSION

This article provides arguments for the claim that the Dominance-based Rough Set Approach (DRSA) is a proper way of handling monotonically ordered data in granular computing. Referring to some ideas of Leibniz, Frege, Boole and Łukasiewicz, DRSA represents fundamental concepts of rough set theory in terms of a generalization that takes into account ordinal properties of data, permitting to deal with the graduality of fuzzy sets. DRSA in the context of ordinal classification, its fuzzy extension, and a rough probabilistic model of DRSA (Variable Consistency − Dominance-based Rough Set Approach) have been presented. Moreover, dominance-based rough approximation of a fuzzy set has been discussed, which infers the most cautious conclusions from available imprecise information; otherwise than almost all known fuzzy rough set approaches, the dominance-based rough approximation of a fuzzy set does not require any fuzzy connective which is always arbitrary to some extent.

Knowledge induced from dominance-based rough approximations of fuzzy sets, or more generally, from ordinal data, is represented in terms of gradual decision rules. The dominance-based rough approximations of fuzzy sets generalize the classical rough approximations of crisp sets, as proved by showing that the classical rough set approach is one of its particular cases. Due to considering only ordinal character of the graduality of fuzzy sets, and due to eliminating all fuzzy connectives, the dominance-based rough approximations of fuzzy sets give a new insight into both rough sets and fuzzy sets, and enable further generalizations of both of them. The recently proposed DRSA for fuzzy case-based reasoning is an example of this capacity. This article also exhibits some important merits of DRSA within granular computing, which can be summarized as follows:

- DRSA extends the paradigm of granular computing to problems involving ordered data,
- it specifies a syntax and modality of information granules, defined by means of dominance-based constraints, which are appropriate for dealing with ordered data,
- it provides a methodology for dealing with this type of information granules, which results in a theory of computing with words and reasoning about ordered data,
- it is supported by several robust and meaningful algebraic models and this ensures the solidity of the obtained results.

The granular computing with ordered data is a very general problem, because also other modalities of information constraints, such as veristic, possibilistic and probabilistic modalities, have to deal with ordered value sets (with qualifiers relative to grades of truth, possibility and probability). For this reason, granular computing with ordered data based on DRSA is a very rich and promising research field. There is a great potential in both theoretical investigations, such as extension to DRSA of a topological and logical approaches or further algebraic structures (for a general survey of logic, algebra and topology for rough set theory see Pagliani & Chakraborty (2008); Polkowski (2002)), and practical applications. In fact, there are many possibilities of applying DRSA to real life problems. The non-exhaustive list of potential applications includes:

- decision support in medicine: in this area there are already many interesting applications (see, e.g., Michałowski et al. (2003, 2005); Pawlak et al. (1986); Wilk et al. (2005)), however, they exploit the classical rough set approach; applications requiring DRSA, which handle ordered value sets of medical signs, as well as monotonic relationship between the value of signs and the degree of gravity of a disease, are in progress;
- customer satisfaction survey: theoretical foundations for application of DRSA in this field are available in Greco et al. (2007a), however, a fully documented application is still missing;
- bankruptcy risk evaluation: this is a field of many potential applications, as can be seen from promising results reported, e.g., by Greco et al. (1998); Słowiński & Zopounidis (1995); Słowiński et al. (1997), however, a wider comparative study involving real data sets is needed;
- operational research problems, such as location, routing, scheduling or inventory management: these are problems formulated either in terms of classification of feasible solutions (see, e.g., Gorsevski & Jankowski (2008)), or in terms of interactive multiobjective optimization, for which the IMO-DRSA (Greco et al., 2008c) procedure is suitable;
- finance: this is a domain where DRSA for decision under uncertainty has to be combined with interactive multiobjective optimization using IMO-DRSA; some promising results going in this direction have been presented by Greco et al. (2007c);
- ecology: assessment of the impact of human activity on the ecosystem is a challenging problem for which the presented methodology is suitable; the up to date applications are based on the classical rough set concept (see, e.g., Flinkman et al. (2000); Rossi et al. (1999)), however, it seems that DRSA handling ordinal data has a greater potential in this field (for some first results see Boggia et al. (2007)).

## ACKNOWLEDGMENT

The third author wishes to acknowledge financial support from the Ministry of Science and Higher Education, grant N N519 314435.

## REFERENCES

Bargiela, A., & Pedrycz, W. (2008). Toward a theory of granular computing for human-centered information processing. *IEEE Transactions on Fuzzy Systems, 16*(2), 320–330.

Boggia, A., Greco, S., & Nuciarelli, N. (2007). Assessing rural sustainable development potentialities by Dominance-based Rough Set Approach. Invited paper presented at the *22nd European Conference on Operational Research (EURO XXII)*, Prague, Czech Republic.

Cattaneo, G., & Ciucci, D. (2004). Algebraic structures for rough sets. In Transactions on Rough Sets II, (volume 3135 of Lecture Notes in Computer Science, pp. 208-252). Berlin, Germany: Springer.

Cattaneo, G., & Nisticó, G. (1989). Brouwer-Zadeh posets and three-valued Łukasiewicz posets. *Fuzzy Sets and Systems, 33*(2), 165–190.

Dubois, D., & Prade, H. (1990). Rough fuzzy sets and fuzzy rough sets. *Internet. J. General Systems, 17*, 191–209.

Dubois, D., & Prade, H. (1992). Putting rough sets and fuzzy sets together. In Słowiński, R. (Ed.), *Intelligent Decision Support - Handbook of Applications and Advances of the Rough Sets Theory* (pp. 203–232). Boston: Kluwer Academic Publishers.

Dubois, D., Prade, H., Esteva, F., Garcia, P., Godo, L., & Lopez De Mantaras, R. (1998). Fuzzy set modelling in case-based reasoning. *International Journal of Intelligent Systems, 13*(4), 345–373.

Fan, T. F., Liu, D. R., & Tzeng, G. H. (2007). Rough set-based logics for multicriteria decision analysis. *European Journal of Operational Research, 182*(1), 340–355.

Flinkman, M., Michałowski, W., Nilsson, S., Słowiński, R., Susmaga, R., & Wilk, S. (2000). Use of rough sets analysis to classify siberian forest ecosystems according to net primary production of phytomass. *INFOR, 38*(3), 145–161.

Fodor, J., & Roubens, M. (1994). *Fuzzy Preference Modelling and Multicriteria Decision Support.* Boston: Kluwer Academic Publishers.

Gilboa, I., & Schmeidler, D. (2001). *A Theory of Case-Based Decisions.* Cambridge, UK: Cambridge University Press.

Gorsevski, P. V., & Jankowski, P. (2008). Discerning landslide susceptibility using rough sets. *Computers, Environment and Urban Systems, 32*(1), 53–65.

Greco, S., Inuiguchi, M., & Słowiński, R. (2002). Dominance-based Rough Set Approach using possibility and necessity measures. In J. J. Alpigini, J. F. Peters, A. Skowron, & N. Zhong (Eds.), Rough Sets and Current Trends in Computing, (volume 2475 of Lecture Notes in Artificial Intelligence, pp. 85-92). Berlin, Germany: Springer-Verlag.

Greco, S., Inuiguchi, M., & Słowiński, R. (2004a). A new proposal for rough fuzzy approximations and decision rule representation. In D. Dubois, J. Grzymała-Busse, M. Inuiguchi, & L. Polkowski (Eds.), Transactions on Rough Sets II: Rough Sets and Fuzzy Sets, (volume 3135 of Lecture Notes in Computer Science, pp. 156-164). Berlin, Germany: Springer.

Greco, S., Inuiguchi, M., & Słowiński, R. (2006a). Fuzzy rough sets and multiple-premise gradual decision rules. *International Journal of Approximate Reasoning, 41*(2), 179–211.

Greco, S., Matarazzo, B., & Słowiński, R. (1998). A new rough set approach to evaluation of bankruptcy risk. In Zopounidis, C. (Ed.), *Operational tools in the management of financial risks* (pp. 121–136). Dordrecht, The Netherlands: Kluwer Academic Publishers.

Greco, S., Matarazzo, B., & Słowiński, R. (1999). The use of rough sets and fuzzy sets in MCDM. In Gal, T., Stewart, T., & Hanne, T. (Eds.), *Advances in Multiple Criteria Decision Making* (pp. 14.1–14.59). Boston: Kluwer Academic Publishers.

Greco, S., Matarazzo, B., & Słowiński, R. (2001a). Rough sets theory for multicriteria decision analysis. *European Journal of Operational Research, 129*(1), 1–47.

Greco, S., Matarazzo, B., & Słowiński, R. (2004b). Dominance-based Rough Set Approach to Knowledge Discovery (I) – General Perspective. In Zhong, N., & Liu, J. (Eds.), *Intelligent Technologies for Information Analysis* (pp. 513–552). Berlin, Germany: Springer-Verlag.

Greco, S., Matarazzo, B., & Słowiński, R. (2004c). Dominance-based Rough Set Approach to Knowledge Discovery (II) – Extensions and Applications. In Zhong, N., & Liu, J. (Eds.), *Intelligent Technologies for Information Analysis* (pp. 553–612). Berlin, Germany: Springer-Verlag.

Greco, S., Matarazzo, B., & Słowiński, R. (2005a). Decision rule approach. In Figueira, J., Greco, S., & Ehrgott, M. (Eds.), *Multiple Criteria Decision Analysis: State of the Art Surveys* (pp. 507–563). Berlin, Germany: Springer-Verlag.

Greco, S., Matarazzo, B., & Słowiński, R. (2005b). Generalizing rough set theory through Dominance-based Rough Set Approach. In D. Ślęzak, J. T. Yao, J. Peters, W. Ziarko, & X. Hu (Eds.), Rough Sets, Fuzzy Sets, Data Mining, and Granular Computing, (volume 3642 of Lecture Notes in Artificial Intelligence, pp. 1-11). Berlin, Germany: Springer-Verlag.

Greco, S., Matarazzo, B., & Słowiński, R. (2006b). Dominance-based Rough Set Approach to Case-based Reasoning. In V. Torra, Y. Narukawa, A. Valls, & J. Domingo-Ferrer (Eds.), Modelling Decisions for Artificial Intelligence, (volume 3885 of Lecture Notes in Artificial Intelligence, pp. 7-18). Berlin, Germany: Springer-Verlag.

Greco, S., Matarazzo, B., & Słowiński, R. (2007a). Customer satisfaction analysis based on rough set approach. *Zeitschrift für Betriebswirtschaft, 16*(3), 325–339.

Greco, S., Matarazzo, B., & Słowiński, R. (2007b). Dominance-based Rough Set Approach as a proper way of handling graduality in rough set theory. In Transactions on Rough Sets VII, (volume 4400 of Lecture Notes in Artificial Intelligence, pp. 36-52). Berlin, Germany: Springer-Verlag.

Greco, S., Matarazzo, B., & Słowiński, R. (2007c). Financial portfolio decision analysis using Dominance-based Rough Set Approach. Invited paper presented at the *22nd European Conference on Operational Research (EURO XXII)*, Prague, Czech Republic.

Greco, S., Matarazzo, B., & Słowiński, R. (2008a). Algebraic structures for Dominance-based Rough Set Approach. In G. Wang, T.-r. Li, J. W. Grzymała-Busse, D. Miao, A. Skowron, & Y. Yao (Eds.), Rough Sets and Knowledge Technology, (volume 5009 of Lecture Notes in Artificial Intelligence, pp. 252-259). Berlin, Germany: Springer.

Greco, S., Matarazzo, B., & Słowiński, R. (2008b). Dominance-based Rough Set Approach and Bipolar Abstract Approximation Spaces. In R. Goebel, J. Siekmann, & W. Wahlster (Eds.), Rough Sets and Current Trends in Computing, (volume 5306 of Lecture Notes in Artificial Intelligence (pp. 31-40). Berlin, Germany: Springer.

Greco, S., Matarazzo, B., & Słowiński, R. (2008c). Dominance-based Rough Set Approach to Interactive Multiobjective Optimization. In Branke, J., Deb, K., Miettinen, K., & Słowiński, R. (Eds.), *Multiobjective Optimization: Interactive and Evolutionary Approaches* (pp. 121–155). Berlin, Germany: Springer.

Greco, S., Matarazzo, B., Słowiński, R., & Stefanowski, J. (2001b). Variable consistency model of dominance-based rough set approach. In W. Ziarko & Y. Yao (Eds.), Rough Sets and Current Trends in Computing, (volume 2005 of Lecture Notes in Artificial Intelligence, pp. 170-181). Berlin, Germany: Springer.

Hume, D. (1748). *An Enquiry Concerning Human Understanding*. Oxford, UK: Clarendon Press.

Inuiguchi, M., Yoshioka, Y., & Kusunoki, Y. (2009). (in press). Variable-precision dominance-based rough set approach and attribute reduction. *International Journal of Approximate Reasoning*.

Klement, E. P., Mesiar, R., & Pap, E. (2000). *Triangular Norms*. Dordrecht, The Netherlands: Kluwer Academic Publishers.

Kolodner, J. (1993). *Case-Based Reasoning*. San Francisco: Morgan Kaufmann.

Leake, D. (1996). CBR in context: The present and future. In Leake, D. (Ed.), *Case-Based Reasoning: Experiences, Lessons, and Future Directions* (pp. 1–30). Menlo Park, CA: AAAI Press.

Lin, T. Y. (1998a). Granular Computing on Binary Relations I: Data mining and Neighborhood Systems. In Skowron, A., & Polkowski, L. (Eds.), *Rough Sets in Knowledge Discovery* (pp. 107–121). Heidelberg, Germany: Physica-Verlag.

Lin, T. Y. (1998b). Granular Computing on Binary Relations II: Rough Set Representations and Belief Functions. In Skowron, A., & Polkowski, L. (Eds.), *Rough Sets in Knowledge Discovery* (pp. 121–140). Heidelberg: Physica-Verlag.

Liu, Y. B., Liu, D. Y., & Gao, Y. (2006). Mining dominance association rules in preference-ordered data. In Liu, G., Tan, V., & Han, X. (Eds.), *Computational Methods* (pp. 1261–1266). Berlin, Germany: Springer.

Loemker, L., & Leibniz, G. W. (1969). Philosophical Papers and Letters. Dordrecht: D. Reidel, 2 edition.

Michałowski, W., Rubin, S., Słowiński, R., & Wilk, S. (2003). Mobile clinical support system for pediatric emergencies. *Journal of Decision Support Systems*, *36*, 161–176.

Michałowski, W., Wilk, S., Farion, K., Pike, J., Rubin, S., & Słowiński, R. (2005). Development of a decision algorithm to support emergency triage of scrotal pain and its implementation in the MET system. *INFOR*, *43*(4), 287–301.

Pagliani, P. (1996). Rough sets and Nelson algebras. *Fundamenta Informaticae*, *27*(2-3), 205–219.

Pagliani, P. (1998). Rough set theory and logic-algebraic structures. In Orłowska, E. (Ed.), *Incomplete Information: Rough Set Analysis* (pp. 109–190). Heidelberg, Germany: Physica-Verlag.

Pagliani, P., & Chakraborty, M. (2008). *A Geometry of Approximation: Rough Set Theory: Logic, Algebra and Topology of Conceptual Patterns*. Berlin, Germany: Springer.

Pawlak, Z. (1982). Rough sets. *International Journal of Computer and Information Sciences*, *11*, 341–356.

Pawlak, Z. (1991). *Rough Sets*. Dordrecht, The Netherlands: Kluwer Academic Publishers.

Pawlak, Z. (2001). Rough Set Theory. *Kunstliche Intelligenz*, *3*, 38–39.

Pawlak, Z., Słowiński, K., & Słowiński, R. (1986). Rough classification of patients after highly selective vagotomy for duodenal ulcer. *International Journal of Man-Machine Studies*, *24*, 413–433.

Polkowski, L. (2002). *Rough set: mathematical foundations*. Heidelberg, Germany: Physica-Verlag.

Pomykała, J., & Pomykała, J. A. (1988). The Stone algebra of rough sets. *Bulletin of the Polish Academy of Sciences. Mathematics*, *36*, 495–508.

Qian, Y., Dang, C., Liang, J., & Tang, D. (2009). Set-valued ordered information systems. *Information Sciences*, *179*, 2809–2832.

Rossi, L., Słowiński, R., & Susmaga, R. (1999). Rough set approach to evaluation of stormwater pollution. *International Journal of Environment and Pollution*, *12*, 232–250.

Sai, Y., Yao, Y. Y., & Zhong, N. (2001). Data analysis and mining in ordered information tables. In *Proceedings of the 2001 IEEE Int. Conference on Data Mining* (pp. 497-504). Washington, DC: IEEE Computer Society Press.

Słowiński, R., Greco, S., & Matarazzo, B. (2002). Mining decision-rule preference model from rough approximation of preference relation. In *Proceedings of the 26th IEEE Annual Int. Conference on Computer Software & Applications (COMPSAC 2002)* (pp. 1129-1134). Oxford, UK.

Słowiński, R., Greco, S., & Matarazzo, B. (2005). Rough set based decision support. In Burke, E. K., & Kendall, G. (Eds.), *Search Methodologies: Introductory Tutorials in Optimization and Decision Support Techniques* (pp. 475–527). New York: Springer.

Słowiński, R., & Zopounidis, C. (1995). Application of the rough set approach to evaluation of bankruptcy risk. *International Journal of Intelligent Systems in Accounting Finance & Management*, *4*, 27–41.

Słowiński, R., Zopounidis, C., & Dimitras, A. I. (1997). Prediction of company acquisition in Greece by means of the rough set approach. *European Journal of Operational Research, 100,* 1–15.

Vakarelov, D. (1992). Consequence relations and information systems. In Słowiński, R. (Ed.), *Intelligent Decision Support: Handbook of Applications and Advances of the Rough Sets Theory* (pp. 391–399). Boston: Kluwer Academic Publishers.

Wilk, S., Słowiński, R., Michałowski, W., & Greco, S. (2005). Supporting triage of children with abdominal pain in the emergency room. *European Journal of Operational Research, 160,* 696–709.

Yang, X., Yang, J., Wu, C., & Yu, D. (2008). Dominance-based rough set approach and knowledge reductions in incomplete ordered information system. *Information Sciences, 178,* 1219–1234.

Yao, J. (2007). A ten-year review of granular computing. In *Proceedings of the 2007 IEEE International Conference on Granular Computing* (pp. 734-739). Silicon Valley, CA.

Yao, J. (2008a). Recent developments in granular computing: a bibliometric study. In *Proceedings of the IEEE International Conference on Granular Computing* (pp. 74-79). Hangzhou, China.

Yao, J. T., Yao, Y. Y., & Ziarko, W. (2008). Special Section on Probabilistic Rough Sets. *International Journal of Approximate Reasoning, 49,* 253–343.

Yao, Y. Y. (2001). Information granulation and rough set approximation. *International Journal of Intelligent Systems, 16,* 87–104.

Yao, Y. Y. (2008b). Granular computing: past, present and future. In *Proceedings of the IEEE International Conference on Granular Computing* (pp. 80-85). Hangzhou, China.

Zadeh, L. A. (1965). Fuzzy sets. *Information and Control, 8,* 338–353.

Zadeh, L. A. (1979). Fuzzy sets and information granularity. In Gupta, M., Ragade, R. K., & Yager, R. R. (Eds.), *Advances in Fuzzy Set Theory and Applications* (pp. 3–18). Amsterdam: North-Holland Publishing Company.

Zadeh, L. A. (1997). Towards a theory of fuzzy information granulation and its centrality in human reasoning and fuzzy logic. *Fuzzy Sets and Systems, 90,* 111–127.

Ziarko, W. (1993). Variable precision rough sets model. *Journal of Computer and System Sciences, 46,* 39–59.

Ziarko, W. (1998). Rough sets as a methodology for data mining. In Polkowski, L., & Skowron, A. (Eds.), *Rough Sets in Knowledge Discovery (Vol. 1,* pp. 554–576). Heidelberg, Germany: Physica-Verlag.

# Compilation of References

Abelló, A., Samos, J., & Saltor, F. (2006). YAM$^2$: a multidimensional conceptual model extending UML. *Information Systems, 31*(6), 541-567.

Aggarwal, C. (2007). *Data Streams: Models and Algorithms*. Berlin, Germany: Springer.

Alon, N., Spencer, J. H. (2000). *The Probabilistic Method, 2nd Ed*. New York: John Wiley & Sons, Inc.

An, J. J., Wang, G. Y., Wu, Y., & Gan, Q. (2005). A rule generation algorithm based on granular computing, *2005 IEEE International Conference on Granular Computing (IEEE GrC2005)* (pp. 102-107). Beijing, P. R. China.

An, Q. S., Shen, J. Y., & Wang, G. Y. (2003). A clustering method based on information granularity and rough sets. *Pattern Recognition and Artificial Intelligence, 16*(4), 412-417.

Banerjee, M., & Khan, A. (2007). *Propositional Logic from Rough Set Theory, Transactions on Rough Sets VI*, (LNCS 4374, pp. 1-25). Berlin Heidelberg: Spring Verlag.

Bargiela A., & Pedrycz W. (2001, June 113-120). Granular clustering with partial supervision. In *Proceedings of the European Simulation Multiconference,* (ESM2001). Prague, Czech Republic.

Bargiela, A. (2001). *Interval and Ellipsoidal Uncertainty Models* In Pedrycz, W. (ed.), *Granular Computing*. Berlin Heidelberg, Germany: Springer Verlag.

Bargiela, A., & Pedrycz W. (2002). *Granular Computing: An Introduction*. Boston: Kluwer Academic Publishers.

Bargiela, A., & Pedrycz W. (2008). Toward a theory of Granular Computing for human-centered information processing. *IEEE Transactions on Fuzzy Systems, 16,* 320-330.

Bargiela, A., & Pedrycz, W. (2005). Granular mappings. *IEEE Trans. on Systems. Man and Cybernetics SMC-A, 35*(2), 288-301.

Bargiela, A., & Pedrycz, W. (2006, May 10-12). The roots of granular computing. *IEEE International Conference on Granular Computing 2006* (GrC06), (vol. 1, pp. 806-809). Atlanta, GA.

Bargiela, A., & Pedrycz, W. (2008). Toward a theory of granular computing for human-centered information processing. *IEEE Transactions on Fuzzy Systems, 16,* 320-330.

Bargiela, A., Pedrycz, W., & Hirota, K. (2004). Granular prototyping in fuzzy clustering. *IEEE Transactions on Fuzzy Systems, 12*(5), 697-709.

Bargiela, A., Pedrycz, W., & Tanaka, M. (2004). An inclusion/exclusion fuzzy hyperbox classifier. *International Journal of Knowledge based Intelligent Engineering Systems, 8*(2), 91-98.

Barrs, B. J. (2002). The conscious access hypothesis: origins and recent evidence. *Trends in Cognitive Sciences, 6*(1), 47-52.

Barwise, J., & Seligman, J. (1997). *Information Flow: The Logic of Distributed Systems*. Cambridge, UK: Cambridge University Press.

Bateson, G. (1978). *Mind and nature: a necessity unity*. New York: E.P. Dutton.

Bazan, J., & Skowron, A. (2005a). Classifiers based on approximate reasoning schemes. In Dunin-Kęplicz, B., Jankowski, A., Skowron, A., and Szczuka, M., (eds.), *Monitoring, Security, and Rescue Techniques in Multiagent Systems, Advances in Soft Computing,* (pp. 191-202). Heidelberg, Germany: Springer.

Bazan, J., Kruczek, P., Bazan-Socha, S., Skowron, A., and Pietrzyk, J. J. (2006a). Automatic planning of treatment of infants with respiratory failure through rough set modeling. In Greco, S., Hata, Y., Hirano, S., Inuiguchi, M., Miyamoto, S., Nguyen, H. S., and Słowiński, R. (eds.), *Fifth International Conference on Rough Sets and Current Trends in Computing (RSCTC 2006), Kobe, Japan, November 6-8, 2006,* volume 4259 of *Lecture Notes in Artificial Intelligence,* (pp. 418-427). Heidelberg, Germany: Springer .

Bazan, J., Kruczek, P., Bazan-Socha, S., Skowron, A., and Pictrzyk, J. J. (2006, July 2-7). Risk pattern identification in the treatment of infants with respiratory failure through rough set modeling. In *Proceedings of Information Processing and Management under Uncertainty in Knowledge-Based Systems* (IPMU'2006), (no. 3, pp. 2650-2657). Paris, France

Bazan, J., Peters, J. F., & Skowron, A. (2005, September 1-3). Behavioral pattern identification through rough set modelling. In Ślęzak, D., Szczuka, M., Duntsch, I., and Yao, Y., (eds.), *Proceedings of the Tenth International Conference on Rough Sets, Fuzzy Sets, Data Mining, and Granular Computing (RSFDGrC 2005), Regina, Canada* (volume 3642 of Lecture Notes in Artificial Intelligence, pp. 688-697). Berlin: Springer.

Bazan, J., Peters, J. F., Skowron, A., Nguyen, H. S., & Szczuka, M. (2003). Rough set approach to pattern extraction from classifiers. *Electronic Notes in Theoretical Computer Science, 82*(4), 1-10.

Bazan, J., Skowron, A., & Swiniarski, R. (2006b). Rough sets and vague concept approximation: From sample approximation to adaptive learning. *Transactions on Rough Sets V, LNCS 4100*(5), 39-62.

Bellman, R. E., Kalaba, R., Zadeh, L. (1966), Abstraction and pattern classification. *Journal of Math. Anal. Appl., 13*, 1-7.

Bender, A., & Glen, R. C. (2004). Molecular similarity: a key technique in molecular informatics. *Org. Biomol. Chem., 2*, 3204–3218.

Bertino, E., Chin, O. B., Sacks-Davis, R., Tan, K., Zobel, J., & Shidlovsky, B., et al. (1997). *Indexing techniques for advanced database systems.* Amsterdam: Kluwer Academic Publishers Group.

Beveridge, W. I. B. (1967). *The art of scientific investigation.* New York: Vintage Books.

Beynon, M. (2001). Reducts within the variable precision rough sets model: a further investigation. *European Journal of Operational Research, 134*(3), 592-605.

Bezdek, J. C. (1981). *Pattern Recognition with Fuzzy Objective Function Algorithms.* New York: Plenum Press.

Bezdek, J. C., & Pal, S. K. (1992). *Fuzzy Models for Pattern Recognition: Methods that Search for Structures in Data.* New York: IEEE Press

Binder, R. V., (1999). *Testing Object-oriented Systems: Models, Patterns and Tools.* Reading, MA: Addison Wesley Longman.

Birkhoff, G., & MacLane, S. (1967). Algebra. New York: The Macmillan Co.

Bittner, T., & Smith, B. (2003). A Theory of Granular Partitions. In Duckham, M, Goodchild, MF, Worboys, MF (eds.), *Foundations of Geographic Information Science,* (pp. 117-151). London: Taylor & Francis Books.

Bittner, T., & Stell, J. (2003). Stratified rough sets and vagueness, In Kuhn, W., Worboys, M., Timpf, S. (eds.), *Spatial Information Theory. Cognitive and Computational Foundations of Geographic Information Science. International Conference* (COSIT'03), (pp. 286-303).

Bobrowski, L., & Bezdek, J. C. (1991). C-Means clustering with the $l_1$ and $l_w$ norms. *IEEE Trans. on Systems Man and Cybernetics, 21*, 545-554.

Boehm, B, Grünbacher, P., & Kepler, J. (2001, May/June). Developing Groupware for Requirements Negotiation: Lessons Learned. IEEE Software, (pp. 46-55).

Boggia, A., Greco, S., & Nuciarelli, N. (2007). Assessing rural sustainable development potentialities by Dominance-based Rough Set Approach. Invited paper presented at the *22nd European Conference on Operational Research (EURO XXII)*, Prague, Czech Republic.

Boixader, D., Jacas, J., & Recasens, J. (2000). Upper and lower approximations of fuzzy sets. *International Journal General Systems, 29*, 555–568.

Bonikowski, Z., Bryniarski, E., & Wybraniec, U. (1998). Extensions and intentions in the rough set theory. *Information Science, 107*, 149-167.

Borrett, S. R., Bridewell, W., R., P. P. L. K., & Arrigo (2007). A method for representing and developing process models. *Ecological Complexity, 4*(1-2), 1-12.

Bose, R. C., Shrikhande, S. S., & Parker, E. T. (1960). Further results on the construction of mutually orthogonal Latin squares and the falsity of Euler's conjecture. *Canadian J. Math. 12*,189-203.

Breiman, L. (2001). Statistical modeling: the two cultures. *Statistical Science, 16*(3), 199-231.

Breiman, L., Friedman, J. H., Olshen, R. A., & Stone, P. J. (1984). *Classification and regression trees.* Belmont, CA: Wadsworth International Group.

Brena, R. F., & Ramirez, E. Z. (2006). A Soft Semantic Web. In *Proceedings of the 2006 1st IEEE Workshop on Hot Topics in Web Systems and Technologies*, (pp. 1-8).

Brena, R. F., & Ramirez, E. Z. (2006). A Soft Semantic Web. In *Proceedings of the 2006 1st IEEE Workshop on Hot Topics in Web Systems and Technologies*, (pp. 1-8).

Broekhoven, E., van, Adriaenssens, V., & De Baets, B. (2007). Interpretability-preserving genetic optimization of linguistic terms in fuzzy models for fuzzy ordered classification: an ecological case study. *International Journal of Approximate Reasoning, 44*, 65-90.

Bronshtein, I., Semendyayev, K., Musiol, G., & Muehlig, H., (eds.) (2003). *Handbook of Mathematics.* Berlin Heidelberg, Germany: Springer Verlag.

Camossi, E., Bertolotto, M., Bertino, E., & Guerrini, G. (2003, September 23). Issues on Modelling Spatial Granularity. In *Proceedings of the Workshop on fundamental issues in spatial and geographic ontologies.* Ittingen, Switzerland.

Canter, B. (2004). Congruences of finite distributive concept algebras. In *Proceedings of ICFCA' 04* , (pp. 128-141).

Cao, L. B., Schurmann, R., & Zhang, C. Q. (2005). Domain-driven in-depth pattern discovery: a practical methodology, In *Proceedings of Australian Data Mining Conference* (pp. 101-114).

Cariani, P. (1997). Emergence of new signal-primitives in neural systems. *Intellectica, 25*, 95-143.

Cattaneo, G., & Ciucci, D. (2004). Algebraic structures for rough sets. In *Proceedings of Transaction on Rough Sets II*, (volume 3135 of *Lecture Notes in Computer Science*, pp. 208-252). Berlin, Germany: Springer.

Cattaneo, G., & Nisticó, G. (1989). Brouwer-Zadeh posets and three-valued Łukasiewicz posets. *Fuzzy Sets and Systems, 33*(2), 165-190.

Ceberio, M., Ferson, S., Kreinovich, V., Chopra, S., Xiang, G., Murguia, A., & Santillan, J. (2006, February 22-24). How To Take Into Account Dependence Between the Inputs: From Interval Computations to Constraint-Related Set Computations. In *Proceedings of the 2nd Int'l Workshop on Reliable Engineering Computing.* Savannah, Georgia, (pp. 127–154), *Journal of Uncertain Systems, 1*(1), 11–34.

Cendrowska, J. (1987). PRISM: An algorithm for inducing modular rules. *International Journal of Man-Machine Studies, 27*, 349-370.

Cestnik, B., Kononenko, I., & Bratko, I. (1987). ASSISTANT 86: a knowledge-elicitation tool for sophisticated users. In *Proceedings of the 2nd European Working Session on Learning* (pp. 31-45).

Chakraborty, M. K., & Banerjee, M. (1993). Rough logic with rough quantifiers. Warsaw University of Technology. *ICS Research Report, 49*(93).

Chakraborty, M. K., & Samanta, P. (2007). Consistency-degree between knowledges. In *Proceedings of Rough Sets and Intelligent Systems Paradigms* (pp.133-142).

Chang, C. L., & Lee, R. C. T. (1973). *Symbolic logic and machine theorem proving.* New York: Academic Press. Liu, X. H. (1989). *Fuzzy Logic and Fuzzy Reseaning.* Jilin, China: Press. Of Jilin University.

Chang, L. Y., Wang, G. Y., & Wu, Y. (1999). An approach for attribute reduction and rule generation based on rough set theory. *Chinese Journal of Software, 10*(11), 1207-1211.

Chen, D., Wang, X., & Zhao, S. (2007). Attribute Reduction Based on Fuzzy Rough Sets. In Kryszkiewicz, M., Peters, J.F., Rybinski, H., Skowron, A. (Eds.), *Proceedings of the International Conference Rough Sets and Intelligent Systems Paradigms* (RSEISP 2007), (Lecture Notes in Artificial Intelligence vol. *4585*, pp. 381-390). Berlin, Germany: Springer.

Chen, Y. H., & Yao, Y. Y. (2006). Multiview intelligent data analysis based on granular computing. *IEEE International Conference on Granular Computing* (GrC'06), (pp. 281-286). Washington, DC: IEEE Computer Society.

Chen, Y. H., & Yao, Y. Y. (2008). A multiview approach for intelligent data analysis based on data operators. *Information Sciences, 178*(1), 1-20.

Cheng, Y., & Xu, D. (2002). Content-based semantic associative video model. *2002 6th International Conference on Signal Processing,* (vol. 1, pp. 727-730).

Chuchro, M. (1993). A certain conception of rough sets in topological Boolean algebras. *Bulletin of the Section of Logic, 22,* 9–12.

Chuchro, M. (1994). On rough sets in topological Boolean algebras. In W. Ziarko (Ed.), *Rough Sets, Fuzzy Sets and Knowledge Discovery* (pp. 157–160). Berlin, Germany: Springer-Verlag.

Cios, K., Pedrycz, W., & Swiniarski, R. (1998). *Data Mining Techniques.* Boston: Kluwer Academic Publishers.

Clark, P., & Niblett, T. (1989). The CN2 induction algorithm. *Machine Learning, 3*(4), 261-283.

Comer, S. (1991). An algebraic approach to the approximation of information. *Fundamenta Informaticae, 14,* 492–502.

Comer, S. (1993). On connections between information systems, rough sets, and algebraic logic. In C. Rauszer (Ed.), *Algebraic Methods in Logic and Computer Science* (vol. 28, pp. 117–127). Polish Academy of Sciences: Banach Center Publisher.

Cover, T., & Thomas, J. (1991). *Elements of Information theory.* New York: John Wiley & Sons, Inc. Fu, S. K., & Mui, J. K. (1981). A survey on image segmentation. *Pattern Recognition, 13,* 3-16.

Crane, D. (1972). *Invisible colleges, diffusion of knowledge in scientific communities.* Chicago: The University of Chicago Press.

Dai, J. H. (2004). Structure of Rough Approximations Based on Molecular Lattices In *Proceedings of 4th International Conference on Rough Sets and Current Trends in Computing* (RSCTC2004), (pp. 1197-1204). Uppsala, Sweden

Darwin, C. (1839). Zoology Notes and Specimen Lists from H.M.S. Cambridge, UK: Cambridge University Press.

Darwin, C. (1859). On the Origin of the Species by Means of Natural Selection. Oxford, UK: J. Murray.

Davis, P. J. (1975). Interpolation & Approximation. New York: Dover Publications Inc.

Dawyndt, P., De Meyer, H., & De Baets, B. (2006). UPGMA clustering revisited: A weight-driven approach to transitive approximation. *International Journal of Approximate Reasoning, 2006,* 42(3): 174-191.

de Medeiros, A. K. A., Weijters, A. J. M. M., & van der Aalst, W. M. P. P. (2007). Genetic process mining: An experimental evaluation. *Data Mining and Knowledge Discovery, 14,* 245-304.

Degtyarenko, K., & Contrino, S. (2004). COMe: the ontology of bioinorganic proteins. *BMC Structural Biology, 4*(3).

Dijkstra, E. W. (EWD237). A preliminary investigation into computer assisted programming. Retrieved September 22, 2008, from

Dijkstra, E. W. (EWD245). On useful structuring. Retrieved September 22, 2008, from http://www.cs.utexas. edu/users/EWD/ewd02xx/EWD245.pdf

Ding, Y., & Embley, D. W. (2006). Using Data-Extraction Ontologies to Foster Automating Semantic Annotation. In *Proceedings and 22nd International Conference on Data Engineering Workshops*, (pp. 138-146).

Doherty, P., ÃLukaszewicz, W., Skowron, A., & Szałas, A. (2006). *Knowledge Representation Techniques: A Rough Set Approach, volume 202 of Studies in Fuzziness and Soft Computing.* Berlin Heidelberg, Germany: Springer Verlag.

Domingos, PP. (2007). Toward knowledge-rich data mining. *Data Mining and Knowledge Discovery, 15,* 21-28.

Dongrui, M. J., & Wu, D. (2007, November 2-4). Perceptual Reasoning: A New Computing With Words Engine. *IEEE International Conference on Granular Computing* (GrC2007), (pp. 446-451). San Francisco: IEEE Computer Society.

Dorado, A., Pedrycz, W., & Izquierdo, E. (2005). User-driven fuzzy clustering: on the road to semantic classification, In *Proceedings of RSFDGrc 2005* (Vol. LNCS3641, pp. 421-430).

Du, W. L., Miao, D. Q., Li, D. G., & Zhang, N. Q. (2005). *Analysis on relationship between concept lattice and granule partition lattice.* Beijing, China: Computer Science.

Dubois, D., & Prade, H. (1990). Rough fuzzy sets and fuzzy rough sets. *International Journal General Systems, 17,* 191–208.

Dubois, D., & Prade, H. (1992). Putting rough sets and fuzzy sets together. In R. Słowiński (Ed.), *Intelligent Decision Support - Handbook of Applications and Advances of the Rough Sets Theory* (pp. 203-232). Boston: Kluwer Academic Publishers.

Dubois, D., & Prade, H. (1995). Fuzzy relation equations and causal reasoning. *Fuzzy Sets and Systems, 75,* 119-134

Dubois, D., Prade, H., Esteva, F., Garcia, P., Godo, L., & Lopez De Mantaras, R. (1998). Fuzzy set modelling in case-based reasoning. *International Journal of Intelligent Systems, 13*(4), 345-373.

Duda, R., & Hart, P. (1973). *Pattern Classification and Scene Analysis.* New York: Wiley.

Düntsch, I., & Gediaga, G. (1998). Uncertainty measures of rough set prediction. *Artificial Intelligence, 106*(1), 109-137.

E. Orlowska (1985). Semantics of Vague Concepts, In G.Dorn, P. Weingartner (Eds.), Foundations of Logic and Linguistics. Problems and Solutions (pp. 465-482). London: Plenum Press.

Earl, D. (2005). The classical theory of concepts. *Internet Encyclopedia of Philosophy.* Retrieved from http://www.iep.utm.edu/c/concepts.htm

Edmonds, B. (2000). Complexity and Scientific Modelling. *Foundations of Science, 5*(3), 379-390.

Egyed, A, Grünbacher, P. (2004, November/December). Identifying Requirements Conflicts and Cooperation: how quality Attributes and Automated Traceability can help. IEEE Software, (pp. 50-58).

Elmasri, R., Fu, J., & Ji, F. (2007, June 20-22). Multi-level conceptual modeling for biomedical data and ontologies integration. *20th IEEE International Symposium on Computer-Based Medical System*s (CBMS'07), (pp. 589-594). Maribor, Slovenia.

Euzenat, J., & Montanari, A. (2005). Time granularity. In Fisher, M., Gabbay, D., Vila, L. (Eds.), *Handbook of temporal reasoning in artificial intelligence,* (pp59-118). Amsterdam: Elsevier.

Fagin, R., Guha, R., Kumar, R., Novak, J., Sivakumar, D., & Tomkins, A. (2005, June 13-16). Multi-Structural Databases. In *Proceedings of PODS 2005.* Baltimore, MD.

Fan, T. F., Liu, D. R., & Tzeng, G. H. (2007). Rough set-based logics for multicriteria decision analysis. *European Journal of Operational Research, 182*(1), 340-355.

Farinas-del-Cerro, L. (n.d.). Resolution of Modal Logic. In *Proceedings of the Eightth International Conference on Atomata Deduction* (LNCS 170, pp. 153-171).

Feng, J., Jost, J., & Minping, Q. (2007). *Network: From Biology to Theory.* Berlin Heidelberg, Germany: Springer Verlag.

Fent, I. de, Gubiani, D., & Montanari, A. (2005). Granular GeoGraph: a multi-granular conceptual model for spatial data. In Calì, A., Calvanese, D., Franconi, E., Lenzerini, M., Tanca, L. (eds), *Proceedings of the 13th Italian Symposium on Advanced Databases* (SEBD'05), (pp368-379). Rome: Aracne editrice.

Ferson, S., Ginzburg, L., Kreinovich, V., Longpré, L., & Aviles, M. (2002). Computing Variance for Interval Data is NP-Hard. *ACM SIGACT News, 33*(2), 108–118.

Ferson. S. (2002). *RAMAS Risk Calc 4.0.* Boca Raton, FL: CRC Press.

Flinkman, M., Michałowski, W., Nilsson, S., Słowiński, R., Susmaga, R., & Wilk, S. (2000). Use of rough sets analysis to classify siberian forest ecosystems according to net primary production of phytomass. *INFOR, 38*(3), 145-161.

Fodor, J., & Roubens, M. (1994). *Fuzzy Preference Modelling and Multicriteria Decision Support.* Boston: Kluwer Academic Publishers.

Fonseca, F., Egenhofer, M., Davis, C., & Camara, G. (2002). Semantic Granularity in Ontology-Driven Geographic Information Systems. *Annals of Mathematics and Artificial Intelligence, 36* (1-2), 121-151.

Foundations of Logic and Linguistics. (n.d.). Problems and Solutions. London: Plenum.

Frawley, W. J., Piatetsky-Shapiro, G., & Matheus, C. (1991). *Knowledge discovery in databases: an overview.* Cambridge, MA: MIT Press.

Friedman, J. H. (1997). Data mining and statistics. What's the connection? Keynote address. In *Proceedings of the 29th Symposium on the Interface: Computing Science and Statistics*, Houston, TX.

Friske, M. (1985). Teaching proofs: a lesson from software engineering. *American Mathematical Monthly, 92*, 142-144.

Gabrys, B., & Bargiela, A. (2000). General fuzzy min-max neural network for clustering and classification. *IEEE Trans. Neural Networks, 11*, 769-783.

Gan, Q., Wang, G. Y., & Hu, J. (2006). A self-learning model based on granular computing. In *Proceedings of the 2006 IEEE International Conference on Granular Computing* (pp. 530-533). Atlanta, GA.

Ganter, B., & Wille, R. (1999). *Formal concept analysis: Mathematical Foundations.* Berlin, Germany: Springer.

Gath, I., & Geva, A. (1989). Unsupervised optimal fuzzy clustering. *IEEE Trans. Pattern Analysis and Machine Intelligence, 11*(7), 773-781.

Gath, I., Iskoz, A., Cutsem, B., & Van, M. (1997). Data induced metric and fuzzy clustering of non-convex patterns of arbitrary shape. *Pattern Recognition Letters, 18*, 541-553.

Gerbrandy, J., & Groeneveld, W. (1997). Reasoning about information change. *Journal of Logic, Language and Information, 6*(2), 147-169.

Gilboa, I., & Schmeidler, D. (2001). *A Theory of Case-Based Decisions.* Cambridge, UK: Cambridge University Press.

Gilhooly, K. J. (1989). Human and machine problem solving, toward a comparative cognitive science. In: Gilhooly, K. J. (Ed.), *Human and Machine Problem Solving* (pp. 1-13). New York: Plenum Press.

Giunchglia, F., & Walsh, T. (1992). A theory of abstraction. *Artificial Intelligence, 56*, 323-390.

Goldberg, D. (1989). *Genetic Algorithms in Search, Optimization and Machine Learning.* Reading, MA: Addison-Wesley.

Goldin, D., Smolka, S., & Wegner, PP. (2006). *Interactive Computation: The New Paradigm.* Berlin Heidelberg, Germany: Springer Verlag.

Gonzalez, J., Rojas, I., Pomares, H., Ortega, J., & Prieto, A. (2002). A new clustering technique for function approximation. *IEEE Trans. on Neural Networks, 13*, 132-142.

Goodrich, M., & Tamassia, R., (2004). *Algorithm Design: Foundations, Analysis, and Internet Examples,* (2$^{nd}$ ed.) New York: John Wiley & Sons, Inc.

Gorsevski, P. V., & Jankowski, P. (2008). Discerning landslide susceptibility using rough sets. *Computers, Environment and Urban Systems, 32*(1), 53-65.

Gottwald, S. (1995). Approximate solutions of fuzzy relational equations and a characterization of t-norms that define metrics for fuzzy sets. *Fuzzy Sets and Systems, 75,* 189-201

Grätzer, G. (1978). General Lattice Theory. *Pure and Applied Mathematics, 75.* New York: Academic Press, Inc.

Grätzer, G. (2006). *The Congruences of a Finite Lattice. A Proof-by-Picture Approach.* Boston: Birkhäuser.

Grätzer, G., & Lasker, H. (1968). Extension theorems on congruences of partial lattices. *Notices Amer. Math. Soc. 15,* 732-785.

Greco, S., Inuiguchi, M., & Słowiński, R. (2002). Dominance-based Rough Set Approach using possibility and necessity measures. In J. J. Alpigini, J. F. Peters, A. Skowron, & N. Zhong (Eds.), *Rough Sets and Current Trends in Computing,* (volume 2475 of *Lecture Notes in Artificial Intelligence,* pp. 85-92). Berlin, Germany: Springer-Verlag.

Greco, S., Inuiguchi, M., & Słowiński, R. (2004a). A new proposal for rough fuzzy approximations and decision rule representation. In D. Dubois, J. Grzymała-Busse, M. Inuiguchi, & L. Polkowski (Eds.), *Transactions on Rough Sets II: Rough Sets and Fuzzy Sets,* (volume 3135 of *Lecture Notes in Computer Science,* pp. 156-164). Berlin, Germany: Springer.

Greco, S., Inuiguchi, M., & Słowiński, R. (2006a). Fuzzy rough sets and multiple-premise gradual decision rules. *International Journal of Approximate Reasoning, 41*(2), 179-211.

Greco, S., Matarazzo, B., & Słowiński R. (1999). The use of rough sets and fuzzy sets in MCDM. In T. Gal, T. Stewart, & T. Hanne (Eds.), *Advances in Multiple Criteria Decision Making* chapter 14, (pp. 14.1-14.59). Boston: Kluwer Academic Publishers.

Greco, S., Matarazzo, B., & Słowiński, R. (1998). A new rough set approach to evaluation of bankruptcy risk. In C. Zopounidis (Ed.), *Operational tools in the management of financial risks* (pp. 121-136). Dordrecht, The Netherlands: Kluwer Academic Publishers.

Greco, S., Matarazzo, B., & Słowiński, R. (2001a). Rough sets theory for multicriteria decision analysis. *European Journal of Operational Research, 129*(1), 1-47.

Greco, S., Matarazzo, B., & Słowiński, R. (2005a). Decision rule approach. In J. Figueira, S. Greco, & M. Ehrgott (Eds.), *Multiple Criteria Decision Analysis: State of the Art Surveys* chapter 13, (pp. 507-563). Berlin, Germany: Springer-Verlag.

Greco, S., Matarazzo, B., & Słowiński, R. (2005b). Generalizing rough set theory through Dominance-based Rough Set Approach. In D. Ślęzak, J. T. Yao, J. Peters, W. Ziarko, & X. Hu (Eds.), *Rough Sets, Fuzzy Sets, Data Mining, and Granular Computing,* (volume 3642 of *Lecture Notes in Artificial Intelligence,* pp. 1-11). Berlin, Germany: Springer-Verlag.

Greco, S., Matarazzo, B., & Słowiński, R. (2006b). Dominance-based Rough Set Approach to Case-based Reasoning. In V. Torra, Y. Narukawa, A. Valls, & J. Domingo-Ferrer (Eds.), *Modelling Decisions for Artificial Intelligence,* (volume 3885 of *Lecture Notes in Artificial Intelligence,* pp. 7-18). Berlin, Germany: Springer-Verlag.

Greco, S., Matarazzo, B., & Słowiński, R. (2007a). Customer satisfaction analysis based on rough set approach. *Zeitschrift für Betriebswirtschaft, 16*(3), 325-339.

Greco, S., Matarazzo, B., & Słowiński, R. (2007b). Dominance-based Rough Set Approach as a proper way of handling graduality in rough set theory. In *Transactions on Rough Sets VII,* (volume 4400 of *Lecture Notes in Artificial Intelligence,* pp. 36-52). Berlin, Germany: Springer-Verlag.

Greco, S., Matarazzo, B., & Słowiński, R. (2007c). Financial portfolio decision analysis using Dominance-based Rough Set Approach. Invited paper presented at the *22nd European Conference on Operational Research (EURO XXII),* Prague, Czech Republic.

Greco, S., Matarazzo, B., & Słowiński, R. (2008a). Algebraic structures for Dominance-based Rough Set Approach. In G. Wang, T.-r. Li, J. W. Grzymała-Busse, D. Miao, A. Skowron, & Y. Yao (Eds.), *Rough Sets and Knowledge Technology*, (volume 5009 of *Lecture Notes in Artificial Intelligence*, pp. 252-259). Berlin, Germany: Springer.

Greco, S., Matarazzo, B., & Słowiński, R. (2008b). Dominance-based Rough Set Approach and Bipolar Abstract Approximation Spaces. In R. Goebel, J. Siekmann, & W. Wahlster (Eds.), *Rough Sets and Current Trends in Computing*, (volume 5306 of *Lecture Notes in Artificial Intelligence* (pp. 31-40). Berlin, Germany: Springer.

Greco, S., Matarazzo, B., & Słowiński, R. (2008c). Dominance-based Rough Set Approach to Interactive Multiobjective Optimization. In J. Branke, K. Deb, K. Miettinen, & R. Słowiński (Eds.), *Multiobjective Optimization: Interactive and Evolutionary Approaches* (chapter 5, pp. 121-155). Berlin, Germany: Springer.

Greco, S., Matarazzo, B., Słowiński, R., & Stefanowski, J. (2001b). Variable consistency model of dominance-based rough set approach. In W. Ziarko & Y. Yao (Eds.), *Rough Sets and Current Trends in Computing*, (volume 2005 of *Lecture Notes in Artificial Intelligence*, pp. 170-181). Berlin, Germany: Springer.

Greco, S., Pawlak, Z., & Slowinski, R. (2004). Can Bayesian confirmation measures be useful for rough set decision rules. *Engineering Applications of Artificial Intelligence, 17*, 345-361.

Grimmett, G. R., & Stirzaker, D. R. (2001). Probability and Random Processes. Oxford, UK: Oxford University Press.

Grizzi, F., & Chiriva-Internati, M. (2005). The complexity of anatomical systems. *Theoretical Biology and Medical Modelling, 2*(26).

Groenen, P. J. F., & Jajuga, K. (2001), Fuzzy clustering with squared Minkowski distances. *Fuzzy Sets and Systems, 120*, 227-237.

Grzymala-Busse, J. W. (1992). LERS - A system for learning from examples based on rough sets. In R. Slowinski

(Ed.), *Intelligent Decision Support* (pp. 3-18). Boston: Kluwer Academic Publishers.

Grzymala-Busse, J. W. (2005). LERS - A data mining system. In *The Data Mining and Knowledge Discovery Handbook* (pp. 1347-1351). Boston: Kluwer Academic Publishers.

Guerrero, F. (2008). Solving the oil equation by a team of geophysicists and computer scientists. *IEEE Spectrum*, 33-36.

Gustafson, D., & Kessel, W. (1992). Fuzzy clustering with a fuzzy covariance matrix. In J. Bezdek and S. Pal (Eds.), *Fuzzy models for Pattern Recognition: Methods that Search for Structures in Data*. New York: IEEE Press.

Hall, O., Barak, I., & Bezdek, J. C. (1999). Clustering with a genetically optimized approach. *IEEE Trans. Evo. Computation, 3*, 103–112.

Han, J. C., & Dong, J. (2007). Perspectives of granular computing in software engineering. In: Lin, T. Y., Hu, X. H., Han, J. C., Shen, X. J., & Li, Z. J. (Eds.), *Proceedings of 2007 IEEE International Conference on Granular Computing* (pp. 66-71). Los Alamitos, CA: IEEE Computer Society Press.

Han, J., & Dong. J., (2007). Perspectives of Granular Computing in Software Engineering. In Lin, T. Y., Hu, X., Han, J. (Ed.), *Proceedings of IEEE International Conference on Granular Computing* (pp. 66-071). San Jose, CA: IEEE Press.

Haralick, R. M., & Shapiro, L. G. (1985). Image segmentation techniques. *Computer Vision, Graphics, and Image Processing, 29*, 100–132.

Hata, Y., & Mukaidono, M. (1999, May 20-22). On Some Classes of Fuzzy Information Granularity and Their Representations. In *Proceedings of the Twenty Ninth IEEE International Symposium on Multiple-Valued Logic*, (pp. 288-293). Freiburg im Breisgau, Germany.

Hawkins, J., & Blakeslee, S. (2004). *On intelligence*. New York: Henry Holt & Company.

Hedman, S. (2004). *A first course in logic—an introduction to model theory, proof theory, computability, and complexity*. Oxford, UK: Oxford University Press.

Henry, C., & Peters, J. F. (2008). Near set index in an objective image segmentation evaluation framework. In *Geobia 2008, Pixels, Objects, Intelligence: GEOgraphic Object Based Information Analysis for the 21st Century*. Alberta, Canada: University of Calgary.

Henry, C., & Peters, J. F. (2007). Image pattern recognition using approximation spaces and near sets. In *Proceedings of Eleventh Int. Conf. on Rough Sets, Fuzzy Sets, Data Mining and Granular Computing* (RSFDGrC 2007, Joint Symposium JRS 2007), (Springer Lecture Notes in Artificial Intelligence, vol. 4482, pp. 475-482).

Hirota, K., & Pedrycz, W. (1995). D-fuzzy clustering. *Pattern Recognition Letters, 16*, 193-200.

Hobbs, J. R. (1985). Granularity. In: Aravind, K. J. (Ed.), *Proceedings of the Ninth International Joint Conference on Artificial Intelligence* (pp. 432-435). New York: Academic Press.

Hobbs, J. R. (1985). Granularity. *International Joint Conference on Artificial Intelligence (IJCAI85)*, 432-435.

Hobbs, J. R. (1985). Granularity. In Proceedings of IJCAI (pp. 432-435). Los Angeles.

Hobbs, J. R., (1985). Granularity, In Joshi, A. K. (Ed.), *Proceedings. of the 9th International Joint Conference on Artificial Intelligence* (pp. 432-435). San Francisco: Morgan Kaufmann.

Hofestädt, R., & Meinecke, F. (1995). Interactive Modelling and Simulation of Biochemical Networks. *Computers in Biology and Medicine, 25*, 321-334.

Hollinger, F.B., & Kleinman, S. (2003). Transfusion transmission of West Nile virus: a merging of historical and contemporary perspectives. *Transfusion, 43*(8), 992-997.

Hooke, R. (1665). Micrographia or Some Physiological Descriptions of Minute Bodies. New York: Cosimo, Inc.

Horstmann, C. (2007). *Big Java* (3rd ed). New York: John Wiley & Sons, Inc.

Hu, J., Wang, G. Y., & Zhang, Q. H. (2006). Uncertainty measure of covering generated rough set, *2006 IEEE/WIC/ACM International Conference on Web Intelligence and Intelligent Agent Technology (WI-IAT 2006 Workshops) (WI-IATW'06)* (pp. 498-504). Hongkong, China.

Hu, J., Wang, G. Y., Zhang, Q. H., & Liu, X. Q. (2006). *Attribute reduction based on granular computing*. Paper presented at the The Fifth International Conference on Rough Sets and Current Trends in Computing (RSCTC2006), Kobe, Japan.

Hu, Q. H., Xie, Z. X., &Yu, D. R. (2007). Hybrid attribute reduction based on a novel fuzzy rough model and information granulation. *Pattern Recognition, 40*, 3509–3521.

Hu, Q. H., Yu, D. R., & Xie, Z. X. (2006). Information-preserving hybrid data reduction based on fuzzy rough techniques. *Pattern Recognition Letters, 27*, 414–423.

Hu, X. H., & Cercone, N. (1995). Learning in relational database: a rough set approach. *International Journal of Computational Intelligence, 11*(2), 323-338.

Hu, X. H., Liu, Q., Skowron, A., Lin, T. Y., Yager, R. R., & Zhang, B. (2005). *Proceedings of 2005 IEEE International Conference on Granular Computing* (pp. 571-574). Beijing, China.

Hu, X., & Cercone, H. (1996). Mining knowledge rules from databases: a rough set approach, *Proceedings of the Twelfth International Conference on Data Engineering* (pp. 96-105).

Huang, B., Guo, L., & Zhou, X. (2007). Approximation Reduction Based on Similarity Relation. In *Proceedings of the IEEE Fourth International Conference on Fuzzy Systems and Knowledge Discovery* (pp. 124-128).

Huang, B., He, X., & Zhou, X. Z. (2004). Rough entropy based on generalized rough sets covering reduction. *Journal of software, 15*(2), 215-220.

Huang, H., Wang, G. Y., & Wu, Y. (2004). A direct approach for incomplete information systems. In *Proceedings of SPIE In Data Mining and Knowledge Discovery: Theory, Tools, and Technology VI* (, Vol. 5433, pp. 114-121).

Hume, D. (1748). *An Enquiry Concerning Human Understanding*. Oxford, UK: Clarendon Press.

Hunter, P. J., & Borg, T. (2003). Integration from Proteins to Organs: The Physiome Project. *Nature, 4*(3), 237-243.

Huynh, V. N., & Nakamori, Y. (2005). A roughness measure for fuzzy sets. *Information Sciences, 173*, 255-275.

Ilczuk, G., & Wakulicz-Deja, A. (2007$_a$). Data preparation for data mining in medical data sets. *LNCS Transactions on Rough Sets, 6*, 83-93.

Ilczuk, G., & Wakulicz-Deja, A. (2007$_b$). Selection of important attributes for medical diagnosis systems. *LNCS Transactions on Rough Sets, 7*, 70-84.

Inuiguchi, M., Hirano, S., & Tsumoto, S. (Eds.) (2003). *Rough Set Theory and Granular Computing.* Berlin, Germany: Springer.

Inuiguchi, M., Yoshioka, Y., & Kusunoki, Y. (2009). Variable-precision dominance-based rough set approach and attribute reduction. *International Journal of Approximate Reasoning.* (In Press).

Jain, A. K. (1989). *Fundamentals of Digital Image Processing.*Upper Saddle River, NJ: Prentice Hall.

Jankowski, A., & Skowron, A. (2007). A wistech paradigm for intelligent systems. *Transactions on Rough Sets VI, LNCS 4374*(5), 94-132.

Jankowski, A., & Skowron, A. (2008a). Logic for artificial intelligence: The Rasiowa-Pawlak school perspective. In Ehrenfeucht, A., Marek, V., and Srebrny, M., (eds.), *Andrzej Mostowski and Foundational Studies*, (pp. 106-143). Amsterdam: IOS Press.

Jankowski, A., Peters, J., Skowron, A., and Stepaniuk, J. (2008). Optimization in discovery of compound granules. *Fundamenta Informaticae, 85*(1-4), 249-265.

Jaulin, L., Kieffer, M., Didrit, O., & Walter, E. (2001). *Applied Interval Analysis.* London: Springer.

Jelonek, J., Krawiec, K., & Slowinski, R. (1995). Rough set reduction of attributes and their domains for neural networks. *International Journal of Computational Intelligence, 11*(2), 339-347.

Jensen, R., & Shen, Q. (2007). Fuzzy-rough sets assisted attribute selection. *IEEE Transactions on Fuzzy Systems, 15*, 73–89.

Jeon, G., Kim, D., & Jeong, J. (2006). Rough sets attributes reduction based expert system in interlaced video sequences. *IEEE Transactions on Consumer Electronics, 52*, 1348-1355.

Johansson, I. (2004b). The Ontology of temperature. *Philosophical Communications, 32*, 115-124.

Kamble, A. S. (2004). *A Data Warehouse Conceptual Data Model for Multidimensional Information.* (PhD thesis), University of Manchester, UK.

Kaplan, N., Sasson, O., Inbar, U., Friedlich, M., Fromer, M., Fleischer, H., Portugaly, E., Linial, N., & Linial, M. (2005). ProtoNet 4.0: A hierarchical classification of one million protein sequences. *Nucleic Acids Research, 33*, 216-218.

Karyannis, N. B., & Mi, G. W. (1997). Growing radial basis neural networks: merging supervised and unsupervised learning with network growth techniques. *IEEE Trans. on Neural Networks, 8*, 1492-1506.

Keet, C. M. (2006). A taxonomy of types of granularity. In: Zhang, Y.Q., & Lin, T.Y. (Eds.), *Proceeding of 2006 IEEE International Conference on Granular Computing* (pp. 106-111). Piscataway, NJ: Institute of Electrical and Electronics Engineers, Inc.

Keet, C. M. (2006, May 10-12). A taxonomy of types of granularity. *IEEE Conference in Granular Computing* (GrC2006), (vol. 1, pp. 106-111). Atlanta, GA: IEEE Computer Society.

Keet, C. M. (2007, November 2-4). Granulation with indistinguishability, equivalence or similarity. *IEEE International Conference on Granular Computing* (GrC2007), (pp. 11-16). San Francisco: IEEE Computer Society.

Keet, C. M. (2007, September 10-13). Enhancing comprehension of ontologies and conceptual models through abstractions. In Basili, R., Pazienza, M.T. (Eds.), *10th Congress of the Italian Association for Artificial Intelligence* (AIIA 2007), (Lecture Notes in Artificial Intelligence vol. 4733, pp. 814-822). Berlin Heidelberg, Germany: Springer-Verlag,

Keet, C. M. (2008). *A formal theory of granularity*. PhD Thesis, KRDB Research Centre, Faculty of Computer Science, Free University of Bozen-Bolzano, Italy. Retrieved June 8, 2008, from http://www.meteck.org/files/AFormalTheoryOfGranularity_ CMK08.pdf

Keet, C. M. (2008, June 2). Toward cross-granular querying over modularized ontologies. *International Workshop on Ontologies: Reasoning and Modularity* (WORM'08), (CEUR-WS Vol-348, pp. 6-17). Tenerife, Spain.

Keet, C. M. (2008a). *A Formal Theory of Granularity*. (PhD Thesis), KRDB Research Centre, Faculty of Computer Science, Free University of Bozen-Bolzano, Italy.

Keet, C. M. (2009, February 10-12). Structuring GIS information with types of granularity: a case study. In *Proceedings of the 6th International Conference on Geomatics*. La Habana, Cuba

Keet, C. M., & Artale, A. (2008). Representing and Reasoning over a Taxonomy of Part-Whole Relations. *Applied Ontology, 3*(1-2), 91-110.

Keet, C. M., & Kumar, A. (2005, August 28-31). Applying partitions to infectious diseases. In Engelbrecht, R., Geissbuhler, A., Lovis, C. Mihalas, G. (eds.), *XIX International Congress of the European Federation for Medical Informatics* (MIE2005), Geneva, Switzerland.

Kim, E., Park, M., Ji, S., & Park, M. (1997). A new approach to fuzzy modeling, *IEEE Trans. on Fuzzy Systems, 5*, 1997, 328-337.

Kiriyama, T., & Tomiyama, T. (1993, May 16-20). Reasoning about Models across Multiple Ontologies. In *Proceedings of the International Qualitative Reasoning Workshop*. Washington, DC.

Klawonn, F., & Kruse, R. (2004). The Inherent Indistinguishability in Fuzzy Systems. In Lenski, W. (ed.), *Logic versus Approximation: Essays Dedicated to Michael M. Richter on the Occasion of his 65th Birthday*, (Lecture Notes in Computer Science, vol. 3075, pp. 6-17). Berlin Heidelberg, Germany: Springer Verlag.

Kleinberg, J., Papadimitriou, C., & Raghavan, P. P. (1998). A microeconomic view of data mining. *Data Mining and Knowledge Discovery, 2*, 311-324.

Klement, E. P., Mesiar, R., & Pap, E. (2000). *Triangular Norms*. Dordrecht, The Netherlands: Kluwer Academic Publishers.

Klir G., & Yuan, B. (1995). *Fuzzy sets and fuzzy logic: theory and applications*. Upper Saddle River, NJ: Prentice Hall.

Knuth, D. E. (1984). Literate programming. *The Computer Journal, 27*(2), 97-111.

Kolodner, J. (1993). *Case-Based Reasoning*. San Francisco: Morgan Kaufmann.

Komorowski, J., Pawlak, Z., Polkowski, L., & Skowron, A. (1999). Rough sets: a tutuorial. In Pal, S. K., & Skowron, A (Eds.), *Rough fuzzy hybridization: a new trend in decision making* (pp. 3-98). Berlin, Germany: Springer/

Kraft, D., & Bautista, M. (2003). Rules and fuzzy rules in text: Concept, extraction and usage. *International Journal of Approximate Reasoning, 34*, 145–161. doi:10.1016/j.ijar.2003.07.005

Kraft, D., & Bautista, M. (2003). Rules and Fuzzy Rules in Text: Concept, Extraction and Usage. *International Journal of Approximate Reasoning, 34*, 145–161.

Kreinovich, V., Lakeyev, A., Rohn, & J., Kahl, P. (1997). *Computational complexity and feasibility of data processing and interval computations*. Dordrecht, The Netherlands: Kluwer.

Kriegel, H.-P., Borgwardt, K. M., Kroger, P., Pryakhin, A., Schubert, M., & Zimek, A. (2007). Future trends in data mining. *Data Mining and Knowledge Discovery, 15*(1), 87-97.

Kripke, S. (1963). Semantic Analysis of Modal Logic. *Zeitxchrift für Mathematische Logik und Grundlagen der Mathematik*, 67-96.

Kryszkiewicz, M. (1998). Rough set approach to incomplete information systems. *Information Science, 112*, 39-49.

Kryszkiewicz, M. (1999). Rules in incomplete information system. *Information Sciences, 113*(3-4), 271-292.

Kryszkiewicz, M. (2001). Comparative study of alternative type of knowledge reduction in inconsistent systems. *International Journal of Intelligent Systems, 16*, 105-120.

Kumar, A., Smith, B., & Novotny, D. D. (2005). Biomedical Informatics and Granularity. *Comparative and Functional Genomics, 5*(6-7), 501-508.

Kuncheva, L. I. (1992). Fuzzy rough sets: application to feature selection. *Fuzzy Sets and Systems, 51*, 147–153.

Kuntz, P., Guillet, F., Lehn, R., & Briand, H. (2000). A user-driven process for mining association rules. In *Proceedings of the 4th European Conference on Principles of Data Mining and Knowledge Discovery* (Vol. 1910, pp. 483-489).

Lazzerini, B., & Marcelloni, F. Classification based on neural similarity. *Electronics Letters, 38*(15), 810-812.

Leake, D. (1996). CBR in context: The present and future. In D. Leake (Ed.), *Case-Based Reasoning: Experiences, Lessons, and Future Directions* (pp. 1-30). Menlo Park, CA: AAAI Press.

Leron, U. (1983). Structuring mathematical proofs. *American Mathematical Monthly, 90,* 174-185.

Leung, Y., & Li, D. Y. (2003). Maximal consistent block technique for rule acquisition in incomplete information systems. *Information Sciences, 153*, 85-106.

Levitin, A. V., (2002). *Introduction to the Design & Analysis of Algorithms.* Reading, MA: Addison Wesley.

Li, D. Y., & Ma, Y. C. (2000). Invariant characters of information systems under some homomorphisms. *Information Sciences, 129*, 211-220.

Li, D. Y., Zhang, B., & Leung, Y. (2004). On knowledge reduction in inconsistent decision information systems. *International Journal of Uncertainty, Fuzziness and Knowledge-Based Systems, 12*(5), 651-672.

Liang, J. Y., & Li, D. Y. (2005). *Uncertainty and Knowledge Acquisition in Information Systems.* Beijing, China: Science Press.

Liang, J. Y., & Qian, Y. H. (2008). Information granules and entropy theory in information systems. Science in China-Series F (In Press)

Liang, J. Y., & Xu, Z. B. (2002). The algorithm on knowledge reduction in incomplete information systems. *International Journal of Uncertainty, Fuzziness and Knowledge-Based Systems, 24*(1), 95-103.

Liang, J. Y., Chin, K. S., Dang, C. Y., & Richard, C. M. Yam. (2002). A new method for measuring uncertainty and fuzziness in rough set theory. International Journal of General Systems, *31*(4), 331-342.

Liang, J. Y., Qian, Y. H., Chu, C. Y., Li, D. Y., & Wang, J. H. (2005). Rough set approximation based on dynamic granulation. *Lecture Notes in Artificial Intelligence, 3641*, 701-708.

Liang, J. Y., Shi, Z. Z., & Li, D. Y. (2004). The information entropy, rough entropy and knowledge granulation in rough set theory. *International Journal of Uncertainty, Fuzziness and Knowledge-Based Systems, 12*(1), 37-46.

Liang, J. Y., Shi, Z. Z., Li, D. Y., & Wierman, W. J. (2006). The information entropy, rough entropy and knowledge granulation in incomplete information systems. *International Journal of General Systems, 35*(6), 641-654.

Lin, T. Y. (1989). Neighborhood Systems and Approximation in Database and Knowledge Base Systems In Ras, Z. W. & Saitta (Eds.), *Proceedings of the Fourth International Symposium on Methodologies of Intelligent Systems* (pp. 75-86). Amsterdam: Elsevier.

Lin, T. Y. (1997). Granular computing. *Announcement of the BISC Special Interest Group on Granular Computing.*

Lin, T. Y. (1997A). Neighborhood Systems - A Qualitative Theory for Fuzzy and Rough Sets, In Wang, P. (Ed.), *Advances in Machine Intelligence and Soft Computing, Volume IV* (pp. 132-155). Durham: NC: Duke University Press.

Lin, T. Y. (1998). Granular Computing on Binary Relations II: Rough Set Representations and Belief Functions. In A. Skowron and L. Polkowski (eds), *Rough Sets in Knowledge Discovery* (pp. 121-140). Berlin, Germany: Physica Verlag.

Lin, T. Y. (1998a). Granular Computing on Binary Relations I: Data mining and Neighborhood Systems.

In A. Skowron & L. Polkowski (Eds.), *Rough Sets in Knowledge Discovery* (pp. 107-121). Heidelberg, Germany: Physica-Verlag.

Lin, T. Y. (2000). Data mining and machine oriented modeling: a granular computing approach. *Journal of Applied Intelligence, 13*(2), 113-124.

Lin, T. Y. (2003). Granular computing. In *Proceedings of the 9th International Conference of Rough Sets, Fuzzy Sets, Data Mining, and Granular Computing* (LNCS 2639, pp. 16-24).

Lin, T. Y. (2006, July 20-22). Granular Computing on Partitions, Coverings Neighborhood Systems. In Proceedings of International Forum on Theory of GrC from Rough Set Perspective. *Journal of Nanchang Institute of Technology, 25*(2), 22-27.

Lin, T. Y. (2006, May 10-12). Toward a Theory of Granular Computing. *IEEE International Conference on Granular Computing* (GrC06). Atlanta, GA: IEEE Computer Society.

Lin, T. Y., & Liu, Q. (1994) Rough approximate operators: axiomatic rough set theory. In W. Ziarko (Ed.), *Rough Sets, Fuzzy Sets and Knowledge Discovery* (pp. 256–260). Berlin, Germany: Springer.

Lin, T. Y., & Liu, Q. (1996). First-order rough logic I: Approximate reasoning via rough sets. *Fundamenta Informaticae, 27*(2-3), 137-154.

Lin, T. Y., (1997B). Granular computing: From Rough Sets and Neighborhood Systems to Information Granulation and Computing in Words.In *Proceedings of European Congress on Intelligent Techniques and Soft Computing II* (pp. 1602-1606). Aachen, Germany.

Lin, T.Y., Yao, Y.Y. and Zadeh, L.A. (Eds.) *Data Mining, Rough Sets and Granular Computing*, Physica-Verlag, Heidelberg, 2002.

Lipski, W. (1981). On databases with incomplete information. Journal of the ACM, 28, 41-70.

Liu, C., & Zhou, Q. (2003). Class-based semantic cohesion computation. In *Proceedings of the 2003 IEEE International Conference on Systems, Man and Cybernetics,* (vol. 2, pp. 1673- 1678).

Liu, G. L. (2005, July 25-27). The Topological Structure of Rough Sets over Fuzzy Lattices. In *Proceedings of the IEEE International Conference on Granular Computing* (vol. 1, pp. 535-538). Beijing, China.

Liu, G. L. (2008). Axiomatic systems for rough sets and fuzzy rough sets. *International Journal of Approximate Reasoning, 48*, 857–867.

Liu, Q. (1996). Accuracy Operator Rough Logic and Its Reasoning. In *Proceedings of RSFD'96 International Conference* (pp. 55-60). Tokyo, Japan: The University of Tokyo.

Liu, Q. (1998). Operator Rough Logic and its Resolution Principle. *Chinese Journal of Computer,5*(21), 476-480. (In Chinese).

Liu, Q. (1998). The OI-resolution of operator rough logic. In L. Polkowski and A. Skowron (eds), *Lecture Notes in Artificial Intelligence* (1424, pp. 432-435). Berlin, Germany: Springer.

Liu, Q. (2001). Neighborhood Logic and Its Data Reasoning on Neighborhood-Valued Information Table. *Chinese Journal of Computers, 24*(4), 405-410. (In Chinese).

Liu, Q. (2002, November 4-6). Approximate Reasoning Based on Granular Computing in Granular Logic. In *Proceedings of ICMLS2002* (pp. 1258-1262).

Liu, Q. (2003, June). Granules and Reasoning Based on Granular Computing. In *Proceedings of the 16th International Conference on Industrial and Engineering Applications of Artificial Intelligence and Expert Systems* (IEA/AIE 2003), (LNAI 2718, pp. 516-526).

Liu, Q. (2004, April). Granules and Applications of Granular Computing in Logical Reseaning. *Research and Development of Computer, 41*(4), 546-551. (In Chinese).

Liu, Q., & Huang, Z. H. (2004). G-Logic and Resolution Reseaning. *Chinese Journal of Computer,27*(7), 865-873. (In Chinese).

Liu, Q., & Sun, H. (2006, July). Theoretical Study of Granular Computing. In *Proceedings of RSKT2006* (LNAI 4062, pp. 93-102).Hong Kong, China: Springer.

Liu, Q., & Wang, J. Y. (2006, May). Semantic Analysis of Rough Logical Formulas Based on Granular Computing. In *Proceedings of IEEE GrC2005* (pp. 393-396). Washington, DC: IEEE Press.

Liu, Q., Jiang, F., & Deng, D. Y. (2003). *Design and Implement for the Diagnosis Software of Blood Viscosity Syndrome Based on Hemorheology on GrC* (Lecture Notes in AI 2639, pp. 413-420). Berlin, Germany: Springer-Verlag.

Liu, Q., Liu, S. H., & Zheng, F. (2001). Rough Logic and Its Applications in Data Mining. *Journal of Software, 12*(3), 415-419. (In Chinese).

Liu, S. H., Hu, F., Jia, Z. Y., & Shi, Z. Z. (2004). A rough set-based hierarchical clustering algorithm. *Journal of Computer research and Development, 41*(4), 552-557.

Liu, S. H., Sheng, Q. J., Wu, B., Shi, Z. Z., & Hu, F. (2003). Research on efficient algorithms for rough set methods. *Chinese Journal of Computers, 26*(5), 524-529.

Liu, Y. B., Liu, D. Y., & Gao, Y. (2006). Mining dominance association rules in preference-ordered data. In G. Liu, V. Tan, & X. Han (Eds.), *Computational Methods* (pp. 1261-1266). Berlin, Germany: Springer.

Liu, C., & Zhou, Q. (2003). Class-based semantic cohesion computation. In *Proceedings of the 2003 IEEE International Conference on Systems, Man and Cybernetics,* (vol. 2, pp. 1673- 1678).

Loemker, L. & Leibniz, G. W. (1969). *Philosophical Papers and Letters.* Dordrecht: D. Reidel, 2 edition.

Louie, E., & Lin, T. Y. (2000). Finding association rules using fast bit computation: machine-oriented modeling, In *Proceedings of the 12th International Symposium on Methodologies for Intelligent Systems,* (pp. 486-494). Charlotte, NC.

Luck, M., McBurney, P., & Preist, C. (2003). *Agent technology. Enabling next generation computing: A roadmap for agent based computing.* Retrieved from AgentLink.org

Luján-Mora, S., Trujillo, J., & Song, I. (2006). A UML profile for multidimensional modeling in data warehouses. *Data & Knowledge Engineering, 59*(3), 725-769.

MacLeod, M. C., & Rubenstein, E. M. (2005). Universals. *The Internet Encyclopedia of Philosophy.* Retrieved from http://www.iep.utm.edu/u/universa.htm

Maimon, O., Kandel, A., Last, M. (2001), Information-theoretic fuzzy approach to data reliability and data mining. *Fuzzy Sets and Systems, 117,* 183-194.

Malinowski, E., & Zimányi, E. (2006). Hierarchies in a multidimensional model: From conceptual modeling to logical representation. *Data & Knowledge Engineering, 59*(2), 348-377.

Malyszko, D., & Stepaniuk, J. (2008, June 16-18). Granular Multilevel Rough Entropy Thresholding in 2D Domain. IIS 2008. In *Proceedings of the 16th International Conference Intelligent Information Systems* (pp. 151-160). Zakopane, Poland.

Malyszko, D., & Stepaniuk, J. (2008, October 23-25). Standard and Fuzzy Rough Entropy Clustering Algorithm in image segmentation. In *Proceedings of RSCTC 2008* (pp. 409-418). Akron, Ohio.

Malyszko, D., & Stepaniuk, J. (n.d.). *Granular Multilevel Rough Entropy Thresholding* [In Press].

Malyszko, D., Wierzchon S. T. (2007). Standard and genetic k-means clustering techniques in Image Segmentation. In *Proceedings of CISIM* (pp.299–304).

Mani, I. (1998). A theory of granularity and its application to problems of polysemy and underspecification of meaning. In A.G. Cohn, L.K. Schubert, and S.C. Shapiro (eds.), *Principles of Knowledge Representation and Reasoning: Proceedings of the Sixth International Conference,* (KR98), (pp. 245-255). San Francisco: Morgan Kaufmann.

Marczewski, E. (1958). A general scheme of independence in mathematics. *Bulletin de 1 Academie Polonaise des Sciences-Serie des Sciences Mathematiques Astronomiques et Physiques, 6,* 331-362.

Marr, D. (1982). *Vision, a computational investigation into human representation and processing of visual information.* San Francisco: W.H. Freeman & Company.

Martella, R. C., Nelson, R., & Marchard-Martella, N. E. (1999). *Research methods: learning to become a critical research consumer.* Boston: Allyn & Bacon.

Masolo, C., Borgo, S., Gangemi, A., Guarino, N., & Oltramari, A. (2003). *Ontology Library.* WonderWeb Deliverable D18 (ver. 1.0, 31-12-2003). Retrieved from http://wonderweb.semanticweb.org

Maulik, U., & Bandyopadhyay, V. (2000). Genetic algorithm-based clustering technique. *Pattern Recognition 33*, 1455-1465.

McCullough, G. (2007). Manitoba North Basis, south of Long Point, Lake Winnipeg. Retrieved from http://home.cc.umanitoba.ca/%7Egmccullo/LWsat.htm

Mencar, C., Castellanoa, G., & Fanellia, A. M. (2007). Distinguishability quantification of fuzzy sets. *Information Sciences, 177*(1), 130-149.

Mi, J. S., Wu, W. Z., & Zhang, W. X. (2003). Comparative studies of knowledge reductions in inconsistent systems. *Fuzzy Systems and Mathematics, 17*(3), 54-60.

Mi, J.-S., & Zhang, W.-X. (2004). An axiomatic characterization of a fuzzy generalization of rough sets. *Information Sciences, 160*, 235–249.

Mi, J.-S., Leung, Y., Wu, W.-Z. (2005). An uncertainty measure in partition-based fuzzy rough sets. *International Journal of General Systems*, 34, 77–90.

Mi, J.-S., Leung, Y., Zhao, H.-Y., & Feng, T. (2008). Generalized fuzzy rough sets determined by a triangular norn. *Inforamtion Sciences, 178*, 3203–3213.

Miao, D. Q. (2005, August-September). Rough Group, Rough Subgroup and their Properties. In *Proceedings of the 10th International Conference* (RSFDGrC2005), (LNAI 3641, Vol. 1, pp. 104-113). Regina, Canada.

Miao, D. Q., & Hu, G. R. (1999). A heuristic algorithm for reduction of knowledge. *Journal of Computer Research & Development, 36*(6), 681-684.

Miao, D. Q., & Wang, J. (1998). On the relationships between information entropy and roughness of knowledge in rough set theory. *Pattern Recognition and Artificial Intelligence, 11*(1), 34-40.

Michałowski, W., Rubin, S., Słowiński, R., & Wilk, S. (2003). Mobile clinical support system for pediatric emergencies. *Journal of Decision Support Systems, 36*, 161-176.

Michałowski, W., Wilk, S., Farion, K., Pike, J., Rubin, S., & Słowiński, R. (2005). Development of a decision algorithm to support emergency triage of scrotal pain and its implementation in the MET system. *INFOR, 43*(4), 287-301.

Michalski, R., & Larson, J. (1980). *Incremental generation of vll hypotheses: the underlying methodology and the description of program AQ11* (Technical Report ISG 83-5). Urbana-Champaign, IL: Computer Science Department, University of Illinois.

Miller, G. (1985). *WordNet Research.* Retrieved February 8, 2008, from http://wordnet.princeton.edu/

Miller, G. (1985). *WordNet Research.* Retrieved February 8, 2008, from http://wordnet.princeton.edu/

Minsky, M. (2007). *The emotion machine: commonsense thinking, artificial intelligence, and the future of the human mind.* New York: Simon & Schuster Paperbacks.

Mitchell, M. (2007). Complex systems: Network thinking. *Artificial Intelligence, 170*(18), 1194-1212.

Mitchell, T. M. (1978). *Version Spaces: An Approach to Concept Learning* (Ph.D. Thesis). Stanford, CA: Computer Science Department, Stanford University.

Mitzenmacher, M., & Upfal, E. (2005). Probability and Computing. Randomized Algorithms and Probabilistic Analysis. Cambridge, UK: Cambridge University Press.

Mollestad, T., & Skowron, A. (1996). A rough set framework for data mining of propositional default rules. In *Proceedings of the 9th International Symposium on Methodologies for Intelligent Systems. ISMIS* (pp. 448-457).

Mordeson, J. N. (2001). Rough set theory applied to (fuzzy) ideal theory. *Fuzzy Sets and Systems, 121*(2), 315-324.

Morsi, N. N., & Yakout, M. M. (1998). Axiomatics for fuzzy rough sets. *Fuzzy Sets and Systems, 100*, 327–342.

Nakamura, A. (1996). A rough logic based on incomplete information and its applications. *International Journal of Approximate Reasoning, 15*, 367-378.Liu, Q., & Wang, Q. Y. (2005, September). Granular Logic with Closeness Relation and Its Reasoning, (LNAI 3641, pp. 709-711). Berlin, Germany: Springer

Nanda, S., & Majumda, S. (1992). Fuzzy rough sets. *Fuzzy Sets and Systems, 45*, 157–160.

National Geographic (2008). National Geographic, Penguins, Mar. Retrieved from http://animals.nationalgeographic.com/animals/photos/penguins/adelie-penguin_image.html

Newell, A., & Simon, H. A. (1972). *Human problem solving.* New Jersey: Prentice-Hall, Inc.

Nguyen, H. S., & Skowron, A. (2008). A rough granular computing in discovery of process models from data and domain knowledge. *Journal of Chongqing University of Post and Telecommunications, 20*(3), 341-347.

Nguyen, H. S., & Slezak, D. (1999). Approximate reducts and association rules correspondence and complexity results. *Lecture Notes in Artificial Intelligence, 1711,* 137-145.

Nguyen, S. H., Bazan, J., Skowron, A., & Nguyen, H. S. (2004). Layered learning for concept synthesis. *Transactions on Rough Sets I, LNCS 3100*(1), 187-208.

Nguyen, T. T., Paddon, C. P. P. W. D. J., & Nguyen, H. S. (2006). Learning sunspot classification. *Fundamenta Informaticae, 72*(1-3), 295-309.

Nikravesh, M. (2002). *Fuzzy Conceptual-Based Search Engine using Conceptual Semantic Indexing* (pp. 146–151). North American Fuzzy Information Processing Society - The Special Interest Group on Fuzzy Logic and the Internet.

Ning, P., Wang, X. S., & Jajodia, S. (2002). An Algebraic Representation of Calendars. *Annals of Mathematics and Artificial Intelligence, 63*(1-2), 5-38.

O'Docherty, M. (2005). *Object-Oriented Analysis & Design.* New York: John Wiley & Sons, Ltd.

Ohgaya, R., Fukano, K., Taniguchi, K., Takagi, T., Aizawa, A., & Nikravesh, M. (2002). *Conceptual Fuzzy Sets-Based Menu Navigation System for Yahoo* (pp. 274–279). North American Fuzzy Information Processing Society - The Special Interest Group on Fuzzy Logic and the Internet.

Ohgaya, R., Fukano, K., Taniguchi, K., Takagi, T., Aizawa, A., & Nikravesh, M. (2002). *Conceptual Fuzzy Sets-Based Menu Navigation System for Yahoo. North American Fuzzy Information Processing Society - The Special Interest Group on Fuzzy Logic and the Internet,* (pp. 274-279).

Øhrn, A., & Komorowski, J. (1997). ROSETTA: A rough set toolkit for analysis of data. In *Proceeding of the Third International Joint Conference on Information Sciences* (pp. 403-407).

Orłowska, E. (1982). Semantics of Vague Concepts, Applications of Rough Sets. Polish Academy of Sciences Institute for Computer Science, (Report 469).

Orlowska, E. (1985). A logic of indiscernibility relation. In A. Skowron (ed), *Computation Theory,* (Lecture Notes in Computer Science 208, pp. 177-186).

Orłowska, E. (1998). Incomplete Information: Rough Set Analysis. Studies in Fuzziness and Soft Computing, 13, 1-22. Berlin Heidelberg, Germany: Springer Verlag.

Orłowska, E., Pawlak, E. (1984). Representation of nondeterministic information, Theoretical Computer Science 29, 27-39.

Pagliani, P. (1996). Rough sets and Nelson algebras. *Fundamenta Informaticae, 27*(2-3), 205-219.

Pagliani, P. (1998). Rough set theory and logic-algebraic structures. In E. Orłowska (Ed.), *Incomplete Information: Rough Set Analysis* (pp. 109-190). Heidelberg, Germany: Physica-Verlag.

Pagliani, P., & Chakraborty, M. (2008). *A Geometry of Approximation: Rough Set Theory: Logic, Algebra and Topology of Conceptual Patterns.* Berlin, Germany: Springer.

Pal, S. K. (2004). Soft data mining, computational theory of perceptions, and rough-fuzzy approach. *Information Sciences, 163*, 5-12.

Pal, S. K., Bandoyopadhay, S., and Biswas, S., editors (2005, December 18-22). *Proceedings of the First International Conference on Pattern Recognition and Machine Intelligence (PReMI'05), Indian Statistical Institute, volume 3776 of Lecture Notes in Computer Science*, Berlin Heidelberg, Germany. Springer Verlag.

Pal, S. K., Pedrycz, W., Skowron, A., & Swiniarski, R. (2001). Presenting the special issue on rough-neruo computing. *Neurocomputing, 36*, 1-3.

Pal, S. K., Polkowski, L., & Skowron, A., editors (2004). *RoughNeural Computing: Techniques for Computing with Words*. Cognitive Technologies. Springer, Berlin.

Pal, S., K., Shankar, B. U., & Mitra, P. (2005). Granular computing, rough entropy and object extraction, *Pattern Recognition Letters, 26*(16), 2509-2517.

Paliwal, A. V., Adam, N. R., Xiong, H., & Bornhovd, C. (2006). Web Service Discovery via Semantic Association Ranking and Hyperclique Pattern Discovery. In *Proceedings of the 2006 IEEE/WIC/ACM International Conference on Web Intelligence,* (vol. 18, pp. 649-652).

Paliwal, A. V., Adam, N. R., Xiong, H., & Bornhovd, C. (2006). Web Service Discovery via Semantic Association Ranking and Hyperclique Pattern Discovery. In *Proceedings of the 2006 IEEE/WIC/ACM International Conference on Web Intelligence,* (vol. 18, pp. 649-652).

Pancerz, K., & Suraj, Z. (2004). Discovering concurrent models from data tables with the ROSECON. *Fundamenta Informaticae, 60*(1-4), 251-268.

Pandurang N. P., & Levy, A. Y. (1995). A semantic theory of abstractions. In Mellish, C. (ed.), *Proceedings of the International Joint Conference on Artificial Intelligence,* (pp.196-203). San Francisco: Morgan Kaufmann.

Parent, C., Spaccapietra, S., & Zimányi, E. (2006a). *Conceptual modeling for traditional and spatio-temporal applications—the MADS approach*. Berlin Heidelberg, Germany: Springer Verlag.

Parker, E. T. (1959). Orthogonal latin squares. In *Proceedings of the Nat. Acad. Sciences.* (vol. 45, pp. 859–862).

Patil, L., Dutta, D., & Sriram, R. (2005). Ontology-based exchange of product data semantics. *IEEE Transactions on Automation Science and Engineering, 2*(3), 213–225. doi:10.1109/TASE.2005.849087

Patrick, J., Palko, D., Munro, R., & Zappavigna, M. (2002). User driven example-based training for creating lexical knowledgebases, *Australasian Natural Language Processing Workshop, Canberra, Australia* (pp. 17-24). Canberra, Australia.

Pavel, M. (1993). Fundamentals of Pattern Recognition (2nd Ed). New York: Marcel Dekker, Inc.

Pawlak, Z. (1981a). Classification of Objects by Means of Attributes. (Report 429). Institute for Computer Science, Polish Academy of Sciences.

Pawlak, Z. (1981b). Rough Sets. (Report 431). Institute for Computer Science, Polish Academy of Sciences.

Pawlak, Z. (1982). Rough Sets. International Journal of Information and Computer Sciences, 11,1982,341-356.

Pawlak, Z. (1984). On Conflicts. Int. J. of Man-Machine Studies, 21, 127-134.

Pawlak, Z. (1987). On Conflicts (in Polish). Warsaw, Poland: Polish Scientific Publishers.

Pawlak, Z. (1987). Rough Logic. *Bull. Polish Acad. Aci. Tech., 35*(5-6), 253-258.

Pawlak, Z. (1991). *Rough Sets: Theoretical Aspects of Reasoning about Data, volume 9 System Theory, Knowledge Engineering and Problem Solving*. Dordrecht, The Netherlands: Kluwer Academic Publishers.

Pawlak, Z. (1992). Concurrent versus sequential the rough sets perspective. *Bulletin of the EATCS, 48*, 178-190.

Pawlak, Z. (1993). Anatomy of conflict. Bulletin of the European Association for Theoretical Computer Science, 50, 234-247.

Pawlak, Z. (1996, July 1-5)). Rough Sets: Present State and Perspectives. In *Proceedings of the Sixth International Conference on Information Processing and Management of Uncertainty in Knowledge-Based Systems* (IPMU'96), (pp. 1137-1146). Granda, Spain.

Pawlak, Z. (1997). Rough real functions and rough controllers. *Rough sets and data mining: Analysis of imprecise data* (pp. 139-147). Boston: Kluwer Academic Publishers.

Pawlak, Z. (1998). An inquiry into anatomy of conflicts. Journal of Information Sciences, 109, 65-78.

Pawlak, Z. (1998). Granularity of knowledge, indiscernibility and rough sets. In: *Proceedings of 1998 IEEE International Conference on Fuzzy Systems* (pp. 106-110). Piscataway, NJ: Institute of Electrical and Electronics Engineers, Inc.

Pawlak, Z. (1998). Rough set theory and its applications in data analysis. *Cybernetics and Systems, 29*, 661-688.

Pawlak, Z. (1999). Rough sets, rough functions and rough calculus. In Pal, S. & Skowron, A., (eds.), *Rough Fuzzy Hybridization, A New Trend in Decision Making*, (pp. 99-109). Berlin, Germany: Springer

Pawlak, Z. (2001). Rough Set Theory. *Kunstliche Intelligenz, 3*, 38-39.

Pawlak, Z. (2005). Some remarks on conflict analysis. *Information Sciences, 166*, 649-654.

Pawlak, Z., & A. Skowron. (2007b). Rough sets: Some extensions. *Information Sciences, 177*(1), 28-40.

Pawlak, Z., & Munakata, T. (1996). Rough control: Application of Rough Set Theory to control. In *Proceeding of the Fourth European Congress on Intelligent Techniques and Soft Computing* (EUFIT'96), (pp. 209-218).

Pawlak, Z., & Skowron, A. (2007). Rudiments of rough sets. *Information Sciences 177*(1), 3-27.

Pawlak, Z., & Skowron, A. (2007). Rudiments of rough sets; Rough sets: Some extensions; Rough sets and boolean reasoning. *Information Sciences, 177*(1), 3-27; 28-40; 41-73.

Pawlak, Z., & Skowron, A. (2007a). Rudiments of rough sets. *Information Sciences, 177*(1), 3-27.

Pawlak, Z., & Skowron, A. (2007b). Rough sets: Some extensions. Information Sciences 177, 28-40.

Pawlak, Z., & Skowron, Z. (2007). Rough sets and Boolean reasoning. *Information Sciences, 177*, 41-73.

Pawlak, Z., Peters, J. F., Skowron, A., Suraj, Z., Ramanna, S., & Borkowski, M. (2001). Rough measures and integrals: A brief introduction. In Terano, T., Nishida, T., Namatame, A., Tsumoto, S., Ohsawa, Y., and Washio, T., (eds.), *New Frontiers in Artificial Intelligence, Joint JSAI 2001 Workshop Post Proceedings, Lecture Notes in Artificial Intelligence*, (volume 2253, pp. 374-379), Berlin, Germany. Springer.

Pawlak, Z., Słowiński, K., & Słowiński, R. (1986). Rough classification of patients after highly selective vagotomy for duodenal ulcer. *International Journal of Man-Machine Studies, 24*, 413-433.

Pedrycz, W. (1985). Algorithms of fuzzy clustering with partial supervision. *Pattern Recognition Letters, 3*, 13-20.

Pedrycz, W. (1989). *Fuzzy Control and Fuzzy Systems*. New York: Wiley.

Pedrycz, W. (1996). Conditional fuzzy C-Means. *Pattern Recognition Letters, 17*, 625-632. Pedrycz, W. (1998). Conditional fuzzy clustering in the design of radial basis function neural networks. *IEEE Trans. on Neural Networks, 9*, 601-612.

Pedrycz, W. (2002). Relational and directional in the construction of information granules. *IEEE Transactions on Systems, Man, and Cybernetics-Part A: Systems and Humans, 32*(5), 605-614.

Pedrycz, W. (2006). *Granular Computing: An Overview, Applied Soft Computing Technologies: The Challenge of Complexity*. Berlin, Germany: Springer.

Pedrycz, W., & Gomide, F. (2007). *Fuzzy Systems Engineering: Toward Human-Centric Computing*. New York: Wiley Interscience.

Pedrycz, W., & Kwak, K. (2006). Granular models as a framework of user-centric system modeling. *IEEE Trans. on Systems, Mans, and Cybernetics – Part A,* , 727-745.

Pedrycz, W., & Vukovick, G. (2000). Granular worlds: representation and communication problems. *International Journal of Intelligent Systems, 15*, 1015-1026.

Pedrycz, W., & Waletzky, J. (1997). Fuzzy clustering with partial supervision, *IEEE Trans. on Systems, Man, and Cybernetics*, *5*, 787-795.

Pedrycz, W., (ed.) (2001). *Granular Computing*. Berlin/Heidelberg, Germany: Springer/Verlag.

Pedrycz, W., Gomide, F. (1998). *An Introduction to Fuzzy Sets*. Cambridge, MA: MIT Press.

Pedrycz, W., Skowron, A., & Kreinovich, V., (eds.) (2008). *Handbook of Granular Computing*. New York: John Wiley & Sons.

Pedrycz, W., Vasilakos, A. (1999). Linguistic models and linguistic modeling. *IEEE Trans. on Systems, Man and Cybernetics*, *29*, 745-757.

Pei, D. W. (2004). Rough Set Models on Two Universes. *Int. J. General Systems 33*(5), 569-581.

Pei, D. W. (2005). A generalized model of fuzzy rough sets. *International Journal of General Systems*, *34*, 603–613.

Peters, J. F., Henry, C. & Ramanna, S. (2005). Rough ethograms: Study of intelligent system behaviour. In M.A. Kłopotek, S. Wierzcho'n, K. Trojanowski (Eds.), *New Trends in Intelligent Information Processing and Web Mining* (IIS05), (pp. 117-126). Gdansk, Poland.

Peters, J. F. (2009). Tolernance near sets and image correspondence. *Int. J. of Bio-Inspired Computation*, *2*, 1-8. (In Press).

Peters, J. F. & Henry, C. (2006c). Reinforcement Learning with Approximation Spaces. *Fundamenta Informaticae*, *71*, 323–349.

Peters, J. F. (1998). Time and clock information systems: Concepts and roughly fuzzy petri net models. In *Rough Sets in Knowledge Discovery 2: Applications, Case Studies and Software Systems*, of *Studies in Fuzziness and Soft Computing*, (volume 19, pp. 385-418). Berlin/Heidelberg, Germany: Springer/Verlag.

Peters, J. F. (2005). Rough ethology: Towards a biologically-inspired study of collective behavior in intelligent systems with approximation spaces. *Transactions on Rough Sets III, LNCS 3100*(3), 153-174.

Peters, J. F. (2007a). Classification of objects by means of features. In Proceedings of the IEEE Symposium Series on Foundations of Computational Intelligence (IEEE SCCI 2007), (pp. 1-8). Honolulu, HI.

Peters, J. F. (2007b). Classification of perceptual objects by means of features. Int. J. of Info. Technology & Intelligent Computing. In press.

Peters, J. F. (2008). Discovery of perceptually near information granules, Novel Developments in Granular Computing: Applications of Advanced Human Reasoning and Soft Computation. Hershey, PA: Information Science Reference.

Peters, J. F. (2008a). Approximation and perception in ethology-based reinforcement learning. In Pedrycz, W., Skowron, A., Kreinovich, V. (Eds.), *Handbook on Granular Computing*. New York: Wiley.

Peters, J. F. (2008a). Classification of perceptual objects by means of features. *International Journal of Information Technology and Intelligent Computing*, *3*(2), 1-35.

Peters, J. F. (2008b). Affinities between perceptual granules: Foundations and perspectives In A. Bargiela, W. Pedrycz, (Eds.), *Human-Centric Information Processing Through Granular Modelling*. Berlin-Heidelberg, Germany: Springer-Verlag. (In Press).

Peters, J. F. (2008b). Discovery of perceptually near information granules. In Yao, J., (ed.), *Novel Developments in Granular Computing: Applications for Advanced Human Reasoning and Soft Computation*. Hershey, PA: IGI Global.

Peters, J. F., & Pawlak, Z. (2007). Zdzisław Pawlak life and work (1906-2006). Information Sciences, 177, 1-2.

Peters, J. F., & Ramanna, S. (2007). Feature Selection: Near Set Approach. In *Proceedings of MCDM'07*, (LNCS 4484), Springer- Verlag, Berlin 57-71.

Peters, J. F., & Ramanna, S. (2009). Affinities between perceptual information granules: Foundations and perspectives. In: A. Bargiela, W. Pedrycz, (Eds.), *Human-Centric Information Processing Through Granular Modelling. Studies in Computational Intelligence*. Berlin, Germany: Springer.

Peters, J. F., & Skowron, A. (1999). Approximate realtime decision making: Concepts and rough fuzzy petri net models. *International Journal of Intelligent Systems, 14*, 805-839.

Peters, J. F., & Skowron, A. (2006a). Zdzislaw Pawlak: Life and Work, Transactions on Rough Sets, 5, 1-24.

Peters, J. F., & Wasilewski, P. (2008). Foundations of near set theory. Hershey, PA: Information Science Reference.

Peters, J. F., Henry, C., & Ramanna, S. (2005a). Rough Ethograms: Study of Intelligent System Behavior. In M.A. Kłopotek, S. Wierzchoń, K. Trojanowski (Eds.), New Trends in Intelligent Information Processing and Web Mining (IIS05), (pp. 117-126). Gdańsk, Poland.

Peters, J. F., Pawlak, Z., & Skowron, A. (2002). A rough set approach to measuring information granules. In *Proceedings of COMPSAC 2002*, (pp. 1135-1139).

Peters, J. F., Shahfar, S., Ramanna, S., & Szturm, T. (2007a). Biologically-inspired adaptive learning: A near set approach. In *Proceedings of Frontiers in the Convergence of Bioscience and Information Technologies* (FBIT07), (pp. 403-408). Washington, DC: SERSC, IEEE Computer Society.

Peters, J. F., Skowron, A, Stepaniuk, J. (2007). Nearness of objects: Extension of approximation space model. Fundamenta Informaticae, 79, 1-16.

Peters, J. F., Skowron, A. (2007). Zdzisław Pawlak life and work (1906-2006). Information Sciences, 177, 1-2.

Peters, J. F., Skowron, A., & Stepaniuk, J. (2006b). Nearness in approximation spaces. In G. Lindemann, H. Schlilngloff et al. (Eds.), Proceedings of Concurrency, Specification & Programming (CS & P'2006), (pp. 434-445). Informatik-Berichte Nr. 206, Humboldt-Universität zu Berlin.

Peters, J. F., Skowron, A., & Stepaniuk, J. (2007). Nearness of objects: Extension of approximation space model. Fundamenta Informaticae, 79, 1-16.

Peters, J. F., Skowron, A., & Stepaniuk, J. (2007b). Nearness of objects: Extension of approximation space model. *Fundamenta Informaticae, 79*(3-4), 497-512.

Peters, J. F., Skowron, A., Ramanna, S., & Synak, P. (2002). Rough sets and information granulation. In: T.B. Bilgic, D. Baets, and O. Kaynak (eds.), *Proceedings of 10th International Fuzzy Systems Association World Congress*, (Lecture Notes in Artificial Intelligence vol. *2715*, pp. 370-377). Berlin Heidelberg, Germany: Springer-Verlag.

Peters, J. F., Skowron, A., Synak, P., & Ramanna, S. (2003). Rough sets and information granulation. In Bilgic, T., Baets, D., Kaynak, O. (Eds.), Tenth Int. Fuzzy Systems Assoc. World Congress IFSA, (Lecture Notes in Artificial Intelligence 2715, 370-377). Instanbul, Turkey. Berlin, Germany: Springer Verlag.

Pinker, S. (1997). *How the mind works*. New York: W.W. Norton & Company.

Poggio, T., & Smale, S. (2003). The mathematics of learning: Dealing with data. *Notices of the AMS, 50*(5), 537-544.

Poincare, H. (1913). Mathematics and Science: Last Essays, (trans. by J.W. Bolduc). New York: Kessinger Pub.

Polkowski, L. (2002). Rough Sets. Mathematical Foundations. Berlin Heidelberg, Germany: Springer-Verlag.

Polkowski, L. (2006). Rough Mereological Reasoning in Rough Set Theory: Recent Results and Problems. In *Proceedings of Rough Sets and Knowledge Technology* (RSKT 2006), (LNCS vol. 4062, pp. 79-92). Berlin, Germany: Springer

Polkowski, L. (2006, July 20-22). A Calculus on Granules from Rough inclusions in Information Systems. In Proceedings of International Forum on Theory of GrC from Rough Set Perspective, *Journal of Nanchang Institute of Technology, 25*(2), 22-27. Nanchang, China.

Polkowski, L., & Artiemjew, P. (2007). On granular rough computing: factoring classifiers through granulated decision systems. In *Proceedings of the International Conference on Rough Sets and Emerging Intelligent Systems Paradigms* (LNAI 4585, pp. 280–289).

Polkowski, L., Semeniuk-Polkowska, M. (2008). Reasoning about Concepts by Rough Mereological Logics. In *Proceedings of Rough Sets and Knowledge Technology* (RSKT 2008), (Springer LNCS vol. 5009, pp. 205-212).

Pomykała, J. & Pomykała, J. A. (1988). The Stone algebra of rough sets. *Bulletin of the Polish Academy of Sciences, Mathematics, 36,* 495-508.

Pomykala, J. A. (1987). Approximation operations in approximation space. *Bulletin of the Polish Academy of Sciences: Mathematics, 35,* 653–662.

Pontow, C., & Schubert, R. (2006). A mathematical analysis of theories of parthood. *Data & Knowledge Engineering, 59,* 107-138.

Qian, Y. H., & Liang, J. Y. (2006). Combination entropy and combination granulation in incomplete information system. *Lecture Notes in Artificial Intelligence, 4062,* 184-190.

Qian, Y. H., & Liang, J. Y. (2008). Positive approximation and rule extracting in incomplete information systems. *International Journal of Computer Science and Knowledge Engineering, 2*(1), 51-63.

Qian, Y. H., Dang, C. Y., & Liang, J. Y. (2008). Consistency measure, inclusion degree and fuzzy measure in decision tables. *Fuzzy Sets and Systems, 159,* 2353-2377.

Qian, Y. H., Dang, C. Y., Liang, J. Y., Zhang, H. Y., & Ma, J. M. (2008). On the evaluation of the decision performance of an incomplete decision table. *Data & Knowledge Engineering, 65*(3) 373-400.

Qian, Y. H., Liang, J. Y., & Dang, C. Y. (2008). Converse approximation and rule extracting from decision tables in rough set theory. *Computer & Mathematics with Applications, 55*(8), 1754-1765.

Qian, Y. H., Liang, J. Y., Dang, C. Y., Wang, F., & Xu, W. (2007). Knowledge distance in information systems. *Journal of System Sciences and System Engineering, 16*(4), 434-449.

Qian, Y. H., Liang, J. Y., Li, D. Y., Zhang, H. Y., & Dang, C. Y. (2008). Measures for evaluating the decision performance of a decision table in rough set theory. *Information Sciences, 178,* 181-202.

Qian, Y., Dang, C., Liang, J., & Tang, D. (2009). Set-valued ordered information systems. *Information Sciences, 179,* 2809-2832.

Qin, K.Y., & Pei, Z. (2005). On the topological properties of fuzzy rough sets. *Fuzzy Sets and Systems, 151,* 601–613.

Qiu, T., Chen, X., Liu, Q., Huang, H. (2007, November 2-4). A Granular Space Model for Ontology Learning. *IEEE International Conference on Granular Computing* (GrC2007), (pp. 61-65). San Francisco: IEEE Computer Society.

Quafatou, M. (2000). a-RST: a generalization of rough set theory. *Information Sciences, 124,* 301-316.

Quan, X., & Biao, M. (2008). Self-Adaptive Ant Colony Algorithm for Attributes Reduction. In Proceedings of the *IEEE International Conference on Granular Computing* (pp. 686-689).

Quinlan, J. R. (1983). Learning efficient classification procedures and their application to chess end-games. In J.S. Michalski, J.G. Carbonell and T.M. Mitchell (Eds.), *Machine Learning: An Artificial Intelligence Approach* (pp. 463-482). San Francisco: Morgan Kaufmann.

Quinlan, J. R. (1993). *C4.5: Programs for Machine Learning.* San Francisco: Morgan Kaufmann.

Radzikowska, A. M., & Kerre, E. E. (2002). A comparative study of fuzzy rough sets. *Fuzzy Sets and Systems, 126,* 137–155.

Ramanna, S. **(2008).** Conflict analysis in the framework of rough sets and granular computing, *Handbook of Granular Computing.* New York: Wiley.

Ramanna, S., & Skowron, A. (2007c). Requirements Interaction and Conflicts: A Rough Set Approach. In *Proceedings of the IEEE Symposium Series on Foundations of Computational Intelligence* (IEEE SCCI 2007). Honolulu, HI.

Ramanna, S., Peters, J. F., & Skowron, A. (2006a). Approaches to Conflict Dynamics based on Rough Sets, *Fundamenta Informaticae,* (75), 1-16.

Ramanna, S., Peters, J. F., & Skowron, A. (2006b) Generalized conflict and resolution model with approximation spaces. In Iniuguchi, M., Greco, S., Nguyen, H.S. (Eds.), *Proceedings of RSCTC'06,* (LNAI, 4259, pp. 274-283). Berlin Heidelberg, Germnay: Springer-Verlag.

Ramanna, S., Peters, J. F., & Skowron, A. (2007a). Approximate Adaptive Learning During Conflict Resolution. *Journal of Information Technology and Intelligent Computing, 2.*

Ramanna, S., Peters, J. F., & Skowron, A. (2007b). Approximation Space-based Socio-Technical Conflict Model. In *Proceedings of RSKT'07,* (LNCS 4481, pp. 476-483). Berlin Heidelberg, Germany: Springer Verlag.

Ramanna, S., Peters, J. F., Skowron, A. (2006, September 27-29) Analysis of Conflict Dynamics by Risk Patterns. In *Proceedings of the Workshop on Concurrency, Specification and Programming* (CS&P 2006), Berlin, Germany.

Ramsay, J. O., & Silverman, B. W. (2002). *Applied Functional Data Analysis.* Berlin: Springer.

Ras, Z. W., & Wyrzykowska, E. (2007). Extended action rule discovery based on single classification rules and reducts. In Hassanien, A., Suraj, Z., Slezak, D., and Lingras, P., (eds.), *Rough Computing: Theories, Technologies and Applications,* (pp. 175-184). Hershey, PA: IGI Global.

Rasiowa, H., & Skowron, A. (1985). Rough concepts logic. In A.Skowron (ed), *Computation Theory* (Lecture Notes in Comp.Sci.208, pp. 288-297).Liu, Q. (2005). *Rough Sets and Rough Reseaning* (Third). Beijing, China: Science Press. (In Chinese).Hamilton, A. G. (1980). *Logic for Mathematicans.* Cambridge, UK: Cambridge University Press.

Reifer, R. J., (2006). *Software Management,* (7th Edition). New York: Wiley-Interscience.

Ribba, B., Colin, T., & Schnell, S. (2006). A multiscale mathematical model of cancer, and its use in analyzing irradiation therapies. *Theoretical Biology and Medical Modelling, 3*(7).

Rissanen, J. (1985). Minimum-description-length principle. In Kotz, S., & Johnson, N. (eds.), *Encyclopedia of Statistical Sciences,* (pp. 523-527). New York: John Wiley & Sons.

Rodal, A. A., Sokolova, O., Robins, D. B., Daugherty, K. M., Hippenmeyer, S., Riezman, H., Grigorieff, N., & Goode, B. L. (2005). Conformational changes in the Arp2/3 complex leading to actin nucleation. *Nature Structural & Molecular Biology, 12,* 26-31.

Roddick, J. F., Hornsby, K., & Spiliopoulou, M. (2001). An updated bibliography of temporal, spatial and spatio-temporal data mining research. In Roddick, J. F. and Hornsby, K., (eds.), *Post-Workshop Proceedings of the International Workshop on Temporal, Spatial and Spatio-Temporal Data Mining, Lecture Notes in Artificial Intelligence,* (volume 2007, pp. 147-163). Berlin, Germany: Springer.

Rosse, C., & Mejino, J. L.V. (2003). A reference ontology for biomedical informatics: the foundational model of anatomy. *Journal of Biomedical Informatics, 36,* 478-500.

Rossi, L., Słowiński, R., & Susmaga, R. (1999). Rough set approach to evaluation of stormwater pollution. *International Journal of Environment and Pollution, 12,* 232-250.

Sai, Y., Yao, Y. Y., & Zhong, N. (2001). Data analysis and mining in ordered information tables. In *Proceedings of the 2001 IEEE Int. Conference on Data Mining* (pp. 497-504). Washington, DC: IEEE Computer Society Press.

Sakai, H., & Nakata, M. (2006). On Rough sets based rule generation from tables. *International Journal of Innovative Computing, Information and Control, 2,* 3-31.

Sakai, H., & Okuma, A. (2004). Basic algorithms and tools for rough non-deterministic information analysis. Transactions on Rough Sets I, (Springer LNCS 3100, pp. 209-231).

Salthe, S. N. (1985). *Evolving hierarchical systems—their structure and representation.* New York: Columbia University Press.

Salthe, S. N. (2001, November). Summary of the Principles of Hierarchy Theory. Retrieved on October 10, 2005, from http://www.nbi.dk/~natphil/salthe/hierarchy th.html

Samuel, A. L. (1962). Artificial intelligence: a frontier of automation. *The Annals of the American Academy of Political and Social Science, 340*(1), 10-20.

Sankar, K. P., & Mitra, P. (2002). Multispectral image segmentation using the rough-set-initialized EM algorithm. *IEEE Transactions on Geoscience and Remote Sensing, 40*, 2495-2501.

Schank, R. C. (1987). What is AI, anyway? *AI Magazine, 8*(4), 59-65.

Shankar, U. (2007). Novel Classification and segmentation techniques with application to remotely sensed images. *T. Rough Sets, 7*, 295-380.

Shary, S. P. (2003, July 8-9). Parameter partitioning scheme for interval linear systems with constraints In *Proceedings of the International Workshop on Interval Mathematics and Constraint Propagation Methods* (ICMP'03), (pp. 1–12). Novosibirsk, Akademgorodok, Russia. (in Russian).

Shary, S. P. (2004). Solving tied interval linear systems. *Siberian Journal of Numerical Mathematics, 7*(4), 363–376 (in Russian).

Shen, Q., & Chouchoulas, A. (2001). Rough Set-Based Dimensionality Reduction for Supervised and Unsupervised Learning. *Int. J. Appl. Comput. Sci., 11*, 583-601.

Shoham, Y. (1998). *Reasoning about Change*. Cambridge, MA: MIT Press.

Simon, H. A. (1963). The organization of complex systems. In: H. H. Pattee (Ed.), *Hierarchy Theory, the Challenge of Complex Systems* (pp. 1-27). New York: George Braziller.

Simpson, P. K. (1992). Fuzzy min-max neural networks - Part1: Classification. *IEEE Trans. Neural Networks, 3*(5), 776-786.

Simpson, P. K. (1993). Fuzzy min-max neural networks – Part 2: Clustering. *IEEE Trans. Neural Networks, 4*(1), 32-45.

Skowron A., Stepaniuk J., & Peters J. F. (2003) Rough sets and infomorphisms: Towards approximation of relations in distributed environments. *Fundamenta Informaticae, 54*, 263–277.

Skowron, A. (1989). The relationship between the rough set theory and evidence theory. *Bulletin of Polish Academy of Science: Mathematics, 37*, 87–90.

Skowron, A. (1995). Extracting laws from decision tables: a rough set approach. *Computational Intelligence, 11*, 371-388.

Skowron, A. (2001). Toward intelligent systems: calculi of information granules. In Proceedings of International Workshop on Rough Set Theory and Granular Computing (RSTGC- 2001), *Bulleting of International Rough Set Society, 5*(1/2), 9-30.

Skowron, A. (2006, July 20-22). Rough-Granular Computing. In Proceedings of International Forum on Theory of GrC from Rough Set Perspective. *Journal of Nanchang Institute of Technology, 25*(2), 22-27.

Skowron, A., & Peters, J. F. (2003). Rough sets: Trends and challenges -plenary paper. In Wang, G., Liu, Q., Yao, Y., Skowron, A. (eds.), *Proceedings of RSFDGrC 2003: Rough Sets, Fuzzy Sets, Data Mining, and Granular Computing.* (Lecture Notes in Artificial Intelligence vol. *2639*, pp. 25-34). Berlin Heidelberg, Germany: Springer-Verlag,

Skowron, A., & Rauszer, C. (1992). The DiscernibilityMatrices and Functions in Information Systems. In Słowinski, R (ed.), *Intelligent Decision Support - Handbook of Applications and Advances of the Rough Sets Theory, System Theory, Knowledge Engineering and Problem Solving 11*, (pp. 331-362). Dordrecht, The Netherlands: Kluwer.

Skowron, A., & Stepaniuk, J. (1996). Tolerance approximation spaces. *Fundamenta Informaticae, 27*, 245-253.

Skowron, A., & Stepaniuk, J. (2001). Extracting patterns using information granules. In Proceedings of International workshop on Rough Set Theory and Granular Computing (RSTGC-2001), *Bulleting of International Rough Set Society, 5*(1/2), 135-142.

Skowron, A., & Stepaniuk, J. (2001). Information granules: towards foundations of granular computing. *International Journal of Intelligent Systems, 16*(1), 57-85.

Skowron, A., & Stepaniuk, J. (2003). Information granules and rough-neural computing. In Pal, S. K., Polkowski, L., & Skowron, A., editors, *Rough-Neural Computing: Techniques for Computing with Words*, Cognitive Technologies, (pp. 43-84). Berlin, Germany: Springer.

Skowron, A., & Suraj, Z. (1993). Rough sets and concurrency. *Bulletin of the Polish Academy of Sciences, 41*, 237-254.

Skowron, A., & Suraj, Z. (1995). Discovery of concurrent data models from experimental tables: A rough set approach. In *Proceedings of the First International Conference on Knowledge Discovery and Data Mining*, (pp. 288-293), Menlo Park, CA: AAAI Press.

Skowron, A., & Synak, P. P. (2004). Complex patterns. *Fundamenta Informaticae, 60*(1-4), 351-366.

Skowron, A., Peters, J. F. (2008). Rough-granular computing. In Pedrycz, W., Skowron, A., Kreinovich, V. (Eds.), Handbook on Granular Computing. New Yokr: Wiley.

Skowron, A., Ramanna, S., & Peters, J. F. (2006). Conflict Analysis and Information Systems: A Rough Set Approach. In *Proceedings of RSKT'06*, (LNCS 4062, pp. 233-241). Berlin, Heidelberg, Germany: Springer Verlag.

Skowron, A., Stepaniuk, J., & Peters, J. F. (2003). Rough sets and infomorphisms: Towards approximation of relations in distributed environments. *Fundamenta Informaticae, 54*(2-3), 263-277.

Skowron, A., Stepaniuk, J., Peters, J., & Swiniarski, R. (2006). Calculi of approximation spaces. *Fundamenta Informaticae, 72*(1-3), 363-378.

Skrenta, R., & Truel, B. (1998). *Open Directory Project*. Retrieved February 10, 2008, from http://www.dmoz.org/

Skrenta, R., & Truel, B. (1998). *Open Directory Project*. Retrieved February 10, 2008, from http://www.dmoz.org/

Slezak, D. (1996). Approximate reducts in decision tables. In: Bouchon-Meunier, B., Delgado, M., Verdegay, J. L., Vila, M. A., & Yager, R (Eds.), *Proceeding of IPMU'96* (Vol. 3. pp. 1159- 1164). Granada, Spain.

Ślęzak, D. (2002). Approximate entropy reducts. *Fundamenta Informaticae, 53*(3-4), 365-387.

Slowinski, R., & Vanderpooten, D. (2000). A Generalized definition of rough approximations based on similarity. *IEEE Transactions on Knowledge and Data Engineering, 12*, 331–336.

Słowiński, R., & Zopounidis, C. (1995). Application of the rough set approach to evaluation of bankruptcy risk. *International Journal of Intelligent Systems in Accounting, Finance and Management, 4*, 27-41.

Słowiński, R., Greco, S., & Matarazzo, B. (2002). Mining decision-rule preference model from rough approximation of preference relation. In *Proceedings of the 26th IEEE Annual Int. Conference on Computer Software & Applications (COMPSAC 2002)* (pp. 1129-1134). Oxford, UK.

Słowiński, R., Greco, S., & Matarazzo, B. (2005). Rough set based decision support. In E. K. Burke & G. Kendall (Eds.), *Search Methodologies: Introductory Tutorials in Optimization and Decision Support Techniques* (chapter 16, pp. 475-527). New York: Springer.

Słowiński, R., Zopounidis, C., & Dimitras, A. I. (1997). Prediction of company acquisition in Greece by means of the rough set approach. *European Journal of Operational Research, 100*, 1-15.

Smith, B. (2004). Beyond Concepts, or Ontology as Reality Representation. In Varzi, A., Vieu, L. (eds.), *Formal Ontology and Information Systems. Proceedings of the Third International Conference* (FOIS 2004), (pp. 73-84). Amsterdam: IOS Press.

Sommerville, I., (2007). *Software Engineering*, (7th ed). Reading, MA: Addison-Wesley.

Sontag, E.D. (2004). Some new directions in control theory inspired by systems biology. *Systems Biology, 1*(1), 9-18.

Sossinsky, A. B. (1986). Tolerance space theory and some applications. Acta Applicandae Mathematicae: An International Survey Journal on Applying Mathematics and Mathematical Applications, 5(2), 137-167.

Sowa, J. F. (2000). *Knowledge representation: logical, philosophical, and computational foundations*. Beijing, China: China Machine Press.

Spencer, J. (1994). Ten Lectures on the Probabilistic Method, 2nd Ed. Society for Industrial and Applied Mathematics (SIAM), Philadelphia.

Stepaniuk J. (2008). *Rough - Granular Computing in Knowledge Discovery and Data Mining, Series: Studies in Computational Intelligence.* Berlin, Germany: Springer.

Sternberg, R. J., & Frensch, P. A. (Eds.). (1991). *Complex problem solving, principles and mechanisms.* Mahwah, NJ: Lawrence Erlbaum Associates.

Stevens, R., Brook, P., Jacksona, K., & Arnold, S. (1998). *Systems Engineering. Coping with Complexity.* London: Prentice-Hall.

Straccia, U. (2006). A Fuzzy Description Logic for the Semantic Web. In Sanchez, E. (ed.), *Capturing Intelligence: Fuzzy Logic and the Semantic Web.* Amsterdam: Elsevier.

Sudha, R., Rajagopalan, M. R., Selvanayaki, M., & Selvi, S. T. (2007). Ubiquitous Semantic Space: A context-aware and coordination middleware for Ubiquitous Computing. In *Proceedings of COMSWARE 2007 and 2nd International Conference on Communication Systems Software and Middleware.* (pp. 1-7).

Sudha, R., Rajagopalan, M. R., Selvanayaki, M., & Selvi, S. T. (2007). Ubiquitous Semantic Space: A context-aware and coordination middleware for Ubiquitous Computing. In *Proceedings of COMSWARE 2007 and 2nd International Conference on Communication Systems Software and Middleware.* **(pp. 1-7).**

Sugeno, M., & Yasukawa, T. (1993). A fuzzy-logic-based approach to qualitative modeling. *IEEE Trans. on Fuzzy Systems, 1,* 7-31.

Sugiyama, K., Hatano, K., & Yoshikawa, M. (2004). Adaptive Web Search Based on User Profile Constructed Without any Effort from Users. In Feldman, S., Uretsky, M., Najork, M. & Wills, C. (Ed.), *Proceedings of the 13th International Conference on World Wide Web,* (pp. 675-684). ACM Press.

Sugiyama, K., Hatano, K., & Yoshikawa, M. (2004). Adaptive Web Search Based on User Profile Constructed Without any Effort from Users. In Feldman, S., Uretsky, M., Najork, M. & Wills, C. (Ed.), *Proceedings of the 13th International Conference on World Wide Web,* pp. 675-684. ACM Press.

Sun, R., (ed.) (2006). *Cognition and Multi-Agent Interaction. From Cognitive Modeling to Social Simulation.* Cambridge, UK: Cambridge University Press.

Suraj, Z. (2000). Rough set methods for the synthesis and analysis of concurrent processes. In Polkowski, L., Lin, T., & Tsumoto, S., editors, *Rough Set Methods and Applications: New Developments in Knowledge Discovery in Information Systems, Studies in Fuzziness and Soft Computing,* (volume 56, pp. 379-488). Heidelberg, Germany: Springer.

Suvorov, P. Yu. (1980). On the recognition of the tautological nature of propositional formulas, *J. Sov. Math., 14,* 1556–1562.

Takagi, T., & Sugeno, M. (1985). Fuzzy identification of systems and its applications to modeling and control. *IEEE Trans. on Systems, Man, and Cybernetics, 15,* 116-132.

Tange, H. J., Schouten, H. C, Kester, A. D. M., & Hasman, A. (1998). The Granularity of Medical Narratives and Its Effect on the Speed and Completeness of Information Retrieval. *Journal of the American Medical Informatics Association, 5*(6), 571-582.

The national academy of engineering (2008). *Grand challenges for engineering.* Retrieved September 19, 2008, from http://www.engineeringchallenges.org

Thiele, H. (2001a). On axiomatic characterisation of fuzzy approximation operators II, the rough fuzzy set based case. In *Proceedings of the 31st IEEE International Symposium on Multiple-Valued Logi* (pp. 330–335).

Thiele, H. (2001b). On axiomatic characterization of fuzzy approximation operators III the fuzzy diamond and fuzzy box cases. In *The 10th IEEE International Conference on Fuzzy Systems* (vol. 2, pp. 1148–1151).

Tsumoto, S. (2007). Mining Diagnostic Taxonomy and Diagnostic Rules for Multi-Stage Medical Diagnosis from Hospital Clinical Data. *IEEE International Conference on Granular Computing* (GrC2007), (pp. 611-616). Washington, DC: IEEE Computer Society.

UCI (n.d.). *UCI machine learning repository*. Retreived from http://mlearn.ics.uci.edu/MLRepositroy.html

Unnikrishnan, K. P., Ramakrishnan, N., S., Sastry, P., & Uthurusamy, R., (eds.) (2006). *Proceedings of 4th KDD Workshop on Temporal Data Mining: Network Reconstruction from Dynamic Data at KDD 2006 Conference*, Philadelphia. ACM SIGKDD.

Vakarelov, D. (1992). Consequence relations and information systems. In R. Słowiński (Ed.), *Intelligent Decision Support: Handbook of Applications and Advances of the Rough Sets Theory* (pp. 391-399). Boston: Kluwer Academic Publishers.

van Benthem, J. (2007). Cognition as interaction. In Bouma, G., KrÄamer, I., and Zwarts, J., editors, *Cognitive Foundations of Interpretation*, (pp. 27-38). Amsterdam, KNAW.

van Benthem, J. (2008). Logic games: From tools to models of interaction. In Gupta, A., Parikh, R., and van Benthem, J., (editors.), *Logic at the Crossroads*, (pp. 283-317). Mumbai, India: Allied Publishers. To appear.

Vapnik, V. (1998). *Statisctical Learning Theory*. New York: John Wiley & Sons.

Varzi, A. C. (2004). Mereology. In Zalta, E.N. (ed.), *The Stanford Encyclopedia of Philosophy*. Retrieved from http://plato.stanford.edu/archives/fall2004/entries/mereology/

Varzi, A. C. (2007). Spatial reasoning and ontology: parts, wholes, and locations. In Aiello, M., Pratt-Hartmann, I. & van Benthem, J. (eds.), *Handbook of Spatial Logics* (pp. 945-1038). Berlin, Germany: Springer.

Vernieuwe, H., Verhoest, N. E. C., De Baets, B., Hoeben, R., & De Troch, F. P. (2007). Cluster-based fuzzy models of groundwater transport. *Advances in Water Resources*, *30*(4), 701-714.

Wang, G. Y. (2001). *Rough set theory and knowledge acquisition*. Xi'an, China: Xi'an Jiaotong University Press.

Wang, G. Y. (2002). Extension of rough set under incomplete information systems. *Journal of Computer Research and Development*, *39*(10), 1238-1243.

Wang, G. Y. (2006). Domain-oriented data-driven data mining based on rough sets. *Journal of Nanchang Institute of Technology*, *25*(2), 46.

Wang, G. Y. (2007). Domain-oriented data-driven data mining (3dm): simulation of human knowledge understanding, *WImBI 2006* (Vol. LNCS 4845, pp. 278-290).

Wang, G. Y., Hu, F., Huang, H., & Wu, Y. (2005). A granular computing model based on tolerance relation. *The Journal of China Universities of Posts and Telecommunications*, *12*(3), 86-90.

Wang, G. Y., Yu, H., & Yang, D. C. (2002). Decision table reduction based on conditional information entropy. *Chinese Journal of Computers*, *25*(7), 759-766.

Wang, G. Y., Yu, H., Yang, D. C., & Wu, Z. F. (2001). Knowledge reduction based on rough set and information entropy. In *Proceedings of the 5th World Multiconference on Systemics, Cybernetics and Informatics* (pp. 555-560). Orlando, FL: IIIS.

Wang, G. Y., Zhao, J., An, J. J., & Wu, Y. (2004). Theoretical study on attribute reduction of rough set theory: comparison of algebra and information views. In *Proceedings of the 3rd International Conference on Cognitive Informatics(ICCI'04)* (pp. 148-155).

Wang, X. J. (1982). *Introduction for mathematical logic*. Beijing, China: Beijing, Press.

Watt, D., & Brown, D., (2001). *Java Collections*. New York:John Wiley & Sons, Inc.

Widell, A., Elmud, H., Persson, M. H., & Jonsson, M. (1996). Transmission of hepatitis C via both erythrocyte and platelet transfusions from a single donor in serological window-phase of hepatitis C. *Vox Sang, 71*(1), 55-57.

Wikipedia (n.d.). *Wiki article on Interaction*. Retrieved from http://en.wikipedia.org/wiki/Interaction

Wilk, S., Słowiński, R., Michałowski, W., & Greco, S. (2005). Supporting triage of children with abdominal pain in the emergency room. *European Journal of Operational Research*, *160*, 696-709.

Wille, R. (1982). Restructuring lattice theory: An approach based on hierarchies of concepts. In *Proceedings of Rival I, ed. Ordered Sets* (pp. 445-470). Boston: Reidel.

Wille, R. (1992). Concept lattices and conceptual knowledge systems. *Computers Mathematics with Applications, 23*, 493-515.

Wille, R. (2000). Boolean concept logic, In B. Canter and G. W. Mineau (Eds.), *Conceptual Structures: Logical, Linguistic, and Computational Issues* (LNAI 1867). Berlin, Germany: Springer

Wimsatt, W. C. (1995). The ontology of complex systems: Levels of Organization, Perspectives, and Causal Thickets. *Canadian Journal of Philosophy, 20*, 207-274.

Wing, J. M. (2006). Computational thinking. *Communication of the ACM, 49*(3), 33-35.

Wiweger, R. (1989) On topological rough sets. *Bulletin of Polish Academy of Sciences: Mathematics, 37*, 89–93.

Woleński, J. (2001). Review of S. Leśniewski, Collected Works, Vols. 1-II. Modern Logic, 8(3 & 4), 195-201.

Wróblewski, J. (1995). Finding minimal reducts using genetic algorithms. In *Proceedings of Second International Joint Conference on Information Science* (pp. 186-189).

Wu, C., & Yang, X., (2005). Information Granules in General and Complete Coverings. In Hu, X., Liu, Q., Skowron, A., Lin, T. Y., Yager, R. R., & Zhang, B., (Eds.), Proceedings of IEEE International Conference on Granular Computing (pp. 675-678). Beijing, China, IEEE Press.

Wu, F.-X. (2007). Inference of gene regulatory networks and its validation. *Current Bioinformatics, 2*(2), 139-144.

Wu, W. Z. (2006, May 10-12). Rough Set Approximations vs. Measurable Space. In *Proceedings of the 2005 IEEE International Conference on Granular Computing* (pp. 329-332). Atlanta, GA.

Wu, W. Z., Zhang, M., Li, H. Z., & Mi, J. S. (2005). Knowledge reduction in random information systems via Dempster-Shafer theory of evidence. *Information Sciences, 174*, 143-164.

Wu, W.-Z., & Zhang, W.-X. (2002). Neighborhood operator systems and approximations. *Information Sciences, 144*, 201–217.

Wu, W.-Z., & Zhang, W.-X. (2004) Constructive and axiomatic approaches of fuzzy approximation operators. *Information Sciences, 159*, 233–254.

Wu, W.-Z., Leung, Y., & Mi, J.-S. (2005). On characterizations of (I, T)-fuzzy rough approximation operators. *Fuzzy Sets and Systems, 154*(1), 76–102.

Wu, W.-Z., Leung, Y., & Zhang, W.-X. (2002). Connections between rough set theory and Dempster-Shafer theory of evidence. *International Journal of General Systems, 31*, 405–430.

Wu, W.-Z., Mi, J.-S., & Zhang, W.-X. (2003). Generalized fuzzy rough sets. *Information Sciences, 151*, 263–282.

Wybraniec-Skardowska, U. (1989). On a generalization of approximation space. *Bulletin of the Polish Academy of Sciences: Mathematics, 37*, 51–61.

Xie, Y., Katukuri, J., Raghavan, V. V., & Johnsten, T. (2008). Examining granular computing from a modeling perspective. In: *Proceedings of 2008 Annual Meeting of the North American Fuzzy Information Processing Society* (pp. 1-5). Piscataway, NJ: Institute of Electrical and Electronics Engineers, Inc.

Xu, R., & Wunsch, D. (2005). Survey of clustering algorithms. *IEEE Transactions on Neural Networks, 16*, 645–678

Xu, Z. B., Liang, J. Y., Dang, C. Y., & Chin, K. S. (2002). Inclusion degree: a perspective on measures for rough set data analysis. *Information Sciences, 141*, 229-238.

Yang, X., Yang, J., Wu, C., & Yu, D. (2008). Dominance-based rough set approach and knowledge reductions in incomplete ordered information system. *Information Sciences, 178*, 1219-1234.

Yang, X.-P. (2007). Minimization of axiom sets on fuzzy approximation operators. *Information Sciences, 177*, 3840–3854.

Yang, X.-P., & Li, T.-J. (2006). The minimization of axiom sets characterizing generalized approximation operators. *Information Sciences, 176*, 887–899.

Yao, J. (2007). A ten-year review of granular computing. In *Proceedings of the 2007 IEEE International*

*Conference on Granular Computing* (pp. 734-739). Silicon Valley, CA.

Yao, J. (2008a). Recent developments in granular computing: a bibliometric study. In *Proceedings of the IEEE International Conference on Granular Computing* (pp. 74-79). Hangzhou, China.

Yao, J. T. (2005). Information granulation and granular relationships. In *Proceedings of the IEEE - Conference on Granular Computing*, (pp.326-329).

Yao, J. T. (2007). A ten-year review of granular computing. *IEEE International Conference on Granular Computing 2007* (GrC'07), (pp. 734-739). IEEE Computer Society.

Yao, J. T. (2008). Recent Developments in Granular Computing. In *Proceedings of the 2008 IEEE International Conference on Granular Computing*, (pp. 74-79).

Yao, J. T., & Yao, Y. Y. (2002). A granular computing approach to machine learning. In *Proceedings of the 1st International Conference on Fuzzy Systems and Knowledge Discovery (FSKD'02)* (pp. 732-736). Singapore.

Yao, J. T., & Yao, Y. Y. (2002). Induction of classification rules by granular computing. In *Proceedings of the 3rd International Conference on Rough Sets and Current Trends in Computing* (Vol. 2475, pp. 331-338).

Yao, J. T., (2006). Information Granulation and Granular Relationships. In Zhang, Y. & Lin, T. Y. (Eds.), *Proceedings of IEEE International Conference on Granular Computing* (pp. 326-329), Atlanta, GA: IEEE Press.

Yao, J. T., Yao, Y. Y., & Ziarko, W. (2008). Special Section on Probabilistic Rough Sets. *International Journal of Approximate Reasoning, 49*, 253-343.

Yao, J. T., Yao, Y.Y., & Zhao, Y. (2005). Foundations of classification. In Lin, T.Y., Ohsuga, S., Liau, C.J. and Hu, X. (Eds.), *Foundations and Novel Approaches in Data Mining* (pp. 75-97). Berlin, Germany Springer.

Yao, J.T. (2007). A ten-year review of granular computing. In *Proceedings of the 3rd IEEE International Conference on Granular Computing* (pp. 734-739).

Yao, Y. Y. (2000). Granular computing: basic issues and possible solution. *Proceedings of the 5th Joint Conference on Information Sciences* (pp. 186-189). Durham, NC: Association for Intelligent Machinery, Inc.

Yao, Y. Y. (1996). Two views of the theory of rough sets in finite universes. *International Journal of Approximate Reasoning, 15*, 291–317.

Yao, Y. Y. (1997). Combination of rough and fuzzy sets based on alpha-level sets. In Lin, T. Y., & Cercone, N. (Eds.), *Rough Sets and Data Mining: Analysis for Imprecise Data* (pp. 301–321). Boston: Kluwer Academic Publishers.

Yao, Y. Y. (1998a). Constructive and algebraic methods of the theory of rough sets. *Journal of Information Sciences, 109*, 21–47.

Yao, Y. Y. (1998b). Generalized rough set model. In L. Polkowski, & A. Skowron (Eds.), *Rough Sets in Knowledge Discovery 1. Methodology and Applications* (pp. 286–318). Berlin Heidelberg, Germany: Springer Verlag.

Yao, Y. Y. (1998c). Relational interpretations of neighborhood operators and rough set approximation operators. *Information Sciences, 111*, 239–259.

Yao, Y. Y. (2001). Information granulation and rough set approximation. *International Journal of Intelligent Systems, 16*(1), 87-104.

Yao, Y. Y. (2001). Modeling data mining with granular computing. In *Proceedings of COMPSAC 2001*, (pp. 638-643).

Yao, Y. Y. (2004). A partition model of granular computing. *Lecture Notes in Computer Science Transactions on Rough Sets*, (vol. 1, pp. 232-253).

Yao, Y. Y. (2004b). Granular computing. *Computer Science (Ji Suan Ji Ke Xue), 31,* 1-5.

Yao, Y. Y. (2005). Perspectives of Granular Computing. *IEEE Conference on Granular Computing* (GrC2005), (vol. *1*, pp. 85-90).

Yao, Y. Y. (2005). Perspectives of granular computing. In: Hu, X.H., Liu, Q., Skowron, A., Lin, T.Y., Yager, R.R., & Zhang, B. (Eds.), *Proceedings of 2005 IEEE*

*International Conference on Granular Computing* (pp. 85-90). Piscataway, NJ: Institute of Electrical and Electronics Engineers, Inc.

Yao, Y. Y. (2006, July 20-22). Three Perspectives of Granular Computing. In Proceedings of International Forum on Theory of GrC from Rough Set Perspective. *Journal of Nanchang Institute of Technology, 25*(2), 22-27.

Yao, Y. Y. (2007). Neighborhood systems and approximate retrieval. *Information Sciences, 174,* 143-164.

Yao, Y. Y. (2007). The art of granular computing. In *Proceeding of the International Conference on Rough Sets and Emerging Intelligent Systems Paradigms* (LNAI 4585, pp. 101-112).

Yao, Y. Y. (2007). The art of granular computing. In *Proceedings of International Conference on Rough Sets and Emerging Intelligent System Paradigms* (RSEISP'07), (LNAI 4585, pp. 101-112).

Yao, Y. Y. (2007b). Structured writing with granular computing strategies. In: Lin, T.Y., Hu, X.H., Han, J.C., Shen, X.J., & Li, Z.J. (Eds.), *Proceedings of 2007 IEEE International Conference on Granular Computing* (pp. 72-77). Los Alamitos, CA: IEEE Computer Society.

Yao, Y. Y. (2008, August). Granular Computing: Past, Present, and Future. *IEEE Conference on Granular Computing 2008,* (GrC'08). Beijing, China: IEEE Computer Society (in press).

Yao, Y. Y. (2008b). The rise of granular computing. *Journal of Chongqing University of Posts and Telecommunications (Natural Science Edition), 20,* 299-308.

Yao, Y. Y., & Liau, C.- J. (2002). A generalized decision logic language for granular computing. In *Proceedings of FUZZ-IEEE'02,* (pp. 1092-1097).

Yao, Y. Y., & Lin, T. Y. (1996). Generalization of rough sets using modal logic. *Intelligent Automation and Soft Computing, 2,* 103–120.

Yao, Y. Y., & Lingras, P. J. (1998). Interpretations of belief functions in the theory of rough sets. *Information Sciences, 104,* 81–106.

Yao, Y. Y., & Liu, Q. (1999, September 11). *A Generalized Decision Logic in Interval-Set-Valued Information table,* (LNAI 1711, pp. 285-294). Berlin, Germany: Springer.

Yao, Y. Y., & Yao, J. T. (2002). Granular computing as a basis for consistent classification problems. In *Proceedings of PAKDD Workshop on Toward the Foundation of Data Mining, 5*(2), 101-106.

Yao, Y. Y., & Zhou, B. (2007). A logic language of granular computing. In *Proceedings of the 6th IEEE International Conference on Cognitive Informatics* (pp. 178-185).

Yao, Y. Y., (2004). A partition model of granular computing. *LNCS Transactions on Rough Sets, 1,* 232-253.

Yao, Y. Y., (2007). Structured Writing with Granular Computing Strategies. In Lin, T. Y., Hu, X., Han, J. (Eds.), *Proceedings of IEEE International Conference on Granular Computing* (pp. 72-77). San Jose, CA, IEEE Press.

Yao, Y. Y., Liau, C.-J., & Zhong, N. (2003). Granular computing based on rough sets, quotient space theory, and belief functions. In *Proceedings of ISMIS'03,* (pp. 152-159).

Yao, Y. Y., Wang, F. Y., Wang, J., & Zeng, D. (2005). Rule + exception strategies for security information analysis. *IEEE Transactions on Intelligent Systems, 20,* 52-57.

Yao, Y. Y., Zhao, Y., & Yao, J. T. (2004). Level construction of decision trees in a partition-based framework for classification. In *Proceedings of Software Engineering and Knowledge Engineering* (pp. 199-205).

Yeung, D. S., Chen, D. G., Tsang, E. C. C. et al. (2005). On the generalization of fuzzy rough sets. *IEEE Transactions on Fuzzy Systems, 13*(3), 343–361.

Yixian,Y. (2006). *Theory and applications of higher-dimensional Hadamard Matrices*. Beijin, China: Science Press.

Yun, G., & Yuanbin, H. (2004). Application of Rough Set Theory on system modeling. In *Proceedings of the IEEE - 5ʰ World Congress on Intelligent Control and Automation* (pp. 2352-2354).

Zadeh, L. A. (1965). Fuzzy sets. *Information and Control, 8*(3), 338-353.

Zadeh, L. A. (1979).Fuzzy Sets and Information Granularity. In M. Gupta, R. Ragade, and R. Yager (eds.), *Advances in Fuzzy Set Theory and Applications* (pp. 3-18). Amsterdam.

Zadeh, L. A. (1996). Fuzzy logic computing with words. *IEEE Trans. Fuzzy Syst. 4*(2) 103-111.

Zadeh, L. A. (1997). Towards a theory of fuzzy information granulation and its centrality in human reasoning and fuzzy logic. *Fuzzy Sets and Systems, 90,* 111-127.

Zadeh, L. A. (1998). Some reflections on soft computing, granular computing and their roles in the conception, design and utilization of information/intelligent systems. *Soft Computing, 2*(1), 23-25.

Zadeh, L. A. (2001). A new direction in AI - toward a computational theory of perceptions. *AI Magazine, 22*(1), 73-84.

Zadeh, L. A. (2002). From computing with numbers to computing with words—from manipulations of measurements to manipulation of perceptions. *International Journal of applied mathematics and computer science, 12*(3), 307-324.

Zadeh, L. A. (2006). Generalized theory of uncertainty (GTU) - principal concepts and ideas. *Computational Statistics & Data Analysis, 51*(1), 15-46.

Zadeh, L. A., (1979). Fuzzy sets and information granularity. In Gupta, M., Ragade, R., & Yager, R. (Eds.), *Advances in Fuzzy Set Theory and Applications* (pp. 3-18). Amsterdam: North-Holland Publishing Co.

Zadeh, L. A., (1997). Towards a theory of fuzzy information granulation and its centrality in human reasoning and fuzzy logic. *Fuzzy Sets and Systems, 19,* 111-127.

Zakowski, W. (1982). On a concept of rough sets. *Demonstratio Mathematica, 15,* 1129–1133.

Zhang, B., & Zhang, L. (1990). *Theory and Applications for Problem Solving.* Tsinghua, China: Publisher of Tsinghua University. (In Chinese).

Zhang, C. Q., & Cao, L. B. (2006). Domain-driven data mining: methodologies and applications. In *Proceedings of the 4th International Conference on Active Media Technology.*

Zhang, J., Silvescu, A., & Honavar, V. (2002). *Ontology-Driven Induction of Decision Trees at Multiple Levels of Abstraction.* (Technical Report ISU-CS-TR 02-13), Computer Science, Iowa State University. Retrieved from http://archives.cs.iastate.edu/documents/disk0/00/00/02/91/

Zhang, L., & Zhang, B. (2005). Fuzzy reasoning model and under quotient space structure. *Information Sciences, 173,* 353-364.

Zhang, L., & Zhang, B. (Eds.). (2007). *Theory and application of problem solving – theory and application of granular computing in quotient spaces (in Chinese), 2nd edition.* Beijing, China: Tsinghua University Press.

Zhang, P., Germano, R., Arien, J., Qin, K. Y., & Xu, Y. (2006). Interpreting and extracting fuzzy decision rules from fuzzy information systems and their inference. *Information Sciences, 176,* 1869-1897.

Zhang, Q. H., Wang, G. Y., Hu, J., & Liu, X. Q. (2006). Incomplete information systems processing based on fuzzy-clustering. In *Proceedings of the 2006 IEEE/WIC/ACM International Conference on Web Intelligence and Intelligent Agent Technology* (WI-IAT 2006 Workshops), (pp. 486-489). Hong Kong, China.

Zhang, W. X., Wu, W. Z., Liang, J. Y., & Li, D. Y. (2001). *Theory and method of rough sets.* Beijing, China: Science Press.

Zhang, W.-X., Leung, Y., & Wu, W.-Z. (2003). *Information Systems and Knowledge Discovery.* Beijing, China: Science Press.

Zhang, Y. Q., & Lin, T. Y. (Eds.). (2006). *Proceedings of 2006 ieee international conference on granular computing.* Atlanta, GA.

Zhao, Y., & Yao, Y. Y. (2005). Interactive user-driven classification using a granule network. In *Proceedings of the Fifth International Conference of Cognitive Informatics* **(pp. 250-259).**

Zheng, Z., Hu, H., Shi, Z. (2005). *Tolerance granular space and its applications*. Washington, DC: IEEE Press.

Zhou, J., Zhang, Q. L., & Chen, W. S. (2004). Generalization of covering rough set. *Journal of Northeastern University(Natural Science)*, *25*(10), 954-956.

Zhou, Y., Young, J. A., Santrosyan, A., Chen, K., Yan, S. F., & Winzeler, E. A. (2005). In silico gene function prediction using ontology-based pattern identification. *Bioinformatics*, *21*(7), 1237-1245.

Zhu, H. B. (2008). Granular problem solving and software engineering. In: Lin, T.Y., Hu, X.H., Han, J.C., Shen, X.J., & Li, Z.J. (Eds.), *Proceedings of 2008 IEEE International Conference on Granular Computing* (pp. 859-864) Piscataway, NJ: Institute of Electrical and Electronics Engineers, Inc.

Zhu, W., & Wang, F. Y. (2003). Reduction and axiomization of covering generalized rough sets. *Information Science*, *152*, 217-230.

Zhu, W., & Wang, F.-Y. (2007). On three types of covering rough sets. *IEEE Transactions on Knowledge and Data Engineering*, *19*, 1131–1144.

Ziarko, W. (1993). Variable precision rough sets model. *Journal of Computer and Systems Sciences*, *46*, 39-59.

Ziarko, W. (1993). Variable precision rough set model. Journal of Computer and System Science, *46*, 39-59.

Ziarko, W. (1998). Rough sets as a methodology for data mining. In L. Polkowski & A. Skowron (Eds.), *Rough Sets in Knowledge Discovery*, (vol. 1, pp. 554-576). Heidelberg, Germany: Physica-Verlag.

Ziarko, W., & Katzberg, J. D. (1993). Rough sets approach to system modeling and control algorithm acquisition. In *Proceedings of the IEEE - Communications, Computers and Power in the Modern Environment* (pp. 154-164).

# About the Contributors

**JingTao Yao** is an associate professor of Computer Science at the University of Regina. He taught in the Department of Information Systems at the Massey University, New Zealand, the Department of Information Systems at the National University of Singapore, Singapore,and the Department of Computer Science and Engineering at Xi'an Jiaotong University, China. He received his Ph.D. degree at the National University of Singapore. He did a B.Eng. degree and an M.Sc. degree at Xi'an Jiaotong University. His research interests include softcomputing, data mining, forecasting, neural networks, computational finance, electronic commerce, Web intelligence, and Web-based support systems.

***

**Andrzej Bargiela** is Professor and member of the Automated Scheduling and Planning research group in the School of Computer Science at the University of Nottingham. Since 1978 he has pursued research focused on processing of uncertainty in the context of modelling and simulation of various physical and engineering systems. His current research falls under the general heading of Computational Intelligence and involve mathematical modelling, information abstraction, parallel computing, artificial intelligence, fuzzy sets and neurocomputing. Bargiela has published over 180 research papers and has co-authored two books: Granular Computing – An Introduction, Kluwer 2002 and Introduction to Fuzzy Logic, AI and Neurocomputing, SOFT, 2005. He is Editor-in-Chief of the Simulation and Modelling in Engineering, serves as Editor of IEEE Transactions on Systems, Man and Cybernetics, SMCA and serves as member of Editorial Board of five international journals. He is editor of a book series on Computer Modelling and Simulation published by J.Wiley and was member of the Editorial Board of the Encyclopedia of Life Support Systems. Dr Bargiela served as Chairman of the European Council for Modelling and Simulation for two terms of office (2002-2006) and has been a member of International Programme Committees of numerous conferences. He also serves as member of the Peer Review College of the Engineering and Physical Sciences Research Council (UK) and served as Specialist Assessor for the Deutsche Forschungsgemeinschaft (DFG-Germany).

**Barnabas Bede** received his BSc.(1998) and MSc(1999) from the University of Oradea, Romania, received PhD in Mathematics from "Babes-Bolyai" University, Cluj Napoca Romania. Currently he is Assistant Professor in the Department of Mathematics, at the University of Texas-Pan American, Edinburg, Texas. His research interests include Fuzzy Differential Equations, Fuzzy Numbers and

Fuzzy Arithmetic, Soft Computing in Image Processing, Nonlinear Approximation, Pseudo-Analysis. Publications include: Generalizations of the differentiability of fuzzy-number-valued functions with pplications to fuzzy differential equations, Fuzzy Sets and Systems, 151(2005) 581-599 (with S.G. Gal), Approximation by pseudo-linear operators, Fuzzy Sets and Systems, 159(2008), 804-820 (with: H. Nobuhara, M. Daňková, A. Di Nola).

**Otávio Augusto Salgado Carpinteiro** was born in Rio de Janeiro, RJ, Brazil. He has a B.Sc. degree in Mathematics, a B.Sc. in Music and a M.Sc. in System and Computing Engineering, all from the Federal University of Rio de Janeiro, Brazil. He has a PhD degree in Cognitive and Computer Science from the University of Sussex, UK. He has worked as a system analyst for many years, and presently he is an associate professor at the Federal University of Itajubá – MG, Brazil, where he has done research, supervised graduate students, and taught courses in Computing Engineering.

**Martine Ceberio** received her M.Sc in Mathematics from the Department of Mathematics of the University of Nantes, France, in 1997, and her Ph.D. from the Department of Computer Science of the University of Nantes, France, in 2003. Her Ph.D. was related to continuous constraint solving techniques, including contributions to interval computations and to soft constraint modeling and solving. After graduating from her Ph.D., Martine Ceberio joined the Computer Science Department of the University of Texas at El Paso, as a visiting assistant professor in 2003, and became a tenure-track assistant professor in 2004. Her work has been focused on techniques for decision making under uncertainty, including the use of interval computations and their combination with multi-criteria decision making techniques. She has also developed applications of constraints to several fields, such as bio-medical engineering, automotive industry.

**Yan Chen** is currently a Ph.D student of the Computer Science Department at Georgia State University, Atlanta, USA. His research interests include semantic computing, data mining and information retrieval.

**Fernando Gomide** received the B.Sc. degree in electrical engineering from the Polytechnic Institute of the Pontifical Catholic University of Minas Gerais, Brazil, the M.Sc. degree in electrical engineering from the University of Campinas (UNICAMP), Brazil, and the PhD degree in systems engineering from Case Western Reserve University (CWRU) Cleveland, Ohio, USA. He is professor of the Department of Computer Engineering and Automation (DCA), FEEC – UNICAMP, since 1983. His interest areas include fuzzy systems, neural and evolutionary computation, modeling, control and optimization, logistics, multi agent systems, decision-making and applications. He was past vice-president of IFSA, member of the editorial board of IEEE Transactions on SMC-B. Currently he serves the board of NAFIPS and the editorial boards of Fuzzy Sets and Systems, Intelligent Automation and Soft Computing, IEEE Transactions on SMC-A, Fuzzy Optimization and Decision Making, International Journal of Fuzzy Systems, and Mathware and Soft Computing. He is a past editor of the Brazilian Society for Automatics – SBA. He is on the Advisory Board of the International Journal of Uncertainty, Fuzziness and Knowledge-Based Systems, Journal of Advanced Computational Intelligence, and Intelligent Automation and Soft Computing and member of the IEEE Task Force on Adaptive Fuzzy Systems, IEEE Emergent Technology Technical Committee.

**Salvatore Greco** is full professor at the Faculty of Economics of Catania University since 2001. His main research interests are in the field of multiple criteria decision aiding (MCDA), in the application of the rough set approach to decision analysis, in the axiomatic foundations of the MCDA methodology, and in the fuzzy integral approach to MCDA. In these fields he cooperates with many researchers of different countries. He received the Best Theoretical Paper Award by the Decision Sciences Institute (Athens, 1999). Together with Benedetto Matarazzo, he organized the 7th International Summer School on MCDA (Catania, 2000). He is author of many articles published in major international journals and specialized books. Together with José Figueira and Matthias Ehrgott he edited the most recent and updated state of art in MCDA. One of his articles, written together Benedetto Matarazzo and Roman Słowiński, has been included in the list of the thirty most influential articles of the European Journal of Operational Research. He has been invited professor at Poznań University of Technology, at the University of Paris Dauphine, and at Ecole Centrale in Paris. He has been invited speaker at international conferences in his field. He has also been referee of the most relevant journals in the field of decision analysis.

**Jianchao Han** is currently an associate professor of computer science at the California State University, Dominguez Hills, Carson, California, USA. He received his Ph.D. degree in Computer Science from the University of Waterloo, Canada, 2001. His research interests include machine learning, knowledge discovery and data mining, data mining applications in bioinformatics and computer security, data, information and knowledge visualization, granular computing and soft computing, fuzzy sets and rough sets, network computing and security, as well as object-oriented software engineering. He has published more than 60 peer-reviewed academic articles in various international conferences and journals. He is the executive editor of International Journal of Granular Computing, Rough Sets and Intelligent Systems.

**Jun Hu**, bore in 1977. Received his B.Eng. Degree and M.Eng. DegreeUniversity of Geosciences in 2000 and 2003 respectively. Now he iscandidate in the school of electronic Engineering of Xidian University.research interests include granular computing, rough set theory, knowledgeetc.

**Andrzej Jankowski** received a Ph.D. from Warsaw University where he workedfor more than 15 years in pioneering research on the algebraic approach toknowledge representation and reasoning structures based on topos theory andevolution of hierarchies of metalogics. He has worked for three years as avisiting professor in the Department of Computer Science in the Universityof North Carolina, Charlotte, USA. He has the unique experience in managingcomplex IT projects in Central Europe: he is the designer and the projectmanager of such complex IT projects as POLTAX, one of the biggest taxmodernization IT projects in Central Europe, executed for the Polishgovernment), as well as e-POLTAX (e-forms for tax system in Poland). Heaccumulated an extensive experience in the government, corporate, industry,and finance sectors (he was executive vice President of BGŻ bank). He alsosupervised several AI-based commercial projects such as intelligent frauddetection for Bank of America and PKN ORLEN, intelligent search engine forUNCC and Duke Energy, data mining projects for Ford and General Motors.

Andrzej Jankowski is one of the founders of the Polish-Japanese Institute ofInformation Technology where he served for five years as its Vice Chancellorfor Research and Teaching. He has also founded Knowledge TechnologyFoundation.

**C. Maria Keet** is Assistant Professor at the Faculty of Computer Science at the Free University of Bozen-Bolzano, where she received her PhD in Computer Science in 2008. Her main research foci are logic-based knowledge representation, ontology and Ontology, and its applications to biological data and knowledge. In addition to having obtained an MSc in Microbiology from Wageningen University and Research Centre (1998), an MA 1st class in Peace & Development Studies from Limerick University (2003), and a BSc(hons) 1st class in IT & Computing from the Open University UK (2004), she has worked for 3.5 years as systems engineer in the IT industry.

**Vladik Kreinovich** received his M.Sc. in Mathematics and ComputerScience from St. Petersburg University, Russia, in 1974, and Ph.D. fromThe Institute of Mathematics, Soviet Academy of Sciences, Novosibirsk, in1979. In 1975-80, worked with the Soviet Academy of Sciences, in particular, in 1978-80, with the Special Astrophysical Observatory (representation and processing of uncertainty in radioastronomy). In 1982-89, worked on error estimation and intelligent information processing for the National Institute for Electrical Measuring Instruments, Russia. In 1989, he was a Visiting Scholar at Stanford. Since 1990, he is with the University of Texas at El Paso. Served as an Invited professor in Paris, Hong Kong, St. Petersburg, Russia, and Brazil. His main interests include representation and processing of uncertainty, especially interval computations. Published 3 books, 6 edited books, and more than 700 papers. He is a member of the editorial board of the international journal "Reliable Computing" and several other journals. Co-maintainer of the interval computations website http://www.cs.utep.edu/interval-comp

**Deyu Li** is a professor of School of Computer and Information Technology of Shanxi University. He received his M.S. degree in Mathematics from Shanxi University in 1998, and his Ph.D degree in Information Science from Xi'an Jiaotong University in 2002. His current research interests include rough set theory, granular computing, data mining and knowledge discovery. He has published more than 10 articles in international journals.

**Jiye Liang** is a professor of School of Computer and Information Technology and Key Laboratory of Computational Intelligence and Chinese Information Processing of Ministry of Education at Shanxi University. He received the Ph.D degree in Information Science from Xi'an Jiaotong University, and was engaged on Postdoctoral research about computer science and technology in the Institute of Computing Technology, the Chinese Academy of Sciences. His research interests include artificial intelligence, granular computing data mining and knowledge discovery. In recent years, he has published over 40 papers in his research fields.

**Qing Liu** is a professor at department of computer science in Nanchang university. In the academic year 1993-1994, as a visiting scholar , to visit in Stanford University and San Jose State University in USA and Lakehead University in Canada. His research interest include Artificial Intelligence, Expert System, Rough Sets, Granular Computer, Logic and Its Reasoning. Once he organized "1th -8th Chinese Conference on Rough Sets and Soft Computing" and 9 th Chinese Conference on Artificial Intelligence for Institute of Higher Education in China. He is invited serve as a member of program committee for international conference on Rough Sets and Current Trends in Computing and Rough Sets, Fuzzy Sets, Data Mining and Granular Computing more. He is invited also serve as a reviewer of papers of many Chinese Journal on Computer Science.He had published over 100 papers in international Journals, Conference and Chinese Journals.

**Xianquan Liu**, born in 1974, received the B.Sc. degree from Chongqing Normal University in 1998 and M.Sc. degree in systematic theory from Chongqing Normal University in 2003. Now, he is Ph.D. degree candidate in computer information processing and technology of Southwest Jiaotong University. His current research interests include fuzzy set theory, rough set theory, quotient space theory, feature selection, pattern recognition, granular computing, etc.

**Zhangang Liu**, born in 1970, received his B.A. degree from Beijing Printing Institute and he is M.A. candidate in the School of Computer Science and Engineering, University of Science and Technology Liaoning China, His current research interests include Formal Concept Analysis and Knowledge Engineering.

**B. Isaías Lima Lopes** obtained his D.Sc. degree in electrical engineering from Federal University of Itajubá, Brazil in 2004. His work includes researches and tests in equipments at the Laboratory of Telecommunications (LTET-LEPCH/Brazil) and Network Technology and Information Theory. He is currently at the Federal University of Itajubá, Brazil, as Associate Professor of the Institute of Engineering of Systems and Information Technologies. He is member of the Research Group on Engineering and Computational Systems (GPESC/UNIFEI). He is professor and associated member of the after-graduation courses in Science and Technology of the Computation. Researcher in the areas of computer networks, software engineering and applications of artificial neural networks in similar areas.

**Yuan Ma**, born in 1941, Professor and M.A. supervisor in the School of Computer Science and Engineering, University of Science and Technology Liaoning China, He was a member of standing commissioner of Rough sets and Soft computing professional committee of Chinese Association for Artificial Intelligence. He was an experts who have made outstanding contribution and enjoys special government allowances from the State Council for life and was an advanced scientific and technological employee in Liaoning province, His main research interests include the theory of database, knowledge discovery, the theory of Rough set, formal concept analysis.

**Dariusz Malyszko** received his Master's degree in Computer Science from Bialystok Technical University in 2004. Ph.D student from 2005. Research area focuses on rough sets, fuzzy sets and evolutionary computation employed in image processing algorithms. Publications in the subject of rough sets and evolutionary computation applied to image analysis problems, mainly image clustering and segmentation routines. Research interests are focused on the application of rough sets in image analysis and evolutionary versions of k-means clustering, comparative assessment of evolutionary k-means clustering, rough entropy in the context of image segmentation evaluation and classification, development and improvement of robust clustering algorithmic schemes.

**Benedetto Matarazzo** is full professor at the Faculty of Economics of Catania University. His research interests are in the area of operational research, and, particularly, in multiple criteria decision aiding (MCDA) and rough sets. He has been invited professor at and co-operates with several universities in Europe. He has also been invited speaker at many scientific conferences. He is member of the editorial boards of the European Journal of Operational Research, Journal of Multi-Criteria Decision Analysis, and Foundations of Computing and Decision Sciences. He has been chairman of the Programme Committee of EURO XVI Conference (Brussels, 1998). He received the Best Theoretical Paper Award by the Decision Sciences Institute (Athens, 1999). One of his articles, written together Salvatore Greco and Roman Słowiński, has been included in the list of the thirty most influential articles of the European Journal of Operational Research. He received the Gold Medal of International Society on Multiple Criteria Decision Making (Chengdu, 2009). He is member of the Organizing Committee of the International Summer School on MCDA, of which he organized the first (Catania, 1983) and the 7th (Catania, 2000) editions.

**Hung Son Nguyen** holds the assistant professor position at Warsaw University. He is a member of International Rough Set Society. He received his M.S. and Ph.D. from Warsaw University in 1994 and 1997, respectively. His main research interests are foundations and applications of rough set theory, data mining, text mining, granular computing, bioinformatics, intelligent multiagent systems, soft computing, and pattern recognition. On these topics he has published more than 80 research papers in edited books, international journals and conferences. Dr Hung Son Nguyen has delivered many invited talks and tutorial during international conferences. He received the "IEEE/WIC/ACM International Conference on Web Intelligence (WI 2005) Best Paper Award". Dr. Hung Son Nguyen is a member of the Editorial Board the following international journals: „Transaction on Rough Sets", „Data mining and Knowledge Discovery" and "ERCIM News" and the assistant to the Editor in Chief of "Fundamenta Informaticae". He has served as a program co-chair of RSCTC'06, as a PC member and a reviewer of various other conferences and journals.

**Witold Pedrycz** received the M.Sc., and Ph.D., D.Sci. all from the Silesian University of Technology, Gliwice, Poland. He is a Professor and Canada Research Chair (CRC) in Computational Intelligence in the Department of Electrical and Computer Engineering, University of Alberta, Edmonton, Canada. He is also with the Polish Academy of Sciences, Systems Research Institute, Warsaw, Poland. His research interests encompass Computational Intelligence, fuzzy modeling, knowledge discovery and data mining, fuzzy control including fuzzy controllers, pattern recognition, knowledge-based neural networks, granular and relational computing, and Software Engineering. He has published numerous papers in these areas. He is also an author of 12 research monographs. Witold Pedrycz has been a member of numerous program committees of IEEE conferences in the area of fuzzy sets and neurocomputing. He serves as Editor-in-Chief of IEEE Transactions on Systems Man and Cybernetics-Part A and Associate Editor of IEEE Transactions on Fuzzy Systems. He is also an Editor-in-Chief of Information Sciences. He is a co-editor in chief of the extended handbook of Granular Computing published in 2008. Dr. Pedrycz is a recipient of the prestigious Norbert Wiener award from the IEEE Society of Systems, Man, and Cybernetics and an IEEE Canada Silver Medal in Computer Engineering.

**James F. Peters** is Co-Founder and Research Group Leader in the Computational Intelligence Laboratory (http://wren.ece.umanitoba.ca/) and Full Professor in the Department of Electrical and Computer Engineering (ECE) at the University of Manitoba. He received a Ph.D. in Constructive Specification of Communicating Processes (1991, Kansas State University) and was a Postdoctoral Fellow, Syracuse University, and Rome Laboratories (1991), Assistant Professor, University of Arkansas and Researcher in the Mission Sequencing and Telecommunications Divisions at the Jet Propulsion Laboratory/Caltech, Pasadena, California (1992-1994). He is currently Co-Editor-in-Chief of the Transactions on Rough Sets published by Springer and he is on the Editorial Board of a number of other journals. In 2002, he collaborated with Zdzisław Pawlak on a descriptive view of the nearness of physical objects. In 2006, he introduced near sets, a generalization of rough sets. This has led to feature-based solutions to the image correspondence problem. In April 2008, he received the International Journal of Intelligent Computing and Cybernetics best journal article award and 2007 Springer JRS2008 Best paper award. His current research interests are in tolerance spaces, perception-based image analysis, finite lattices, fuzzy sets, near sets, especially tolerance near sets, rough sets, and perceptual morphology.

**Carlos A. M. Pinheiro** received the B.Sc. degree in electrical engineering from the Federal Engineering School of Itajubá (EFEI), Brazil, the M.Sc. degree in power systems from the Federal Engineering School of Itajubá, and D.Sc. degree in control systems from the State University of Campinas (UNICAMP), Brazil. He has been professor at the Federal University of Itajubá, Brazil, since 1983. His interest areas include control systems, identification and modeling of dynamic systems, digital processing, power electronics, applications of artificial intelligence (fuzzy logic, neural networks and evolutionary computation). He is author of papers and books on topics related with modeling and control of dynamic systems. He is a member of IEEE Control Systems Society and of SBA – Brazilian Society of Automatic.

**Andrzej Pownuk** received his M.Sc in Applied Mechanics (Fundamental Technological Research) from Department of Mathematics and Physics, the Silesian University of Technology in Gliwice, Poland in 1995, and Ph.D. form the Department of Civil Engineering, the Silesian University of Technology in Gliwice, Poland, in 2001. His Ph.D. was related to modeling of uncertainty in civil engineering. In 2002 he was working as a researcher for Chevron Oil Company in San Ramon, California, USA. His research was related to modeling of uncertainty in oil engineering.In 2003 he was working for Vienna University in Vienna, Austria. During that time his research was related to interval finite element and optimization.Since 2006 he is working for the department of Mathematical Sciences, The University of Texas at El Paso as assistant professor of mathematics.Complete list of his papers (approximately 70) can be found at his web page http://andrzej.pownuk.com.

**Yuhua Qian** graduated from Department of Computer Science, Shanxi University, China in 2000, and then joined Agriculture Development Bank of China. In 2002, he came to School of Computer and Information Technology, Shanxi University, and got MS degree there. Now He is an Assistant Professor and is pursuing PhD degree in Key Laboratory of Computational Intelligence and Chinese Information Processing of Ministry of Education. His main interests are in granular computing, rough sets, fuzzy sets, data mining, intelligent decision-making, uncertain measuring and information theory. He has published more than 10 articles in international journals.

**Sheela Ramanna** is a Full Professor and Past Head of the Applied Computer Science Department at the University of Winnipeg. She received a Ph.D. in Computer Science from Kansas State University in 1991 and a B.E in Electrical Engineering and M.Tech in Computer Science and Engineering from India. She serves on the Editorial Board of the Transactions on Rough Sets Journal (TRS) published by Springer-Verlag, and is current member of the Steering Committee, International Rough Sets Society(IRSS), and current member of the Executive Board of IRSS. She also serves on the Editorial Board on International Journal of Fuzzy Systems and Rough Systems (IJFSRS) and International Journal of Computer and Systems Engineering (IJCSE). She served as Program Co-Chair for JRS2007 held in Toronto. Her paper on rough control co-authored with James F. Peters received the IFAC Best Paper Award in 1998. She has served on numerous Program Committees for International Conferences and is a reviewer for several journals. She has published numerous articles on the theory and application of computational intelligence techniques (rough, fuzzy and neural networks) in journals, conferences, books and edited volumes. Her research interests include theory and application of Rough Sets, Methodologies for Intelligent Systems and Knowledge Discovery and Data Mining (KDD) of Software Engineering Data. She is a member of the Computational Intelligence Laboratory at the University of Manitoba.

**Andrzej Skowron** holds a Ph.D. degree and Doctor of Science (Habilitation) degree in Mathematical Foundations of Computer Science from the University of Warsaw in Poland. In 1991 he received the Scientific Title of Professor. He is Full Professor in the Faculty of Mathematics, Computer Science and Mechanics at Warsaw University. Andrzej Skowron is the author or co-author of more than 350 scientific publications. He was a supervisor of 20 PhD Theses and more than 100 M.Sc. theses.He is on Editorial Boards of many others journals including Knowledge Discovery and Data Mining. He is Editor-in-Chief of Fundamenta Informaticae and co-editor-in-chief of LNCS Transactions on Rough Sets.Andrzej Skowron has served on the program committees of over 100 international conferences. He has delivered numerous invited talks at international conferences including a plenary talk at the 16-th IFIP World Computer Congress (Beijing, 2000).His areas of expertise include reasoning with incomplete information, soft computing methods and applications, rough sets, rough mereology, granular computing, data mining including process mining, decision support systems, intelligent agents, adaptive systems and wisdom technology. He was involved in several national and international research and commercial projects related, e.g., to data mining (fraud detection, web mining), control of unmanned vehicles, decision support systems and approximate reasoning in distributed environments, as well as financial prediction in Forex.

**Roman Słowiński** is professor and founding head of the Laboratory of Intelligent Decision Support Systems within the Institute of Computing Science, Poznań University of Technology, Poland. Since 2002 he holds, moreover, professor's position at the Systems Research Institute of the Polish Academy of Sciences in Warsaw. He has done extensive research on methodology and techniques of Operational Research and Computational Intelligence. He is laureate of the EURO Gold Medal (Aachen, 1991), and Doctor Honoris Causa of Polytechnic Faculty of Mons (2000), University of Paris Dauphine (2001) and Technical University of Crete (2008). In 2004, he was elected member of the Polish Academy of Sciences, a corporation of 350 outstanding Polish scholars. He holds, moreover, the Edgeworth-Pareto Award, by International Society on Multiple Criteria Decision Making (Cape Town, 1997). In 2005, he received the Annual Prize of the Foundation for Polish Science, regarded as the most prestigious scientific award in Poland. Since 1999, he is editor, and since 2007 co-ordinating editor, of the European Journal of Operational Research. He is on editorial board of twenty other scientific journals. He organized the First International Workshop on Rough Set Theory and Applications in Poznań, in 1992. His record of publications includes fourteen monographs, and over three hundred scientific articles in major international journals and edited volumes. He supervised twenty three Ph.D. theses in Operational Research and Computational Intelligence.

**Jaroslaw Stepaniuk** holds a Ph.D. degree in Mathematical Foundations of Computer Science from the University of Warsaw in Poland, Doctor of Science (Habilitation) degree in Computer Science from the Institute of Computer Science Polish Academy of Sciences. Jaroslaw Stepaniuk is Associate Professor in the Faculty of Computer Science at Bialystok University of Technology. Actually he is the author of more than 130 scientific publications. His areas of expertise include reasoning with incomplete information, approximate reasoning, soft computing methods and applications, rough sets, granular computing, synthesis and analysis of complex objects, intelligent agents, knowledge discovery systems, and advanced data mining techniques.

**Marcin Szczuka** received his M. Sc. in Mathematics and Ph.D. in Computer Science (with honours) in 1995 and 2000, respectively, from the From the Faculty of Mathematics, Informatics and Mechanics, the University of Warsaw, Poland. Since 1995 he is working as researcher at the University of Warsaw. He has worked as a visiting scholar in several higher education institutions in Japan, Sweden, and Canada. He authored over 30 research papers, edited several books and conference proceedings. He is a member of editorial boards of several international journals. He organised and chaired several international workshops, conferences and seminars. In the past he was involved in several national and international research projects, including research programmes of the European Union.Currently, the main research interests of Marcin Szczuka are concerned with complex decision support systems construction based on knowledge discovery and interactions, elements of granular computing and rough set theory, as well as knowledge discovery and knowledge utilisation for heterogeneous, complex data sources.

**Athanasios T. Vasilakos** is a Professor at the department of Computer and Telecommunications Engineering, University of Western Macedonia, Greece, and a Visiting Professor at the Graduate Programme of the department of Electrical and Computer Engineering, National Technical University of Athens (NTUA). He is the coauthor (with W.Pedrycz) of the books Computational Intelligence in

Telecommunications Networks (CRC press, USA, 2001), Ambient Intelligence, Wireless Networking, Ubiquitous Computing (Artech House, USA, 2006), coauthor (with M.Parashar, S.Karnouskos, W.Pedrycz) Autonomic Communications (Springer, in press), Arts and Technologies (MIT Press, in press), coauthor (with M.Anastasopoulos) Game Theory in Communication Systems (IGI Inc., USA, in press), coauthor with Yan Zhang, Thrasyvoulos Spyropoulos) Delay Tolerant Networking (CRC press, in press). He has published more than 200 articles in top international journals and conferences. He is the Editor-in-Chief of the inderscience publishers journals: International Journal of Adaptive and Autonomous Communications Systems (IJAACS, http://www.inderscience.com/ijaacs ), International Journal of Arts and Technology (IJART, http://www.inderscience.com/ijart). He was or he is at the Editorial Board of more than 20 international journals including: IEEE Communications Magazine (19992002 and 2008), IEEE Transactions on Systems, Man and Cybernetics (SMC, Part B, 2007), IEEE Transactions on Information Technology in Biomedicine (2008), IEEE Transactions on Wireless Communications (invited), ACM Transactions on Autonomous and Adaptive Systems (invited), EURASIP WCN, and ACM/Springer WINET. He is Chairman of the Telecommunications Task Force of the Intelligent Systems Applications Technical Committee (ISATC) of the IEEE Computational Intelligence Society (CIS). He is a Member of the IEEE and ACM.

**Guoyin Wang**, born in Chongqing, China, in 1970. He received the bachelor's degree in computer software, the master's degree in computer software, and the Ph.D. degree in computer organization and architecture from Xi'an Jiaotong University, Xi'an, China, in 1992, 1994, and 1996, respectively. He worked at the University of North Texas, USA, and the University of Regina, Canada, as a visiting scholar during 1998-1999. Since 1996, he has been working at the Chongqing University of Posts and Telecommunications, where he is currently a professor and PhD supervisor, the Chairman of the Institute of Computer Science and Technology (ICST), and the Dean of the College of Computer Science and Technology. He is also a part-time professor with the Xi'an Jiaotong University, Shanghai Jiaotong University, Southwest Jiaotong University, Xidian University, and University of Electronic Science and Technology of China. Professor Wang is the Chairman of the Advisory Board of International Rough Set Society (IRSS), Chairman of the Rough Set Theory and Soft Computation Society, Chinese Association for Artificial Intelligence. He serves as a program committee member for many international conferences and editorial board member of several international journals. Professor Wang has been awarded several government medals, and was named as a national excellent teacher and a national excellent university key teacher by the Ministry of Education, China, in 2001 and 2002 respectively. In 2004, Professor Wang was elected into the Program for New Century Excellent Talents in University by the Ministry of Education of P R China. In 2008, he won the award of the funding for excellent youth scientists from Chongqing city. He has given many invited talks at international and national conferences, and has given many seminars in many universities in USA, Canada, Poland, and China. The institute (ICST) directed by Professor Wang was elected as one of the top ten outstanding youth organizations of Chongqing, China. Professor Wang is the author of 2 books, the editor of many proceedings of international and national conferences, and has over 200 research publications. His research interests include data mining, machine learning, rough set, soft computing, knowledge technology, etc.

**Wei-Zhi Wu** received his B.Sc degree in Mathematics from Zhejiang Normal University in 1986, M.Sc degree in Mathematics from the East China Normal University in 1992, and Ph.D. degree in Applied Mathematics from Xi'an Jiaotong University, P. R. China in 2002. From 2003 and 2004, he was a postdoctoral researcher in the School of Management, Xi'an Jiaotong University. From June 2005 to March 2006, he was a postdoctoral fellow in Department of Geography and Resource Management, The Chinese University of Hong Kong. He is currently a Professor of Mathematics with the School of Mathematics, Physics, and Information Science, Zhejiang Ocean University. He has published 2 monographs and more than 60 articles in international journals and book chapters. His current research interests include approximate reasoning, rough sets, random sets, formal concept analysis, and granular computing. Dr. Wu serves in the editorial boards of several international journals.

**Yiyu Yao** is a professor of computer science in the Department of Computer Science, University of Regina, Regina, Saskatchewan, Canada. His research interests include information retrieval, rough sets, interval sets, granular computing, Web intelligence, data mining and fuzzy sets. He has published over 200 journal and conference papers. He is an area editor of International Journal of Approximate Reasoning, a member of the editorial boards of the Web Intelligence and Agent Systems journal, Transactions on Rough Sets, Journal of Intelligent Information Systems, Journal of Chongqing University of Posts and Telecommunication, The International Journal of Cognitive Informatics & Natural Intelligence (IJCiNi), International Journal of Software Science and Computational Intelligence (IJSSCI). He has served and is serving as a program co-chair of several international conferences. He is a member of ACM and IEEE.

**Qinghua Zhang**, was born in 1974, Ph. D. candidate in the school of information and technology of Southwest Jiaotong University. His current main researchm include intelligent information processing and granular computing, etc.

**Wen-Xiu Zhang** received his B.Sc degree in Mathematics from Nankai University, P.R. China, in 1964 and M.Sc degree in Information Theory, Probability, and Statistics from Nankai University in 1967. He is currently Professor of Research Centre of Applied Mathematics at Xi'an Jiaotong University. He is the author and coauthor of more than 140 academic journal papers and 16 textbooks and research monographs. His research interests include applied probability theory, set-valued stochastic process, and computer reasoning in artificial intelligence. He serves as a vice-editor-in-chief of the Journal of Engineering Mathematics (in Chinese) and a vice-editor-in-chief of Fuzzy System and Mathematics. He is also a member of the standing council of mathematics society of China and a member of IFSA.

**Xuedong Zhang**, born in 1963, received his Ph. D from School of Information Science and Enginerring in Northeastern University China, Professor and M.A. supervisor. He was director of the School of Computer Science and Engineering, University of Science and Technology Liaoning China and was director of Image and Graphics Institute, His main research interests include multi-dimensional data signal processing, computer vision, biological information to identify, embedded system.

**Yanqing Zhang** is currently an Associated Professor of the Computer Science Department at Georgia State University, Atlanta, USA. His research interests include hybrid intelligent systems, computational intelligence, machine learning, neural networks, fuzzy logic, evolutionary computation, kernel machines, granular computing, data mining, Yin-Yang computation, natural Computing, bioinformatics, computational Web intelligence, intelligent agents for e-Business and e-Security, intelligent grid computing and intelligent wireless mobile computing.

**Yan Zhao** received her B. Eng. from the Shanghai University of Engineering and Science, People's Republic of China, in 1994, and M.Sc. and Ph.D. from the University of Regina, Canada in 2003 and 2007, respectively. She is a current post doctoral research fellow in the Department of Computer Science, University of Regina. Her research interests include data mining, human-computer interaction, machine learning, granular computing and rough sets.

**JiaQing Zhou**, born in 1969. Received his B.Eng. Degree from Southwest Normal University in 1991 and M.Eng. Degree from Southwest Jiaotong University in 2001. Now he is Ph.D. degree candidate in the school of information science andtechnology of Southwest Jiaotong University . His current research interests includegranular computing, rough set theory, knowledge acquisition, computer network, etc

# Index